	ECHO	Echocardiography
	EEG	Electroencephalogram
	EGD	Esophagogastroduodenoscopy
	ELISA	Enzyme-linked immunosorbent assay
	EMG	Electromyography
	ENG	Electroneurography
	EP	Evoked potential
	EPS	Electrophysiologic study
	ER	Estrogen receptor
	ERCP	Endoscopic retrograde cholangiopancrea-tography
	ESR	Erythrocyte sedimentation rate
	EUG	Excretory urography
F	FBS	Fasting blood sugar
	FDPs	Fibrin degradation products
	Fe	Iron
	FSH	Follicle-stimulating hormone
	FSPs	Fibrin split products
	FTA-ABS	Fluorescent treponemal antibody absorption test
	FTI	Free thyroxine index
	FUT	Fibrinogen uptake test
G	G-6-PD	Glucose-6-phosphate dehydrogenase
	GB series	Gallbladder series
	GE reflux	Gastroesophageal reflux scan
	GGT	Gamma-glutamyl transferase
	GGTP	Gamma-glutamyl transpeptidase
	GH	Growth hormone
	GHb, GHB	Glycosylated hemoglobin
	GI series	Gastrointestinal series
	GTT	Glucose tolerance test
H	HAA	Hepatitis-associated antigen
	HAV	Hepatitis A virus
	Hb, Hgb	Hemoglobin
	HB_cAb	Hepatitis B core antibody
	HB_cAg	Hepatitis B core antigen
	HBV	Hepatitis B virus
	HCG	Human chorionic gonadotropin
	HCO_3^-	Bicarbonate
	HCS	Human chorionic somatomammotropin
	Hct	Hematocrit
	HDL	High-density lipoprotein
	HIV	Human immunodeficiency virus
	HSV-2	Herpes simplex virus, type 2
I	Ig	Immunoglobulin
	INR	International normalization ratio
	IVC	Intravenous cholangiography

Mosby's

Diagnostic and

Laboratory

Test Reference

Mosby's
Diagnostic and Laboratory Test Reference

Third Edition

Kathleen Deska Pagana, PhD, RN

Associate Professor
Department of Nursing
Lycoming College
Williamsport, Pennsylvania

Timothy James Pagana, MD, FACS

Surgical Oncologist
Williamsport, Pennsylvania

Illustrated

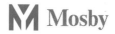 Mosby

St. Louis Baltimore Boston Carlsbad Chicago Naples New York
Philadelphia Portland London Madrid Mexico City Singapore
Sydney Tokyo Toronto Wiesbaden

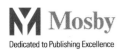

Dedicated to Publishing Excellence

A Times Mirror
Company

Vice President and Publisher: Nancy L. Coon
Editor: Loren S. Wilson
Developmental Editor: Brian Dennison
Project Manager: Deborah L. Vogel
Senior Production Editor: Judith Bange
Designer: E. Rohne Rudder
Manufacturing Manager: Theresa Fuchs
Illustrator: Mark Swindle
Cover Art: Teresa Breckwoldt

Printed in the United States of America
Composition by Clarinda Company
Printing/binding by R.R. Donnelley & Sons Company

Mosby-Year Book, Inc.
11830 Westline Industrial Drive
St. Louis, Missouri 63146

Library of Congress Cataloging in Publication Data

Pagana, Kathleen Deska
    Mosby's diagnostic and laboratory test reference / Kathleen Deska
  Pagana, Timothy James Pagana.—3rd ed.
        p.   cm.
    Includes bibliographical references and index.
    ISBN 0-8151-4327-3
    1. Diagnosis, Laboratory—Handbooks, manuals, etc.   2. Nursing-
  -Handbooks, manuals, etc.   I. Pagana, Timothy James
  II. Title.
    [DNLM: 1. Diagnosis, Laboratory—handbooks.   2. Nursing Care-
  -handbooks.   QY 39 P128m 1996]
    RB37.P24   1996
    616.07′5—dc20
    DNLM/DLC
  for Library of Congress

96 97 98 99 00/9   8   7   6   5   4   3   2   1

Consultants

Leonard R. Collins, MD
Obstetrics and Gynecology
Williamsport, Pennsylvania

Daniel R. Gandy, DO
Nephrology,
Williamsport, Pennsylvania

Edward C. Keating, MD
Cardiologist
Heart and Lung Center
The Williamsport Hospital and
    Medical Center
Williamsport, Pennsylvania

Gary L. Lattimer, MD
Infectious Diseases
Williamsport, Pennsylvania

**Edwina A. McConnell, PhD,
RN**
Consultant
Madison, Wisconsin;
Professor
Texas Tech University
Lubbock, Texas

Warren L. Robinson, MD
Oncology,
Williamsport, Pennsylvania

Robert E. St. John, RN, RRT
Cardiopulmonary Nurse Clinician
Jewish Hospital at Washington
    University Medical Center
St. Louis, Missouri

Keith N. Shenberger, MD
Rheumatology,
Williamsport, Pennsylvania

William R. Somers, MD
Susquehanna Gastroenterology,
Williamsport, Pennsylvania

**Pamela Becker Weilitz,
MSN(R), RN**
Barnes Hospital at Washington
    University Medical Center
St. Louis, Missouri

We lovingly dedicate this book to our daughters

Jocelyn Marie Pagana

Denise Kathleen Pagana

Theresa Noel Pagana

Mosby's Diagnostic and Laboratory Test Reference provides the user with an up-to-date, essential reference that allows easy access to 647 clinically relevant laboratory and diagnostic tests. A unique feature of this handbook is its consistent format, which allows for quick reference without sacrificing the depth of detail necessary for a thorough understanding of diagnostic and laboratory testing. All tests begin on a new page and are listed in alphabetical order by their complete name. The alphabetical format is a strong feature of the book; it allows the user to locate tests quickly without having to place tests in an appropriate category or body system. New to this edition is a User's Guide to Test Preparation and Procedures. This guide should eliminate test repetition because of problems in patient preparation, test procedures, and/or collection techniques. Every feature of this book is geared to provide pertinent information in a sequence that best simulates priorities in the clinical setting.

The following information is provided, whenever possible, for effective diagnostic and laboratory testing:

Name of test. Tests are listed by their complete name. A complete list of abbreviations and alternate test names follows each main entry.

Type of test. This section identifies whether the test is, for example, an x-ray procedure, ultrasound, nuclear scan, blood test, urine test, sputum test, or microscopic examination of tissue. This section helps the reader identify the source of the laboratory specimen or location of the diagnostic procedure.

Normal findings. Normal values are listed, when applicable, for the infant, child, adult, and elderly person. Also, where appropriate, values are separated into male and female. It is important to realize that normal ranges of laboratory tests vary from institution to institution. This variability is even more obvious among the various laboratory textbooks. For this reason, we have deliberately chosen *not* to add a table of normal values as an appendix, and we encourage the user to check the normal values at the institution where the test is performed. This should be relatively easy, since most laboratory reports indicate normal values.

Possible critical values. These values give an indication of results that are well outside the usual range of normal. These results generally require immediate intervention.

Test explanation and related physiology. This section provides a concise, yet comprehensive description of each test. This explanation includes fundamental information about the test itself, specific indications for the test, how the test is performed, what disease or disorder the various results may show, how it will affect the patient or client, and relevant pathophysiology that will enhance understanding of the test.

Contraindications. These data are crucial because they alert the user to patients who should not have the test. Patients frequently highlighted in this section include those who are pregnant, are allergic to iodinated or contrast dyes, or have bleeding disorders.

Potential complications. This section alerts the user to potential problems that will necessitate astute assessments and interventions. For example, if a potential complication is renal failure, the implication may be to hydrate the patient before the test and force fluids after the test. A typical potential complication for many x-ray procedures is allergy to iodinated dye. Patient symptoms and appropriate interventions are described in detail.

Interfering factors. This section contains pertinent information because many factors can invalidate the test or make the test results unreliable. An important feature of this section is the inclusion of drugs that can interfere with test results. Drugs that increase or decrease test values are always listed at the end of this section for consistency and quick access. A drug symbol (🍷) is used to emphasize these drug interferences.

Procedure and patient care. This section emphasizes the role of nurses and other health care providers in diagnostic and laboratory testing by addressing psychosocial and physiologic interventions. Patient education and rationales are included. For quick access to essential information, this section is divided into *before, during,* and *after* time sequences.

Before. This section addresses the need to explain the procedure and to allay patient concerns or anxieties. If a consent is usually required, this is listed as a bulleted item in this section. Other important features of this section include requirements such as fasting, obtaining baseline values, and performing bowel preparations.

During. This section gives specific directions for clinical specimen studies (e.g., urine and blood studies). An estimate of the approximate amount of a specimen is sometimes given; however, this amount may vary from institution to institution. This section describes pointers that students may not realize or health care providers may forget. Diagnostic procedures and their variations are described in a numbered, usually step-by-step format. Important information, such as who performs the test, where the study is performed, patient sensation, and duration of the procedure, is bulleted for emphasis. The duration of the procedure is very helpful for patient teaching because it indicates the time generally allotted for each study.

After. This section includes vital information that the nurse or other health care provider should heed or convey following the test. Examples include factors such as maintaining bed rest, comparing pulses with baseline values, encouraging fluids, and observing for signs and symptoms of sepsis.

Abnormal findings. As the name implies, this section lists the abnormal findings for each study. Increased or decreased values are listed when appropriate.

Notes. The blank spaces at the end of tests facilitate individualizing the studies according to the institution performing the test. Variations in any area of the test (e.g., patient preparation, test procedure, normal values, postprocedural care) can be noted.

This logical format emphasizes clinically relevant information; the clarity of this format will facilitate a quick understanding of content essential to both students and health care providers. Color has been used to help locate tests and highlight critical information (e.g., possible critical values). Color is also used in the numerous illustrations that are included to enhance the reader's understanding of many diagnostic procedures (e.g., bronchoscopy, fetoscopy, ERCP, pericardiocentesis, TEE). Many tables are used to simplify complex material on topics such as autoimmune diseases, hepatitis testing, and protein electrophoresis. Extensive cross-referencing exists throughout the book. This permits full understanding and helps the user tie together or locate related studies, such as those on the cardiac enzymes (CPK, LDH, AST).

For easy access, a listing of abbreviations for test names is included on the book's endpapers. Appendix A includes a list of studies according to *body systems.* This listing may familiarize the user with other related studies the patient or client may need or the user may want to review. This should be especially useful for students and health care providers working in specialized areas.

Appendix B provides a listing of studies according to *test type*. This listing may help the user read and learn about similarly performed tests and procedures (e.g., x-rays of the skull, chest, and abdomen). Appendix C provides a list of typical abbreviations and units of measurement. Finally, a comprehensive index includes the names of all tests and their synonyms and any other relevant terms found within the tests.

Many new studies, such as biophysical profile, apolipoprotein, and antineutrophil cytoplasmic antibody studies, have been added. All other studies have been revised and updated. Outdated studies have been eliminated. We are most appreciative of the excellent reviewers, and we thank them all. We sincerely thank our editors for their enthusiasm and continual support.

We are most grateful to the many students, nurses, and other health care providers who made the first two editions of this book so successful. This success validated the need for a user-friendly and quick reference approach to laboratory and diagnostic testing.

We invite additional comments from users of this book so that we may continue to provide useful, relevant diagnostic and laboratory test information to users of future editions.

Contents

Health care economics demand that laboratory and diagnostic testing be performed accurately and in the least amount of time possible. Tests should not have to be repeated because of problems in patient preparation, test procedure, and/or specimen collection technique. The following guidelines delineate the responsibilities for health care providers to ensure safety for test procedures and accuracy in test results. Guidelines are described for the following major types of tests: blood, urine, stool, x-ray, nuclear scanning, ultrasound, and endoscopy.

Blood tests

Overview

Blood studies are used to assess a multitude of body processes and disorders. Common studies include enzymes, serum lipids, electrolyte levels, red and white blood cell counts, clotting factors, hormone levels, and levels of breakdown products such as blood urea nitrogen.

Guidelines

- Observe universal precautions in collecting a blood specimen.
- Check whether fasting is required. Many studies (such as fasting blood sugar and cholesterol levels) require the patient to fast for a designated time.
- If ordered, withhold medications until the blood is drawn.
- Note the time of day that the blood test is drawn. Some blood test results (such as those for cortisol) vary according to a diurnal pattern, and this must be considered when blood levels are interpreted.
- Note the patient's position for certain tests. For example, renin levels are affected by body position.
- Collect the blood in the proper color-coded test tube. Blood collection tubes have color-coded stoppers to indicate the presence or absence of different types of additives (preservatives and anticoagulants). A preservative prevents change in the specimen, and an anticoagulant inhibits clot formation or coagulation. Charts are available from the laboratory indicating the type of tube needed for the particular blood test.

- Follow the recommended "order of draw" when collecting tubes. Draw specimens into nonadditive tubes (e.g., red-top) before drawing them into tubes with additives. Fill the tubes in the following order:
  1. Blood culture tubes (to maintain sterility)
  2. Nonadditive tubes (e.g., red-top)
  3. Coagulation tubes (e.g., blue-top)
  4. Heparin tubes (e.g., green-top)
  5. Ethylenediaminetetraacetic acid–K3 (EDTA-K3) tubes (e.g., lavender-top)
  6. Oxalate/fluoride tubes (e.g., gray-top)
- To obtain valid results, do not fasten the tourniquet for longer than 1 minute. Prolonged tourniquet application can cause stasis and hemoconcentration.
- Collect the blood specimen from the arm without an intravenous (IV) device, if possible. IV infusion can influence test results.
- Do not use the arm bearing a dialysis arteriovenous (AV) fistula for venipuncture unless the physician specifically authorizes it.
- Because of the risk of cellulitis, do not take specimens from the side on which a mastectomy or axillary lymph node dissection was performed.
- Follow the unit guidelines for drawing blood from an indwelling venous catheter, such as a triple-lumen catheter. Guidelines will specify the amount of blood to be drawn from the catheter and discarded before blood is collected for laboratory studies. The guidelines will also indicate the amount and type of solution needed to flush the catheter after drawing the blood to prevent it from being clogged by blood.
- Do not shake the blood specimen. Hemolysis may result from vigorous shaking and invalidate test results.
- Collect blood cultures before the initiation of antibiotic therapy. Blood cultures are often drawn when the patient manifests a fever. Often, two or three cultures are taken at 30-minute intervals from different venipuncture sites.
- Skin punctures can be used for blood tests on capillary blood. Common puncture sites include the fingertips, earlobes, and heel surfaces. Fingertips are often used for small children, and the heel is the most commonly used site for infants.

- Record the exact time when the specimen was collected. Indicate any drugs that the patient is taking.
- Ensure that the blood tubes are correctly labeled and delivered to the laboratory.
- After the specimen is drawn, apply pressure or a pressure dressing to the venipuncture site. Assess the site for bleeding.
- If the patient fasted before the blood test, reinstitute appropriate diet.

Urine tests

Overview

Urine tests are easy to obtain and provide valuable information about many body system functions, such as kidney function, glucose metabolism, and various hormone levels. The ability of the patient to obtain specimens appropriately should be assessed to determine the need for assistance.

Guidelines

- Observe universal precautions in collecting a urine specimen.
- Use the first morning specimen for routine urinalysis because it is more concentrated. To collect a first morning specimen, have the patient void before going to bed and collect the first urine specimen immediately on rising.
- *Random* urine specimens can be collected at any time. They are usually obtained during daytime hours and without any prior patient preparation.
- If a *culture and sensitivity* (C&S) study is required, or if the specimen is likely to be contaminated by vaginal discharge or bleeding, collect a "clean-catch" or "midstream" specimen. This requires meticulous cleansing of the urinary meatus with an iodine preparation to reduce contamination of the specimen by external organisms. Then the cleansing agent must be completely removed, since it may contaminate the specimen. Obtain the midstream collection by:
  1. Having the patient begin to urinate in a bedpan, urinal, or toilet and then stop urinating (This washes the urine out of the distal urethra.)
  2. Correctly positioning a sterile urine container, into which the patient voids 3 to 4 ounces of urine
  3. Capping the container
  4. Allowing the patient to finish voiding

- One-time *composite urine specimens* are collected over a period that may range anywhere from 2 to 24 hours. To collect a timed specimen, instruct the patient to void and discard the first specimen. This is noted as the "start time" of the test. Instruct the patient to save all subsequent urine in a special container for the designated period of time. Remind the patient to void before defecating so that urine is not contaminated by feces. Also, instruct the patient not to put toilet paper in the collection container. A preservative is usually used in the collection container. At the end of the specified time period, have the patient void and then add this urine to the specimen container, thus completing the collection process.

- Collection containers for 24-hour urine specimens should hold 3 to 4 L of urine and have tight-fitting lids. They should be labeled with the patient's name, the starting collection date and time, the ending collection date and time, the name of the test, the preservative, and storage requirements during collection.

- Many urine collections require preservatives to maintain their stability during the collection period. Some specimens are best preserved by being kept on ice or under refrigeration.

- *Urinary catheterization* may be needed for patients unable to void. This procedure is not preferred, because of the risk of introducing organisms and because of patient discomfort.

- For patients with an *indwelling urinary catheter,* obtain a specimen by attaching a small-gauge (e.g., 25-gauge) needle to a syringe and aseptically inserting the needle into the catheter at a point distal to the sleeve leading to the balloon. Aspirate urine and then place it in a sterile urine container. The urine that accumulates in the plastic reservoir bag should never be used for a urine test.

- Urine specimens from infants and young children are usually collected in a disposable pouch called a *U bag.* This bag has an adhesive backing around the opening to attach to the child. Once the bag is in place, check the child every 15 minutes to see if an adequate specimen has been collected. Remove the specimen as soon as possible after the collection, and then label it and transport it to the laboratory.

- Indicate on the laboratory slip any medications that may affect test results.

Stool tests

Overview

The examination of feces provides important information that aids in the differential diagnosis of various gastrointestinal disorders. Fecal studies may also be used for microbiologic studies, chemical determinations, and parasitic examinations.

Guidelines

- Observe universal precautions in collecting a stool specimen.
- Collect stool specimens in a clean container that has a fitted cover.
- Do not mix urine and toilet paper with the stool specimen. Both can contaminate the specimen and alter the results.
- Fecal analysis for occult blood, white blood cells, or qualitative fecal fat requires only a small amount of a randomly collected specimen.
- Quantitative tests for daily fecal excretion of a particular substance require a minimum of a 3-day fecal collection. This collection is necessary because the daily excretion of feces does not correlate well with the amount of food ingested by the patient in the same 24-hour period. Refrigerate specimens or keep them on ice during the collection period. Collect stool in a 1-gallon container.
- Some fecal collections require dietary restrictions before the collection (e.g., tests for occult blood).
- A small amount of fecal blood that is not visually apparent is termed *occult blood*. Chemical tests using commercially prepared slides are routinely employed to detect fecal blood. Numerous commercial slide tests use guaiac as the indicator. These guaiac tests are routinely done on nursing units in the hospital.
- Consider various factors (such as other diagnostic tests and medications) in planning the stool collection. For example, if the patient is scheduled for x-ray studies using barium sulfate, collect the stool specimen first. Various medications (e.g., tetracyclines and antidiarrheal preparations) affect the detection of intestinal parasites.
- Correctly label and deliver stool specimens to the laboratory within 30 minutes after collection. If you are unable to deliver the specimen within 30 minutes, it may be refrigerated for up to 2 hours.

X-ray studies

Overview

Because of the ability of x-rays to penetrate human tissue, x-ray studies provide a valuable picture of body structures. X-ray studies can be as simple as a routine chest x-ray film or as complex as dye-enhanced cardiac catheterization. With the increasing concern about radiation exposure, it is important to realize that the patient may want to know if the proposed benefit outweighs the risk involved.

Guidelines

- Assess the patient for any similar or recent x-ray procedures or allergies to iodine dye.
- Women in their childbearing years should have x-ray examinations during menses or 10 to 14 days after the onset of menses to avoid possible exposure to a fetus.
- Pregnant women should not have x-ray procedures, if possible, because of the risk of damage to the fetus.
- Note if other x-ray studies are being planned; schedule them in the appropriate sequence. For example, x-ray examinations that do not require contrast material should precede examinations that do require contrast material. X-ray studies using barium should be scheduled after ultrasonography studies.
- Note the necessary dietary restrictions. Studies such as a barium enema and intravenous pyelogram (IVP) are more accurate if the patient is kept NPO for several hours before the test.
- Determine if bowel preparations are necessary. For example, barium enemas and IVPs require bowel-cleansing regimens.
- Determine if signed consent forms are required. These are necessary for most invasive x-ray procedures.
- Remove metal objects such as necklaces and watches because they can hinder visualization of the x-ray field.
- Patient aftercare is determined by the type of x-ray procedure. For example, a patient having a simple chest x-ray study will not require postprocedure care. However, invasive x-ray procedures involving contrast dyes (such as cardiac catheterization) require extensive nursing measures to detect potential complications.
- Many types of contrast media are used in radiographic studies. For example, organic iodides and iodized oils are fre-

quently used. Patients who receive contrast media should be carefully evaluated for allergic reactions, which can range from mild nausea and vomiting to severe anaphylaxis.

Nuclear scanning

Overview

With the administration of a radionuclide and subsequent detection of the measurement of radiation of a particular organ, functional abnormalities of various body areas (such as the brain, heart, lung, and bones) can be detected. Because the half-lives of the radioisotopes are short, only minimal radiation exposure occurs.

Guidelines

- Radiopharmaceuticals concentrate in target organs by various mechanisms. For example, some labeled compounds such as hippuran are cleared from the blood and excreted by the kidneys. Some phosphate compounds concentrate in the bone and infarcted tissue. Lung function can be studied by imaging the distribution of inhaled gases or aerosols.
- Note whether the patient has had any recent exposure to radionuclides. The previous study could interfere with the interpretation of the current study.
- Note the patient's age and current weight. This information is used to calculate the amount of radioactive substance to be administered.
- Nuclear scans are contraindicated in pregnant women and nursing mothers.
- Many of the scanning procedures do not require special preparation. However, a few have special requirements. For example, in bone scanning, the patient is encouraged to drink several glasses of water between the time of the injection of the isotope and the actual scanning. For some studies, blocking agents may need to be given to prevent other organs from taking up the isotope.
- For most nuclear scans, a small amount of an organ-specific radionuclide is given orally or injected intravenously. After the radioisotope concentrates in the desired area, the area is scanned. The scanning procedure usually takes place in the nuclear medicine department.
- Instruct the patient to lie still during the scanning.
- Usually, encourage the patient to drink extra fluids to enhance excretion of the radionuclide after the test is finished.

- Although the amount of radionuclide excreted in the urine is very low, rubber gloves are sometimes recommended if the urine must be handled. Some hospitals may advise the patient to flush the toilet several times after voiding.

Ultrasound studies

Overview

In diagnostic ultrasonography, harmless high-frequency sound waves are emitted and penetrate the organ being studied. The sound waves bounce back to the sensor and are electronically converted into a picture of the organ. Ultrasonography is used to assess a wide variety of body areas, including the pelvis, abdomen, heart, and pregnant uterus.

Guidelines

- Most ultrasound procedures require little or no preparation. However, the patient having a pelvic sonogram needs a full bladder, and the patient having an ultrasound examination of the gallbladder must be kept NPO before the procedure.
- Ultrasound examinations are usually performed in an ultrasound room; however, they can be performed on the patient unit.
- Apply a greasy paste to the skin overlying the desired organ. This paste is used to enhance sound transmission and reception because air impedes transmission of sound waves to the body.
- Because of the noninvasive nature of ultrasonography, no special nursing measures are needed after the study except for helping the patient remove the ultrasound paste.
- Ultrasound examinations have no radiation risk.
- Ultrasound examinations can be repeated as many times as necessary without being harmful to the patient. No cumulative effect has been seen.
- Barium has an adverse effect on the quality of abdominal studies. For this reason, schedule ultrasound of the abdomen before barium studies.
- Large amounts of gas in the bowel will not permit visualization of the bowel. This is because bowel gas is a reflector of sound.

Endoscopy procedures

Overview

With the help of a lighted, flexible instrument, internal structures of many areas of the body (such as the stomach, colon, joints, bronchi, urinary system, and biliary tree) can be directly viewed. The specific purpose and procedure should be reviewed with the patient.

Guidelines

- Preparation for an endoscopic procedure varies with the internal structure being examined. For example, examination of the stomach (gastroscopy) will require the passage of an instrument through the esophagus to the stomach. The patient is kept NPO for 8 to 12 hours before the test to prevent gagging, vomiting, and aspiration. For colonoscopy, an instrument is passed through the rectum and into the colon. Therefore the bowel must be cleansed and free of fecal material to afford proper visualization. Arthroscopic examination of the knee joint is usually done with the patient under general anesthesia, which necessitates routine preoperative care.

- Schedule endoscopic examinations before barium studies.

- Obtain a signed consent for endoscopic procedures.

- Endoscopic procedures are preferably performed in a specially equipped endoscopy room or in the operating room by a physician. However, some kinds can safely be performed at the bedside.

- Air is instilled into the bowel during colon examinations to maintain patency of the bowel lumen and to afford better visualization. This sometimes causes gas pains.

- In addition to visualization of the desired area, special procedures can be performed. Biopsies can be obtained, and bleeding ulcers can be cauterized. Also, knee surgery can be performed during arthroscopy.

- Specific postprocedure interventions are determined by the type of endoscopic examination performed. All procedures have the potential complication of perforation and bleeding. Most procedures use some type of sedation; safety precautions should be observed until the effects of the sedatives have worn off.

- After colonoscopy and similar studies, the patient may complain of rectal discomfort. A warm tub bath may be soothing.

- Usually, keep the patient NPO for 2 hours after endoscopic procedures of the upper gastrointestinal system. Be certain that swallow, gag, and cough reflexes are present before permitting fluids or liquids to be ingested orally.

List of figures

Mosby's

Diagnostic and

Laboratory

Test Reference

abdominal ultrasound (Abdominal sonogram; Echogram; Ultrasound of the kidney, liver, pancreatobiliary system, gallbladder, pancreas, biliary tree)

Type of test Ultrasound

Normal findings Normal abdominal aorta, liver, gallbladder, bile ducts, pancreas, kidneys, ureters, and bladder

Test explanation and related physiology

Through use of reflected sound waves, ultrasonography provides accurate visualization of the abdominal aorta, liver, gallbladder, pancreas, bile ducts, kidneys, ureters, and bladder. The technique of ultrasonography requires the emission of high-frequency sound waves from the transducer to penetrate the particular organ being studied. The sound waves are bounced back to the transducer and then electronically converted into a pictorial image. A realistic Polaroid or x-ray film of the image is then obtained.

The *kidney* is ultrasonographically evaluated in order to diagnose and locate renal cysts, to differentiate renal cysts from solid renal tumors, to demonstrate renal and pelvic calculi, to document hydronephrosis, and to guide a percutaneously inserted needle for cyst aspiration or biopsy. One advantage of a kidney sonogram over intravenous pyelography (see p. 487) is that it can be performed on patients with impaired renal function because no intravenous contrast is required.

Another use of sonography is in the assessment of the *abdominal aorta* for aneurysmal dilation. Sonographic evidence of an aortic aneurysm greater than 5 cm or any size aneurysm that is documented to be significantly enlarging is an indication for abdominal aorta aneurysm resection. Ultrasound is also an ideal way to follow aneurysms before and after surgery.

Ultrasound is used in detecting cystic structures of the *liver* (e.g., benign cysts, hepatic abscesses, dilated hepatic ducts) and solid intrahepatic tumors (primary and metastatic). Hepatic ultrasound can also be performed intraoperatively by using a sterile probe. This technique allows for accurate location of small, nonpalpable hepatic tumors or abscesses. The *gallbladder and extrahepatic ducts* can be visualized and are examined for evidence of gallstones, polyps, or dilation secondary to obstructive strictures or tumors. The *pancreas* is examined for evidence of tumor, pseudocysts, acute inflammation, chronic inflammation, or pancreatic abscess. Ultrasound of the pancreas is frequently performed serially to document and demonstrate resolution of acute pancreatic inflammatory processes.

Because this study requires no contrast material and has no associated radiation, it is especially useful in patients who are allergic to contrast and in those who are pregnant. While fasting may be preferred, it is not mandatory. (See discussion of pelvic ultrasonography [p. 608] for sonographic evaluation of pelvic organs.)

Interfering factors

- Barium or gas will distort the sound waves and alter test results. This test should be performed before any x-ray testing with barium.

Procedure and patient care

Before

- Explain the procedure to the patient.
- Tell the patient that fasting may or may not be required depending on the organ to be examined. No fasting is required for ultrasonography of the abdominal aorta, kidney, liver, spleen, or pancreas. Fasting, however, is preferred for ultrasound of the gallbladder and biliary tree.

During

- Note the following procedural steps:
  1. The patient is placed on the ultrasonography table in the prone or supine position depending on the organ to be studied.
  2. A greasy conductive paste is applied to the patient's skin. This paste is used to enhance sound wave transmission and reception.
  3. A transducer is placed over the skin.
  4. Pictures are taken of the reflections from the organs being studied.
- The test is completed in approximately 20 minutes, usually by an ultrasound technologist, and interpreted by a radiologist.
- Tell the patient that no discomfort is associated with the procedure.

After

- Remove the coupling agent (grease) from the patient's abdomen or back.
- Note that if a biopsy is done, refer to biopsy of the specific organ (e.g., liver biopsy or kidney biopsy).

Abnormal findings

Kidney
Renal cysts
Renal tumor
Renal calculi
Hydronephrosis
Ureteral obstruction
Perirenal abscess
Glomerulonephritis
Pyelonephritis
Perirenal hematoma

Gallbladder
Polyps
Tumor
Gallstone

Liver
Tumor
Abscess
Intrahepatic dilated bile ducts

Pancreas
Tumor
Cysts
Pseudocysts
Abscess
Inflammation

Bile ducts
Gallstone
Dilation
Stricture
Tumor

Abdominal aorta
Aneurysm

notes

acetylcholine receptor antibody (AChR Ab, (Anti–acetylcholine receptor antibody)

Type of test Blood

Normal findings ≤0.03 nmol/L or negative

Test explanation and related physiology

This antibody may cause a block in neuromuscular transmission by interfering with the binding of AChR sites on the muscle membrane, thereby preventing muscle contraction. Antibodies to AChR occur in over 85% of patients with acquired myasthenia gravis (MG). Lower levels are seen in patients with only ocular MG. The presence of this antibody is virtually diagnostic of MG, but a negative test does not exclude the disease. The measured titers do not correspond well with the severity of MG in different patients. In an individual patient, however, antibody levels are particularly useful in monitoring response to therapy. As the patient improves, antibody titers decrease.

There are three different AChR antibodies. The *AChR-binding antibody* is most commonly used. If this test is negative and the diagnosis of MG is highly suspected, the *AChR-modulating antibody* is used and may be more sensitive. Furthermore, a positive modulating antibody test may indicate subclinical MG, contraindicating the use of curare-like drugs. The *AChR-blocking antibody* is less sensitive but can be quantitated more accurately. The most commonly used assay for AChR antibody is radioimmunoassay.

Interfering factors

- False-positive results may occur in patients with amyotrophic lateral sclerosis who have been treated with cobra venom.
- False-positive results may be seen in patients with penicillamine-induced, myasthenia-like symptoms.
- ☝ Drugs that may cause *increased* levels include muscle paralytic medicines (succinylcholine) and snake venom.

Procedure and patient care

Before

- Explain the procedure to the patient.
- Tell the patient that no fasting is required.

During

- Collect a venous blood sample in a red-top tube.
- List on the laboratory slip all medications that the patient has taken in the last few days.

After

- Apply pressure or a pressure dressing to the venipuncture site.
- Assess the venipuncture site for bleeding.

Abnormal finding

Positive

Myasthenia gravis

notes

acid-fast bacilli smear (AFB)

Type of test Sputum

Normal findings No bacilli seen

Test explanation and related physiology

The most clinically significant acid-fast bacilli is *Mycobacterium tuberculosis*. This is the causative agent in tuberculosis (TB). After taking up a dye such as fuchsin, *M. tuberculosis* is not decolorized by acid alcohol (i.e., it is acid-fast). It is seen under the microscope as a red, rod-shaped organism. If this bacillus is seen, the patient may have active TB. However, other species of mycobacteria, *Nocardia,* and some fungi are acid-fast. The acid-fast bacilli smear is most commonly performed on sputum. However, other specimens, such as cerebrospinal fluid (CSF), tissue, and synovial fluid, may be used. Smears may be negative as much as 50% of the time even with positive cultures. See p. 829 for discussion of TB cultures.

Procedure and patient care

Before

- Explain to the patient the procedure for sputum collection.
- Remind the patient that the sputum must be coughed up from the lungs and that saliva is not sputum.
- Hold antibiotics until after the sputum has been collected.
- Give the patient a sterile sputum container the night before the sputum is to be collected so that the morning specimen may be obtained when the patient awakens.
- Instruct the patient to rinse out his or her mouth with water before the sputum collection to decrease contamination by particles in the oropharynx. Remind the patient not to use mouthwash.

During

- For best results, obtain sputum collection when the patient awakens in the morning.
- Collect at least 1 teaspoon of sputum in a sterile sputum container.
- Obtain sputum by having the patient cough after taking several deep breaths.
- If the patient is unable to produce a sputum specimen,

stimulate coughing by lowering the head of the patient's bed or by giving the patient an aerosol administration of a warm hypertonic solution.
- Note that other methods to collect sputum, such as endotracheal aspiration, fiberoptic bronchoscopy, and transtracheal aspiration, may be used if necessary.
- For AFB determinations, collect sputum on three separate occasions.

After
- Avoid personal contamination and wear gloves when handling all patient secretions.
- Inform the patient to notify the nurse as soon as the specimen is collected.
- Label the specimen and send it to the laboratory as soon as possible.
- Inform the patient that culture results may take 3 weeks or longer.

Abnormal finding
Tuberculosis

notes

acid phosphatase (Prostatic acid phosphatase [PAP], Tartrate-resistant acid phosphatase [TRAP])

Type of test   Blood

Normal findings

Adult/elderly: 0.11-0.60 U/L (Roy, Brower, Hayden; 37° C)
    or 0.11-0.60 U/L (SI units)
Child: 8.6-12.6 U/ml (30° C)
Newborn: 10.4-16.4 U/ml (30° C)

Test explanation and related physiology

Acid phosphatase is found in many tissues, including liver, red blood cells, bone marrow, and platelets. Highest levels are found in the prostate gland. Determination of the acid phosphatase level is primarily used to diagnose and stage prostatic carcinoma and to monitor the efficacy of treatment. Elevated levels are seen in patients with prostatic cancer that has metastasized beyond the capsule to other parts of the body, especially bone. If the tumor is successfully treated by surgery, acid phosphatase levels decrease in several days. If the tumor is treated by estrogen therapy, enzyme levels return to normal in several weeks. Rising levels of acid phosphatase may indicate a poor prognosis. Several isoenzymes of acid phosphatase can be determined by electrophoresis. The most clinically significant isoenzyme is the prostatic acid phosphatase (PAP). It is more accurate than total acid phosphatase in the prostatic cancer patient but less accurate than the prostate-specific antigen (PSA) (see p. 668).

Acid phosphatase is also found at high concentrations in seminal fluid; therefore, acid phosphatase tests may be performed on vaginal secretions to investigate alleged acts of rape.

High levels of acid phosphatase exist in white blood cells (mostly monocytes and lymphocytes). This is helpful in identifying lymphoproliferative diseases, especially hairy-cell leukemia. In general, acid phosphatase is identified by cellular hydrolysis of naphthol phosphoric acid. The optimum pH for this reaction is on the acid side. When tartaric acid is added to the solution, hydrolysis of the substance by acid phosphatase is inhibited in prostate cells but not in the cells of hairy-cell leukemia. The identification of tartrate-resistant acid phosphatase (TRAP) is therefore very helpful in the diagnosis of hairy-cell leukemia. It is important to note, however, that the specimens of 5% of patients with hairy-cell leukemia are not tartrate resistant.

Interfering factors

- Falsely high levels of acid phosphatase may occur in males after a digital examination or after instrumentation of the prostate (e.g., cystoscopy) because of prostatic stimulation.
- Drugs that may cause *elevated* levels include androgens (in females) and clofibrate (Atromid S).
- Drugs that may cause *decreased* levels include fluorides, phosphates, oxalates, and alcohol.

Procedure and patient care

Before

- Explain the procedure to the patient.
- Tell the patient that no food or drink restrictions are associated with this test.
- Remember that some laboratories request they be notified before the blood sample is drawn so that immediate attention (<1 hr) can be given to the sample.

During

- Collect approximately 5 to 10 ml of blood in a red-top tube.
- Avoid hemolysis. Red blood cells contain acid phosphatase.
- Note on the laboratory slip if the patient has had a prostatic examination or instrumentation of the prostate within the last 24 hours.

After

- Apply pressure or a pressure dressing to the venipuncture site.
- Assess the venipuncture site for bleeding.
- Have the test performed without delay or freeze the specimen.
- Do *not* leave the specimen at room temperature for 1 hour or longer, because the enzyme is heat and pH sensitive and its activity will decrease.

Abnormal findings

▲ **Increased levels**

Prostatic carcinoma
Multiple myeloma
Paget's disease
Sickle cell crisis
Gaucher's disease
Renal impairment
Recent prostate manipulation

Benign prostatic hypertrophy
Prostatitis
Cancer of the breast and bone
Cirrhosis
Hyperparathyroidism
Thrombocytosis
Cancer metastasis to the bone

notes

adrenal venography

Type of test X-ray with contrast dye

Normal findings Normal adrenal veins and normal adrenal vein hormone assay

Test explanation and related physiology

Adrenal venography is a radiologic test performed to obtain blood samples from the adrenal vein and to allow localization of adrenal pathology. Once the vein is identified, a catheter can be placed in the vein and blood selectively obtained from each adrenal vein.

In patients with Cushing's syndrome, the blood is analyzed for plasma cortisol. If the plasma cortisol level in the blood obtained from one side is much higher than that of the other, a unilateral adrenal tumor is causing Cushing's syndrome. If, on the other hand, plasma cortisol levels are bilaterally elevated, one can safely conclude that Cushing's syndrome is caused by bilateral adrenal hyperplasia.

In patients with a pheochromocytoma, the adrenal venous blood is analyzed for catecholamines. If the catecholamine level on one side is much higher than that of the other, a unilateral pheochromocytoma exists on the side with the elevated levels. If blood obtained from both sides is equally elevated, the patient probably has bilateral adrenal pheochromocytoma. If the adrenal venous blood samples are not elevated on either side in a patient who has elevated peripheral blood catecholamine levels, the pheochromocytoma exists outside the adrenal gland (i.e., extraadrenal pheochromocytoma).

The venous blood also can be evaluated for aldosterone, androgens, and other substances.

Contraindications

- Patients with allergies to shellfish or iodinated dye
- Patients with bleeding disorders

Potential complications

- Allergic reaction to iodinated dye
  Allergic reactions may vary from mild flushing, itching, and urticaria to severe, life-threatening anaphylaxis (evidenced by respiratory distress, drop in blood pressure, or shock). In the

unusual event of anaphylaxis, the patient is treated with diphenhydramine (Benadryl), steroids, and epinephrine. Oxygen and endotracheal equipment should be on hand for immediate use.

- Adrenal hemorrhage or necrosis caused by the pressure of the dye injection
  This may cause Addison's disease (adrenal insufficiency).
- Cellulitis
- Thrombophlebitis
- Bacteremia

Procedure and patient care

Before

- Explain the procedure to the patient.
- Ensure that a written and informed consent for this procedure has been obtained.
- Assess the patient for allergies to iodine dye. Inform the radiologist if an allergy to iodinated contrast is suspected. The radiologist may prescribe a Benadryl-and-steroid preparation to be administered before testing. Usually, hypoallergenic nonionic contrast will be used during the test.
- Administer propranolol (Inderal), a beta-adrenergic blocker, and phenoxybenzamine (Dibenzyline), an alpha-adrenergic blocker, for the patient with a suspected pheochromocytoma. This prevents a potentially fatal catecholamine-induced hypertensive episode.

During

- Bring the fasting patient to the angiography laboratory (usually in the radiology department).
- Place the patient in the supine position on the x-ray table.
- Note the following procedural steps:
  1. The patient's groin is prepared and draped in a sterile manner.
  2. After the venipuncture site is locally anesthetized, the femoral vein is catheterized.
  3. The catheter is passed into the adrenal vein.
  4. Dye is injected to visualize the adrenal veins and to ensure that the catheter is in the adrenal vein.
  5. Blood is obtained and sent to the chemistry laboratory for assays.
- Note that this procedure is usually performed by an angiographer (radiologist) in approximately 1 hour.

- Tell the patient that the only discomfort is the groin puncture necessary for venous access.

A

After

- Evaluate the patient's vital signs frequently for signs of bleeding or hemorrhage.
- Assess the patient with a suspected pheochromocytoma for signs and symptoms of a hypertensive episode. If such an episode occurs, notify the physician immediately to obtain an order for appropriate alpha- and beta-adrenergic blocking agents.
- Assess the groin site for redness, pain, swelling, and bleeding with each vital sign check.
- Apply cold compresses to the puncture site if needed to reduce discomfort or swelling.

Abnormal findings

Unilateral adrenal tumor
Bilateral adrenal tumor
Unilateral pheochromocytoma
Bilateral pheochromocytoma
Extraadrenal pheochromocytoma

notes

adrenocorticotropic hormone (ACTH, Corticotropin)

Type of test Blood

Normal findings

AM: 15-100 pg/ml or 10-80 ng/L (SI units)
PM: <50 pg/ml or <50 ng/L (SI units)

Test explanation and related physiology

The serum ACTH study is a test of anterior pituitary gland function that affords the greatest insight into the causes of either Cushing's syndrome or Addison's disease. In the patient with Cushing's syndrome, an elevated ACTH level can be caused by a pituitary ACTH-producing tumor, or a nonpituitary (ectopic) ACTH-producing tumor, usually in the lung, pancreas, thymus, or ovary. ACTH levels over 200 pg/ml usually indicate ectopic ACTH production. If the ACTH level is below normal in a patient with Cushing's syndrome, an adrenal adenoma or carcinoma is probably the cause of the hyperfunction.

In patients with Addison's disease, an elevated ACTH level indicates primary adrenal gland failure, as in adrenal gland destruction caused by infarction, hemorrhage, or autoimmunity; surgical removal of the adrenal gland; congenital enzyme deficiency; or adrenal suppression after prolonged ingestion of exogenous steroids. If the ACTH level is below normal in a patient with adrenal insufficiency, hypopituitarism is most probably the cause of the hypofunction.

One must be aware that there is a diurnal variation of ACTH levels. Levels in evening samples are usually one half to two thirds those of morning specimens. ACTH is accurately measured by radioimmunoassay.

Interfering factors

- Stress (trauma, pyrogens, or hypoglycemia) and pregnancy can increase levels.
- Recently administered radioisotope scans can affect levels.
- Drugs that may cause *increased* levels include estrogens, ethanol, vasopressin, aminoglutetimide, amphetamines, insulin, metyrapone, and spironolactone.
- Corticosteroids may *decrease* ACTH levels.

Procedure and patient care

A

Before

- Explain the procedure to the patient. Allow plenty of time to answer questions so that the patient's stress is diminished as much as possible.
- Keep the patient NPO after midnight the day of the test.
- Evaluate the patient for stress factors that would invalidate the test results.
- Evaluate the patient for sleep pattern abnormalities. With a normal sleep pattern, the ACTH level is highest between 4 AM and 8 AM and lowest around 9 PM.

During

- Collect approximately 20 ml of heparinized venous blood in a green-top tube.
- Chill the blood tube to prevent enzymatic degradation of ACTH.

After

- Place the specimen in ice water and send it to the chemistry laboratory immediately. ACTH is a very unstable peptide in plasma and should be stored at minus 20° C to prevent artificially low values.
- Apply pressure or a pressure dressing to the venipuncture site.
- Assess the venipuncture site for bleeding.

Abnormal findings

▲ **Increased levels**

Addison's disease (primary adrenal insufficiency)

Cushing's disease (pituitary-dependent adrenal hyperplasia)

Ectopic ACTH syndrome

Stress

Adrenogenital syndrome (congenital adrenal hyperplasia)

▼ **Decreased levels**

Secondary adrenal insufficiency (pituitary insufficiency)

Cushing's syndrome

Hypopituitarism

Adrenal adenoma or carcinoma

Steroid administration

adrenocorticotropic hormone stimulation test (ACTH stimulation test, Cortisol stimulation test, Cosyntropin test)

Type of test Blood

Normal findings

Rapid test: cortisol levels increase more than 7 μg/dl above
  baseline
24-hour test: cortisol levels greater than 40 μg/dl
3-day test: cortisol levels greater than 40 μg/dl

Test explanation and related physiology

Exogenous ACTH is given to the patient, and the ability of
the adrenal glands to respond to ACTH stimulation is measured
by plasma cortisol levels. Patients with cushingoid symptoms
caused by bilateral adrenal hyperplasia will have an exaggerated
response to the ACTH stimulation. Hyperfunctioning adrenal
tumors, however, which are usually autonomous and relatively
insensitive to changes in ACTH levels, are associated with little
or no increase in cortisol levels over baseline values in these patients.

This test is even more valuable in the patient suspected of having adrenal insufficiency. An appropriate increase in plasma cortisol levels after the infusion of ACTH shows that the adrenal
gland is capable of functioning if stimulated. The cause of the
adrenal insufficiency would lie within the pituitary gland (hypopituitarism, which is secondary adrenal insufficiency). If either
little or no rise in cortisol levels occurs, the adrenal gland cannot secrete cortisol because of primary adrenal pathology (Addison's disease), which may be caused by adrenal hemorrhage,
infarction, autoimmunity, metastatic tumor, surgical removal of
the adrenal glands, or congenital adrenal enzyme deficiency.

The rapid stimulation test is only a screening test. A normal
response excludes primary or secondary adrenal insufficiency. To
substantiate the diagnosis of adrenal insufficiency and to differentiate primary insufficiency from secondary insufficiency, a
3-day test is essential. It should be noted that the adrenal gland
can also be stimulated by insulin. When insulin is the stimulant,
cortisol levels and glucose levels are measured.

Interfering factors

☛ Drugs that may cause artificially *increased* cortisol levels include corticosteroid, estrogens, and spironolactone.

Procedure and patient care

Before

- Keep the patient NPO after midnight the day of the test.

During

Rapid test

- Obtain a baseline plasma cortisol level. This should be done within 30 minutes of cosyntropin (ACTH-like drug) administration.
- Administer an IV injection of cosyntropin over a 2-minute period.
- Measure plasma cortisol levels 30 and 60 minutes after drug administration.

24-hour test

- Obtain a baseline plasma cortisol level.
- Start an IV infusion of synthetic cosyntropin in 1 L of normal saline.
- Administer the solution at the rate of 2 U/hr for 24 hours.
- After 24 hours, obtain another plasma cortisol level.

3-day test

- Obtain a baseline plasma cortisol level.
- Administer 25 U of cosyntropin IV over an 8-hour period on 2 to 3 consecutive days.
- The plasma cortisol is then measured at 12, 24, 36, 48, 60, and 72 hours after the start of the test.
- Collect plasma for cortisol levels in a red-top tube.

After

- Apply pressure or a pressure dressing to the venipuncture site.
- Check the venipuncture site for bleeding.

Abnormal findings

Adrenal insufficiency
  Increase above normal response (secondary adrenal insufficiency)
    Hypopituitarism
  Normal or below normal response (primary adrenal insufficiency)
    Addison's disease

    Adrenal infarction/hemorrhage
    Metastatic tumor to the adrenal gland
    Congenital enzyme adrenal insufficiency
    Surgical removal of the adrenal gland
Cushing's syndrome
  Increased above normal response
    Bilateral adrenal hyperplasia
  Normal or below normal response
    Adrenal adenoma
    Adrenal carcinoma
    ACTH-producing tumor
    Chronic steroid ingestion

notes

agglutinins, febrile/cold

Type of test Blood

Normal findings

Febrile (warm) agglutinins: no agglutination in titers $\leq 1:80$
Cold agglutinins: no agglutination in titers $\leq 1:16$

Test explanation and related physiology

Febrile agglutinins serologic studies are used to diagnose infectious diseases such as salmonellosis, rickettsial diseases, brucellosis, and tularemia. Neoplastic diseases such as leukemias and lymphomas are also associated with febrile agglutinins. Appropriate antibiotic treatment of the infectious agent is associated with a drop in the titer activity of febrile agglutinins.

Cold agglutinins occur in patients who are infected by other agents, most notably *Mycoplasma pneumoniae*. Other diseases include influenza, mononucleosis, rheumatoid arthritis, and lymphomas.

The febrile and cold agglutinins are antibodies that cause red blood cells (RBCs) to aggregate at high or low temperatures, respectively. Normally, agglutination may occur in concentrated serum ($<1:32$ dilution). Agglutination occurring at titers greater than $1:16$ for cold agglutinins and $1:80$ for febrile agglutinins is considered abnormal and diagnostic of the infectious agent the agglutinins represent.

Temperature regulation is important for the performance of these tests. For *cold agglutinins,* the red-top tube is previously warmed to over 37°C; for *febrile agglutinins,* the red-top tube is cooled. The specimen is immediately taken to the laboratory so that no hemolysis will occur. Under no circumstances should the cold agglutinin specimen be refrigerated or the febrile agglutinin be heated. At the laboratory, the cold agglutinin specimen is chilled and evaluated for agglutination of RBCs. The febrile agglutinin specimen is heated and also inspected for agglutination of RBCs. Serial dilutions are performed to detect the dilution at which agglutination occurs.

Procedure and patient care

Before
- Explain the procedure to the patient.
- Tell the patient that no fasting is required.

During
- Collect approximately 7 ml of venous blood in a red-top tube (warmed or cooled; see previous discussion).

After
- Apply pressure or a pressure dressing to the venipuncture site.
- Observe the venipuncture site for bleeding.
- Transport the specimen immediately to the laboratory.

Abnormal findings

▲ **Increased febrile agglutinins**

Salmonellosis infection
Rickettsial disease
Brucellosis
Tularemia
Leukemia
Lymphoma

▲ **Increased cold agglutinins**

Mycoplasma pneumoniae infection
Viral illness
Infectious mononucleosis
Multiple myeloma
Scleroderma
Cirrhosis
Staphylococcemia
Thymic tumor
Influenza
Rheumatoid arthritis
Lymphoma

notes

AIDS serology (Acquired immunodeficiency serology, AIDS screen, Human immunodeficiency virus (HIV) antibody test, Western blot test for HIV and antibody, Enzyme-linked immunosorbent assay [ELISA] for HIV and antibody)

Type of test Blood

Normal findings No evidence of HIV antigen or antibodies

Test explanation and related physiology

Tests used to detect the antibody to HIV, which is the virus that causes acquired immunodeficiency syndrome (AIDS), were first licensed by the Food and Drug Administration (FDA) in 1985 for the screening of blood and plasma donors. The HIV virus is also known as human T-lymphotrophic virus, type III (HTLV-III), or the lymphadenopathy-associated virus (LAV). Since 1985, millions of HIV antibody tests have been performed in laboratories of blood and plasma collection centers, in counseling centers, and in clinical screening facilities. Those at high risk for AIDS include sexually active male homosexuals and bisexual men and women with multiple partners, IV drug abusers, persons receiving blood products containing HIV, and infants exposed to the virus during gestation and delivery. Accurate test results require attention to both the intrinsic quality of the tests and the technical ability of the technician performing them.

Because of the medical and social significance of a positive test for HIV antibody, test results must be accurate and their interpretation correct. Therefore the U.S. Public Health Service has emphasized that an individual can be said to have serologic evidence of HIV infection only after an enzyme immunoassay (EIA) screening test is repeatedly reactive and another test, such as Western blot or immunofluorescence assay, validates the results.

The enzyme-linked immunosorbent assay (ELISA), which tests for antibodies to HIV in serum or plasma, is the most widely used serologic test for AIDS. It is important to note that ELISA detects *antibodies* to HIV. Because it does not detect viral antigens, it cannot detect infection in its earliest stage, before antibodies are formed. ELISA is used for clinical diagnosis, screening blood and blood products, and testing individuals who believe they may be infected with HIV.

The sensitivity (i.e., probability that the test results will be reactive if the specimen is a true positive) of the ELISA test is approximately 99% for blood from persons infected with HIV for 12 weeks or more. The probability of a false-negative test is remote except during the first few weeks after infection, before detectable antibodies appear.

The specificity (probability that test results will be nonreactive if the specimen is a true negative) of the ELISA test is approximately 99% when repeatedly reactive tests are considered. To increase the specificity of serologic tests further, a supplemental test (most often the Western blot) is done to validate repeatedly reactive ELISA results. Sensitivity of the blot test is comparable to or greater than a repeatedly reactive ELISA. The testing sequence of a repeatedly reactive ELISA and a positive Western blot test is highly predictive of HIV infection.

The diagnostic test described above detects HIV infection based on demonstration of *antibodies* to HIV. Recently it has become possible to diagnose HIV infection by the direct detection of HIV or one of its components. New tests are now available in the research laboratory, and are of considerable help when the Western blot results are indeterminate. The simplest of these tests is the *p24 antigen capture assay*. This is an ELISA-type assay that detects the viral protein p24 in the peripheral blood of HIV-infected individuals, where it exists either as a free antigen or complexed to anti-p24 antibodies.

The p24 antigen may be detectable as early as 2 to 6 weeks after infection. Throughout the course of HIV infection, an equilibrium exists between p24 antigen and anti-p24 antibodies. During the first few weeks of infection, before the development of an immune response, there is a sharp increase in p24 antigen levels. These levels decline after the development of anti-p24 antibodies. Later in HIV disease, p24 antigen levels become detectable again.

The p24 antigen test is currently being used to assess the antiviral activity of experimental HIV therapies. The p24 antigen test can also be used to diagnose neonatal HIV infection, detect HIV before seroconversion, and determine the progression of AIDS.

Interfering factors

- False-positive results can occur in patients who have autoimmune disease, lymphoproliferative disease, leukemia, lymphoma, syphilis, or alcoholism.
- False-negative results can occur in the early incubation stage or end stage of AIDS.

Procedure and patient care

Before

- Explain the procedure to the patient.
- Obtain an informed consent if required by the institution.
- Tell the patient that no fasting or preparation is required.
- Maintain a nonjudgmental attitude toward the patient's sexual practices and allow the patient ample time to express his or her concerns regarding the results.

During

- Observe universal blood and body precautions. Wear gloves when handling blood products from all patients.
- Collect 7 ml of peripheral venous blood in a red-top tube. The blood is usually sent to an outside laboratory for testing.
- If the patient wishes to remain anonymous, use a number with the patient's name and record it accurately.
- Note that if the ELISA test is repeatedly reactive (i.e., test is positive twice consecutively), the Western blot test is performed on the same blood sample.
- If the Western blot test is equivocal, collect a second serum specimen 2 to 4 months later for testing.

After

- Apply pressure or a pressure dressing to the venipuncture site.
- Assess the site for bleeding.
- Inform the patient to observe the venipuncture site for infection. Patients with AIDS are immunocompromised and susceptible to infection.
- Follow the institution's policy regarding test result reporting. Do not give results over the telephone. Remember that positive results may have devastating consequences.
- Explain to the patient that a positive Western blot test merely implies exposure to and presence of the AIDS virus within the body. It does not mean that the patient has clinical AIDS. Not all patients with positive antibodies will acquire the disease.
- Encourage patients testing positive to identify their sexual contacts so that they can be informed and tested.
- Inform the patient that subsequent sexual contact will put new partners at high risk for contracting AIDS.
- Provide patient education regarding safe sexual practices.

Abnormal findings

▲ **Increased levels**
AIDS
AIDS-related complex (ARC)

notes

AIDS T-lymphocyte cell markers (CD4 marker, CD4/CD8 ratio, CD4 percentage)

Type of test Blood

Normal findings Total CD4 count greater than 1000 cells/mm^3

Test explanation and related physiology

The test used to detect the antibody to HIV, which is the virus that causes AIDS, is explained on p. 21. The pathogenesis of AIDS is largely attributed to a decrease in the T lymphocyte that bears the CD4 receptor. Progressive depletion of CD4 T lymphocytes is associated with an increased likelihood of clinical complications from AIDS. Therefore CD4 measurement is a prognostic marker that can indicate whether a patient infected with HIV is at risk for developing opportunistic infections. The measurement of CD4 cell levels is used for deciding the timing of initiating *Pneumocystis carinii* pneumonia prophylaxis and the use of antiviral therapy and for determining the prognosis of patients with HIV infection.

There are three related measurements of CD4 T lymphocytes. The first measurement is the *total CD4 cell count*. This is measured in whole blood and is the product of the white blood cell count, the lymphocyte differential count, and the percentage of lymphocytes that are CD4 T cells. The second measurement, the *CD4 percentage,* is a more accurate prognostic marker. It measures the percentage of CD4 lymphocytes in the whole blood sample by using immunophenotyping with flow cytometry. This procedure relies on detecting specific antigenic determinants on the surface of the CD4 lymphocyte by antigen-specific monoclonal antibodies labeled with a fluorescent dye. The third prognostic marker, which is also more reliable than the total CD4 count, is the *ratio of CD4 cells to CD8 (T-suppresser) cells.*

Of the three T-cell measurements, total CD4 count is the most variable. There is substantial diurnal variation in this count. Because it is a calculated measurement, the combination of laboratory error and personal fluctuation can result in wide variations in test results. With the CD4 percentage and CD4/CD8 ratios, very little diurnal variation and laboratory error exist. The Multicenter AIDS Cohort Study suggests that the latter two measurements are more accurate than the total CD4 count. Because the total CD4 cell count was originally thought to be the best marker, however, this test was used in many of the studies that now form the basis for practice recommendations. It will take time before the more accurate measurements find clinical pertinence in practice recommendations.

The U.S. Public Health Service has recommended that CD4 prognostic markers be monitored every 3 to 6 months in all persons infected with HIV. Because the CD4 counts gradually fall in virtually all such patients, periodic review of the count can be emotionally stressful for both the patient and physician. The patient confronts his or her mortality as the health care provider confronts his or her ultimate powerlessness against the relentlessly advancing infections.

As the CD4 cell measurements decrease, the percentage of persons developing AIDS increases. Forty-eight percent of patients can be expected to develop AIDS within 6 months when their CD4 count is 100 cells/mm^3.

It is recommended that antiviral therapy be started in patients whose CD4 count is less than 500 to 600 cells/mm^3. *Pneumocystis carinii* pneumonia prophylaxis should start when the CD4 count is less than 200 to 300 cells/mm^3.

CD4 prognostic markers also can be useful in guiding the approach to the patient's symptoms. Complaints such as cough and headache are common in most people; however, in patients infected with HIV, these symptoms often raise concerns about opportunistic infections. If the CD4 cell count was over 500 cells/mm^3 in the past 6 months, there is a very low probability that these symptoms result from opportunistic infections. Knowing this, the patient and physician can feel comfortable with routine care.

Contraindications

- Patients who are not emotionally prepared for the prognosis that the results may indicate

Interfering factor

- Diurnal variation

Procedure and patient care

Before

- Explain the procedure to the patient.
- Tell the patient that no fasting or preparation is required.
- Maintain a nonjudgmental attitude toward the patient's

sexual practices. Allow the patient ample time to express his or her concerns regarding the results.

During

- Record the time of day when the blood specimen is being obtained.
- Observe universal body and blood precautions. Wear gloves when handling blood products from all patients.
- Never recap needles. Dispose of needles and syringes required for obtaining the blood specimen in a puncture-proof container designed for this purpose.
- Obtain 10 ml of blood in a large green-top tube (containing sodium heparin).
- Obtain 5 ml of blood in a small purple-top tube (containing ethylenediaminetetraacetic acid [EDTA]).

After

- Keep the specimen at room temperature. Do not refrigerate.
- The specimen must be evaluated within 24 hours.
- Most specimens are sent to a central laboratory. Be sure to draw the blood immediately before the courier's departure to the central laboratory.
- Apply pressure or a pressure dressing to the venipuncture site.
- Assess the puncture site for bleeding.
- Instruct the patient to observe the venipuncture site for infection. Patients with AIDS are immunocompromised and susceptible to infection.
- Encourage the patient to discuss his or her concerns regarding the prognostic information that may be obtained by these results.

Abbnormal findings

▼ **Decreased levels**
Increased risk for clinical symptoms from AIDS
Increased risk for opportunistic infections

notes

alanine aminotransferase (ALT, Serum glutamic-pyruvic transaminase [SGPT])

Type of test Blood

Normal findings

Adult/child: 5-35 IU/L or 8-20 U/L (SI units)
Elderly: may be slightly higher than adult
Infant: may be twice as high as adult

Test explanation and related physiology

Alanine aminotransferase is found predominantly in the liver; lesser quantities are found in the kidneys, heart, and skeletal muscle. Injury or disease affecting the liver parenchyma will cause a release of this hepatocellular enzyme into the bloodstream, thus elevating serum ALT levels. Generally, most ALT elevations are caused by liver dysfunction. Therefore this enzyme is not only sensitive but also quite specific in indicating hepatocellular disease. In hepatocellular disease other than viral hepatitis, the ALT/AST ratio (DeRitis ratio) is less than 1. In viral hepatitis, the ratio is greater than 1. This is helpful in the diagnosis of viral hepatitis.

Interfering factors

- Previous IM injections may cause elevated levels.
- Drugs that may cause *increased* ALT levels include acetaminophen, allopurinol, aminosalicylic acid (PAS), ampicillin, azathioprine, carbamazepine, cephalosporins, chlordiazepoxide, chlorpropamide, clofibrate, cloxacillin, codeine, dicumarol, indomethacin, isoniazid (INH), methotrexate, methyldopa, nafcillin, nalidixic acid, nitrofurantoin, oral contraceptives, oxacillin, phenothiazines, phenylbutazone, phenytoin, procainamide, propoxyphene, propranolol, quinidine, salicylates, tetracyclines, and verapamil.

Procedure and patient care

Before

- Explain the procedure to the patient.
- Tell the patient that no fasting is required.

During

- Collect approximately 7 to 10 ml of blood in a red-top tube and send it to the laboratory for analysis.
- Indicate on the laboratory slip any medications that might affect the test results.

After

- Apply pressure or a pressure dressing to the venipuncture site.
- Assess the venipuncture site for bleeding. Patients with liver dysfunction often have prolonged clotting times.

Abnormal findings

▲ **Increased levels**

Hepatitis
Cirrhosis
Hepatic necrosis
Cholestasis
Hepatic ischemia

Hepatic tumor
Hepatotoxic drugs
Obstructive jaundice
Myositis
Pancreatitis

notes

aldolase

Type of test Blood

Normal findings

Adult: 3.0-8.2 Sibley-Lehninger U/dl or 22-59 mU at 37° C
  (SI units)
Child: approximately two times the adult values
Newborn: approximately four times the adult values

Test explanation and related physiology

Serum aldolase is very similar to the enzymes aspartate aminotransferase (AST, SGOT) (see p. 117) and creatine phosphokinase (CPK) (see p. 293). Aldolase is an enzyme used in the glycolytic breakdown of glucose. As with AST and CPK, aldolase exists throughout the body in most tissues. This test is most useful in indicating muscular or hepatic cellular injury or destruction. The serum aldolase level is very high in patients with muscular dystrophies, dermatomyositis, and polymyositis. Levels also are increased in patients with gangrenous processes, muscular trauma, and muscular infectious diseases (e.g., trichinosis). Elevated levels are also noted in chronic hepatitis, obstructive jaundice, and cirrhosis.

Neurologic diseases causing weakness can be differentiated from muscular causes of weakness with this test. Normal values are seen in patients with such neurologic diseases as poliomyelitis, myasthenia gravis, and multiple sclerosis. Elevated aldolase levels are seen in the primary muscular disorders.

Interfering factors

- Previous IM injections may cause *elevated* levels.
- ✗ Drugs that may cause *increased* aldolase levels include hepatotoxic agents.
- ✗ Drugs that may cause *decreased* levels include phenothiazines.

Procedure and patient care

Before

- Explain the procedure to the patient.
- Note that a short period of fasting usually will provide more accurate results.

A

During

- Collect 7 to 10 ml of blood in a red-top tube.
- Indicate on the laboratory slip any drugs that may affect test results.

After

- Apply pressure or pressure dressing to the venipuncture site.
- Observe the venipuncture site for bleeding.

Abnormal findings

▲ **Increased levels**

Hepatocellular diseases (e.g., hepatitis)
Muscular diseases (e.g., muscular dystrophy, dermatomyositis, polymyositis)
Muscular trauma (e.g., severe crush injuries)
Muscular infections (e.g., trichinosis)
Gangrenous processes (e.g., gangrene of the bowel)

▼ **Decreased levels**

Late muscular dystrophy
Hereditary fructose intolerance

notes

aldosterone assay

Type of test   Blood, urine (24-hour)

Normal findings

Blood

Supine: 3-10 ng/dl or 0.08-0.30 nmol/L (SI units)
Upright
   Female: 5-30 ng/dl or 0.14-0.80 nmol/L (SI units)
   Male: 6-22 ng/dl or 0.17-0.61 nmol/L (SI units)
Newborn: 5-60 ng/dl

1 week-1 year: 1-160 ng/dl	5-7 years: <5-50 ng/dl
1-3 years: 5-60 ng/dl	7-11 years: 5-70 ng/dl
3-5 years: <5-80 ng/dl	11-15 years: <5-50 ng/dl

Urine

2-80 µg/24 hr or 5.5-72.0 nmol/24 hr (SI units)

Test explanation and related physiology

Aldosterone, a hormone produced by the adrenal cortex, is a potent mineralocorticoid. Production of this enzyme is regulated primarily by the renin-angiotensin system and secondarily by adrenocorticotropic hormone (ACTH) or plasma sodium or potassium concentration. Aldosterone stimulates the renal tubules to absorb increased amounts of sodium (which causes water retention) and to secrete potassium. In this way, it regulates sodium, potassium, and water balance based on the body's needs.

Increased aldosterone levels are a major diagnostic finding in primary aldosteronism, in which a tumor of the adrenal cortex (Conn's syndrome) or bilateral adrenal hyperplasia causes increased production of aldosterone. The typical pattern for primary aldosteronism is an increased aldosterone level and a decreased renin level. The renin level is low because the increased aldosterone level "turns off" the renin-angiotensin mechanism. Patients with primary aldosteronism characteristically have hypertension and hypokalemia. Increased aldosterone levels are also present in secondary aldosteronism (caused by renal vascular occlusion or other renal disease, diuretics, laxative abuse, hypovolemia, or pregnancy), but renin levels are high.

The aldosterone assay can be done on a 24-hour urine specimen or a plasma blood sample. The advantage of the 24-hour urine sample is that short-term fluctuations are eliminated. Plasma values are more convenient to sample, but they are affected by the short-term fluctuations. For example, lower aldosterone values occur in the afternoon. Having the patient in an upright position greatly increases the plasma aldosterone level. Twenty-four-hour urine collection is much more reliable by avoiding the effect of those interfering factors. Levels of both urine and plasma are increased by low-sodium diets and are decreased by high-sodium diets. Hypokalemia inhibits aldosterone secretion.

Primary aldosteronism can be diagnosed by demonstrating very little or no rise in renin with aldosterone stimulation using salt restriction. Further aldosterone secretion will not be suppressed with saline infusion in these patients. Aldosterone can be measured in blood obtained from adrenal venous sampling (see p. 11). In this situation, high levels from the right and left adrenal veins are diagnostic of bilateral adrenal hyperplasia. Unilateral high aldosterone levels are found in tumors of the adrenal gland.

Interfering factors

- Strenuous exercise and stress can stimulate adrenocortical secretions and increase aldosterone levels.
- Excessive licorice ingestion can cause decreased levels, because it produces an aldosterone-like effect.
- Values are influenced by posture, diet, and pregnancy.
- ✖ Drugs that may cause *increased* levels include diazoxide (Hyperstat), hydralazine (Apresoline), nitroprusside (Nipride), diuretics, laxatives, potassium, and spironolactone.
- ✖ Drugs that may cause *decreased* levels include fludrocortisone (Florinef), propranolol (Inderal), and angiotensin-converting inhibitor (e.g., captopril), as well as licorice.

Procedure and patient care

Before

- Explain the procedure for the blood collection to the patient. Hospitalized patients will usually have the blood drawn before getting out of bed. Inform nonhospitalized patients when to arrive at the laboratory and how the amount of time in the upright position affects the test.
- Tell the patient that no fasting is necessary.
- Explain the procedure for collecting a 24-hour urine sample.

- Give the patient verbal and written instructions regarding dietary and medication restrictions.
- Instruct the patient to maintain a normal sodium diet (approximately 3 g/day) for at least 2 weeks before the blood or urine collection.
- Have the patient ask the physician whether drugs that alter sodium, potassium, and fluid balance (e.g., diuretics, antihypertensives, steroids, oral contraceptives) should be withheld. Test results will be more accurate if these are suspended at least 2 weeks before either the blood or the urine test.
- Inform the patient that renin inhibitors (e.g., propranolol) should not be taken 1 week before the test.
- Tell the patient to avoid licorice for at least 2 weeks before the test because of its aldosterone-like effect.

During blood collection

- Collect approximately 5 to 10 ml of venous blood in a red- or green-top tube.
- For hospitalized patients, draw the sample with the patient in the supine position *before* he or she arises.
- Note that sometimes a second specimen (upright sample) is collected 4 hours later, after the patient has been up and moving.
- Indicate on the laboratory slip if the patient was supine or standing during the venipuncture.
- Handle the blood specimen gently. Rough handling may cause hemolysis and alter the test results.
- Transport the specimen on ice to the laboratory.
- List on the laboratory slip any medications that can affect test results.

During urine collection

- Instruct the patient to begin the 24-hour urine collection after urinating.
- Discard this specimen and note this time as the start of the 24-hour collection.
- Collect urine passed over the next 24 hours.
- Instruct the patient to void before defecating so that the urine is not contaminated by feces.
- Remind the patient not to put toilet paper in the collection container.
- Use a preservative with this 24-hour specimen.

- Keep the urine specimen on ice or refrigerated during the 24 hours.
- Collect the last specimen as close as possible to the end of the 24 hours. Add this urine to the container.

After blood collection

- Apply pressure or a pressure dressing to the venipuncture site.
- Assess the venipuncture site for bleeding.

After urine collection

- Transport the urine specimen promptly to the laboratory.

Abnormal findings

▲ **Increased levels**

Primary aldosteronism
Hyponatremia
Hyperkalemia
Stress
Cushing's syndrome
Malignant hypertension
Generalized edema (from congestive heart failure, nephrotic syndrome, cirrhosis)
Renal arterial stenosis
Bartter's syndrome
Pregnancy
Oral contraceptives
Diuretics
Steroid therapy

▼ **Decreased levels**

Patients on a high-sodium diet
Hypernatremia
Hypokalemia
Addison's disease
Toxemia of pregnancy
Antihypertensive therapy
Diabetes mellitus

notes

alkaline phosphatase (ALP)

Type of test Blood

Normal findings

Adult: 30-85 ImU/ml or 42-128 U/L (SI units)
Elderly: slightly higher than adults
Child/adolescent
    <2 years: 85-235 ImU/ml
    2-8 years: 65-210 ImU/ml
    9-15 years: 60-300 ImU/ml
    16-21 years: 30-200 ImU/ml

Test explanation and related physiology

Although ALP is found in many tissues, the highest concentrations are found in the liver, biliary tract epithelium, and bone. The intestinal mucosa and placenta also contain ALP. This phosphatase enzyme is called *alkaline* because its function is increased in an alkaline environment. Detection of this enzyme is important for determining liver and bone disorders. Within the liver, ALP is present in Kupffer's cells. These cells line the biliary collecting system. Enzyme levels of ALP are greatly increased in both extrahepatic and intrahepatic obstructive biliary disease and cirrhosis. Other liver abnormalities, such as hepatic tumors, hepatoxic drugs, and hepatitis, cause lesser elevations in ALP levels.

Bone is the most frequent extrahepatic source of ALP; new bone growth is associated with elevated ALP levels. Pathologic new bone growth occurs with osteoblastic metastatic (e.g., breast, prostate) tumors. Paget's disease, healing fractures, rheumatoid arthritis, hyperparathyroidism, and normal-growing bones are sources of elevated ALP levels as well.

Isoenzymes of ALP are also used to distinguish between liver and bone diseases. These isoenzymes are most easily differentiated by the heat stability test and electrophoresis. The isoenzyme of liver origin (ALP_1) is heat stable; the isoenzyme of bone origin (ALP_2) is inactivated by heat.

Interfering factors

- Recent ingestion of a meal can increase ALP levels.
- Drugs that may cause *elevated* ALP levels include albumin made from placental tissue, allopurinol, antibiotics, azathio-

prine, colchicine, fluorides, indomethacin, isoniazid (INH), methotrexate, methyldopa, nicotinic acid, phenothiazine, probenecid, tetracyclines, and verapamil.

☛ Drugs that may cause *decreased* levels include arsenicals, cyanides, fluorides, nitrofurantoin, oxalates, and zinc salts.

Procedure and patient care

Before

- Explain the procedure to the patient.
- Tell the patient that no fasting is usually required. Overnight fasting may be required for isoenzymes.

During

- Collect approximately 7 to 10 ml of blood in a red-top tube.
- List on the laboratory slip any medications that can affect test results.

After

- Apply pressure or a pressure dressing to the venipuncture site.
- Assess the venipuncture site for bleeding. Patients with liver dysfunction often have prolonged clotting times.

Abnormal findings

▲ **Increased levels**

Cirrhosis

Intrahepatic or extrahepatic biliary obstruction

Primary or metastatic liver tumor

Normal pregnancy (third trimester, early postpartum)

Intestinal ischemia or infarction

Metastatic tumor to the bone

Healing fracture

Hyperparathyroidism

Paget's disease

Rheumatoid arthritis

Normal bones of growing children

▼ **Decreased levels**

Hypothyroidism

Malnutrition

Milk-alkali syndrome

Pernicious anemia

Hypophosphatemia

Scurvy (vitamin C deficiency)

Celiac disease

Excess vitamin B ingestion

alpha₁-antitrypsin test (A1AT, ATT)

Type of test Blood

Normal findings >250 mg/dl or 0.8-2.1 g/L (SI units)

Test explanation and related physiology

Serum alpha₁-antitrypsin (α_1-antitrypsin) determinations are obtained when an individual has a family history of emphysema, because a familial tendency to have a deficiency of this antienzyme exists. Deficient or absent serum levels of this enzyme are found in some patients with the early onset of emphysema. These people usually develop severe, disabling emphysema. The exact mechanism by which an antitrypsin deficiency produces emphysema, however, is unclear. A similar deficiency is seen in children with cirrhosis and other liver diseases. ATT is also an acute-phase reactant that is elevated in the face of inflammation, infection, or malignancy. It is not specific as to the source of the inflammatory process. Pregnant women in their last trimester have elevated ATT levels.

Deficiencies of ATT can be genetic or acquired. Genetic typing has shown that most persons have two *M* genes, designated as *MM,* and have alpha₁-antitrypsin levels over 250 mg/dl. Z and S genes are typically associated with alterations in serum levels of alpha₁-antitrypsin. Individuals who are homozygous *ZZ* or *SS* always have serum levels below 50 mg/dl and often near zero. Acquired deficiencies in ATT can occur in patients with protein deficiency syndromes (such as malnutrition, liver disease, nephrotic syndrome, and neonatal respiratory distress syndrome). These people develop severe panacinar emphysema in the third or fourth decade of life. Their major clinical symptoms usually include progressive dyspnea with minimal coughing. Chronic bronchitis is prominent in those patients with deficient ATT levels who smoke. Bronchiectasis can also occur in these patients.

Individuals of the heterozygous state *MZ* or *MS* have serum levels of alpha₁-antitrypsin between 50 and 250 mg/dl. Approximately 5% to 14% of the adult population are in the heterozygous state, which is considered to be a risk factor for emphysema. ATT is now qualitatively measured using immunochemical methods. Quantitation is possible but rarely useful with phenotyping. Routine serum protein electrophoresis is a good screening test for ATT deficiency because ATT is the major protein in the alpha₁ globulin region.

Interfering factors

- Serum levels of alpha$_1$-antitrypsin increase during pregnancy.
- Drugs that may cause *increased* levels include oral contraceptives.

Procedure and patient care

Before

- Explain the procedure to the patient.
- Note that no fasting is usually required. Verify this with the laboratory performing the study.

During

- Collect approximately 5 to 10 ml of blood.

After

- Apply pressure or a pressure dressing to the venipuncture site.
- Observe the venipuncture site for bleeding.
- If the results show the patient is at risk for developing emphysema, begin patient teaching. Include such factors as avoidance of smoking, infection, and inhaled irritants; proper nutrition; adequate hydration; and education about the disease process of emphysema.

Abnormal findings

▲ **Increased levels**
Inflammatory disorders
Cancer
Thyroid infections
Stress
Infection

▼ **Decreased levels**
Early onset of emphysema
Cirrhosis
Nephrotic syndrome
Malnutrition
End-stage cancer
Protein-losing enteropathy
Neonatal respiratory distress syndrome

notes

alpha-fetoprotein (AFP, α_1-Fetoprotein)

Type of test Blood

Normal findings

Adult: <40 ng/ml or <40 μg/L (SI units)

Child (<1 yr): <30 ng/ml

Ranges are stratified by weeks of gestation and vary according to different laboratories.

Test explanation and related physiology

AFP is an oncofetal protein normally produced by the fetal liver and yolk sac. It is the dominant fetal serum protein in the first trimester of life and diminishes to very low levels by the age of 1 year. Normally, it is found in very low levels in the adult. Increased serum levels are found in as many as 90% of patients with hepatomas. The higher the AFP level, the greater the tumor burden. A decrease in AFP would be seen if the patient were experiencing a response to antineoplastic therapy. AFP is not specific for hepatomas, although extremely high levels (above 500 ng/ml) are diagnostic for hepatoma. Other neoplastic conditions, such as yolk sac and germ cell tumors of the testicles and ovaries and, to a lesser extent, Hodgkin's disease, lymphoma, and renal cell carcinoma, are also associated with elevated AFP levels. Noncancerous causes of elevated AFP levels occur in patients with cirrhosis or chronic active hepatitis.

AFP is also helpful in the diagnosis of neural tube defects (NTDs), which can vary from a small myelomeningocele to anencephaly. While not widely used in United States, AFP can be used for widespread screening for NTDs. Normally, AFP from fetal sources can be detected in the mother's blood after 10 weeks of gestation. Peak levels occur between 16 and 18 weeks. With NTDs, AFP leaks out of the fetal serum through the neural tube defect and into the amniotic fluid. Maternal serum reflects that change in amniotic AFP levels. When elevated maternal serum AFP levels are identified, further evaluation with repeat serum AFP levels, amniotic fluid AFP levels, and ultrasound is warranted. Elevated serum AFP levels in pregnancy may also indicated multiple pregnancy or intrauterine death. Low AFP levels after correction as to age of gestation, maternal weight, race, and presence of diabetes are found in mothers carrying offspring with trisomy 21 (Down's syndrome).

Interfering factors

- Fetal blood contamination can cause increased AFP levels.
- Multiple pregnancies can cause increased levels.
- Recent administration of radioisotopes can affect values.

Procedure and patient care

Before

- Explain the procedure to the patient.
- Tell the patient that no food or fluid restriction is required.

During

- Collect approximately 7 to 10 ml of blood in a red-top tube.

After

- Apply pressure or a pressure dressing to the venipuncture site.
- Assess the venipuncture site for bleeding.
- Include the gestational age on the laboratory slip.

Abnormal findings

Neural tube defects (e.g., anencephaly, encephalocele, spina bifida, myelomeningocele)
Abortion
Multiple pregnancy
Intrauterine fetal death
Cirrhosis
Hepatitis
Primary hepatocellular cancer
Germ cell or yolk sac cancer of the ovary
Germ cell or yolk sac cancer of the testicle
Lymphoma
Renal cell carcinoma

notes

ammonia level

Type of test Blood

Normal findings

Adult: 15-110 μg/dl or 47-65 μmol/L (SI units)
Child: 40-80 μg/dl
Newborn: 90-150 μg/dl

Test explanation and related physiology

Ammonia, which is a by-product of protein metabolism, is normally converted by the liver into urea and then secreted by the kidneys. With severe liver dysfunction, or when the blood flow to the liver is altered (e.g., in portal hypertension), ammonia cannot be catabolized; the blood levels rise. Congenital enzymatic defects in the urea cycle also can cause a rise in ammonia levels. Finally, impaired renal function diminishes excretion of ammonia, and the blood levels rise. High levels of ammonia can result in encephalopathy and coma.

Interfering factors

▮ Drugs that may cause *increased* ammonia levels include acetazolamide, alcohol, ammonium chloride, barbiturates, narcotics, parenteral nutrition, and diuretics (loop, thiazide).

▮ Drugs that may cause *decreased* levels include broad-spectrum antibiotics (e.g., neomycin), lactulose, levodopa, lactobacillus, and potassium salts.

Procedure and patient care

Before

- Explain the procedure to the patient.
- Note that no fasting is usually required.

During

- Collect approximately 5 to 7 ml of blood in a green-top tube. Note that some institutions require the specimen be sent to the laboratory in an iced container.
- List on the laboratory slip any drugs that can affect test results.
- Avoid hemolysis and send the specimen promptly to the laboratory.

After

- Apply pressure or a pressure dressing to the venipuncture site.
- Assess the venipuncture site for bleeding. Many patients with liver disease have prolonged clotting times.

Abnormal findings

▲ **Increased levels**

Primary hepatic disease
Renal failure
Reye's syndrome
Severe heart failure with congestive hepatomegaly
Hemolytic disease of the newborn (erythroblastosis fetalis)
Hepatic encephalopathy
Hepatic coma
Genetic metabolic disorder of the urea cycle
Portal hypertension

▼ **Decreased levels**

Essential and malignant hypertension

notes

amniocentesis (Amniotic fluid analysis)

Type of test Fluid analysis

Normal findings Vary with the reason for the test

Test explanation and related physiology

Amniocentesis involves the placement of a needle through the patient's abdominal and uterine walls into the amniotic cavity to withdraw fluid for analysis. Studying amniotic fluid is vitally important in assessing the following:

1. *Fetal maturity status,* especially pulmonary maturity (when early delivery is preferred).
2. *Sex of the fetus.* For example, sons of mothers who are known to be carriers of X-linked recessive traits would have a 50:50 chance of inheritance.
3. *Genetic and chromosomal aberrations,* such as hemophilia, Down's syndrome, galactosemia.
4. *Fetal status affected by Rh isoimmunization.* Mothers with Rh isoimmunization will have a series of amniocentesis procedures during the second half of pregnancy to assess the level of bilirubin pigment in the amniotic fluid. The quantity of bilirubin is used to assess the severity of hemolytic anemia in Rh-sensitized pregnancy. The higher the amount of bilirubin, the lower the amount of fetal hemoglobin. Amniocentesis is usually initiated at 24 to 25 weeks. This allows assessment of the severity of the disease and the status of the fetus. Early delivery or blood transfusion may be indicated.
5. *Hereditary metabolic disorders,* such as cystic fibrosis.
6. *Anatomic abnormalities,* such as neural tube closure defects (myelomeningocele, anencephaly, spina bifida).
7. *Fetal distress,* detected by meconium staining of the amniotic fluid. This is caused by relaxation of the anal sphincter. In this case, the normally colorless and pale, straw-colored amniotic fluid may be tinged with green. Other color changes may also indicate fetal distress. For example, a yellow discoloration may indicate a blood incompatibility. A yellow-brown opaque appearance may indicate intrauterine death. A red color indicates blood contamination either from the mother or the fetus.

Fetal maturity is determined by analysis of the amniotic fluid for the following:

1. *Lecithin/sphingomyelin (L/S) ratio.* The L/S ratio is a measure of fetal lung maturity, which is determined by measuring the phospholipids in amniotic fluid. Lecithin is the major constituent of surfactant, an important substance required for alveolar ventilation. If surfactant is insufficient, the alveoli collapse during expiration. This results in atelectasis and respiratory distress syndrome (RDS), which is a major cause of death in immature babies. In the immature fetal lung, the sphingomyelin concentration in amniotic fluid is higher than the lecithin concentration. At 35 weeks of gestation, the concentration of lecithin rapidly increases, whereas sphingomyelin concentration decreases. An L/S ratio of 2:1 (3:1 in mothers with diabetes) or greater is a highly reliable indication that the fetal lung, and therefore the fetus, is mature. In such a case, the infant after birth would be unlikely to develop RDS.

2. *Phosphatidylglycerol (PG).* This is a minor component (about 10%) of lung surfactant phospholipids. However, since PG is almost entirely synthesized by mature lung alveolar cells, it is a good indicator of lung maturity. Since PG appears late in gestation, this test indicates a more mature surfactant than that found in the L/S ratio described above. In healthy pregnant women, PG appears in amniotic fluid after 35 weeks of gestation, and levels gradually increase until term. An advantage of the PG assay is that it is not affected by contamination of amniotic fluid by blood or meconium. These two contaminants cause false-positive and false-negative results for the L/S evaluation. In addition, the presence of PG in the amniotic fluid in the vagina after the membranes are ruptured indicates a low risk for RDS of the newborn. The simultaneous determination of the L/S ratio and the presence of PG is an excellent method of assessing fetal maturity based on pulmonary surfactant.

3. *Lamellar body count.* This new test to determine fetal maturity is also based on the presence of surfactant. Lamellar bodies are concentrically layered structures produced by type II pneumocytes. On cross-section, these small (about 3 microns) structures look like an onion and are called lamellar bodies. These lamellar bodies represent the

storage form of pulmonary surfactant. Because lamellar bodies and platelets are indistinguishable to cell counters, the lamellar body count is obtained by analyzing the amniotic fluid with a cell counter and recording the platelet count. Lamellar body results are calculated in units of particle density per microliter of amniotic fluid. Some researchers have recommended cutoffs of 30,000/µl and 10,000/µl to predict low and high risk for RDS, respectively. If the count is greater than 30,000, the negative predictive value for RDS is 100%. If the lamellar body count is less than 10,000, the probability of RDS is high (67%). Values between 10,000 and 30,000/µl represent intermediate risk for RDS. At this time, not enough information is available on lamellar body count in diabetics to advocate its use in this high-risk group.

There are several advantages of lamellar body counts. One, they are faster, more precise, and more objective, and they require less amniotic fluid than phospholipid analysis. Two, test results are not invalidated by the presence of blood or meconium. Three, the instrumentation required for this test is readily available, thus allowing it to be performed in some laboratories where phospholipid analysis is not available.

Genetic and chromosomal studies performed on cells aspirated within the amniotic fluid can indicate the gender of the fetus (important in sex-linked diseases such as hemophilia) or any of the described genetic and chromosomal aberrations. Increased levels of alpha-fetoprotein (AFP) in the amniotic fluid may indicate a neural crest abnormality (see p. 40). Amniocentesis may be done on the premise that elective abortion should be performed if the fetus is severely defective.

The timing of the amniocentesis varies according to the clinical circumstances. With advanced maternal age and if chromosomal or genetic aberrations are suspected, the test should be done early enough (at 14 to 16 weeks of gestation) to allow a safe abortion. This timing is essential because of the 2 weeks necessary for cell growth to determine the study's results. If information on fetal maturity is sought, performing the study during or after the thirty-fifth week of gestation is best. Placental localization by ultrasonography should be done before amniocentesis to avoid the needle passing into the placenta, possibly interrupting the placenta, and inducing bleeding or abortion.

Contraindications

- Patients with abruptio placentae
- Patients with placenta previa
- Patients with a history of premature labor (before 34 weeks of gestation, unless the patient is receiving antilabor medication)
- Patients with an incompetent cervix

Potential complications

- Miscarriage
- Fetal injury
- Leak of amniotic fluid
- Infection (amnionitis)
- Abortion
- Premature labor
- Maternal hemorrhage with possible maternal Rh isoimmunization
- Amniotic fluid embolism
- Abruptio placentae
- Inadvertent damage to the bladder or intestines

Interfering factors

- Fetal blood contamination can cause falsely elevated AFP levels.
- Hemolysis of the specimen can alter results.
- Contamination of the specimen with meconium or blood may give inaccurate L/S ratios.

Procedure and patient care

Before

- Explain the procedure to the patient. Allay any fears and allow the patient to verbalize her concerns.
- Obtain an informed consent from the patient and her spouse.
- Tell the patient that no food or fluid is restricted.
- Evaluate the mother's blood pressure and the fetal heart rate.
- Follow instructions regarding emptying the bladder, which depend on gestational age. Before 20 weeks of gestation, the bladder may be kept full to support the uterus. After 20 weeks, the bladder may be emptied to minimize the chance of puncture.

- Localize the placenta before the study by ultrasound to permit selection of a site that will avoid placental puncture.

During

- Place the patient in the supine position.
- Note the following procedural steps:
  1. The skin overlying the chosen site is prepared and usually anesthetized locally.
  2. A long needle with a stylet is inserted through the mid-abdominal wall and directed at an angle toward the middle of the uterine cavity (Figure 1).
  3. The stylet is then removed and a sterile plastic syringe attached.
  4. After 5 to 10 ml of amniotic fluid is withdrawn, the needle is removed. (This fluid volume is replaced by newly formed amniotic fluid within 3 to 4 hours after the procedure.)

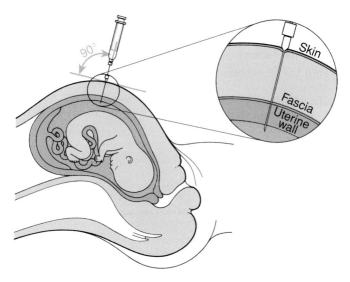

Figure 1 Amniocentesis. Ultrasound scanning is usually used to determine the placental site and to locate a pocket of amniotic fluid. The needle is then inserted. Three levels of resistance are felt as the needle penetrates the skin, fascia, and uterine wall. When the needle is placed within the uterine cavity, amniotic fluid is withdrawn.

5. The specimen is placed in a light-resistant container to prevent breakdown of bilirubin.
6. The site is covered with an adhesive bandage.
7. If the amniotic fluid is bloody, the physician must determine whether the blood is maternal or fetal in origin. Kleinhauer-Boetke stain will stain fetal cells pink. Meconium in the fluid is usually associated with a compromised fetus.

- Note that this procedure takes approximately 20 to 30 minutes.
- Tell the patient that the discomfort associated with amniocentesis is usually described as a mild uterine cramping that occurs when the needle contacts the uterus. Some women may complain of a "pulling" sensation as the amniotic fluid is withdrawn.
- Remember that many women are extremely anxious during this procedure.

After

- Place amniotic fluid in a sterile, siliconized glass container and transport it to a special chemistry laboratory for analysis. Sometimes the specimen may be sent by air mail to another commercial laboratory.
- Inform the patient that the results of this study are usually not available for at least 2 weeks.
- For women who have Rh-negative blood, administer RhoGAM because of the risk of immunization from the fetal blood.
- Assess the fetal heart rate after the test to detect any ill effects related to the procedure. Compare this value with the preprocedural baseline value.
- If the patient felt dizzy or nauseated during the procedure, instruct her to lie on her left side for several minutes before leaving the examining room.
- Observe the puncture site for bleeding or other drainage.
- Instruct the patient to call her physician if she has any fluid loss, bleeding, temperature elevation, abdominal pain or cramping, fetal hyperactivity, or unusual fetal lethargy.

Abnormal findings

Genetic or chromosomal aberrations (e.g., hemophilia, Down's syndrome, galactosemia)

Rh isoimmunization

Hereditary metabolic disorders (e.g., cystic fibrosis, Tay-Sachs disease)

Neural tube closure defects (e.g., myelomeningocele, anencephaly, spina bifida)

Meconium staining (fetal stress)

Immature fetal lungs

Sickle cell anemia

Thalassemia

Sex-linked disorders (e.g., hemophilia)

notes

amylase, blood

Type of test Blood

Normal findings 56-190 IU/L, 80-150 Somogyi units/dl, or 25-125 U/L (SI units). Values may be slightly increased during normal pregnancy and in the elderly.

Possible critical values More than three times the upper limit of normal (depending on the method)

Test explanation and related physiology

Serum amylase is an easily and rapidly performed test that is most specific for pancreatitis. Amylase is normally secreted from the pancreatic acinar cell into the pancreatic duct and then into the duodenum. Once in the intestine, it aids the catabolism of carbohydrates to their component simple sugars. Damage to acinar cells (as in pancreatitis) or obstruction of the pancreatic duct flow (as in pancreatic carcinoma) causes an outpouring of this enzyme into the intrapancreatic lymph system and the free peritoneum. Blood vessels draining the free peritoneum and absorbing the lymph pick up the excess amylase. An abnormal rise in the serum level of amylase occurs within 12 hours of the onset of disease. Because amylase is rapidly cleared by the kidney, serum levels return to normal 48 to 72 hours after the initial insult. Persistent pancreatitis, duct obstruction, or pancreatic duct leak (e.g., pseudocysts) will cause persistent elevated serum amylase levels.

Although serum amylase is a sensitive test for pancreatic disorders, it is not specific. Other nonpancreatic diseases can cause elevated amylase levels in the serum. For example, in a bowel perforation, intraluminal amylase leaks into the free peritoneum and is picked up by the peritoneal blood vessels. This results in an elevated serum amylase level. Also, a penetrating peptic ulcer into the pancreas will cause elevated amylase levels. Duodenal obstruction can be associated with less significant elevations in amylase. Because salivary glands contain amylase, elevations can be expected in patients with parotiditis (mumps). Amylase is also found, in low levels, in the ovaries and skeletal muscles. Ectopic pregnancy and severe diabetic ketoacidosis are also associated with hyperamylasemia.

Patients with chronic pancreatic disorders (e.g., chronic pancreatitis) that have previously resulted in pancreatic cell destruction often do not have high amylase levels associated with the above disorders, because less amylase is made within the pancreas.

Interfering factors

- IV dextrose solutions can cause a false-negative result.
- ⚑ Drugs that may cause *increased* serum amylase levels include aminosalicylic acid (PAS), aspirin, azathioprine, corticosteroids, dexamethasone, ethyl alcohol, glucocorticoids, iodine-containing contrast media, loop diuretics (e.g., furosemide), methyldopa, narcotic analgesics, oral contraceptives, and prednisone.
- ⚑ Drugs that may cause *decreased* levels include citrates, glucose, and oxalates.

Procedure and patient care

Before

- Explain the procedure to the patient.
- Tell the patient that no fasting is required.

During

- Collect 5 to 7 ml of venous blood in a red-top tube.
- Indicate on the laboratory slip any medications that may affect test results.

After

- Apply pressure or a pressure dressing to the venipuncture site.
- Check the venipuncture site for bleeding.

Abnormal findings

▲ Increased levels

Acute pancreatitis
Perforated peptic ulcer
Perforated bowel
Parotiditis (mumps)
Pulmonary infarction
Chronic relapsing pancreatitis

Penetrating peptic ulcer
Necrotic bowel
Acute cholecystitis
Ectopic pregnancy
Diabetic ketoacidosis
Duodenal obstruction

notes

amylase, urine

Type of test Urine (24-hour)

Normal findings 3-35 IU/hr or 6-30 Wohlgemuth units/ml, up to 5000 Somogyi units/24 hr or 6.5-48.1 U/hr (SI units)

Test explanation and related physiology

Amylase is normally secreted from the pancreatic acinar cells into the pancreatic duct and then into the duodenum. Once in the intestine, it aids the catabolism of carbohydrates to their component simple sugars. Destruction of acinar cells (as in pancreatitis) or obstruction to the pancreatic duct flow (as in pancreatitic carcinoma) causes an outpouring of this enzyme into the bloodstream.

Because the kidney rapidly clears amylase, disorders affecting the pancreas cause elevated amylase levels in the urine. The serum levels of amylase rise transiently. They usually return to normal 1 to 2 days after the onset of the disease. Levels of amylase in the urine, however, remain elevated 5 to 7 days after the onset of disease. This is important if one is to diagnose pancreatitis in patients who have had symptoms for 3 days or longer.

As with serum amylase (see p. 51), urine amylase is sensitive but not specific for pancreatitic disorders. Other diseases, such as parotiditis (mumps), cholecystitis, perforated bowel, penetrating peptic ulcer, ectopic pregnancy, and renal infarctions, can cause elevated urine levels; however, urine levels are usually highest with pancreatitis. A comparison of the renal clearance ratio of amylase to creatinine provides more diagnostic information than either the urine amylase level or the serum amylase level alone. When the amylase/creatinine clearance ratio is 5% or more, the diagnosis of pancreatitis can be made with certainty. With ratios less than 5% in a patient having elevated serum and urine amylase levels, nonpancreatic pathologic conditions should be suspected (e.g., perforated bowel, macroamylasemia).

Interfering factors

- IV dextrose solutions can cause a false-negative result.
- Drugs that may cause *increased* serum amylase levels include aminosalicylic acid (PAS), aspirin, azathioprine, corticosteroids, dexamethasone, ethyl alcohol, glucocorticoids, iodine-containing contrast media, loop diuretics (e.g., furosemide),

methyldopa, narcotic analgesics, oral contraceptives, and prednisone.

🖑 Drugs that may cause *decreased* levels include citrates, glucose, and oxalates.

Procedure and patient care

Before

- Explain the procedure to the patient.
- Tell the patient that no fasting is required.
- Record the exact times of urine collection.

During

- Instruct the patient to begin the 24-hour urine collection after urinating. Discard the initial specimen and start the 24-hour timing at that point.
- Collect all urine passed during the next 24 hours.
- A *2-hour spot urine* can be sent instead of the 24-hour urine collection.
- Show the patient where to store the urine specimen.
- Keep the specimen on ice or refrigerated during the collection period. No preservative is needed.
- Post the hours for urine collection in a prominent place to prevent accidental discarding of the specimen.
- Instruct the patient to void before defecating so that urine is not contaminated by stool.
- Remind the patient not to put toilet paper in the urine collection container.
- Collect the last specimen as close as possible to the end of the collection period. Add this urine to the container.
- List on the laboratory slip any medications that may affect test results.

After

- Send the urine specimen to the laboratory promptly.

Abnormal findings

▲   Increased levels

Acute pancreatitis
Perforated peptic ulcer
Perforated bowel
Parotiditis (mumps)
Pulmonary infarction
Chronic relapsing pancreatitis
Penetrating peptic ulcer
Necrotic bowel
Acute cholecystitis
Ectopic pregnancy
Diabetic ketoacidosis

amyloid beta protein precursor, soluble (sBPP)

Type of test CSF analysis

Normal findings >450 U/L

Test explanation and related physiology

Alzheimer's disease is one of the most important of all degenerative neurologic diseases because of its devastating nature and its frequency of occurrence. It has recently been confirmed that the histologic lesions of the brain known as senile plaques (which contain amyloid) and the amyloid in the meningeal blood vessels of patients with Alzheimer's disease consist of this newly described protein. Recent evidence suggests that it may be this protein that exerts neurotoxic effects. The amyloid peptide (beta or A4 peptide) gene is on chromosome 21. This is the same chromosome on which the familial Alzheimer's disease gene has been localized in some families. In some families with familial Alzheimer's disease, there are mutations in the amyloid precursor protein.

This test is used in the diagnosis of Alzheimer's disease. A cerebrospinal fluid (CSF) sample is obtained by lumbar puncture (see p. 526). The soluble BPP is normally found in the CSF of healthy individuals. Low levels may be found in some elderly patients suffering from dementia. Low levels may indicate an alteration in the formation of the amyloid beta protein or its precursors as may be found in Alzheimer's disease.

Procedure and patient care

Before
- Explain the procedure to the patient.
- Refer to the instructions for a lumbar puncture and CSF examination (see p. 526).

During
- Collect a CSF specimen as indicated in the lumbar puncture discussion.

After
- Follow the postprocedure guidelines after a lumbar puncture.

Abnormal finding

▼ **Decreased levels**
Alzheimer's disease

notes

androstenedione

Type of test Blood

Normal findings <250 ng/dl

Possible critical values >1000 ng/dl

Test explanation and related physiology

Androstenedione is a precursor of cortisol, aldosterone, testosterone, and estrogen. The importance of this hormone is in the diagnosis of virilizing syndromes in the female. In the adrenal glands of females, androstenedione is converted to the above-noted hormones. In the female peripheral tissues and ovaries, androstenedione is converted into testosterone and estrogen. Tumors of the adrenal glands (cancers or adenomas) or ovaries (stroma tumors) can secrete large amounts of androstenedione, which is then converted into testosterone. This can cause virilizing symptoms such as hirsutism, change in voice, sterility, etc.

Children with congenital adrenal hyperplasia have enzyme defects in the conversion of androstenedione to cortisol. Excess androstenedione is built up. As adrenocorticotropic (ACTH) levels increase, androstenedione levels increase still further. Again, this hormone is converted into testosterone in the peripheral tissues. Female pseudohermaphroditism results. In the male with similar congenital defects, precocious puberty will be obvious. Female patients with Cushing's syndrome are usually adult and experience virilization through the same pathophysiologic process.

Patients with polycystic ovary syndrome (Stein-Leventhal syndrome) may also have elevated levels of testosterone precursors, including androstenedione.

Interfering factors

- A radioactive scan performed 1 week before the test may invalidate the test results.
- Drugs that may *increase* levels of androstenedione are corticotropin, clomiphene, and metyrapone.
- Steroids may *decrease* levels of androstenedione.

Procedure and patient care

Before
- Explain the procedure to the patient.
- Tell the patient that the specimen should be collected 1 week before or after the menstrual period.

During
- Collect one red-top tube of venous blood.
- Indicate the date of the last menstrual period on the laboratory form.

After
- Apply pressure or a pressure dressing to the venipuncture site.
- Assess the venipuncture site for bleeding.

Abnormal findings

▲ **Increased values**
  Stein-Leventhal syndrome
  Adrenal tumor
  Congenital adrenal hyperplasia
  Ectopic ACTH-producing tumors
  Ovarian tumor
  Cushing's syndrome

▼ **Decreased values**
  Primary or secondary adrenal insufficiency

notes

angiotensin-converting enzyme (ACE, Serum angiotensin-converting enzyme [SACE])

Type of test Blood

Normal findings 23-57 U/ml (over 20 years of age)

Test explanation and related physiology

Angiotensin-converting enzyme is found in pulmonary epithelial cells and converts angiotensin I to angiotensin II (a potent vasoconstrictor). For this reason, the ACE levels may be used in the evaluation of hypertension. Elevated ACE levels are found in a high percentage of patients with sarcoidosis.

This test is primarily used in patients with sarcoidosis to evaluate the severity of disease and the response to therapy. Levels are especially high with active pulmonary sarcoidosis and can be normal with inactive sarcoidosis. Elevated ACE levels also occur in conditions other than sarcoidosis, including Gaucher's disease (a rare familial disorder of fat metabolism), leprosy, alcoholic cirrhosis, active histoplasmosis, tuberculosis, Hodgkin's disease, myeloma, scleroderma, pulmonary embolism, and idiopathic pulmonary fibrosis.

Assay for ACE can be done with spectrophotometry or radioimmunoassay.

Interfering factors

- Patients under 20 years of age normally have very high ACE levels.
- Hemolysis or hyperlipidemia may factitiously *decrease* ACE levels.
- Drugs that may cause *decreased* ACE levels include ACE inhibitor antihypertensives and steroids.

Procedure and patient care

Before
- Explain the procedure to the patient.
- Tell the patient that no fasting is required.

During
- Collect approximately 5 ml of blood in a red-top tube.
- Note on the laboratory slip if the patient is taking steroids.

After
- Apply pressure or a pressure dressing to the venipuncture site.
- Assess the venipuncture site for bleeding.

Abnormal findings

▲ **Increased levels**

Sarcoidosis
Gaucher's disease
Tuberculosis
Leprosy
Alcoholic cirrhosis
Active histoplasmosis
Hodgkin's disease
Myeloma

Idiopathic pulmonary fibrosis
Diabetes mellitus
Primary biliary cirrhosis
Amyloidosis
Hyperthyroidism
Scleroderma
Pulmonary embolism

notes

antegrade pyelography

Type of test X-ray with contrast dye

Normal findings Normal outline, size, and position of the ureters and bladder

Test explanation and related physiology

Occasionally, a kidney with very poor dye excretion following intravenous pyelography (IVP) also cannot be adequately examined by retrograde pyelography, because the ureter is impassable from below (e.g., from obstruction) or a cystoscopic procedure is clinically contraindicated. For this patient, the upper collecting system may be opacified by injection of contrast material via a percutaneous needle puncture of the renal pelvis or calyx. This test is usually performed when attempts at retrograde catheterization (retrograde pyelography) have been unsuccessful. Antegrade pyelography is specifically indicated in the following conditions:

1. Localization of ureteral obstruction caused by a stricture, nonopaque ureteral stone, or tumor
2. Evaluation of ureteral obstruction after a urinary diversion procedure
3. Hydronephrosis in a child with poor IVP dye excretion in order to identify ureteropelvic and ureterovesical obstruction

Potential complications

- Hemorrhage from the needle
  The kidney is a highly vascular organ.
- Allergic reaction to iodinated dye
  This rarely occurs, because the dye is not administered intravenously.

Procedure and patient care

Before

- Explain the procedure to the patient. Allay the patient's fears and allow time for the patient to verbalize concerns.
- Obtain an informed consent.
- Check for allergy to iodine or shellfish and inform the physician.

During

- Place the patient in a prone position.
- Note the following procedural steps:
  1. The renal pelvis is localized by ultrasound or fluoroscopy. A dilated collecting system is more easily identified than a normal collecting system.
  2. Skin overlying the desired site is marked and prepared antiseptically.
  3. With the patient under local anesthesia, the skin is incised and a needle with a stylet is inserted toward the renal pelvis.
  4. With the patient suspending respiration, a smaller, thin-walled needle with a stylet is advanced through the needle into the lumen of the renal pelvis. Flexible tubing connects the syringe to the needle to aspirate urine.
  5. Contrast material is injected to outline the upper collection system to the point of obstruction below.
  6. Posteroanterior, oblique, and anteroposterior x-ray views are taken.
- Note that this test is performed by a radiologist or urologist in less than 1 hour.
- Inform the patient that the only uncomfortable aspect of this test is the local anesthesia used to numb the skin overlying the pelvis.

After

- Apply a small pressure dressing to the incision site.
- Assess the incision site for bleeding.
- Because the kidney is a highly vascular organ, check the vital signs as ordered to detect any evidence of bleeding.
- Note that antibiotic drugs are often recommended for several days to avoid infection, which may be caused by the instrumentation at a level above the ureteral obstruction.
- Evaluate for signs of an allergic reaction to dye (e.g., dyspnea, rash, tachycardia, hives).

Abnormal findings

Ureteral stone

Ureteral obstruction from tumor or adhesions

Ureteropelvic or ureterovesical obstruction from a stone, tumor, or scarring

Congenital or acquired hydronephrosis

anticardiolipin antibodies (aCL antibodies, ACA)

Type of test Blood

Normal findings

Negative
<23 g/L for IgG anticardiolipin antibodies
<11 mg/L for IgM anticardiolipin antibodies

Test explanation and related physiology

Antiphospholipid antibodies, which include anticardiolipin antibodies and the lupus anticoagulant, are present in half of the patients with systemic lupus erythematosus (SLE). Immunoglobulins G and M to cardiolipin are found in approximately 40% of patients with SLE. Spontaneous abortion, placental infarction, thrombotic episodes, and strokes in young adults have been associated with elevated levels of these antibodies. Anticardiolipin antibodies frequently occur in association with the lupus anticoagulant, which may prolong the partial thrombopolastin time (PTT) and is found in about 15% to 30% of SLE patients.

The "antiphospholipid antibody syndrome" (which includes the presence of anticardiolipin antibodies and the lupus anticoagulant) may be a risk factor for clinical findings of venous and arterial thrombosis, neuropsychiatric disorders, recurrent spontaneous abortion, and thrombocytopenia. Both antibodies may be found in drug-induced lupus, in nonautoimmune diseases (e.g., syphilis and acute infection), and in the elderly. Despite the name lupus "anticoagulant," clinically significant bleeding is rare without thrombocytopenia.

Procedure and patient care

Before

- Explain the procedure to the patient.
- Tell the patient that no fasting is required.

During

- Collect a venous blood sample according to the laboratory protocol.

After

- Apply pressure or a pressure dressing to the venipuncture site.

- Assess the venipuncture site for bleeding.

Abnormal findings

▲   **Increased levels**

Systemic lupus erythematosus	Syphilis
Thrombosis	Acute infection
Thrombocytopenia	Elderly
Recurrent fetal loss	

notes

anticentromere antibody test (Centromere antibody)

Type of test Blood

Normal findings Negative (if positive, serum will be titrated)

Test explanation and related physiology

A centromere is the region of the chromosome referred to as the "primary constriction" that divides the chromosome into "arms." During cell division, the centromere exists in the "pole" of the mitotic spindle.

Anticentromere antibodies are found in a very high percentage of patients with CREST syndrome, a variant of scleroderma. CREST is characterized by calcinosis, Raynaud's phenomenon, esophageal dysfunction, sclerodactyly, and telangiectasia. Anticentromere antibodies, on the contrary, are present in only a small minority of patients with scleroderma. No correlation exists between antibody titer and disease activity.

Procedure and patient care

Before
- Explain the procedure to the patient.
- Tell the patient that no fasting is usually required.

During
- Collect one red-top tube of venous blood.

After
- Apply pressure or a pressure dressing to the venipuncture site.
- Assess the venipuncture site for bleeding.

Abnormal finding

Positive
CREST syndrome

notes

antideoxyribonuclease-B titer (Anti-DNase-B [ADB], ADNase-B)

Type of test Blood

Normal findings

Preschool: ≤60 U
School age: ≤170 U
Adult: ≤85 U

Test explanation and related physiology

Like the antistreptolysin O titer (ASO) test (see p. 88), this immunologic test also detects antigens produced by group A streptococci and is elevated in most patients with acute rheumatic fever or poststreptococcal glomerulonephritis. This test is often run concurrently with the ASO; subsequent testing is usually performed to detect differences between the acute and convalescent blood samples. A rise in the titer of two or more dilution increments between acute and convalescent sera is significant and indicates that a streptococcal infection has occurred.

Interfering factors

✴ Drugs that may *decrease* test results include antibiotics.

Procedure and patient care

Before

- Explain the procedure to the patient.
- Inform the patient that no fasting is required.

During

- Collect one red-top tube of venous blood.

After

- Apply pressure to the venipuncture site after the blood is drawn.
- Assess the site for bleeding.

Abnormal findings

▲   Increased levels

Acute rheumatic fever
Poststreptococcal glomerulonephritis

antidiuretic hormone (ADH, Vasopressin)

Type of test Blood

Normal values 1-5 pg/ml or <1.5 ng/L (SI units)

Test explanation and related physiology

Antidiuretic hormone, also known as vasopressin, is formed by the hypothalamus and stored in the posterior pituitary gland. It controls the amount of water reabsorbed by the kidney. ADH release is stimulated by an increase in serum osmolality or a decrease in intravascular blood volume. Physical stress, surgery, and even high levels of anxiety may also stimulate ADH release. With a release of ADH, more water is reabsorbed from the glomerular filtrate at the level of the distal convoluted renal tubule and collecting ducts. This increases the amount of free water within the bloodstream and causes a very concentrated urine. With low ADH levels, water is allowed to be excreted, thereby producing hemoconcentration and a very dilute urine.

Diabetes insipidus (DI) occurs when ADH secretion is inadequate or when the kidney is unresponsive to ADH stimulation. Inadequate ADH secretion is usually associated with central neurologic abnormalities such as trauma, tumor, or inflammation of the brain. Surgical ablation of the pituitary gland will also result in a neurologic form of DI; such patients excrete large volumes of free water within a dilute urine. Therefore the blood is hemoconcentrated, causing the patient to have a strong thirst response.

Primary renal diseases may make the renal collecting system less sensitive to ADH stimulation. Again, in this instance, a dilute urine created by excretion of high volumes of free water may occur (nephrogenic DI). To differentiate ADH deficiency (central DI) from renal resistance to ADH (nephrogenic DI), a water deprivation ADH stimulation test is performed. During this test, water intake is restricted. Urine osmolality is measured. Vasopressin is administered. In central DI, there is no rise in urine osmolality with restriction, but there is a rise with vasopressin. In nephrogenic DI, there is no rise in urine osmolality after water deprivation or vasopressin administration.

High serum ADH levels are associated with the syndrome of inappropriate ADH secretion (SIADH). In response to this inappropriately high level of ADH secretion, water is reabsorbed by the kidneys greatly in excess of normal amounts. Thus the patient becomes very hemodiluted. Blood levels of important serum ions diminish, causing severe neurologic, cardiac, and metabolic alterations. The most frequent cause of SIADH is the paraneoplastic syndrome of ectopic ADH production. The most common tumors associated with SIADH include carcinoma of the lung and thymus, lymphomas, leukemia, and carcinomas of the pancreas, urologic tract, and intestine. SIADH is also associated with pulmonary diseases (e.g., tuberculosis, bacterial pneumonia), severe stress (e.g., surgery, trauma), and brain tumors.

Interfering factors

- Patients with dehydration, hypovolemia, and stress may have increased ADH levels.
- Patients with overhydration, decreased serum osmolality, and hypervolemia may have decreased ADH levels.
- Use of a glass syringe or collection tube causes degradation of ADH.
- ✗ Drugs that *elevate* ADH levels include acetaminophen, barbiturates, cholinergic agents, estrogen, nicotine, oral hypoglycemic agents, some diuretics (e.g., thiazides), cyclophosphamide, narcotics, and tricyclic antidepressants.
- ✗ Drugs that *decrease* ADH levels include alcohol, beta-adrenergic agents, morphine antagonists, and phenytoin (Dilantin).

Procedure and patient care

Before

- Explain the procedure to the patient.
- Ensure that the patient is adequately hydrated. Tell the patient to fast for 12 hours.
- Evaluate the patient for high levels of physical or emotional stress.

During

- Collect approximately 7 ml of venous blood in a *plastic* red-top tube with the patient in the sitting or recumbent position.
- Record on the laboratory slip any drugs that may alter test results.

After

- Apply pressure or a pressure dressing to the venipuncture site.
- Assess the venipuncture site for bleeding.
- Note that the laboratory personnel usually freeze the serum and send it to a reference laboratory for testing.

Abnormal findings

▲ Increased levels

Syndrome of inappropriate ADH secretion

Nephrogenic diabetes insipidus caused by primary renal diseases

Postoperative states

Systemic neoplasm (ectopic ADH)

Severe physical stress (e.g., trauma, pain, prolonged mechanical ventilation)

Central nervous system tumors or infection

Pneumonia

Pulmonary tuberculosis

Brain tumor

Acute porphyria

Hypovolemia

Dehydration

▼ Decreased levels

Neurogenic (or central) diabetes insipidus caused by central nervous system trauma, tumor, or infection

Surgical ablation of the pituitary gland

Overhydration

Decreased serum osmolality

Hypervolemia

Nephrotic syndrome

Psychogenic polydipsia

notes

anti-DNA antibody test (Antideoxyribonucleic acid antibodies, Antibody to double-stranded DNA, Anti-double-stranded DNA, Anti-ds-DNA, DNA antibody, Native double-stranded DNA)

Type of test Blood

Normal findings Low antibody levels or none (units depend on laboratory and methodology)

Test explanation and related physiology

The anti-ds-DNA test is useful for the diagnosis and follow-up of systemic lupus erythematosus (SLE). This antibody is found in approximately 65% to 80% of patients with active SLE and rarely in other diseases. High titers are characteristic of SLE. These antibodies also may be found in some patients with other rheumatic diseases and in those with chronic hepatitis, infectious mononucleosis, and biliary cirrhosis. The anti-DNA titer decreases with successful therapy and increases with an exacerbation of SLE and especially with the onset of glomerulonephritis.

Interfering factors

- A radioactive scan performed within 1 week before the test may alter the test results.
- 🖊 Drugs that may cause *increased* levels include hydralazine and procainamide.

Procedure and patient care

Before

- Explain the procedure to the patient.
- Tell the patient that no fasting is required.

During

- Collect one red-top tube of venous blood.

After

- Apply pressure or a pressure dressing to the venipuncture site.
- Assess the venipuncture site for bleeding.

Abnormal findings

▲ **Increased levels**

Systemic lupus erythematosus   Infectious mononucleosis
Chronic hepatitis   Biliary cirrhosis

notes

anti–extractable nuclear antigens (Anti-ENA, Antibodies to extractable nuclear antigens, Antiribonucleoprotein [anti-RNP], Anti-Smith [anti-SM])

Type of test Blood

Normal findings Negative

Test explanation and related physiology

Anti-ENA is a group of antibodies to certain antigens that consist of RNA and protein. The ENA antigen is extracted from thymus using phosphate-buffered saline and therefore is sometimes referred to as "saline-extracted antigen." The most common ENAs are Smith (SM) and ribonucleoprotein (RNP).

The antinuclear Smith (anti-SM) antibody is present in about 30% of patients with systemic lupus erythematosus (SLE) and in about 8% of patients with mixed connective tissue (MCT) diseases. However, it is not present in patients with most other rheumatoid-collagen diseases.

The antinuclear ribonucleoprotein (anti-RNP) is reported in nearly 100% of patients with mixed connective tissue (MCT) disease and in about 25% of patients with SLE, discoid lupus, and progressive systemic sclerosis (scleroderma). In high titer, anti-RNP is suggestive of MCT.

There are two other antibodies to ENAs. Anti-SS-A and anti-SS-B are described on p. 86 and are used mainly in the diagnostic evaluation of Sjögren's syndrome.

Procedure and patient care

Before

- Explain the procedure to the patient.
- Tell the patient that no fasting is required.

During

- Collect a venous blood sample in a red-top tube.

After

- Apply pressure or a pressure dressing to the venipuncture site.
- Assess the venipuncture site for bleeding.
- Check the venipuncture site for infection. Patients with autoimmune disease have a compromised immune system.

Abnormal findings

▲ **Increased anti-SM antibodies**

Systemic lupus erythematosus

Mixed connective tissue disease

▲ **Increased anti-RNP antibodies**

Mixed connective tissue disease

Systemic lupus erythematosus

Discoid lupus

Scleroderma

notes

antiglomerular basement membrane antibodies
(Anti-GBM antibody, AGBM, Glomerular basement antibody, Goodpasture's antibody)

Type of test Blood or microscopic examination (lung or renal)

Normal findings Negative

Test explanation and related physiology

This test is used to detect the presence of circulating glomerular basement membrane antibodies in Goodpasture's syndrome and occasionally in other forms of glomerulonephritis. Goodpasture's syndrome is an autoimmune disease characterized by the presence of circulating antibodies against the renal glomerular basement membrane and the pulmonary alveolar basement membrane. Patients with this problem usually display a triad of glomerulonephritis, pulmonary hemorrhage, and antibodies to basement membrane antigens.

With the use of immunohistochemistry, and now with radioimmunoassay, antibodies also can be demonstrated in the glomeruli, renal tubular basement membrane, and the pulmonary capillary basement membranes. Therefore, lung or renal biopsies are required to obtain this specimen as well. Serum assays are a faster and more reliable method for diagnosing Goodpasture's syndrome, especially in patients in whom renal or lung biopsy may be difficult or contraindicated. Furthermore, serum levels can be used in monitoring response to therapy (plasmaphoresis or cytotoxic).

Procedure and patient care

Before
- Explain the procedure to the patient.
- Tell the patient to fast for 8 hours before the test. Water is permitted.
- If a lung biopsy (see p. 534) or renal biopsy (see p. 704) will be used to collect the specimen, explain these procedures to the patient.

During
- Collect one red-top tube of venous blood.

After
- Apply pressure or a pressure dressing to the venipuncture site.
- Assess the venipuncture site for bleeding.

Abnormal findings

Positive

Goodpasture's syndrome
Glomerulonephritis

notes

antimitochondrial antibody and anti–smooth muscle antibody tests (AMA and ASMA)

Type of test Blood

Normal findings

No antimitochondrial antibodies (AMAs) at titers >1:5
No anti–smooth muscle antibodies (ASMAs) at titers >1:20

Test explanation and related physiology

The AMA and ASMA tests are used primarily to diagnose primary biliary cirrhosis and autoimmune chronic active hepatitis (CAH), respectively. Jaundice from extrahepatic biliary duct obstruction is not associated with the high elevations of these antibody levels. Intrahepatic cholestasis is often associated with elevated levels of these antibodies. Normally, the serum does not contain AMAs at a titer greater than 1:5 and ASMAs at a titer greater than 1:20.

Antimitochondrial antibodies are found in less than 1% of normals and are associated with liver and bile duct autoimmune diseases. AMA appears in 94% of patients with primary biliary cirrhosis; these patients also have greatly elevated liver enzyme levels and a normal cholangiogram. Their liver biopsy is compatible with primary liver cirrhosis. AMA reactivity is seen in 25% of patients with CAH. For the AMA test, immunofluorescent assay or enzyme-linked immunosorbent assay (ELISA) techniques are used. False-positive results occur in patients with scleroderma, systemic lupus erythematosus (SLE), or syphilis.

Anti–smooth muscle antibodies are present in only about 30% of patients with primary biliary cirrhosis; however, 94% of patients with chronic hepatitis have ASMAs. ASMA titers do not appear to be predictive of prognosis or of response to therapy for CAH. False-positive ASMA tests may be caused by infectious mononucleosis, viral hepatitis, multiple sclerosis, or hepatomas. For the ASMA test, immunofluorescence is used to detect reactivity.

Procedure and patient care

Before

- Explain the procedure to the patient.

- Tell the patient that no fasting or special preparation is required.

During

- Collect 7 to 10 ml of venous blood in a red-top tube.

After

- Apply pressure or a pressure dressing to the venipuncture site.
- Check the venipuncture site for bleeding. Patients with jaundice often have bleeding disorders associated with vitamin K deficiency.

Abstract findings

▲ **Increased levels**

AMA	*ASMA*
Primary biliary cirrhosis	Chronic active hepatitis
Chronic active hepatitis	Primary biliary cirrhosis
Scleroderma (CREST syndrome)	Viral hepatitis
	Infectious mononucleosis
Systemic lupus erythematosus	Some malignant tumors
Syphilis	Intrinsic asthma

notes

antimyocardial antibodies (AMA)

Type of test Blood

Normal findings Negative (if positive, serum will be titrated)

Test explanation and related physiology

An immunologic basis for rheumatic heart disease has been suspected for a long time. Research has now documented the presence of serum antibodies against myocardial components and deposition of immunoglobulin and complement in lesional areas. Antibodies against heart muscle are found in 20% to 40% of post–cardiac surgery patients, with higher levels noted in the smaller number with post–cardiac injury clinical syndrome.

Antimyocardial antibodies may be detected in rheumatic heart disease, cardiomyopathy, postthoracotomy syndrome, and post–myocardial infarction. This test is used in the detection of an autoimmune cause for these conditions and for monitoring their response to treatment. This test is performed by indirect immunofluorescent technique. Positive results are reported in titers.

Procedure and patient care

Before
- Explain the procedure to the patient.
- Tell the patient that no fasting or special preparation is necessary.

During
- Collect a venous blood sample in a red-top tube of blood.

After
- Apply pressure or a pressure dressing to the venipuncture site.
- Check the venipuncture site for bleeding.

Abnormal findings

▲ Increased values

Rheumatic heart disease   Post–myocardial infarction
Cardiomyopathy   Rheumatic fever
Postthoracotomy syndrome   Streptococcal infection

antineutrophil cytoplasmic antibody (ANCA)

Type of test Blood

Normal findings Negative

Test explanation and related physiology

Wegener's granulomatosis (WG) is a regional systemic vasculitis in which the small arteries of the kidneys, lungs, and upper respiratory tract are damaged by a necrotizing inflammation. Diagnosis can be made by biopsy of clinically affected areas. Recently, serologic testing has begun to play a key role in the diagnosis of WG and other systemic vasculitis syndromes. Most patients with WG have circulating autoantibodies against neutrophil cytoplasm, which are useful in the diagnosis.

Antineutrophil cytoplasmic antibodies (ANCAs) are antibodies directed against cytoplasmic components of neutrophils. There are two types of antineutrophil cytoplasmic antibodies. The C-ANCA pattern is highly specific (95% to 99%) for WG and gives diffuse granular staining of the cytoplasm. The P-ANCA pattern produces a perinuclear staining of neutrophils. Although the P-ANCA pattern is found in patients with WG, it also occurs in other conditions, especially those with microscopic polyarteritis. This blood test may be useful to follow the course of the disease, to monitor the response to therapy, and to provide early detection of relapse.

Procedure and patient care

Before
- Explain the procedure to the patient.
- Tell the patient that no fasting is required.

During
- Collect venous blood in a tube as determined by the laboratory performing the test.

After
- Apply pressure or a pressure dressing to the venipuncture site.
- Observe the venipuncture site for bleeding.

Abnormal findings

▲ **Increased levels**

Wegener's granulomatosis	Idiopathic crescentic glomerulonephritis
Microscopic polyarteritis	

antinuclear antibody (ANA)

Type of test Blood

Normal findings No ANA detected in a titer with a dilution >1:32

Test explanation and related physiology

Many abnormal antibodies exist in patients with autoimmune (rheumatic) diseases. ANA is a protein antibody that reacts against cellular nuclear material. ANA is quite sensitive in detecting systemic lupus erythyematosus (SLE). Positive results occur in approximately 95% of patients with this disease; however, many other rheumatic diseases and drugs can cause a false-positive ANA test. ANA, therefore, is not a specific test for SLE. When a patient has a positive LE cell prep and a positive ANA test, SLE is strongly suspected. Often, the ANA test is used to screen patients with suspected SLE. If the ANA test is negative, the patient probably does not have SLE.

The test is usually performed by combining the patient's serum with nuclear material derived from a rat's liver or other such tissue. Fluorescein-labeled antihuman serum is then mixed with the patient's serum and the rat's nuclear material. If positive, the radiolabeled antihuman antibody should attach to the patient's ANA. This fluorescein will then be seen under the ultraviolet microscope. The patient's serum is serially diluted, and the ANA test is carried out with each dilution. The most dilute serum in which ANA is detected is called the *titer*. The test is considered positive if ANA is found in a titer with a dilution of greater than 1:32.

There are many specific patterns of ANA reactivity that have been detected by immunofluorescence, enzyme-linked immunosorbent assay (ELISA), and enzyme immunoassay (EIA). These patterns are the basis for establishing a series of subtypes of ANA antibodies (Table 1). ANA antibodies are positive in many different types of autoimmune diseases (Table 2).

Interfering factors

☞ Drugs that may cause a false-positive ANA test include acetazolamide, aminosalicyclic acid, chlorprothixene, chlorothia-

A

TABLE 1 Antinuclear antibodies/fluorescent patterns

Homogeneous	Antideoxynucleoprotein
Peripheral	Anti–native (double-stranded)
Nuclear membrane	DNA
Speckled	Anti–single-stranded DNA
Pseudo-ACA	Antihistone
Anticentromere	Anti-Smith
Nucleolar	Antiribonucleoprotein
Mitotic spindle	Anti–SSA, SSB, SSC
Cytoplasmic	Antinucleolar
Antinuclear lamins	Anti–Scl-70
Antiribosomal	Anti–proliferating cell nuclear
Anti–centriole/centrosome/	antigen
midbody	Anti–mitotic spindle

TABLE 2 Autoimmune disease and positive antibodies

Autoimmune disease	Positive antibodies
SLE	ANA, SLE prep, dsDNA, ssDNA, anti-DNP, SS-A
Drug-induced SLE	ANA
Sjögren's syndrome	RF, ANA, SS-A, SS-B
Scleroderma	ANA, Scl-70, RNA, dsDNA
Raynaud's disease	ACA, Scl-70
Mixed connective tissue disease	ANA, RNP, RF, ssDNA
Rheumatoid arthritis	RF, ANA, RANA, RAP,
Primary biliary cirrhosis	AMA
Thyroiditis	Antimicrosomal, antithyroglobulin
Chronic active hepatitis	ASMA

---

zides, griseofulvin, hydralazine, penicillin, phenylbutazone, phenytoin sodium, procainamide, streptomycin, sulfonamides, and tetracyclines.

▼ Drugs that may cause a false-negative test include steroids.

Procedure and patient care

Before
- Explain the procedure to the patient.
- Tell the patient that no fasting or preparation is required.

During
- Collect 7 to 10 ml of venous blood in a red-top tube.
- Indicate on the laboratory slip any drugs that may affect the test results.

After
- Apply pressure or a pressure dressing to the venipuncture site.
- Assess the venipuncture site for bleeding.
- Because they are usually immunocompromised, instruct patients with an autoimmune disease to check for signs of infection at the venipuncture site. These patients often take steroids that further compromise their immune system.

Abnormal findings

▲ **Increased levels**

Systemic lupus erythematosus
Rheumatoid arthritis
Chronic hepatitis
Periarteritis (polyarteritis) nodosa
Dermatomyositis
Scleroderma

Infectious mononucleosis
Raynaud's disease
Sjögren's syndrome
Other immune diseases
Leukemia
Myasthenia gravis
Cirrhosis

notes

antiscleroderma antibody (Scl-70 antibody, Scleroderma antibody)

Type of test Blood

Normal findings Negative

Test explanation and related physiology

This antibody is diagnostic for scleroderma (progressive systemic sclerosis) and is present in 20% to 30% of patients with that disease. This is a multisystem disorder characterized by fibrosis of the skin, blood vessels, and visceral organs, including the heart, lungs, kidneys, and gastrointestinal tract.

The absence of this antibody does not exclude the diagnosis of scleroderma. The antibody is only occasionally seen in other rheumatic diseases, such as systemic lupus erythematosus, mixed connective tissue disease (MCTD), Sjögren's syndrome, polymyositis, and rheumatoid arthritis.

Interfering factors

☒ Drugs that may cause *increased* levels include aminosalicylic acid, isoniazid, methyldopa, penicillin, propylthiouracil, streptomycin, and tetracycline.

Procedure and patient care

Before
- Explain the procedure to the patient.
- Tell the patient that no fasting is required.

During
- Collect a venous sample of blood in a red-top tube.

After
- Apply pressure or a pressure dressing to the venipuncture site.
- Assess the venipuncture site for bleeding.

Abnormal findings

Positive
Scleroderma
CREST syndrome

antispermatozoal antibody (Sperm agglutination and inhibition, Sperm antibodies, Antisperm antibodies, Infertility screen)

Type of test Fluid analysis; blood

Normal findings Negative

Test explanation and related physiology

The antispermatozoal antibody test is an infertility screening test used to detect the presence of sperm antibodies. Antibodies directed toward sperm antigens can result in diminished fertility. In addition to a semen specimen, the serum of both partners should be studied for sperm antibodies, because a relationship may exist between spermatozoal antibodies in women's serum and unexplained fertility.

Antisperm antibodies may be found in men with blocked efferent ducts in the testes and in 70% of those who have had a vasectomy. The reabsorption of sperm from the blocked ducts may result in the formation of autoantibodies to sperm.

Procedure and patient care

Before

- Explain the procedure to the patient.
- Inform the man that a semen specimen should be collected after avoiding ejaculation for at least 3 days.
- Give the male patient the proper container for the sperm collection.
- If the specimen is to be collected at home, be certain the patient is told that it must be taken to the laboratory for testing within 2 hours after collection.

During

- Collect a venous blood sample of approximately 7 to 10 ml from both the male and the female patient in red-top tubes.

After

- Apply pressure or a pressure dressing to the venipuncture sites.
- Check the venipuncture sites for bleeding.
- Instruct the couple when and how to obtain the test results.

Abnormal findings

Infertility
Blocked efferent ducts in the testes
Vasectomy

notes

anti-SS-A (Ro), anti-SS-B (La), and anti-SS-C antibody (Anti-Ro, Anti-La, Sjögren's antibodies)

Type of test   Blood

Normal findings   Negative

Test explanation and related physiology

This test is used to detect anti-SS-A (Ro), anti-SS-B (La), and anti-SS-C antibodies produced in Sjögren's syndrome, an immunologic abnormality characterized by progressive destruction of the exocrine glands leading to mucosal and conjunctival dryness. This disease can occur by itself (primary) or in association with other autoimmune diseases, such as systemic lupus erythematosus (SLE), rheumatoid arthritis, and scleroderma. In the latter case, it is referred to as *secondary Sjögren's syndrome.*

Anti-SS-A antibodies may be found in approximately 60% to 70% of patients with primary Sjögren's syndrome and in 30% to 40% of patients with SLE. Anti-SS-B antibodies may be found in approximately 50% to 60% of patients with primary Sjögren's syndrome and in 10% to 15% of patients with SLE. Patients with both Sjögren's syndrome and rheumatoid arthritis may have neither anti-SS-A nor anti-SS-B antibodies. Therefore this test is useful in the differential diagnosis of Sjögren's syndrome, SLE, and mixed connective tissue diseases. This test is particularly useful in "ANA (antinuclear antigen)–negative" cases of SLE, because these antibodies are present in the majority of such patients.

Procedure and patient care

Before

- Explain the procedure to the patient.
- Tell the patient that no fasting is required.

During

- Collect a venous blood sample in a red-top tube.

After

- Apply pressure or a pressure dressing to the venipuncture site.
- Assess the venipuncture site for bleeding.
- Check the venipuncture site for infection. Patients with autoimmune disease have a compromised immune system.

Abnormal findings

A

Positive

Sjögren's syndrome
Scleroderma

Antinuclear antibody (ANA)–
   negative lupus
Neonatal lupus

notes

antistreptolysin O titer (ASO titer)

Type of test Blood

Normal findings

Adult/elderly: ≤160 Todd units/ml
Newborn: similar to mother's value
    6 months-2 years: ≤50 Todd units/ml
    2-4 years: ≤160 Todd units/ml
    5-12 years: 170-330 Todd units/ml

Test explanation and related physiology

The ASO titer is a serologic procedure demonstrating the reaction of the body to infection caused by group A streptococci bacteria. It is used primarily in detecting poststreptococcal diseases, such as glomerulonephritis, rheumatic fever, bacterial endocarditis, and scarlet fever.

The streptococcus organism produces an enzyme called *streptolysin O*, which has the ability to destroy (lyse) red blood corpuscles. Because streptolysin O is antigenic, the body reacts by producing ASO, a neutralizing antibody. ASO appears in the serum 1 week to 1 month after the onset of a streptococcal infection; a high titer is not specific for a certain type of poststreptococcal disease but merely indicates that a streptococcal infection is or has been present. When the ASO elevation is seen in a patient with glomerulonephritis or endocarditis, one can safely assume that the disease was caused by streptococcal infection. Subsequent testing may be done to detect the difference between the acute and convalescent blood sample.

Another immunologic test, *antideoxyribonuclease B (anti-DNase B)* (see p. 66), also detects antigens produced by group A streptococci. The anti-DNase B level is elevated in most patients with acute rheumatic fever and poststreptococcal glomerulonephritis.

Interfering factors

- Increased beta-lipoprotein levels inhibit streptolysin O and give a falsely high ASO titer.
- Drugs that may cause *decreased* ASO levels include antibiotics and adrenocorticosteroids.

Procedure and patient care

Before
- Explain the procedure to the patient.
- Tell the patient that no fasting is required.

During
- Collect approximately 5 to 10 ml of blood in a red-top tube.
- Avoid hemolysis of the blood specimen.
- Note on the laboratory slip any medications that may affect the test results.

After
- Apply pressure or a pressure dressing to the venipuncture site.
- Observe the venipuncture site for bleeding.
- Note that repeat ASO testing may be done to determine the highest level of increase.

Abnormal findings

▲ **Increased levels**
Streptococcal infection
Acute rheumatic fever
Acute glomerulonephritis

Bacterial endocarditis
Scarlet fever

notes

antithrombin III (AT-III, Functional antithrombin III assay, Heparin cofactor, Immunologic antithrombin III, Serine protease inhibitor)

Type of test Blood

Normal findings

Plasma: >50% of control value
Serum: 15% to 34% lower than plasma value
Immunologic: 17-30 mg/dl
Functional: 80% to 120%
(Values vary according to laboratory methods)

Test explanation and related physiology

This test helps to detect hypercoagulable states associated with episodes of venous thrombosis. AT-III inhibits coagulation through an inactivation of thrombin and other clotting factors. The action of AT-III is catalyzed by heparin. In normal coagulation, homeostasis results from a balance between AT-III and thrombin. A deficiency of AT-III increases coagulation or the tendency toward thrombosis.

This test is used to evaluate both response to heparin therapy and hypercoagulable and fibrinogenolytic states. It also can test for a hereditary deficiency of AT-III, which is characterized by a predisposition toward thrombus formation. Acquired AT-III deficiency may be seen in patients with cirrhosis, liver failure, advanced carcinoma, nephrotic syndrome, disseminated intravascular coagulation (DIC), and acute thrombosis. Asymptomatic individuals with an antithrombin deficiency should receive prophylactic anticoagulation to raise their antithrombin levels before any medical/surgical circumstances in which inactivity increases the risk of thrombosis. Increased levels of AT-III may occur in patients with acute hepatitis, obstructive jaundice, vitamin K deficiency, and kidney transplantation.

Interfering factors

▪ Drugs that may cause *increased* levels include anabolic steroids, androgens, oral contraceptives (containing progesterone), and sodium warfarin.
▪ Drugs that may cause *decreased* levels include fibrinolytics, heparin, L-asparaginase, and oral contraceptives (containing estrogen).

Procedure and patient care

Before

- Explain the procedure to the patient.
- Tell the patient that no fasting is required.

During

- Collect a venous blood sample in a blue- or red-top tube.

After

- Apply pressure or a pressure dressing to the venipuncture site.
- Assess the venipuncture site for bleeding.
- Send the specimen to the laboratory immediately after collection.

Abnormal findings

▲ **Increased levels**

Kidney transplant
Acute hepatitis
Obstructive jaundice
Vitamin K deficiency

▼ **Decreased levels**

Disseminated intravascular coagulation
Hypercoagulation states (e.g., deep vein thrombosis)
Hepatic disorders (especially cirrhosis)
Nephrotic syndrome
Protein-wasting diseases (malignancy)
Hereditary familial deficiency of AT-III

notes

antithyroglobulin antibody (Thyroid autoantibody, Thyroid antithyroglobulin antibody, Thyroglobulin antibody)

Type of test Blood

Normal findings Titer <1:100

Test explanation and related physiology

The serum antithyroglobulin titer evaluation detects the presence of thyroid antibodies formed in response to thyroglobulin released from the thyroid gland in certain destructive thyroid disorders. These autoantibodies combine with thyroglobulin and cause inflammation in the thyroid gland. These thyroid antibodies indicate the presence of an autoimmune disease, and they may be responsible for further destruction of the thyroid gland. This test is usually used in conjunction with the antithyroid microsomal antibody test (see p. 94).

This test is primarily used in the differential diagnosis of thyroid diseases such as Hashimoto's thyroiditis. The level must be extremely high to confirm the diagnosis of Hashimoto's thyroiditis. This antibody is present in only about 50% of patients with Hashimoto's thyroiditis.

Interfering factors

- Normal individuals, especially elderly women, may have antithyroglobulin antibodies.

Procedure and patient care

Before
- Explain the procedure to the patient.
- Tell the patient that no fasting is required.

During
- Collect approximately 3 to 5 ml of blood in a red-top tube.

After
- Apply pressure or a pressure dressing to the venipuncture site.
- Assess the venipuncture site for bleeding.

Abbnormal findings

▲ **Increased levels**

Hashimoto's thyroiditis
Rheumatoid arthritis
Rheumatoid-collagen disease
Pernicious anemia

Thyrotoxicosis
Hypothyroidism
Thyroid carcinoma
Myxedema

notes

antithyroid microsomal antibody (Antimicrosomal antibody, Microsomal antibody, Thyroid autoantibody, Thyroid antimicrosomal antibody)

Type of test Blood

Normal findings Titer <1:100; present in 5% to 10% of healthy people

Test explanation and related physiology

This test is used to detect thyroid microsomal antibodies, which are found in 70% to 90% of patients with Hashimoto's thyroiditis. Microsomal antibodies are produced in response to microsomes escaping from the epithelial cells surrounding the thyroid follicle. These escaped microsomes then act as antigens and give rise to antibodies. These immune complexes initiate inflammatory and cytotoxic effects on the thyroid follicle. This test is usually performed in conjunction with the antithyroglobulin antibody test (see p. 92).

Procedure and patient care

Before
- Explain the procedure to the patient.
- Tell the patient that no fasting is required.

During
- Collect approximately 3 to 5 ml of venous blood in a red-top tube.

After
- Apply pressure or a pressure dressing to the venipuncture site.
- Assess the venipuncture site for bleeding.

Abnormal findings

▲ **Increased values**

Hashimoto's thyroiditis   Thyroiditis
Myxedema   Nontoxic nodular goiter
Thyroid carcinoma

apolipoproteins (Apolipoprotein A-I [Apo A-I], Apolipoprotein B [Apo B], Lipoprotein (a) [Lp (a)])

Type of test Blood

Normal findings

Apo A-I
Adult/elderly
  Male: 75-160 mg/dl
  Female: 80-175 mg/dl
Child
  Newborn
    Male: 41-93 mg/dl
    Female: 38-106 mg/dl
  6 months-4 years
    Male: 67-167 mg/dl
    Female: 60-148 mg/dl
  5 to 17 years: 83-151 mg/dl

Apo B
Adult/elderly
  Male: 50-125 mg/dl
  Female: 45-120 mg/dl
Child
  Newborn: 11-31 mg/dl
  6 months-3 years: 23-75 mg/dl
  5-17 years:
    Male: 47-139 mg/dl
    Female: 41-132 mg/dl

Apo A-I/apo B ratio
Male: 0.85-2.24
Female: 0.76-3.23

Lipoprotein (a)
Caucasian (5th-95th percentile)
  Male: 2.2-49.4 mg/dl
  Female: 2.1-57.3 mg/dl
African-American (5th-95th percentile)
  Male: 4.6-71.8 mg/dl
  Female: 4.4-75.0 mg/dl

Test explanation and related physiology

The protein component of lipoproteins, which plays an important role in lipid transport, is composed of several specific polypeptides called apolipoproteins. Apolipoproteins are also involved in binding lipoproteins to lipoprotein receptors at the cell surface, thus facilitating lipid uptake by cells.

Apolipoprotein A (apo A) is the major polypeptide component of high-density lipoprotein (HDL). Apo A has two major forms: apo A-I, which constitutes about 75% of the apo A in HDL, and apo A-II, which constitutes about 20% of the total HDL protein. In general, as HDL levels increase, apo A-I values increase. Since apo A-I reflects the HDL content of the serum and HDL levels are greater in females, apo A-I values are also higher in women than in men. Apo A-I has been proposed to be a better index of atherogenic risk than is HDL assay.

Apolipoprotein B (apo B) is the major polypeptide component of low-density lipoprotein (LDL) and makes up about 80% of that protein. Forty percent of the protein portion of very-low-density lipoprotein (VLDL) is composed of apo B. Apo B has been shown to exist in two forms: apo B-100 and apo B-48. Apo B-100 is synthesized in the liver and found in lipoproteins of endogenous origin (VLDL and LDL). Apo B-100 is the principal transport mechanism for endogenous cholesterol. Apo B-100 has an affinity for the LDL receptor located on cell surfaces in peripheral tissues and is involved with cellular deposition of cholesterol. Because of this, some believe that apo B-100 may be a better indicator of atherosclerotic heart disease than is LDL. The second apo B component is apo B-48, which is of intestinal origin and found mainly in chylomicrons. Apo B-48 serves to transport ingested lipids through the intestines and into the bloodstream.

Lipoprotein (a) [Lp(a)] (referred to as "lipoprotein little a") is another lipoprotein. The two polypeptide components of Lp(a) are apo (a) and an LDL-like protein containing apo B-100. Recent research has suggested that increased levels of Lp(a) may be an independent risk factor for atherosclerosis. It has been shown that apo (a) is a deformed relative of plasminogen, the precursor of the proteolytic enzyme plasmin, which is responsible for dissolving fiber clots. This strong resemblance between an apolipoprotein and plasminogen may provide a link between lipids, the clotting mechanism, and atherogenesis. Microthrombi containing fibrin on the vessel wall become incorporated into the atherosclerotic plaque. It is suggested that, following endothelial damage, Lp(a) may insinuate itself into the arterial wall, inhibiting the cleavage of fibrin in microthrombi by competing with plasminogen for access for fibrin. Atherosclerotic damage of the arterial wall soon follows, leading to occlusive disease or aneurysm.

Quantification of apolipoproteins is beginning to be performed as a routine clinical procedure. However, there are many unsolved methodologic problems in apolipoprotein immunoassays, creating significant variability. Several studies have indicated that apo A-I and apo B are better determinants of atherosclerotic disease than are lipid or lipoprotein determinants. Decreased levels of apo A-I and increased levels of apo B-100 are associated with increased risk of coronary heart disease. Reports also indicate that a low ratio of apo A-I to apo B may be a good predictor of coronary heart disease. Individuals with increased concentrations of Lp(a) appear to have a significantly higher risk for coronary heart disease.

These and other apolipoproteins are associated with the identification of other maladies. For example, the apo E4 gene has been proposed as a risk factor for Alzheimer's disease. Familial hypercholesterolemia, some forms of renal failure, nephrotic syndrome, and estrogen depletion in women over the age of 50 may be associated with increased levels of Lp(a).

Interfering factors

Apo A-I

- Physical exercise may increase apo A-I levels.
- Smoking may decrease levels.
- Diets high in carbohydrates or polyunsaturated fats may decrease apo A-I levels.
- Drugs that may *increase* apo A-I levels include carbamazepine, estrogens, ethanol, lovastatin, niacin, oral contraceptives, phenobarbital, pravastatin, and simvastatin.
- Drugs that may *decrease* apo A-I levels include androgens, beta blockers, diuretics, and progestins.

Apo B

- Diets high in saturated fats and cholesterol may increase apo B levels.
- Drugs that may *increase* apo B levels may include androgens, beta blockers, diuretics, ethanol abuse, and progestins.

☛ Drugs that may *decrease* apo B levels include cholestyramine, estrogen (postmenopausal women), lovastatin, simvastatin, neomycin, niacin, and thyroxine.

Lipoprotein (a)

☛ Drugs that may *decrease* Lp(a) include estrogens, niacin, neomycin, and stanozolol.

Procedure and patient care

Before

- Explain the procedure to the patient.
- Instruct the patient to fast for 12 to 14 hours before testing. Only water is permitted.
- Inform the patient that smoking is prohibited.

During

- Collect venous blood in a red-top tube.
- Indicate on the laboratory slip any drugs that may affect test results.

After

- Apply pressure or a pressure dressing to the venipuncture site.
- Observe the venipuncture site for bleeding.

Abnormal findings

▲ **Increased apo A-I**
Familial hyperalpha-
  lipoproteinemia
Pregnancy
Weight reduction

▼ **Decreased apo A-I**
Coronary artery disease
Ischemic coronary dis-
  ease
Myocardial infarction
Familial hypoalpha-
  lipoproteinemia
Fish eye disease
Uncontrolled diabetes
  mellitus
Tangier disease
Nephrotic syndrome
Chronic renal failure
Cholestasis
Hemodialysis

▲ **Increased apo B**

Hyperlipoproteinemia
(types IIa, IIb, IV, V)
Nephrotic syndrome
Pregnancy
Hemodialysis
Biliary obstruction
Coronary artery disease
Diabetes
Hypothyroidism
Anorexia nervosa

▲ **Increased levels of Lp(a)**

Premature coronary artery disease
Stenosis of cerebral arteries
Uncontrolled diabetes mellitus
Severe hypothyroidism
Familial hypercholesterolemia
Chronic renal failure
Estrogen depletion

▼ **Decreased apo B**

Tangier disease
Hyperthyroidism
Malnutrition
Inflammatory joint disease
Chronic pulmonary disease
Weight reduction
Chronic anemia
Reye's syndrome

▼ **Decreased levels of Lp(a)**

Alcoholism
Malnutrition
Chronic liver hepatocellular disease

notes

arteriography (Angiography)

Type of test X-ray with contrast dye

Normal findings Normal arterial vasculature

Test explanation and related physiology

With the injection of radiopaque contrast material into arteries, blood vessels can be visualized to determine arterial anatomy, vascular disease, or neoplasms. With a catheter usually placed through the femoral and into the desired artery, radiopaque contrast is rapidly injected while x-ray films are obtained. Blood flow dynamics, abnormal blood vessels, vascular anomalies, normal and abnormal vascular anatomy, and tumors are easily seen. With the use of digital subtraction angiography (DSA), bony structures can be obliterated from the picture.

DSA is a sophisticated type of computerized fluoroscopy that, when used with arterial angiography, can better visualize the arteries of the body, especially the carotid and cerebral arteries. DSA enables small differences in x-ray absorption between an artery and the surrounding tissues to be converted to digital information and stored. It is especially useful when adjacent bone inhibits visualization of the blood vessel to be evaluated. For DSA, an image (mask) is made of the area of clinical interest and stored in the computer program. After intraarterial injection of contrast material, subsequent images are made. The computer then subtracts the preinjection "mask" image from the postinjection image. This removes all the undesired images (e.g., bone) and leaves the arterial image of high contrast and quality.

While nearly all major blood vessels can be visualized through the technique of arteriography, the kidneys, adrenal glands, brain, and abdominal aorta (with lower extremities) are most usually visualized. Coronary arteriography is described under cardiac catheterization (see p. 196).

Renal angiography permits evaluation of blood flow dynamics, demonstration of abnormal blood vessels, and differentiation of a vascular renal cyst from hypervascular renal cancers. Arteriosclerotic narrowing (stenosis) of the renal artery is best demonstrated with this study. The angiographic location of the stenotic area is helpful for the vascular surgeon considering repair. Complete transection of the renal artery by blunt or penetrating trauma can also be seen as total vascular obstruction. Highly vascular renal cancers can produce a "blush" of contrast material during angiography.

The adrenal gland and its arterial system can also be visualized by *adrenal arteriography*. Both benign and malignant tumors of the adrenal gland can be detected easily by this technique. Bilateral adrenal hyperplasia can also be identified.

Cerebral angiography provides radiographic visualization of the cerebral vascular system with the injection of radiopaque dye into the carotid or vertebral arteries. With this procedure, abnormalities of the cerebral circulation, such as aneurysms, occlusions, stenosis, or arteriovenous (AV) malformations, can be identified. A vascular tumor is seen as a mass containing small, abnormal blood vessels. A nonvascular tumor, abscess, or hematoma appears as a mass distorting the normal vascular contour.

Lower extremity arteriography allows for accurate identification and location of occlusions within the abdominal aorta and lower extremity arteries. After the catheter is placed in the aorta or more selectively into the femoral artery, radiopaque dye is injected. X-ray films are taken in timed sequence to allow radiographic visualization of the arterial system of the lower extremities. Total or near-total occlusion of the flow of dye is seen in arteriosclerotic vascular occlusive disease. Emboli are seen as total occlusions of the artery. Arterial traumas such as lacerations or intimal tears (laceration of the arterial inner lining) likewise appear as total or near-total obstruction of the flow of dye. Aneurysmal dilatation of the arteries or its branches also can be seen. Unusual arterial disorders such as Buerger's disease and fibromuscular dysplasia have the classic arterial "beading," which is pathognomonic.

Lower extremity arteriography is usually performed electively on patients with symptoms and signs of peripheral vascular disease. Emergency arteriography, however, is needed when the blood flow to an extremity has ceased suddenly. Immediate surgical therapy is then needed and is most effective when the surgeon has knowledge of the etiology and location of this sudden occlusion. This knowledge can only be obtained by arteriography.

Contraindications

- Patients with allergies to shellfish or iodinated dye
- Patients who are uncooperative or agitated
- Patients who are pregnant

- Patients with renal disorders, because iodinated contrast is nephrotoxic
- Patients with a bleeding propensity
- Patients with unstable cardiac disorders
- Patients who are dehydrated, because they are especially susceptible to dye-induced renal failure

Potential complications

- Allergic reaction to iodinated dye

  These reactions may vary from mild flushing, itching, and urticaria to severe, life-threatening anaphylaxis (evidenced by respiratory distress, drop in blood pressure, and shock). In the unusual event of anaphylaxis, diphenhydramine (Benadryl), steroids, and epinephrine are added to routine resuscitative efforts. Oxygen and endotracheal equipment should be on hand for immediate use.
- Hemorrhage from the arterial puncture site used for arterial access
- Arterial embolism from dislodgment of an arteriosclerotic plaque
- Soft tissue infection around the puncture site
- Renal failure, especially in elderly patients who are chronically dehydrated or have a mild degree of renal failure
- Dissection of the intimal lining of the artery causing complete or partial arterial occlusion
- Pseudoaneurysm development as a result of failure of the puncture site to seal
- With adrenal angiography, fatal hypertensive crisis may occur in patients with pheochromocytoma. Propranolol (Inderal), a beta-adrenergic blocker, and phenoxybenzamine (Dibenzyline), an alpha-adrenergic blocker, are given for several days before the study to avoid precipitation of a malignant hypertensive episode.
- In adrenal angiography, hemorrhage of the adrenal gland can occur. This may lead to adrenal insufficiency.

Procedure and patient care

Before

- Explain the procedure to the patient. Allay any fears and allow the patient to verbalize concerns.
- Ensure that written and informed consent for this procedure is in the patient's chart.

- Inform the patient that a warm flush may be felt when the dye is injected.
- Assess the possibility of allergies to iodinated dye. Inform the radiologist if an allergy to iodinated contrast is suspected. The radiologist may prescribe diphenhydramine (Benadryl) and steroid preparation to be administered before the test. Usually hypoallergenic nonionic contrast will be used during the test.
- Determine if the patient has been taking anticoagulants.
- Keep the patient NPO for at least 2 to 8 hours before testing.
- Mark the site of the patient's peripheral pulses with a pen before arterial catheterization. This will permit assessment of the peripheral pulses after the procedure.
- If the patient does not have peripheral pulses before arteriography, document that fact so that arterial occlusion will not be suspected on the postangiogram assessment.
- Administer preprocedural medications as ordered.
- If the patient is suspected of having pheochromocytoma, administer propranolol and phenoxybenzamine as ordered to prevent a potentially fatal hypertensive episode.
- Ensure that the appropriate coagulation studies have been performed and are normal.
- For cerebral angiograms, perform a baseline neurologic assessment in order to compare subsequent assessments. This is to potentially diagnose any strokes that may be precipitated by cerebral arteriography.
- Remove all valuables and dental prostheses.
- Instruct the patient to void before the study because the iodinated dye can act as an osmotic diuretic.
- Inform the patient that bladder distention may cause some discomfort during the study.

During

- Note the following preprocedural steps:
  1. The patient may be sedated before being taken to the angiography room, which is usually within the radiology department.
  2. The patient is placed on the x-ray table in the supine position.
  3. If the femoral artery is to be used, the groin is shaved, prepared, and draped in a sterile manner.
  4. The femoral artery is cannulated, and a wire is threaded

up that artery and into or near the opening of the desired artery to be examined (Figure 2).

5. A catheter is then placed over that wire. The wire and catheter are both placed under fluoroscopic visualization. Because the catheter and wire have a curled tip at the end, both can be manipulated directly into the artery to be studied. The wire is removed.

6. Through the catheter, iodinated contrast material is injected by the use of an automated injector at a preset, controlled rate. This occurs over several seconds.

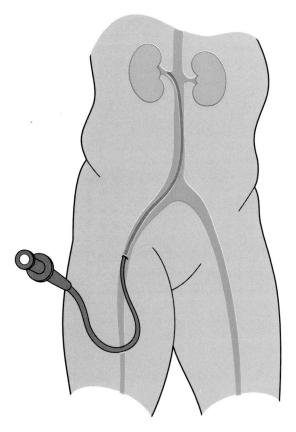

Figure 2 Catheter insertion for a renal angiogram.

7. Serial x-ray films are taken in timed sequence to show the arterial injection, and subsequent x-ray films are taken to show the venous phase of the injection.

- Note that this procedure is usually performed by an angiographer (radiologist) in approximately 1 to 2 hours.
- During the dye injection, remind the patient that an intense, burning flush may be felt throughout the body but lasts only a few seconds.
- Tell the patient that the only discomfort is the groin puncture necessary for arterial access.
- Remind the patient of the discomfort of lying on a hard x-ray table for a long period of time.
- During adrenal angiography, monitor blood pressure for evidence of malignant hypertensive storm.

After

- X-ray studies are completed, the catheter is removed, and a pressure dressing is applied to the puncture site.
- Monitor the patient's vital signs for indications of hemorrhage.
- Assess the peripheral arterial pulse in the extremity used for vascular access and compare it with the preprocedural baseline values.
- Perform a neurologic assessment for any signs of catheter-induced embolic stroke syndrome if cerebral arteriography is performed.
- Observe the arterial puncture site frequently for signs of bleeding or hematoma.
- Maintain pressure at the puncture site with a 1- to 2-pound sandbag or an IV bag.
- Keep the patient on bed rest for about 8 hours following the procedure to allow for complete sealing of the arterial puncture site.
- Assess the patient's extremities for signs of loss of blood supply (e.g., loss of pulses, numbness, pallor, tingling, pain, loss of sensory/motor function).
- Note and compare the color and temperature of the extremity with that of the uninvolved extremity.
- Administer mild analgesics for minor discomfort at the arterial puncture site.
- Notify the physician if the patient has severe, continuous pain.

- Have the patient drink fluids to prevent dehydration caused by the diuretic action of the dye.
- Evaluate the patient for delayed allergic reaction to the dye (dyspnea, rashes, tachycardia, hives). This usually occurs within 2 to 6 hours after the test. Treat the patient as described above.

Abnormal findings

Adrenal angiography

Pheochromocytoma
Adrenal adenoma

Adrenal carcinoma
Bilateral adrenal hyperplasia

Arteriography of the lower extremity

Arteriosclerotic occlusion
Embolus occlusion
Primary arterial diseases (e.g., fibromuscular dysplasia, Buerger's disease)

Aneurysm
Aberrant arterial anatomy
Tumor neovascularity
Neoplastic arterial compression

Brain arteriography

Vascular aneurysm
Vascular occlusion or stenosis
Vascular AV malformations
Tumor

Abscess
Hematoma
Cerebral vascular thrombosis

Kidney arteriography

Anatomic aberrant blood vessels
Renal cyst
Renal solid tumor

Arthrosclerotic narrowing of the renal artery
Renal vascular causes of hypertension

notes

arthrocentesis with synovial fluid analysis (Synovial fluid analysis, Joint aspiration)

Type of test Fluid analysis

Normal findings

Synovial fluid: clear and straw colored with few white blood cells (WBCs), no crystals, and a good mucin clot

Chemical test values (e.g., glucose determination): approximating those found in the bloodstream

Test explanation and related physiology

Arthrocentesis is performed by inserting a sterile needle into a joint space, usually the knee, to obtain a specimen of synovial fluid, a liquid found in small amounts in the joints. Aspiration (withdrawal of the fluid) may be performed on any major joint, such as the knee, shoulder, hip, elbow, wrist, or ankle.

Arthrocentesis is performed for many different reasons, such as to establish the diagnosis of infection, crystal-induced arthritis, synovitis, or neoplasms involving the joint. This procedure is also used to identify the cause of joint effusion, to follow the progression of joint disease, and to inject antiinflammatory medications (usually corticosteroids) into a joint area.

A culture of the sample of synovial fluid is taken; the sample is also examined microscopically and chemically. Normal joint fluid is clear, straw colored, and quite viscous because of hyaluronic acid. Viscosity is reduced in patients with inflammatory arthritis and can be grossly evaluated by forcing synovial fluid from a syringe. Fluid of high viscosity forms a "string" several inches long; fluid of low viscosity drips similar to water.

The *mucin clot test* correlates with the viscosity. This test is performed by adding acetic acid to joint fluid. The formation of a tight, ropy clot indicates qualitatively good mucin and the presence of adequate molecules of intact hyaluronic acid. The mucin clot is poor in quality and quantity in inflammatory joint diseases, such as rheumatoid arthritis. Synovial fluid should not form a fibrin clot, because normal joint fluid does not contain fibrinogen. The fluid will clot only if blood entered the joint during the aspiration or trauma, or if an inflammatory effusion is present.

The synovial fluid glucose value is usually within 10 ml/dl of the serum glucose value. For proper interpretation, the synovial fluid glucose and serum glucose samples should be drawn simultaneously after the patient has fasted for 6 hours. The synovial fluid glucose level falls with increasing inflammation. In septic arthritis, the synovial fluid glucose value may be less than 50% of the serum glucose value. A low synovial glucose level also may be seen in patients with rheumatoid arthritis. Occasionally, the synovial fluid is tested for protein, uric acid, and lactate levels.

Cell counts should be performed on the synovial fluid as well. Normally, the joint fluid contains less than 200 WBCs/mm^3 and 2000 red blood cells (RBCs)/μl. A very high percentage of neutrophils (over 75%) is found in most patients with acute bacterial infectious arthritis. Leukocytes can also occur in other conditions, such as acute gouty arthritis and rheumatoid arthritis. Usually, the differential white cell count will indicate monocytosis or lymphocytosis with these later-mentioned diseases.

Acid-fast stains for tubercle bacilli are also performed on the synovial fluid. Bacterial and fungal cultures are obtained when these diseases are suspected. Gonococci are a cause of joint infection; however, previous antibiotic therapy reduces the possibility of diagnosis by culture. Synovial fluid is also examined under polarized light for the presence of crystals, which permits differential diagnosis between gout and pseudogout.

The synovial fluid also can be analyzed for complement levels. The complement level may be decreased in patients with systemic lupus erythematosus or rheumatoid arthritis. Decreased joint complement levels may be caused by consumption of the complement by the antigen-antibody complexes within the joint cavity.

One of the most important tests routinely performed on synovial fluid is the microscopic examination for crystals. For example, urate crystals indicate gouty arthritis. Calcium pyrophosphate crystals are found in pseudogout. Cholesterol crystals occur in rheumatoid arthritis.

Contraindications

- Patients with skin or wound infections in the area of the needle puncture because of the risk of sepsis

Potential complications

- Joint infection
- Hemorrhage in the joint area

Procedure and patient care

Before
- Explain the procedure to the patient.
- Obtain an informed consent if this is the institution's policy.
- Keep the patient NPO after midnight on the day of the test. This is done to prevent alterations of the chemical determinations (e.g., glucose) that may be performed with the study. However, this study may be done more conveniently in a physician's office without the patient fasting.

During
- Have the patient lie on his or her back with the joint fully extended.
- Note the following procedural steps:
  1. The skin is locally anesthetized to minimize pain.
  2. The area is aseptically cleansed, and a needle is inserted through the skin and into the joint space.
  3. Fluid is obtained for analysis. The joint area sometimes may be wrapped with an elastic bandage to compress free fluid within a certain area, thereby ensuring maximal collection of fluid.
  4. If a corticosteroid is to be administered, a syringe containing the steroid preparation is attached to the needle and the drug is injected.
  5. The needle is removed, and a pressure dressing may be applied to the site.
  6. Sometimes a peripheral venous blood sample is taken to compare chemical tests on the blood with chemical studies on the synovial fluid.
- Note that a physician performs this procedure in an office or at the patient's bedside in approximately 10 minutes.
- Tell the patient that the only discomfort associated with this test is the injection of the local anesthetic.
- Be aware that joint-space pain may worsen after fluid aspiration, especially in patients with acute arthritis.

After
- Assess the joint for any pain, fever, or swelling, which may indicate infection.
- Apply ice to decrease pain and swelling.
- Keep a pressure dressing on the joint to avoid recollection of joint fluid or development of a hematoma.

- Tell the patient to avoid strenuous use of the joint for the next several days.

Abnormal findings

Infection   Septic arthritis
Arthritis   Systemic lupus erythematosus
Synovitis   Rheumatoid arthritis
Neoplasm   Gout
Joint effusion   Pseudogout

notes

A

arthrography (Arthrogram)

Type of test X-ray with contrast dye

Normal findings Normal bursae, menisci, ligaments, and articular cartilage of the joint

Test explanation and related physiology

Arthrography affords radiographic visualization of a joint after the injection of a radiopaque substance, air, or both into the joint cavity to outline the soft tissue structures not normally seen on routine x-ray films. Bones, meniscus, cartilage, and ligaments are clearly visualized with this procedure. Joint derangement and synovial cysts are also diagnosed with arthrography.

Arthrography is usually performed on the knee and shoulder joints; however, it can also be done on other joints, such as the ankles, hips, wrists, or temporomandibular joint. This procedure is usually performed on patients with persistent, unexplained joint pain, swelling, or dysfunction.

Contraindications

- Patients who are pregnant
- Patients with active arthritis
- Patients with joint infection

Potential complications

- Infection at the puncture site
- Allergic reaction to the iodinated dye
  This rarely occurs, because the dye is not administered intravenously.

Procedure and patient care

Before
- Explain the procedure to the patient.
- Obtain an informed consent if required by the institution.
- Tell the patient that no fasting or sedation is required.

During
- Place the patient in the supine position on the examining table.
- Note the following procedural steps:
  1. The skin overlying the joint is aseptically cleansed and anesthetized.

2. A needle is inserted into the joint space.
3. Fluid is aspirated to minimize dilution of the contrast material, which could diminish the quality of the x-ray films.
4. With the needle still in place, the aspirating syringe is removed and a syringe containing dye is inserted.
5. The contrast agent is injected.
6. The needle is removed, and the joint is manipulated to help distribute the contrast material. The patient may be asked to walk several steps or to pass the joint through range-of-motion exercises.
7. X-ray films are taken with the joint held in various positions.

- Note that the physician performs this procedure in approximately 30 minutes.
- Tell the patient that pressure or a tingling sensation may be felt as the contrast medium is injected and that some discomfort in the joint may occur.

After

- Assess the joint for swelling after the test. Apply ice if necessary.
- Administer a mild analgesic (e.g., aspirin, acetaminophen) if the patient has mild discomfort.
- Report any increase in pain or swelling to the physician.
- Inform the patient that crepitant noises (crackling tissue-paper sounds) in the joint may be heard after the test. These symptoms are normal and usually disappear in 1 to 2 days. The sounds are caused by the air injected into the joint during the procedure.

Abnormal findings

Joint derangement
Cysts
Arthritis
Fractured knee meniscus
Muscle tendon tears

Cartilaginous diseases (e.g., chondromalacia)
Ligamentous injury
Synovial tumor
Synovitis

notes

arthroscopy

Type of test Endoscopy

Normal findings Normal ligaments, menisci, and articular surfaces of the joint

Test explanation and related physiology

Arthroscopy is an endoscopic procedure that allows examination of a joint interior with a specially designed endoscope. Endoscopy is a highly accurate test, because it allows direct visualization of the anatomic site (Figure 3). Although this technique can visualize many joints of the body, it is most often used to evaluate the knee for meniscus cartilage or ligament tears. It is also used in the differential diagnosis of acute and chronic disorders of the knee.

Physicians can now perform corrective surgery on the knee through the endoscope. Arthroscopy provides a safe, convenient

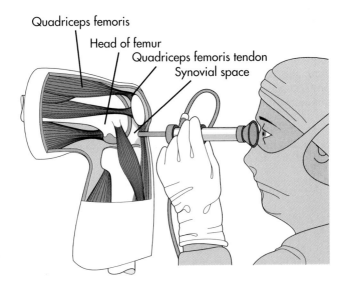

Figure 3 Arthroscopy.

alternative to open surgery (arthrotomy), because surgical instruments can be passed directly through the arthroscope.

Arthroscopy is also used to monitor the progression of disease and the effectiveness of therapy. Visual findings may be recorded by attaching a video camera to the arthroscope.

Contraindications

- Patients with ankylosis, because it is almost impossible to maneuver the instrument into a joint stiffened by adhesions
- Patients with local skin or wound infections because of the risk of sepsis

Potential complications

- Infection
- Hemarthrosis
- Swelling
- Thrombophlebitis
- Joint injury
- Synovial rupture

Procedure and patient care

Before

- Explain the procedure to the patient.
- Ensure that the physician has obtained written consent for this procedure.
- Follow the routine, preoperative procedure of the institution.
- Keep the patient NPO after midnight on the day of the test.
- Instruct the patient who will use crutches after the procedure regarding the appropriate crutch gait. The patient should use crutches after arthroscopy until he or she can walk without limping.
- Shave the hair in the area 6 inches above and below the joint before the test (as ordered).

During

- Place the patient on his or her back on an operating room table.
- Note the following procedural steps:
    1. Local or general anesthesia is used.
    2. The leg is carefully scrubbed, elevated, and wrapped with an elastic bandage from the toes to the lower thigh to drain as much blood from the leg as possible.
    3. A tourniquet is placed on the patient's leg. If the tour-

niquet is not used, a fluid solution may be instilled into the patient's knee immediately before insertion of the arthroscope to distend the knee and to help reduce bleeding.

4. The foot of the table is lowered so that the patient's knee is at a 45-degree angle.
5. A small incision is made in the skin around the knee.
6. The arthroscope (a lighted instrument) is inserted into the joint space to visualize the inside of the knee joint.
7. Although the entire joint can be viewed from one puncture site, additional punctures for better visualization are often necessary.
8. After the area is examined, biopsy or appropriate surgery can be performed.
9. Before removing the arthroscope, the joint is irrigated. Pressure is then applied to the knee to remove the irrigating solution.
10. After a few stitches are placed into the skin, a pressure dressing is applied over the incision site.

- Note that this procedure is performed in the operating room by an orthopedic surgeon in approximately 15 to 30 minutes.
- Tell the patient receiving local anesthesia that he or she may have transient discomfort from the injection of the local anesthetic and the pressure of the tourniquet on the leg.
- Inform the patient that a thumping sensation may be felt as the arthroscope is inserted into the joint and that the joint may be painful for several days.

After
- Assess the patient's neurologic and circulatory status.
- Assess vital signs and observe the patient for signs of infection, including fever, swelling, increased pain, and redness or drainage at the incision site.
- Instruct the patient to elevate the knee when sitting and to avoid overbending the knee so that swelling is minimized.
- Inform the patient that he or she can usually walk with the assistance of crutches; however, this depends on the extent of the procedure and the physician's protocol.
- Tell the patient to minimize use of the joint for several days.
- Examine the incision site for bleeding.
- Apply ice to reduce pain and swelling.
- Inform the patient that the sutures will be removed in approximately 7 to 10 days.

Abnormal findings

Torn cartilage

Torn ligament

Patellar disease

Patellar fracture

Chondromalacia

Osteochondritis dissecans

Cyst (e.g., Baker's)

Synovitis

Osteoarthritis

Rheumatoid arthritis

Degenerative arthritis

Meniscal disease

Osteochondromatosis

Trapped synovium

notes

aspartate aminotransferase (AST; formerly called Serum glutamic-oxaloacetic transaminase [SGOT])

Type of test Blood

Normal findings
Adult: 8-20 U/L, 5-40 IU/L, or 8-20 U/L (SI units);
   females tend to have slightly lower values than males
Elderly: values slightly higher than adult
Child: values similar to adult
Newborn/infant: 15-60 U/L

Test explanation and related physiology

The AST/SGOT enzyme is one of the enzymes tested in the cardiac enzyme series. This enzyme is found in very high concentrations within the heart muscle, liver cells, skeletal muscle cells, and to a lesser degree in the kidneys and pancreas. Although not specific for myocardial injury, when observed with the enzymes creatine phosphokinase (CPK, see p. 293) and lactic dehydrogenase (LDH, see p. 501), it is useful in diagnosis, quantitative analysis, and determination of timing of a recent myocardial infarction (MI). The AST level rises within 6 to 10 hours after MI, peaks at 12 to 48 hours, and returns to normal in 3 to 4 days assuming further cardiac injury does not occur. Myocardial injuries such as angina, pericarditis, or rheumatic carditis do not increase the AST level.

As with CPK, serial determinations of AST are helpful in determining the timing, initiation, and resolution of MI. Unlike the isoenzyme CPK-MB, however, it is much less specific for infarction of myocardial muscle cells.

Because AST also exists within the liver cells, diseases that affect the hepatocyte will cause elevated levels of this enzyme. Serum AST levels are often compared with alanine aminotransferase (ALT, see p. 28) levels. The AST/ALT ratio is usually greater than 1.0 in patients with alcoholic cirrhosis, liver congestion, and metastatic tumor of the liver. Ratios less than 1.0 may be seen in patients with acute hepatitis, viral hepatitis, or infectious mononucleosis.

Patients with acute pancreatitis, acute renal diseases, musculoskeletal diseases, or trauma may have a transient rise in serum AST. Patients with red blood cell abnormalities such as acute hemolytic anemia and severe burns also can have elevations of this enzyme. AST levels may be decreased in patients with beriberi or diabetic ketoacidosis and in patients who are pregnant.

Interfering factors

- Pregnancy may cause decreased AST levels.
- Exercise may cause increased levels.
- ✓ Drugs that may cause *increased* levels include antihypertensives, cholinergic agents, coumarin-type anticoagulants, digitalis preparations, erythromycin, isoniazid, methyldopa, oral contraceptives, opiates, salicylates, hepatotoxic medications, and verapamil.

Procedure and patient care

Before

- Explain the procedure to the patient.
- Discuss with the patient the need and reason for frequent venipunctures in diagnosing MI.
- Avoid giving the patient any IM injection.
- If possible, hold drugs that could interfere with test results for 12 hours before the test.

During

- Collect a venous sample of blood in a red-top tube. This is usually done daily for 3 days and then again in 1 week. Rotate the venipuncture site.
- Avoid hemolysis.
- Indicate on the laboratory slip any drugs that may cause false-positive results.
- Record the time and date of any IM injection given.
- Record the exact time and date when the blood test is performed. This aids in the interpretation of the temporal pattern of enzyme elevations.

After

- Apply pressure or a pressure dressing to the venipuncture site.
- Observe the venipuncture site for bleeding.

Abnormal findings

▲ **Increased levels**
Myocardial infarction
Cardiac operations
Cardiac catheterization
  and angioplasty
Hepatitis
Hepatic cirrhosis
Drug-induced liver injury
Hepatic metastasis
Acute pancreatitis
Skeletal muscle trauma
Recent noncardiac sur-
  gery
Multiple trauma
Hepatic necrosis
Severe, deep burn
Acute hemolytic anemia
Progressive muscular dys-
  trophy
Infectious mononucleosis
  with hepatitis
Recent convulsions
Hepatic infiltrative pro-
  cess (e.g., tumor)
Primary muscle diseases
  (e.g., myopathy, myosi-
  tis)
Acute renal disease
Heat stroke

▼ **Decreased levels**
Beriberi
Diabetic ketoacidosis
Pregnancy

notes

barium enema (BE, Lower GI series)

Type of test X-ray with contrast dye

Normal findings

Normal filling, contour, patency, and positioning of barium in the colon

Normal filling of the appendix and terminal ileum

Test explanation and related physiology

The BE study consists of a series of x-ray films visualizing the colon. It is used to demonstrate the presence and location of polyps, tumors, and diverticula. Anatomic abnormalities (e.g., malrotation) also can be detected. Therapeutically, the BE may be used to reduce nonstrangulated ileocolic intussusception in children. Bleeding from diverticula can cease with barium enema.

The BE is occasionally used to assess filling of the appendix. When the clinical picture suggests possible appendicitis, failure of the appendix to fill with barium may support the diagnosis. Although the colon is the main organ evaluated by a BE, reflux of barium into the terminal ileum also will allow adequate visualization of the distal portion of the small intestine. Diseases that affect the terminal ileum, especially Crohn's disease (regional enteritis), can be identified. Inflammatory bowel disease involving the colon can be detected with BE. Fistulas involving the colon can be demonstrated by BE.

In many instances, air is insufflated into the colon after the instillation of barium. This provides an air contrast to the barium. With air contrast, the colonic mucosa can be much more accurately visualized. This is called an *air-contrast barium enema*. It is used especially when small polyps are suspected. The accuracy of the regular BE in detecting small colonic tumors is approximately 60%; however, the accuracy of an air-contrast BE in detecting small colonic tumors exceeds 85%.

Contraindications

- Patients suspected of a perforation of the colon
  In these patients, diatrizoate (Gastrografin), a water-soluble contrast medium, is used.
- Patients who are unable to cooperate
  This test requires the patient to hold the barium in the rectum and colon. This is especially difficult for elderly patients.

B

Potential complications

- Colonic perforation, especially when the colon is weakened by inflammation, tumor, or infection
- Barium fecal impaction

Interfering factors

- Barium within the abdomen from previous barium tests
- Significant residual stool within the colon
  This precludes adequate visualization of the entire bowel wall. Stool may be confused for polyps.
- Spasm of the colon
  Spasm can mimic the radiographic signs of a cancer. The use of IV glucagon minimizes spasm.

Procedure and patient care

Before

- Explain the procedure to the patient. Encourage the patient to verbalize questions and fears.
- Assist the patient with the bowel preparation, which varies among institutions. In elderly patients, this preparation can be exhaustive and even cause severe dehydration. A typical preparation for most adults would include the following actions.

Day before examination

- Give the patient clear liquids for lunch and supper (no dairy products).
- Have the patient drink one glass of water or clear fluid every hour for 8 to 10 hours.
- Administer one full bottle (10 ounces) of magnesium citrate or X-Prep (extract of senna fruit) at 2 PM.
- Administer three 5-mg bisacodyl (Dulcolax) tablets at 7 PM.
- Keep the patient NPO after midnight the day of the test.

Day of examination

- Keep the patient NPO.
- Administer a bisacodyl suppository at 6 AM and/or a cleansing enema.
- Note that pediatric patients will have individualized bowel preparations.
- Note that special preparations will be ordered for patients with an ileostomy or colostomy.
- Determine whether the bowel is adequately cleansed.
  When the fecal return is similar to clear water, preparation is adequate; if large, solid fecal waste is still being evacuated,

preparation is inadequate. Notify the radiologist, who may want to extend the bowel preparation.

- Suggest that the patient take reading material to the x-ray department to occupy the time while expelling the barium.

During

- Note the following procedural steps:
    1. The test begins with placement of a balloon rectal catheter.
    2. The balloon on the catheter is inflated tightly against the anal sphincter to hold the barium within the colon.
    3. The patient is asked to roll in the lateral, supine, and prone positions.
    4. The barium is dripped into the rectum by gravity.
    5. The barium flow is monitored fluoroscopically.
    6. The colon is thoroughly examined as the barium flow progresses through the large colon and into the terminal ileum.
    7. The barium is drained out.
    8. If an air-contrast BE has been ordered, air is insufflated into the large bowel.
    9. The patient is asked to expel the barium, and a postevacuation x-ray film is taken.
    10. The standard procedure for administering the barium through a colostomy is to instill the contrast medium through an irrigation cone placed in the stoma. When the x-ray series is completed, the barium is allowed to be expelled from the stoma. A gentle stream of clean water for irrigation is helpful in expelling residual barium.
- Note that this test is usually performed in the radiology department by a radiologist in approximately 45 minutes.
- Inform the patient that abdominal bloating and rectal pressure will occur during instillation of barium.

After

- Ensure that the patient defecates as much barium as possible.
- Inform the patient that bowel movements will be white. When all the barium has been expelled, the stool will return to normal color.
- Suggest the use of soothing ointments on the anal area to minimize any anorectal pain that may result from the aggressive test preparation.

- Encourage ingestion of fluids to avoid dehydration caused by the cathartics.
- Encourage rest after the procedure. The cleansing regimen and BE procedure may be exhausting.
- Note that laxatives may be ordered to facilitate evacuation of barium.

Abnormal findings

Malignant tumor

Polyps

Diverticula

Inflammatory bowel diseases (e.g., ulcerative colitis, Crohn's disease)

Colonic stenosis secondary to ischemia, infection, or previous surgery

Perforated colon

Colonic fistula

Appendicitis

Extrinsic compression of the colon from extracolonic tumors (e.g., ovarian)

Extrinsic compression of the colon from an abscess

notes

barium swallow

Type of test X-ray with contrast dye

Normal findings Normal size, contour, filling, patency, and positioning of the esophagus

Test explanation and related physiology

This barium contrast study is a more thorough examination of the esophagus than that provided by most upper GI series (see p. 834). As in most barium contrast studies, defects in normal filling and narrowing of the barium column indicate tumor, strictures, or extrinsic compression from extra-esophageal tumors or an abnormally enlarged heart and great vessels. Varices also can be seen as serpiginous, linear-filling defects. Anatomic abnormalities such as hiatal hernia, Shatzski's rings, and diverticula (Zenker's or epiphrenic) can be seen as well.

In patients with esophageal reflux, the radiologist may identify reflux of the barium from the stomach back into the esophagus. Muscular abnormalities such as achalasia, as well as diffuse esophageal spasm, can be easily detected by a barium swallow. If perforations or rupture of the esophagus is suspected, it is best not to use barium. A water-soluble x-ray contrast should be used.

Contraindications

- Patients with evidence of bowel obstruction
  Barium may create a stonelike impaction.
- Patients with a perforated viscus
  If barium were to leak, the degree and duration of infection would be much worse. Usually, when perforation is suspected, diatrizoate (Gastrografin), a water-soluble contrast medium, is used.
- Patients whose vital signs are unstable
- Patients who are unable to cooperate for the test

Potential complication

- Barium-induced fecal impaction

Interfering factor

- Food within the esophagus, which prevents adequate visualization

Procedure and patient care

Before

- Explain the procedure to the patient.
- Instruct the patient not to take anything by mouth for at least 8 hours before the testing. Usually, the patient is kept NPO after midnight on the day of the test.
- Assess the patient's ability to swallow. If the patient tends to aspirate, inform the radiologist.
- Accompany the hospitalized patient to the x-ray department if vital signs are not stable and the test still needs to be performed.

During

- Note the following procedural steps:
  1. The fasting patient is asked to swallow the contrast medium. Usually, this is barium sulfate in a milkshake-like substance; however, if a perforated viscus is possible, Gastrografin is used.
  2. As the patient drinks the contrast through a straw, the x-ray table is tilted to the near-erect position.
  3. The patient is asked to roll into various positions so that the entire esophagus can be adequately visualized.
  4. With fluoroscopy, the radiologist follows the barium column through the entire esophagus.
- Note that this procedure is usually performed in the radiology department by a radiologist in approximately 15 to 20 minutes.
- Tell the patient that no discomfort is associated with this test.

After

- Inform the patient of the need to evacuate all the barium. Cathartics are recommended. Initially, stools will be white but should return to normal color with complete evacuation.

Abnormal findings

Total or partial esophageal
  obstruction
Cancer
Scarred strictures
Lower esophageal rings
Peptic esophageal ulcers
Varices
Peptic or corrosive esophagitis
Achalasia

Esophageal motility disorders
  (e.g., presbyesophagus, diffuse esophageal spasm)
Diverticula
Chalasia
Extrinsic compression from
  extraesophageal tumors, car-
  diomegaly, or aortic aneurysm

notes

Barr body analysis (Sex chromatin body, Chromatin-positive body)

Type of test Microscopic examination

Normal findings Depend on the gender of the child

Test explanation and related physiology

Barr body (or Barr chromatin body) analysis studies may be performed when ambiguity of the newborn's genitalia makes assigning a gender to the infant difficult. This test is also done to detect sex chromosomal abnormalities such as Turner's syndrome and Klinefelter's syndrome.

The Barr body is a chromatin mass derived from one of the X chromosomes. That is the inactive sex chromosome. The Barr body is seen as a nucleolar satellite on histologic preparations. The number of Barr bodies is one less than the total number of X chromosomes in the cell nucleus. Therefore females (XX) normally have one Barr body and are considered to be chromatin positive; normal males (XY) have no Barr bodies and are chromatin negative. A female with Turner's syndrome (XO) would have no Barr body. These females are characterized by ovarian dysgenesis, amenorrhea, and the lack of secondary sexual maturation. A male with Klinefelter's syndrome (XXY) would have one Barr body. Klinefelter's syndrome is the most common form of male hypogonadism, which is caused by a chromosomal abnormality resulting in primary testicular failure. An XXX female would have two Barr bodies.

Scoring Barr bodies in the buccal mucosal cells is less costly than karyotype analysis, but the technical limitations of the test are considerable. For example, Y chromosome abnormalities cannot be identified. Because of the obvious benefit of a full cytogenic study, sex chromatin studies have fallen out of favor.

Interfering factors

- Buccal smear specimens may show false lowering of sex chromatin bodies if specimens are taken during the first week of life or during adrenocorticosteroid or estrogen therapy.
- Poor slide preparation can obscure the test results.

Procedure and patient care

Before
- Explain the procedure to the patient or parents.

During
- Note the following procedural steps:
  1. Sex chromatin analysis can be performed using any cell in the body. The most easily obtained cells are from the buccal mucosa. The oral mucosa is scraped, and the cells are smeared onto a glass slide.
  2. After chemical fixation and staining, the cells are studied.
  3. Assessment of the results, together with the secondary sexual characteristics and the genitalia of the patient, permit presumptive diagnosis of certain sex chromosomal abnormalities.
  4. If necessary, the results can be confirmed by chromosomal *karyotyping* (systematic arrangement of photographed chromosomes to demonstrate structure and number) (see p. 240).
- Note that a buccal smear is performed by a technician in less than 5 minutes. A pathologist studies the slide smear.
- Tell the patient that no or minimal discomfort is associated with this test.

After
- Inform the patient how and when to obtain the test results.

Abnormal findings

Chromosomal abnormalities (e.g., Turner's syndrome, Klinefelter's syndrome)

notes

Bence Jones protein

Type of test Urine

Normal findings No Bence Jones protein present

Test explanation and related physiology

Bence Jones proteins are lightweight immunoglobulins found in one half of the patients with multiple myeloma. These proteins are most notably made by the plasma cells in these patients. They also may be associated with tumor metastases to the bone, chronic lymphocytic leukemias, lymphoma, macroglobulinemia, and amyloidosis. These immunoglobulins are rapidly cleared by the kidney and are excreted into the urine. Because the Bence Jones protein is rapidly cleared from the blood by the kidney, it is very difficult to detect in the blood; therefore only urine is used for this study. Normally, urine should contain no Bence Jones proteins.

Routine urine testing for proteins using reagent strips often does not reflect the type or amount of proteins in the urine. In fact, the strip may even show a completely negative result despite large amounts of Bence Jones globulins. Urine electrophoresis and immunophoresis are the procedures of choice, especially when the amount of proteins needs to be quantitated. There are other temperature-dependent studies that are available for testing.

Interfering factor

- Dilute urine may yield a false-negative result.

Procedure and patient care

Before
- Explain the procedure to the patient.
- Instruct the patient not to contaminate the urine specimen with toilet paper or stool.

During
- Instruct the patient to collect an early morning specimen of at least 50 ml of uncontaminated urine in a container. It may be helpful to know the amount of these proteins excreted over 24 hours. If so, a 24-hour collection is ordered.

After

- Immediately transport the specimen to the laboratory.
  If it cannot be taken to the laboratory immediately, refrigerate the specimen, because heat-coagulable proteins can decompose, causing a false-positive test.

Abnormal findings

▲   **Increased levels**

Multiple myeloma (plasmacytoma)
Various metastatic tumors
Chronic lymphocytic leukemia

Amyloidosis
Lymphoma
Macroglobulinemia

notes

B

Type of test   Blood

Normal findings

Adult/elderly/child

Total bilirubin: 0.1-1.0 mg/dl or 5.1-17.0 μmol/L (SI units)

Indirect bilirubin: 0.2-0.8 mg/dl or 3.4-12.0 μmol/L (SI units)

Direct bilirubin: 0.1-0.3 mg/dl or 1.7-5.1 μmol/L (SI units)

Newborn total bilirubin: 1-12 mg/dl or 17.1-20.5 μmol/L (SI units)

Test explanation and related physiology

Bile, which is formed in the liver, has many constituents, including bile salts, phospholipids, cholesterol, bicarbonate, water, and bilirubin. Bilirubin metabolism begins with the breakdown of red blood cells (RBCs) in the reticuloendothelial system (Figure 4). Hemoglobin is released from RBCs and broken down to heme and globin molecules. Heme is then catabolized to form biliverdin, which is transformed to bilirubin. This form of bilirubin is called *unconjugated* (indirect) bilirubin. In the liver, indirect bilirubin is conjugated with a glucuronide, resulting in *conjugated* (direct) bilirubin. The conjugated bilirubin is then excreted from the liver cells and into the intrahepatic canaliculi, which eventually lead to the hepatic ducts, the common bile duct, and the bowel.

Jaundice is the discoloration of body tissues caused by abnormally high blood levels of bilirubin. This yellow discoloration is recognized when the total serum bilirubin exceeds 2.5 mg/dl. Jaundice results from a defect in the normal metabolism or excretion of bilirubin. This defect can occur in any stage of heme catabolism.

Physiologic jaundice of the newborn occurs if the newborn's liver is immature and does not have enough conjugating enzymes. This results in a high circulating blood level of unconjugated bilirubin, which can pass through the blood-brain barrier and deposit in the brain cells of the newborn. This can cause encephalopathy *(kernicterus)*.

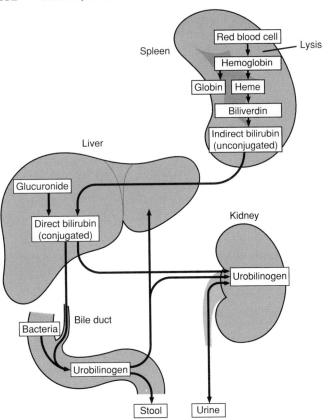

Figure 4 Bilirubin metabolism and excretion.

If the defect in bilirubin metabolism occurs after glucuronide addition, *conjugated (direct) hyperbilirubinemia* will result. Obstruction of the bile duct by a gallstone is the classic example of obstructed bilirubin excretion causing a direct hyperbilirubinemia.

Once the jaundice is recognized either clinically or chemically, it is important (for therapy) to differentiate whether it is predominantly caused by unconjugated or conjugated bilirubin. This in turn will help differentiate the etiology of the defect. In general, jaundice caused by hepatocellular dysfunction (e.g., hepatitis) results in elevated levels of unconjugated bilirubin.

Jaundice resulting from extrahepatic obstruction of the bile ducts (e.g., gallstones or tumor blocking the bile ducts) results in elevated conjugated bilirubin levels; this type of jaundice usually can be resolved surgically or endoscopically.

The total serum bilirubin level is the sum of the conjugated (direct) and unconjugated (indirect) bilirubin. Normally, the unconjugated bilirubin makes up 70% to 85% of the total bilirubin. In patients with jaundice, when more than 50% of the bilirubin is conjugated, it is considered a conjugated hyperbilirubinemia from gallstones, tumor, inflammation, scarring, or obstruction of the extrahepatic ducts. Unconjugated hyperbilirubinemia exists when less than 15% to 20% of the total bilirubin is conjugated. Diseases that typically cause this form of jaundice include accelerated erythrocyte (RBC) hemolysis, hepatitis, or drugs.

Delta bilirubin is a form of bilirubin that is covalently bound to albumin. It has a longer half-life than the other bilirubins; therefore it remains elevated during the convalescent phases of hepatic disorders when the conjugated bilirubin would have already returned to normal. It can be derived by the following calculation: total bilirubin minus conjugated bilirubin plus unconjugated bilirubin.

Interfering factors

- Blood hemolysis and lipemia can produce erroneous results.
- Drugs that may cause *increased* levels of total bilirubin include allopurinol, anabolic steroids, antibiotics, antimalarials, ascorbic acid, azathioprine, chlorpropamide (Diabinese), cholinergics, codeine, dextran, diuretics, epinephrine, meperidine, methotrexate, methyldopa, monoamine oxidase inhibitors, morphine, nicotinic acid (large doses), oral contraceptives, phenothiazines, quinidine, rifampin, salicylates, steroids, sulfonamides, theophylline, and vitamin A.
- Drugs that may cause *decreased* levels of total bilirubin include barbiturates, caffeine, penicillin, and salicylates (high dose).

Procedure and patient care

Before

- Explain the procedure to the patient.
- Note that fasting requirements vary among different laboratories. Some require keeping the patient NPO after midnight the day of the test except for water.

During

- Collect 5 to 7 ml of venous blood in a red-top tube.
- Use a heel puncture for blood collection in infants.
- Prevent hemolysis of blood during phlebotomy.
- Do *not* shake the tube because inaccurate test results may occur.
- Protect the blood sample from bright light. Prolonged exposure (over 1 hour) to sunlight or artificial light can reduce bilirubin content.
- List on the laboratory slip any drugs that may affect test results.

After

- Apply pressure or a pressure dressing to the venipuncture site.
- Assess the venipuncture site for bleeding. Patients who are jaundiced can have prolonged clotting times.

Abnormal findings

▲ **Increased levels of conjugated (direct) bilirubin**

Gallstones
Extrahepatic duct obstruction (tumor, inflammation, gallstone, scarring, or surgical trauma)
Extensive liver metastasis
Cholestasis from drugs
Dubin-Johnson syndrome
Rotor's syndrome

▲ **Increased levels of unconjugated (indirect) bilirubin**

Erythroblastosis fetalis
Hemolytic jaundice
Large-volume blood transfusion
Resolution of a large hematoma
Hepatitis
Sepsis
Neonatal hyperbilirubinemia
Hemolytic anemia
Crigler-Najjar syndrome
Gilbert syndrome
Pernicious anemia
Cirrhosis
Transfusion reaction
Sickle cell anemia

bilirubin, urine

Type of test Urine

Normal findings No bilirubin in urine

Test explanation and related physiology

Bile, which is formed in the liver, has many constituents, including bile salts, phospholipids, cholesterol, bicarbonate, water, and bilirubin. Bilirubin metabolism begins with the breakdown of red blood cells (RBCs) in the reticuloendothelial system (see Figure 4, p. 132). Hemoglobin is released from RBCs and broken down to heme and globin molecules. Heme is then catabolized to form biliverdin, which is transformed to bilirubin. This form of bilirubin is called *unconjugated* (indirect) bilirubin. In the liver, indirect bilirubin is conjugated with a glucuronide, resulting in *conjugated* (direct) bilirubin. The conjugated bilirubin is then excreted from the liver cells and into the intrahepatic canaliculi, which eventually lead to the hepatic ducts, the common bile duct, and the bowel.

Jaundice is the discoloration of body tissues caused by abnormally high blood levels of bilirubin. This yellow discoloration is recognized when the total serum bilirubin exceeds 2.5 mg/dl. Jaundice results from a defect in the normal metabolism or excretion of bilirubin. This defect can occur in any stage of heme catabolism.

Physiologic jaundice of the newborn occurs if the newborn's liver is immature and does not have enough conjugating enzymes. This results in a high circulating blood level of unconjugated bilirubin, which can pass through the blood-brain barrier and deposit in the brain cells of the newborn. This can cause encephalopathy *(kernicterus)*.

If the defect in bilirubin metabolism occurs after glucuronide addition, *conjugated (direct) hyperbilirubinemia* will result. Obstruction of the bile duct by a gallstone is the classic example of obstructed bilirubin excretion causing a direct hyperbilirubinemia.

Once the jaundice is recognized either clinically or chemically, it is important (for therapy) to differentiate whether it is predominantly caused by unconjugated or conjugated bilirubin. This in turn will help differentiate the etiology of the defect. In general, jaundice caused by hepatocellular dysfunction (e.g., hepatitis) results in elevated levels of unconjugated bilirubin. This usually cannot be repaired surgically. On the other hand, jaundice resulting from extrahepatic dysfunction (e.g., gallstones or tumor blocking the bile ducts) results in elevated levels of conjugated bilirubin; this type of jaundice usually can be resolved surgically or endoscopically.

When the defect in bilirubin metabolism occurs after conjugation, elevated levels of conjugated bilirubin occur. Unlike the unconjugated form, conjugated bilirubin is water soluble and can be excreted into the urine. Therefore bilirubin in urine suggests disease affecting bilirubin metabolism after conjugation or defects in excretion (e.g., gallstones).

Interfering factors

- Bilirubin is not stable in urine, especially when exposed to light.
- Drugs that may cause *increased* bilirubin levels include allopurinol, antibiotics, barbiturates, chlorpromazine, diuretics, ethoxazene (Serenium), oral contraceptives, phenazopyridine (Pyridium), steroids, and sulfonamides.
- Drugs that can cause *false-negative results* include indomethacin (Indocin) and ascorbic acid (vitamin C).

Procedure and patient care

Before
- Explain the procedure to the patient.
- Tell the patient that no food or drink restrictions are necessary.

During
- Note that this is a spot urine test.
- Collect at least 10 ml of urine for quick, simple testing.
- Use reagent strips (e.g., Multistix) or tablets (e.g., Icotest) for quick, simple testing.

Multistix
- Note that this is a firm, plastic strip with seven separate areas for testing pH, protein, glucose, ketones, bilirubin, blood, and urobilinogen.
- For testing bilirubin, obtain a fresh urine specimen and examine it as soon as possible.
- Immerse the dipstick in the well-mixed urine, then remove immediately to avoid dissolving other reagents.

- Tap the dipstick against the rim of the urine container to remove excess urine.
- Hold the strip horizontally and compare it with the color chart on the label of the bottle after 20 to 30 seconds, according to directions. Results are given in the range of 0 to +3.

Icotest tablets
- Place 5 drops of urine on the special test mat.
- Add 2 drops of water. The bilirubin test is positive if the mat turns blue or purple within 30 seconds.
- Note that this test is considered more sensitive than reagent strips for detecting bilirubin.

After
- Do not reuse reagent strips or Icotest tablets.
- Whether using strips or tablets or if sending the urine to the laboratory, list any medications that may affect test results.

Abnormal findings

▲   **Increased levels of conjugated (direct) bilirubin**

Gallstones
Extrahepatic duct obstruction (tumor, inflammation, gallstone, scarring, or surgical trauma)

Extensive liver metastasis
Cholestasis from drugs
Dubin-Johnson syndrome
Rotor's syndrome

notes

biophysical profile (BPP, Fetal biophysical profile)

Type of test Ultrasound, fetal activity study

Normal findings Score of 8-10 points (if amniotic fluid volume is adequate)

Possible critical values Less than 4 may necessitate immediate delivery.

Test explanation and related physiology

The BPP is a method of evaluating fetal status during the antepartal period based on five variables originating within the fetus: fetal heart rate, fetal breathing movement, gross fetal movements, fetal muscle tone, and amniotic fluid volume. Fetal heart rate reactivity is measured by the nonstress test (see p. 571), and the other four parameters are measured by ultrasound scanning.

The major premise behind the BPP is that variable assessments of fetal biophysical activity are more reliable than an examination of a single parameter (such as fetal heart rate). Indications for this test include factors such as postdate pregnancy, maternal hypertension, diabetes mellitus, vaginal bleeding, maternal Rh sensitization, maternal history of stillbirth, and premature rupture of membranes. The BPP is probably more useful in identifying a fetus that is in jeopardy than in predicting future fetal well-being.

The five parameters are briefly described here. Each parameter is scored and contributes either a 2 or a 0 to the score. Therefore 10 is the perfect score, and 0 is the lowest score.

1. *Fetal heart rate reactivity.* This is measured and interpreted in the same way as the nonstress test (see p. 571). The fetal heart rate is considered reactive when there are movement-associated fetal heart rate accelerations of at least 15 beats/min above baseline and 15 seconds in duration over a 20-minute period. A score of 2 is given for reactivity, and a score of 0 indicates that the fetal heart rate is nonreactive.

2. *Fetal breathing movements.* This parameter is assessed based on the assumption that fetal breathing movements indicate fetal well-being and their absence may indicate hypoxemia. Fetal breathing becomes increasingly regular in frequency and uniformity after the thirty-sixth week of

gestation. To earn a score of 2, the fetus must have at least one episode of fetal breathing lasting at least 60 seconds within a 30-minute observation. Absence of this breathing pattern is scored a 0 on the BPP. It is important to note that several factors can alter fetal breathing movements. For example, fetal breathing movements increase during the second and third hours after maternal meals and also at night. Fetal breathing movements may decrease in conditions such as hypoxemia, hypoglycemia, nicotine use, and alcohol ingestion.

3. *Fetal body movements.* Fetal activity is a reflection of neurologic integrity and function. The presence of at least three discrete episodes of fetal movements within a 30-minute observation period is given a score of 2. A score of 0 is given with two or fewer fetal movements in this time period. It is important to note that fetal activity is greatest 1 to 3 hours after the mother has consumed a meal. For this reason, it is often suggested that this test be arranged in relation to mealtime.

4. *Fetal tone.* In the uterus, the fetus is normally in a position of flexion. However, the fetus also stretches, rolls, and moves in the uterus. The arms, legs, trunk, and head may be flexed and extended. A score of 2 is earned when there is at least one episode of active extension with return to flexion. An example of this would be the opening and closing of the hand. A score of 0 is given for slow extension with a return to only partial flexion; fetal movement not followed by return to flexion; limbs or spine in extension; and an open fetal hand.

5. *Amniotic fluid volume.* Amniotic fluid volume has been demonstrated to be an effective method of predicting fetal distress. Oligohydramnios (too little amniotic fluid) has been associated with fetal anomalies, with uterine growth retardation, and with postterm pregnancy. Immediate delivery is recommended for a postterm client with oligohydramnios because of the high risk of associated problems, such as umbilical cord compromise. A score of 2 is given for this parameter when there is at least one pocket of amniotic fluid that measures 1 cm in two perpendicular planes. A score of 0 indicates either that fluid is absent in most areas of the uterine cavity or that the largest pocket measures 1 cm or less in the vertical axis.

A score of 8 or 10 with a normal amount of amniotic fluid indicates a healthy fetus. A score of 8 with oligohydramnios or a score of 4 to 6 is equivocal. An equivocal test result is interpreted as possibly abnormal. Some clinicians would recommend repeating the test within 24 hours. However, others may advocate extending testing after any equivocal or abnormal test result. A score of 0 or 2 is abnormal and indicates the need for assessment of immediate delivery.

Although the BPP is fairly new, it has already been modified. Some physicians omit the nonstress test if the ultrasound parameters are normal. Some physicians have added placental grading as a sixth parameter.

Interfering factors

- Central nervous system stimulants such as catecholamines and hyperglycemia can increase BPP activities.
- Hypoxemia and trauma may decrease fetal biophysical activities.
- Drugs that may *decrease* BPP include analgesics, anesthetics, and sedatives.

Procedure and patient care

Before

- Explain the procedure to the patient.
- Inform the patient that no fasting is required.

During

- Fetal heart rate reactivity is measured and interpreted from a nonstress test (see p. 571).
- Fetal breathing movements, fetal body movements, fetal tone, and amniotic fluid volume are determined by ultrasound imaging (see obstetric ultrasonography, p. 608)

After

- If the test results are abnormal or equivocal, support the patient in the next phase of the fetal evaluation process.

Abnormal findings

Fetal asphyxia
Congenital anomalies
Oligohydramnios
Intrauterine growth retardation
Postterm pregnancy

bleeding time (Ivy bleeding time)

B

Type of test Blood

Normal findings 1-9 minutes (Ivy method)

Possible critical values >12 minutes

Test explanation and related physiology

The bleeding time test is used to evaluate the vascular and platelet factors associated with hemostasis. When vascular injury occurs, the first hemostatic response is a spastic contraction of the lacerated microvessels. Next, platelets adhere to the wall of the vessel at the area of laceration in an attempt to plug the hole. Failure of either process results in a prolonged bleeding time.

For this study, a small, standard superficial incision is made in the forearm, and the time required for the bleeding to stop is recorded. This is called the *bleeding time*. Normal values vary according to the method used; the method most often used today is the Ivy bleeding time test.

Prolonged values occur in the following:
1. Patients with decreased platelet counts (see p. 631) or function
2. Patients with disseminated intravascular coagulation (DIC) resulting from consumption of platelets
3. Patients with uremia, because such patients' platelets are reduced in number and function
4. Patients with warfarin (Coumadin) overdosage
5. Increased capillary fragility secondary to collagen vascular disease, Cushing's disease, or Henoch-Schönlein syndrome (purpura)
6. Ingestion of antiinflammatory drugs (e.g., aspirin, indomethacin)

Contraindications

- Patients with low platelet counts
- Patients who are unable to cooperate
- Patients who cannot have a blood pressure cuff placed on the arm (e.g., those with cellulitis)
- Patients with a history of keloid formation
- Patients with senile skin changes

- Patients who have had a mastectomy
  Avoid the arm on that side.

Potential complications

- Skin infection
- Excessive bleeding from test site

Interfering factors

▮ Drugs that may cause *increased* bleeding times include anti-coagulants, dextran, indomethacin, salicylates, streptokinase, allopurinol, some antibiotics, halothane, nonsteroidal antiin-flammatory drugs, urokinase, and warfarin.

Procedure and patient care

Before

- Explain the procedure to the patient.
- Obtain a consent form if required by the institution.
- Tell the patient that no fasting is required.
- Obtain a drug history to detect if the patient has recently had aspirin, anticoagulants, or any other medications that may affect test results.

During

- Note the following procedural steps:
  1. The skin of the inner part of the forearm is cleansed with alcohol or povidone-iodine (Betadine).
  2. A blood pressure cuff is applied on the arm above the elbow, inflated to 40 mm Hg, and maintained at this pressure during the study.
  3. A small laceration is then made 1-mm deep into the skin, and the time is recorded.
  4. Bleeding ensues, and the blood is wiped clean at 30-second intervals.
  5. When no new bleeding occurs, the time is again noted.
  6. The interval from the beginning to the end of bleeding is calculated. This is the bleeding time.
  7. The blood pressure cuff is then removed, and an adhesive dressing is applied to the patient's arm.
  8. If bleeding persists more than 10 minutes, the test is stopped and a pressure dressing is applied.
- Indicate on the laboratory slip any medications that may affect test results.
- Note that this test is usually performed by a laboratory technician in less than 10 minutes.

- Inform the patient that minor discomfort may occur with this test because of the skin laceration.

After

- Apply pressure or pressure dressing to the puncture site.
- Assess the puncture site for bleeding.

Abnormal findings

▲ **Prolonged times or increased values**

Bone marrow failure
Primary or metastatic tumor infiltration of bone marrow
Disseminated intravascular coagulation
Thrombocytopenia
Hypersplenism
von Willebrand's disease
Collagen vascular disease
Cushing's disease
Henoch-Schönlein syndrome
Severe liver disease
Clotting factor deficiency
Capillary fragility
Leukemia
Uremia
Bernard-Soulier syndrome
Connective tissue disorder
Hereditary telangiectasia
Glanzmann's thrombasthenia

notes

blood culture and sensitivity

Type of test Blood

Normal findings Negative

Test explanation and related physiology

Blood cultures are obtained to detect the presence of bacteria in the blood. Bacteremia can be intermittent and transient, except in endocarditis or suppurative thrombophlebitis. Bacteremia is usually accompanied by chills and fever; thus the blood culture should be drawn when the patient manifests these signs. It is important that at least two culture specimens be obtained from two different sites. If one produces bacteria and the other does not, it is safe to assume that the bacteria in the first culture may be a contaminant and not the infecting agent. When both cultures grow the infecting agent, bacteremia exists. If the patient is receiving antibiotics, the laboratory should be notified. The blood culture specimen should be taken shortly before the next dose of the antibiotic is administered; a resin that binds antibiotics can be added to the specimen, thereby allowing the growth and identification of any bacteria in the laboratory.

Culture specimens drawn through an IV catheter are frequently contaminated, and tests using them should not be performed unless catheter sepsis is suspected. In these situations, blood culture specimens drawn through the catheter help to identify the causative agent more accurately than a culture specimen from the catheter tip.

All cultures preferably should be performed before antibiotic therapy is initiated. Otherwise, the antibiotic may interrupt the organism's growth in the laboratory. Often, however, the physician will want to institute antibiotic therapy before the culture results are reported. In these instances, a *Gram stain* of the specimen smeared on a slide is most helpful and can be reported in less than 10 minutes. Overwhelming bacteremia must be present to identify bacteria on a blood specimen Gram stain. All forms of bacteria are grossly classified as *gram positive* (blue staining) or *gram negative* (red staining). Knowledge of the organism's shape (e.g., spheric or rod shaped) also can be very helpful in its identification. With knowledge of the Gram stain results, the physician can institute a reasonable antibiotic regimen based on past experience as to which organism might be present. Most organisms require approximately 24 hours to grow in the laboratory, and a preliminary report can be given at that time. Often, 48 to 72 hours are required for growth and identification of the organism. Anaerobic organisms may take longer to grow. Cultures may be repeated after antibiotic therapy to assess resolution of the infection.

Interfering factors

- Contamination of the blood specimen, especially by skin bacteria, may occur.
- Drugs that may alter test results include antibiotics.

Procedure and patient care

Before

- Explain the procedure to the patient.
- Tell the patient that no fasting is required.

During

- Carefully prepare the proposed venipuncture site with povidone-iodine (Betadine). Allow the skin to dry.
- Clean the tops of the vacutainer tubes or culture bottles with povidone-iodine and allow them to dry. Some laboratories suggest cleaning with 70% alcohol after cleaning with Betadine and air drying.
- Collect approximately 10 to 15 ml of venous blood by venipuncture from each site in a 20-ml syringe.
- Discard the needle on the syringe and replace with a second, sterile needle before injecting the blood sample into the culture bottle.
- Inoculate the anaerobic bottle first if both anaerobic and aerobic cultures are needed.
- Mix gently after inoculation.
- Label the specimen with the patient's name, date, time, and tentative diagnosis.
- Indicate on the laboratory slip any medications that may affect test results.

After

- Transport the culture bottles immediately to the laboratory (or at least within 30 minutes).
- Notify the physician of any positive results so that appropriate antibiotic therapy can be initiated.

Abnormal finding

Bacteremia

blood gases (Arterial blood gases [ABGs])

Type of test Blood

Normal findings

pH
Adult/child: 7.35-7.45
Newborn: 7.32-7.49
2 months-2 years: 7.34-7.46

Pco_2
Adult/child: 35-45 mm Hg
Child <2 years: 26-41 mm Hg

HCO_3^-
Adult/child: 21-28 mEq/L
Newborn/infant: 16-24 mEq/L

Po_2
Adult/child: 80-100 mm Hg
Newborn: 60-70 mm Hg

O_2 saturation
Adult/child: 95% to 100%
Elderly: 95%
Newborn: 40% to 90%

Possible critical values

pH: <7.25, >7.55
Pco_2: <20, >60
HCO_3^-: <15, >40
Po_2: <40
O_2 saturation: 75% or lower

Test explanation and related physiology

Measurement of ABGs provides valuable information in assessing and managing a patient's respiratory and metabolic (renal) disturbances.

pH

The pH is inversely proportional to the actual hydrogen ion concentration. Therefore, as the hydrogen ion concentration decreases, the pH increases, and vice versa. The pH is a measure of alkalinity (pH >7.4) and acidity (pH <7.35). In respiratory or metabolic alkalosis, the pH is elevated; in respiratory or metabolic acidosis, the pH is decreased.

P_{CO_2}

The P_{CO_2} is a measure of the partial pressure of CO_2 in the blood. P_{CO_2} is referred to as the *respiratory* component in acid-base determination, because this value is primarily controlled by the lungs. As the CO_2 level increases, the pH decreases. Therefore the CO_2 level and the pH are inversely proportional.

The P_{CO_2} level is elevated in primary respiratory acidosis and decreased in primary respiratory alkalosis (Table 3). Because the lungs compensate for primary metabolic acid-base derangements, P_{CO_2} levels are affected by metabolic disturbances as well. In metabolic acidosis, the lungs attempt to compensate by "blowing off" CO_2 to raise pH. In metabolic alkalosis, the lungs attempt to compensate by retaining CO_2 to lower pH (Table 4).

HCO_3^-

The bicarbonate ion (HCO_3^-) is a measure of the *metabolic* (renal) component of the acid-base equilibrium. This ion can be measured directly by the bicarbonate value or indirectly by the CO_2 content (see p. 190). As the HCO_3^- level increases, the pH also increases; therefore the relationship of bicarbonate to pH is directly proportional. HCO_3^- is elevated in metabolic alkalosis and decreased in metabolic acidosis (Table 3). The kidneys also are used to compensate for primary respiratory acid-base derangements. For example, in respiratory acidosis the kidneys attempt to compensate by reabsorbing increased amounts of HCO_3^-. In respiratory alkalosis, the kidneys excrete HCO_3^- in increased amounts in an attempt to lower pH through compensation (Table 4).

P_{O_2}

This is an indirect measure of the oxygen content of the arterial blood. P_{O_2} is a measure of the tension (pressure) of oxygen dissolved in the plasma. The P_{O_2} level is decreased in:

1. Patients who are unable to oxygenate the arterial blood because of O_2 diffusion difficulties (e.g., pneumonia, shock lung)
2. Patients who have premature mixing of venous blood with arterial blood (e.g., in congenital heart disease)
3. Patients who have underventilated and overperfused pulmonary alveoli (pickwickian syndrome; i.e., obese patients

TABLE 3 Normal values for arterial blood gases and abnormal values in uncompensated acid-base disturbances

Acid-base disturbances	pH	P_{CO_2} (mm Hg)	HCO_3^- (mEq/L)	Common cause
None (normal values)	7.35-7.45	35-45	22-26	
Respiratory acidosis	↓	↑	Normal	Respiratory depression (drugs, central nervous system trauma) Pulmonary disease (pneumonia, chronic obstructive pulmonary disease, respiratory underventilation)
Respiratory alkalosis	↑	↓	Normal	Hyperventilation (emotions, pain, respirator overventilation)
Metabolic acidosis	↓	Normal	↓	Diabetes, shock, renal failure, intestinal fistula
Metabolic alkalosis	↑	Normal	↑	Sodium bicarbonate overdose, prolonged vomiting, nasogastric drainage

TABLE 4 Acid-base disturbances and compensatory mechanisms

Acid-base disturbance	Mode of compensation
Respiratory acidosis	Kidneys will retain increased amounts of HCO_3^- to increase pH.
Respiratory alkalosis	Kidneys will excrete increased amounts of HCO_3^- to lower pH.
Metabolic acidosis	Lungs "blow off" CO_2 to raise pH.
Metabolic alkalosis	Lungs retain CO_2 to lower pH.

who cannot ventilate properly when in the supine position)

O_2 saturation

Oxygen saturation is an indication of the percentage of hemoglobin saturated with O_2. When 92% to 100% of the hemoglobin carries O_2, the tissues are adequately provided with O_2. As the Po_2 level decreases, the percentage of hemoglobin saturation also decreases. This decrease (see an oxyhemoglobin dissociation curve) is linear to a certain value. However, when the Po_2 level drops below 60 mm Hg, small decreases in the Po_2 level will cause large decreases in the percentage of hemoglobin saturated with O_2. At O_2 saturation levels of 70% or lower, the tissues are unable to extract enough O_2 to carry out their vital functions.

Procedure and patient care

Before

- Explain the procedure to the patient.
- Notify the laboratory before drawing ABGs so that the necessary equipment can be calibrated before the blood sample arrives.
- Perform the Allen test to assess collateral circulation before performing the arterial puncture on the radial artery.
- To perform the Allen test, make the patient's hand blanch by obliterating both the radial and the ulnar pulses, and then release the pressure over the ulnar artery only. If flow through the ulnar artery is good, flushing will be seen immediately. The Allen test is then positive, and the radial artery can be used for puncture.

- If the Allen test is negative (no flushing), repeat it on the other arm.
- If both arms give a negative result, choose another artery for puncture.
- Note that the Allen test ensures collateral circulation to the hand if thrombosis of the radial artery should follow the puncture.

During

- Note that arterial blood can be obtained from any area of the body where strong pulses are palpable, usually from the radial, brachial, or femoral artery.
- Cleanse the arterial site.
- Attach a 20-gauge needle to a syringe containing approximately 0.2 ml of heparin.
- After drawing 3 to 5 ml of blood, remove the needle and apply pressure to the arterial site for 3 to 5 minutes.
- Expel any air bubbles in the syringe.
- Cap the syringe and gently rotate to mix the blood and heparin.
- Indicate on the laboratory slip if the patient is receiving oxygen therapy or is attached to a ventilator.
- Note that an arterial puncture is performed by laboratory technicians, respiratory-inhalation therapists, nurses, or physicians in approximately 10 minutes.
- Tell the patient that the arterial puncture is associated with more discomfort than a venous puncture.

After

- Place the arterial blood on ice and immediately take it to the chemistry laboratory for analysis.
- Apply pressure or a pressure dressing to the arterial puncture site for 3 to 5 minutes to avoid hematoma formation.
- Assess the puncture site for bleeding. Remember that an artery rather than a vein has been stuck.
- If the patient has an abnormal clotting time or is taking anticoagulants, apply pressure for a longer period (approximately 15 minutes).

Abnormal findings

See Table 3.

Type of test Blood

Normal findings

Normal quantity of red and white blood cells (RBCs, WBCs) and platelets

Normal size, shape, and color of RBCs

Normal WBC differential count

Test explanation and related physiology

When adequately prepared and examined microscopically by an experienced technologist, a smear of peripheral blood is the most informative of all hematologic tests. All three hematologic cell lines (RBCs, WBCs, platelets) can be examined.

Microscopic examination of the RBCs can reveal variation in RBC size (anisocytosis), shape (poikilocytosis), color, or intracellular content. Classification of RBCs according to these variables is most helpful in identifying the causes of anemia.

RBC size

   Microcytes (small RBCs)

      Iron deficiency

      Hereditary spherocytosis

      Thalassemia

   Macrocytes (larger size)

      Vitamin B_{12} or folic acid deficiency

      Reticulocytosis secondary to increased erythropoiesis (RBC production)

      Occasional liver disorder

      Postsplenectomy anemia

RBC shape

   Spherocytes (small and round)

      Hereditary spherocytosis

      Acquired immunohemolytic anemia

   Elliptocytes (crescent or sickle shaped)

      Hereditary elliptocytosis

      Sickle cell anemia

   Leptocytes, or "target cells" (thin and with less hemoglobin)

   Hemoglobinopathies

   Thalassemia

Spicule cell
  Uremia
  Liver disease
  Bleeding ulcer
RBC color
  Hypochromic (pale)
    Iron deficiency
    Thalassemia
    Cardiac disease
  Hyperchromasia (more colored)
    Concentrated hemoglobin, usually caused by dehydration
RBC intracellular structure
  Nucleus (Because the RBC maturation process results in loss
    of the nucleus, nucleated RBCs [normoblasts] seen in the
    peripheral smear indicate increased RBC production.)
    "Normal" for infant's blood
    Physiologic response to RBC deficiency (as in hemolytic
      anemias, sickle cell crisis, transfusion reaction, and
      erythroblastosis fetalis)
    Physiologic response to hypoxemia (as in congenital heart
      disease and congestive heart failure)
    Marrow-occupying neoplasm or fibrotic tissue (as in my-
      eloma and leukemia)
  Basophilic stippling (refers to bodies enclosed or included in
    the cells)
    Lead poisoning
    Reticulocytosis
  Howell-Jolly bodies (small, round remnants of nuclear mate-
    rial)
    Postsplenectomy
    Hemolytic anemia
    Megaloblastic anemia
  Heinz bodies (small, irregular particles of hemoglobin)
    Drug-induced RBC injury
    Hemoglobinopathies
    Hemolytic anemia
The WBCs are examined for total quantity, differential count,
and degree of maturity. An increased number of immature WBCs
may indicate leukemia. A decreased WBC count indicates failure
of marrow to produce WBCs, resulting from drugs, chronic disease, neoplasia, or fibrosis.

Finally, an experienced cell examiner also can estimate platelet
number (see p. 631) on a peripheral blood smear.

Procedure and patient care

Before

- Explain the procedure to the patient.
- Tell the patient that no fasting is required.

During

- Collect a drop of blood from a finger stick or heel stick and place it on a slide.
- If necessary, perform a venipuncture and collect the blood in a lavender-top tube.
- Note that a blood smear is first studied with an automated calculator programmed to recognize abnormal blood cell shapes and so on. A more accurate smear is performed by a technologist. Low counts may be "hand counted" to ensure accuracy. The most accurate smear requires review by a pathologist.

After

- Apply pressure or a pressure dressing to the venipuncture site.
- Assess the venipuncture site for bleeding.

Abnormal findings

See listing under Test Explanation and Related Physiology.

notes

blood typing

Type of test Blood

Normal findings Compatibility

Test explanation and related physiology

With blood typing, ABO and Rh antigens can be detected in the blood of prospective blood donors and potential blood recipients. This test is also used to determine the blood type of expectant mothers and newborns. Human blood is grouped according to the presence or absence of these antigens. The two major antigens, A and B, form the basis of the ABO system. Group A red blood cells (RBCs) contain A antigens; group B RBCs contain B antigens; group AB RBCs have both A and B antigens; and group O RBCs have neither A nor B antigens (Table 5). The presence or absence of Rh antigens on the RBCs determines the classification of Rh positive or Rh negative.

All patients who are pregnant should have blood typing and Rh-factor determination. If the patient's blood is Rh negative or type O (the most common type), the husband's blood should also be typed. If his blood is Rh positive or type AB, the woman's blood should be examined for the presence of Rh antibodies (by the indirect Coombs' test, see p. 283). If the initial screening is negative (no antibodies to Rh found), the test is repeated at weeks 30 and 36 of pregnancy. If these tests are also negative, no risk is involved to the fetus; if the test is positive, the fetus has been affected by maternal hemolysis of the fetal RBCs. The severity of the hemolytic anemia is then evaluated by the quantity of bilirubin in the amniotic fluid (see amniocentesis, p. 44).

TABLE 5 Blood typing

Blood type	Antigen	Antibody
Group A	A	B
Group B	B	A
Group AB (universal receiver)	A, B	None
Group O (universal donor)	None	A, B

ABO and Rh typing also is performed during pregnancy to advise the mother whether she is a candidate for RhoGAM (Rh immunoglobulin) after the delivery. RhoGAM will prevent any further fetal hemolytic problems during subsequent pregnancies.

Blood transfusions are actually transplantations of tissue (blood) from one person to another. It is important that the recipient does not have antibodies to the donor's RBCs, and that the donor does not have antibodies to the recipient's RBCs. If either of these conditions exists, there will be a hypersensitivity reaction, which can vary from mild fever to anaphylaxis with severe intravascular hemolysis. Although typing for the major ABO and Rh antigens does not guarantee that no reaction will occur, it does greatly reduce the possibility of such a reaction.

Many potential minor antigens are not routinely detected during blood typing. If allowed to go unrecognized, these minor antigens also can initiate a blood transfusion reaction. Therefore blood is not only typed but also crossmatched to identify a mismatch of blood caused by minor antigens. Crossmatching consists of the mixing of the recipient's serum with the donor's RBCs in saline solution followed by the addition of Coombs' serum (indirect Coombs' test, see p. 283).

Procedure and patient care

Before

- Explain the procedure to the patient.
- Tell the patient that no fasting is required.

During

- Collect approximately 7 to 14 ml of venous blood in a red-top tube. (This may vary among laboratories.)
- Avoid hemolysis.
- Appropriately label the blood tube before sending it to the laboratory.

After

- Apply pressure or a pressure dressing to the venipuncture site.
- Assess the venipuncture site for bleeding.

Abnormal findings

None

bone marrow biopsy (Bone marrow examination, Bone marrow aspiration)

Type of test Microscopic examination of tissue

Normal findings Active erythroid cell line, myeloid and lymphoid cell lines, and megakaryocyte (platelet) production

Test explanation and related physiology

By examination of a bone marrow specimen, the hematologist can fully evaluate hematopoiesis. Examination of the bone marrow reveals the number, size, and shape of the red and white blood cells (RBCs, WBCs) and megakaryocytes (platelet precursors) as these cells evolve through their various stages of development in the bone marrow. Samples of the bone marrow can be obtained by either aspiration or surgical removal. Microscopic examination includes estimation of cellularity, determination of the presence of fibrotic tissue or neoplasms (both primary and metastatic), and estimation of iron storage.

For the estimation of cellularity, the specimen is examined and the relative quantity of each cell type determined. This is more accurately performed on a biopsy specimen than on an aspirate, because the aspirate may not be truly representative of the entire marrow. Leukemias or leukemoid drug reactions are suspected when increased numbers of leukocyte precursors are present. Physiologic marrow leukemoid compensation for infection also will be recognized by finding an increased number of leukocyte precursors. Decreased numbers of marrow leukocyte precursors occur in patients with myelofibrosis, metastatic neoplasia, or agranulocytosis; in elderly patients; and following radiation therapy or chemotherapy.

Increased numbers of marrow RBC precursors occur with polycythemia vera or as physiologic compensation to hemorrhagic or hemolytic anemias. Decreased numbers of marrow RBC precursors occur with erythroid hypoplasia following chemotherapy, radiation therapy, administration of other toxic drugs, iron deficiency, or marrow replacement by fibrotic tissue or neoplasms.

Increased numbers of platelet precursors (megakaryocytes) are seen in the marrow of patients following acute hemorrhage or some forms of chronic myeloid leukemia. This increase also may be compensatory in patients with secondary hypersplenism associated with portal hypertension or other conditions. Decreased numbers of megakaryocytes occur in patients who have had radiation therapy, chemotherapy, or other drug therapy and in patients with neoplastic or fibrotic marrow infiltrative diseases. Patients with aplastic anemia also have decreased numbers of megakaryocytes.

Increased numbers of lymphocyte precursors occur in chronic or viral infections (e.g., mononucleosis), lymphocytic leukemia, and lymphoma. Plasma cells (plasmocytes) are increased in number in patients with multiple myelomas, Hodgkin's disease, hypersensitivity states, rheumatic fever, and other chronic inflammatory diseases.

Estimation of cellularity also can be expressed as a ratio of myeloid (WBC) to erythroid (RBC) cells (M/E ratio). The normal M/E ratio is approximately 3:1. The M/E ratio is greater than normal in those diseases mentioned previously in which increased leukocyte precursors are present or erythroid precursors are decreased. The M/E ratio is below normal when either leukocyte precursors are decreased or erythroid precursors are increased. A more detailed listing of diseases affecting the M/E ratio can be found in most hematology textbooks.

Drug-induced or idiopathic myelofibrosis can be detected by examination of the bone marrow. Using special stains, one can estimate iron stores with a marrow biopsy. Although fibrosis or neoplasia occasionally can be detected in aspiration studies, biopsy is the best method. Leukemias, multiple myelomas, and polycythemia vera can easily be detected in biopsy specimens. Similarly, lymphomas and other metastatic tumors (e.g., cancers of the breast, kidney, and lung) can be seen.

Contraindications

- Patients with acute coagulation disorders because of the risk of excessive bleeding
- Patients who cannot cooperate and remain still during the procedure

Potential complications

- Hemorrhage, especially if the patient has a coagulopathy
- Infection, especially if the patient is leukopenic
- Inadvertent puncture of the heart or great vessels when the test is performed on the sternum

Procedure and patient care

Before

- Explain the procedure to the patient.
- Obtain a written and informed consent for this procedure.
- Encourage the patient to verbalize fears, because many patients are anxious concerning this study.
- Assess the coagulation studies. Report any evidence of coagulopathy to the physician.
- Obtain an order for sedatives if the patient appears extremely apprehensive.
- Remind the patient to remain very still throughout the procedure.

During

- Note the following procedural steps for *bone marrow aspiration,* which is performed on the sternum, iliac crest, anterior or posterior iliac spines, and proximal tibia (in children):
  1. The procedure is usually performed at the patient's bedside using local anesthesia.
  2. A preferred site is the posterior iliac crest, with the patient placed prone or on the side.
  3. The area overlying the bone is prepared and draped in a sterile manner.
  4. The overlying skin and soft tissue, along with the periosteum, is infiltrated with lidocaine.
  5. A large-bore needle containing a stylus is slowly advanced through the soft tissue and into the outer table of the bone.
  6. Once inside the marrow, the stylus is removed and a syringe is attached.
  7. One half to 2 ml of bone marrow is aspirated, smeared on slides, and allowed to dry.
  8. The slides are sprayed with a preservative and taken to the pathology laboratory.
- Note the following procedural steps for *bone marrow biopsy:*
  1. The skin and soft tissues overlying the bone are incised.
  2. A core biopsy instrument is "screwed" into the bone.
  3. The biopsy specimen is obtained and sent to the pathology laboratory for analysis.
- Note that aspiration is performed by a trained nurse or physician. Bone marrow biopsy–specimen removal is usually per-

formed by a physician. The duration of these studies is approximately 20 minutes.

- Inform the patient that he or she may have some apprehension when pressure is applied to puncture the outer table of the bone during biopsy specimen removal or aspiration.
- Tell the patient that he or she probably will feel pain during lidocaine infiltration and pressure when the syringe plunger is withdrawn for aspiration.

After

- Apply pressure to the puncture site to arrest minimal bleeding. Apply an adhesive bandage.
- Observe the puncture site for bleeding. Ice packs may be used to help control bleeding.
- Assess for tenderness and erythema, which may indicate infection. Report this to the physician.
- Evaluate the patient for signs of shock (increased pulse rate, decreased blood pressure) and pain.
- Normally, place the patient on bed rest for 30 to 60 minutes after the test.
- Note that some patients complain of tenderness at the puncture site for several days after this study. Mild analgesics may be ordered.

Abnormal findings

Neoplasm
Infection
  Viral
  Bacterial
  Fungal
Myelofibrosis
Agranulocytosis
Polycythemia vera
Multiple myelomas
Hodgkin's disease

Hypersensitivity states
Acute hemorrhagic marrow
  hyperplasia
Anemia
Lymphoma
Chronic inflammatory disease
Leukemia
Rheumatic fever
AIDS

notes

bone scan

Type of test Nuclear scan

Normal findings No evidence of abnormality

Test explanation and related physiology

The bone scan permits examination of the skeleton by a scanning camera after IV injection of a radionuclide material. The degree of radionuclide uptake is related to the metabolism of the bone. Normally, a uniform concentration should be seen throughout the bones of the body. An increased uptake of isotope is abnormal and may represent tumor, arthritis, fracture, degenerative bone and joint changes, osteomyelitis, bone necrosis, osteodystrophy, and Paget's disease. These areas of concentrated radionuclide uptake are often called *hot spots* and are detectable months before an ordinary x-ray film can reveal the pathology. Hot spots occur because new bone growth is usually stimulated around areas of pathology. If pathology exists and there is no new bone formation around the lesion, the scan will not pick up the abnormality.

The major reason a bone scan is performed is to detect metastatic cancer to the bone. All malignancies capable of metastasis may reach the bone, especially those of the prostate, breast, lung, kidney, urinary bladder, and thyroid gland. Bone scans may be serially repeated to document the tumor's response to antineoplastic therapy.

Bone scans also provide valuable information in the evaluation of patients with trauma or unexplained pain. Bone scanning is much more sensitive than routine x-ray films in detecting small and difficult-to-find fractures, especially in the spine, ribs, face, and small bones of the extremities. Bone scans are used to determine the age of a fracture as well. If a fracture is seen on a plain x-ray film and the uptake around that fracture is not increased on a bone scan, the injury is said to be an "old" fracture, exceeding several months in age.

Although the bone scan is extremely sensitive, it unfortunately is not very specific. Fractures, infections, tumors, and arthritic changes all appear similar in this scan.

Contraindications

- Patients who are pregnant because of the risk of fetal damage
- Patients who are lactating because of the risk of contaminating the infant

Procedure and patient care

Before

- Explain the procedure to the patient.
- Assure patients they will not be exposed to large amounts of radioactivity, because only tracer doses of the isotope are used.
- Tell the patient that no fasting or sedation is required.

During

- Note the following procedural steps:
  1. The patient receives an IV injection of an isotope, usually sodium pertechnetate (technetium-99m) in a peripheral vein.
  2. The patient is encouraged to drink several glasses of water between the time of radioisotope injection and the scanning. This facilitates renal clearance of the circulating tracer not picked up by the bone. The waiting period before scanning is approximately 1 to 3 hours.
  3. The patient is instructed to urinate.
  4. The patient is positioned in the supine position on the scanning table in the nuclear medicine department.
  5. A radionuclide detector is placed over the patient's body and records the radiation emitted by the skeleton.
  6. This information is translated into a two-dimensional view of the skeleton, which is then visualized on Polaroid or x-ray film.
  7. The patient is repositioned in the prone and lateral positions during the test.
- Note that this scan is performed by a nuclear medicine technician in 30 to 60 minutes. It is interpreted by a physician trained in nuclear medicine imaging.
- Tell the patient that the injection of the radioisotope causes slight discomfort.
- Inform patients in significant pain that lying on the hard scanning table can be uncomfortable.

After
- Because only tracer doses of radioisotope are used, remember that no precautions need to be taken to prevent radioactive exposure to other personnel or family present.
- Assure the patient that the radioactive substance is usually excreted from the body within 6 to 24 hours.
- Encourage the patient to drink fluids to aid in the excretion of the radioactive substance.
- Observe the injection site for redness or swelling.

Abnormal findings

Primary or metastatic tumor of the bone
Fracture
Degenerative arthritis
Rheumatoid arthritis
Osteomyelitis
Bone necrosis
Renal osteodystrophy
Paget's disease
Osteomyelitis

notes

brain scan (Cisternal scan, Cerebral blood flow)

Type of test Nuclear scan

Normal findings No areas of increased radionuclide uptake within the brain

Test explanation and related physiology

Brain scanning allows for the detection of pathologic cerebral conditions by nuclear counter scanning of the patient's cranial contents after IV administration of a radioisotope. This study is performed in patients with frequent and severe headaches, stroke (cerebrovascular accident [CVA]) syndrome, seizure complaints, or other neurologic complaints. Normally, the blood-brain barrier does not allow blood to come in direct contact with brain tissue. Frequently used isotopes (e.g., technetium-99m pertechnetate, mercury-201, radioiodinated albumin) are unable to cross this blood-brain barrier. In localized pathologic conditions, however, this normal barrier is disrupted. The isotopes are then preferentially localized or concentrated in abnormal regions of the brain.

The precise cause of the disruption of the blood-brain barrier can be any of various pathologic processes. Unfortunately, the brain scan is not a specific indicator of the exact pathologic process. Study of the location, size, and shape of the abnormality, along with the timing of the scan, may help specify the pathologic process.

The timing of brain scanning in relation to the onset of CVA-like symptoms is usually significant. For example, in cerebral infarction, scanning performed soon after the onset of symptoms may be normal and then become abnormal 2 weeks later; this combination is virtually pathognomonic of infarction. Scanning patients with cerebral thrombosis without infarction may never reveal abnormalities. Tumors and abscesses will show abnormalities on the initial scan.

The injection of isotopes followed by immediate scanning can be used to detect changes in the dynamics of cerebral blood flow by comparing one side of the brain with the other. For example, cerebrovascular occlusive disease is characterized by a decreased flow, in contrast to an arteriovenous (AV) malformation, which is associated with an increased flow rate.

Cisternal scans may be performed by injecting radioactive material into the subarachnoid space and then taking serial scans of the head. These scans are useful in evaluating ventricular size and patency of the cerebrospinal fluid (CSF) pathways and reabsorbtion. Because only a small amount of CSF enters the ventricles, their uptake of radioactive material normally should be minimal. Blocks in the CSF pathways may prevent this reabsorption, however, and thus large amounts of isotopes may appear in the ventricles. Cisternal scans also may be used to evaluate CSF leakage in patients with recurrent meningitis and to evaluate hydrocephalus.

In general, computed tomography scans, magnetic resonance imaging scans, and carotid duplex scans have replaced the brain scan in diagnostic neurology.

Contraindications

- Patients who are pregnant
- Patients who cannot cooperate during the testing

Procedure and patient care

Before

- Explain the procedure to the patient.
- Administer blocking agents as ordered before scanning. For example, potassium chloride prevents an inordinate amount of technetium uptake by the choroid plexus, which would simulate a pathologic cerebral condition. Similar solutions (e.g., potassium iodine, Lugol's solution) may be given orally to block thyroid uptake. Blocking agents are not necessary with the use of technetium-99m diethylenetriamine pentaacetic acid.
- Check for allergy to iodine if an iodinated solution will be used.
- Consider having a sedative ordered for agitated patients.

During

- Note the following procedural steps:
  1. After administration of the radioisotope, the patient is placed in the supine, lateral, and prone positions while a counter is placed over the head.
  2. The radioisotope counts are anatomically displayed and photographed while the patient remains very still.
  3. When cerebral flow studies are performed, the counter is immediately placed over the head.

4. The counts are anatomically recorded in timed sequence to follow the isotope during its first flow through the brain.

5. Another scan is obtained 30 minutes to 2 hours later for identification of pathologic tissues.

- Note that this study is performed by a technician in the nuclear medicine department in approximately 35 to 45 minutes.

- Tell the patient that no discomfort is associated with this study other than the peripheral IV puncture required for injection of the radioisotope.

After

- Assure the patient that the radioactive material is usually excreted from the body within 6 to 24 hours.

- Because only tracer doses of radioisotopes are used, remember that no precautions need to be taken to prevent radioactive exposure to other personnel or family present.

- Encourage the patient to drink fluids to aid the excretion of the isotope from the body.

- Observe the injection site for redness and swelling.

Abnormal findings

Cerebral neoplasm
Brain abscess
Acute cerebral infarction
Subdural hematoma
Cerebral thrombosis
Cerebrovascular occlusive disease

Cerebral hemorrhage
Hematoma
AV malformation
Aneurysm
CSF leakage
Hydrocephalus
Cancer metastasis to the brain

notes

---

breast sonogram (Ultrasound mammography)

Type of test Ultrasound

Normal findings No evidence of abnormality

Test explanation and related physiology

Ultrasound mammography is a useful test for differentiating cystic and solid breast lesions, for diagnosing disease in women with very dense breasts, and in the follow-up of women with fibrocystic disease. In diagnostic ultrasound, harmless high-frequency sound waves are emitted and penetrate the breast. The sound waves are bounced back to the sensor and arranged in a pictorial image by electronic conversion. The equivalent of a realistic Polaroid or x-ray film picture of the breast tissue is then obtained.

Ultrasound of the breast is also useful in the examination of women who are pregnant and have a newly palpable breast mass. Young women under the age of 21 may experience greater risk of radiation from x-ray mammography. Ultrasound is often used to evaluate symptomatic women in this age group. Ultrasound also may be used to evaluate women who have silicone prosthesis–augmented breasts. The prosthesis can be penetrated by the ultrasound beam. Ordinarily, these prostheses would obscure residual tissue on physical examination and x-ray mammography.

Ultrasound examination is also a viable alternative for women who refuse to have x-ray mammography because of unreasonable fear of diagnostic radiation. Ultrasound is especially useful in patients with an abnormal mass on a mammogram. The intrinsic nature (cystic vs. solid) can be determined. Most cysts are benign. Diagnostic accuracy is improved when breast ultrasound is combined with x-ray mammography (see p. 553).

When a breast abnormality cannot be seen well enough on a mammogram for localization biopsy, ultrasound can be used to localize the abnormality for biopsy or aspiration.

Procedure and patient care

Before

- Explain the procedure to the patient. Assure the patient that no discomfort is associated with this study.
- Inform the patient that no fasting or sedation is required

before the tests. Instruct the patient not to apply any lotions or powders to the breasts on the examination day.

During

- Note the following procedural steps:
  1. The patient lies in the prone position on the examining table, which contains a tank that holds heated and chlorinated water.
  2. One breast at a time is immersed in the water.
  3. The transducer that produces the ultrasound waves and detects their echoes is positioned at the bottom of the water tank.
  4. Alternatively, the patient is placed in the supine position, and the transducer is directly applied to the breast using contact gel to improve sound transmission.
- Note that this test is performed by an ultrasound technician in approximately 15 minutes.
- Although there is no discomfort associated with this procedure, women with back problems or limited flexibility may have difficulty maintaining the position for this procedure.
- Some laboratories use a hand-held transducer that can be placed on the skin overlying the breast after using a conductive paste.

After

- After the test is completed, the breasts are dried or the conductive paste is removed.

Abnormal findings

Cyst	Fibroadenoma
Hematoma	Fibrocystic disease
Cancer	Abscess

notes

bronchography (Bronchogram, Laryngography)

Type of test X-ray with contrast dye

Normal findings Normal tracheobronchial tree

Test explanation and related physiology

A bronchogram is an x-ray examination of the tracheobronchial tree produced after the instillation of an iodinated dye into the bronchi via a catheter or bronchoscope. Positioning of the patient and the catheter allows the radiopaque material to coat all portions of the tracheobronchial tree so that their outline can be recorded on a chest x-ray film. X-ray films are taken to demonstrate the outline and structure of the trachea, bronchi, and entire tracheobronchial tree.

Bronchography is indicated to diagnose bronchiectasis, to identify obstruction in the distal bronchi, and to detect congenital or acquired forms of tracheobronchial malformation and fistula. Bronchography may be used in the evaluation of patients for possible surgery and of those with recurring, localized pneumonia or severe hemoptysis. Bronchography should not be performed when patients have an exacerbation of cough or sputum production. The test should be performed after the symptoms are treated and when mucous secretions are minimal. Because of the alterations in pulmonary function, as well as occasional inflammatory reactions induced by this procedure, studying one lung at a time is safer than studying both. The indications for bronchography have diminished since the development of flexible fiberoptic bronchoscopy, which has provided direct visualization of the tracheobronchial tree.

Contraindications

- Patients who are pregnant
- Patients with acute infections
- Patients with respiratory insufficiency

Potential complications

- Bronchospasm or laryngospasm
- Allergic reaction to iodinated dye
  This rarely occurs, because the dye is not administered intravenously.

Interfering factors

- Excessive coughing or sputum production can inhibit bronchiolar filling and cause premature expulsion of the contrast
material.

Procedure and patient care

Before

- Explain the procedure to the patient. Allay any concerns and
allow the patient to express any fears.
- Obtain informed consent if required by the institution.
- Check for allergies to iodine dye and shellfish.
- Keep the patient NPO after midnight the day of the test.
- Instruct the patient to perform thorough mouth care the
night before and the morning of the test to minimize the risk
of introducing bacteria into the lungs during the procedure.
- Consider postural drainage to promote expulsion of mucus
or exudate from the lungs.
- Remove and safely store the patient's dentures, glasses, or
contact lenses.
- Administer the preprocedural medications as ordered. Medications may include atropine to decrease secretions and to
minimize vagally induced bradycardia and diazepam (Valium) for its sedative effect.
- Instruct the patient not to swallow the local anesthetic
sprayed into the throat. Provide an emesis basin for expectoration.
- Ask the patient to make every effort to suppress coughing
during the procedure. Coughing will prevent adequate
bronchiolar filling and also expel the contrast substance before the test is completed. Rapid, shallow breathing will help
to suppress the cough reflex. If the patient has a productive
cough, an expectorant is administered and postural drainage
is performed for 1 to 3 days before the procedure.

During

- Place the patient in a sitting position.
- Note the following procedural steps:
  1. After spraying a local anesthetic into the patient's nose or
  mouth to suppress the gag reflex, a catheter or bronchoscope is passed into the trachea.
  2. The pharynx, larynx, and major bronchi are anesthetized
  before introduction of the radiopaque dye.

3. The position of the patient and the placing of the catheter allow the radiologist to fill regions of interest selectively with radiopaque material.

4. The positions assumed by the patient are usually the reverse of those used in postural drainage.

5. Multiple x-ray views are obtained.

- Note that bronchography is performed by a radiologist in approximately 45 minutes.
- Inform the patient of the discomfort usually associated with this test.

After

- If indicated, perform postural drainage to help remove the radiopaque dye from the tracheobronchial tree.
- Instruct the patient not to eat or drink anything until the tracheobronchial anesthesia has worn off and the gag reflex returns, usually in approximately 2 hours.
- Observe the patient closely for evidence of impaired respiration or laryngospasm. Vocal chords may go into spasm after intubation. Emergency resuscitation equipment should be readily available.
- Encourage the patient to cough, which will help clear the tracheobronchial tree.
- Inform the patient that a slight temperature elevation often occurs for 2 to 3 days after the test.
- Inform the patient that a sore throat also often develops. This can be relieved by gargling or by taking throat lozenges.
- Note that follow-up x-ray films may be taken later to ascertain if any dye remains in the tracheobronchial tree.
- Tell the patient that normal activities may usually be resumed 24 hours after the test.

Abnormal findings

Bronchiectasis
Bronchial obstruction
Tracheobronchial fistula

notes

bronchoscopy

Type of test Endoscopy

Normal findings Normal larynx, trachea, bronchi, and alveoli

Test explanation and related physiology

Bronchoscopy permits endoscopic visualization of the larynx, trachea, and bronchi by either a flexible fiberoptic bronchoscope or a rigid bronchoscope. *Diagnostic* uses of bronchoscopy include:

1. Direct visualization of the tracheobronchial tree for abnormalities (e.g., tumors, inflammation, strictures)
2. Biopsy of specimens from observed lesions
3. Aspiration of "deep" sputum for culture and sensitivity and cytology determinations

Therapeutic uses of bronchoscopy include:

1. Aspiration of retained secretions in patients with airway obstruction or postoperative atelectasis
2. Control of bleeding within the bronchus
3. Removal of foreign bodies that have been aspirated
4. Brachytherapy, which is endobronchial radiation therapy using an iridium wire placed via the bronchoscope
5. Palliative laser obliteration of bronchial neoplastic obstruction

The *rigid bronchoscope* is a wide-bore metal tube that permits visualization of only the larger airways. It is mainly used for the removal of large foreign bodies. Its use has radically diminished since the advent of the newer flexible fiberoptic bronchoscope.

Because of its smaller size and its flexibility, the *flexible fiberoptic bronchoscope* has increased the diagnostic reach of bronchoscopy to the smaller bronchi. This newer scope has an accessory lumen through which cable-activated instruments can be used for removing biopsy specimens of pathologic lesions. Also, the collection of bronchial washings (obtained by flushing the airways with saline solution), pulmonary toilet, and the instillation of anesthetic agents can be carried out through this extra lumen. Double-sheathed, plugged-protected brushes also can be passed through this accessory lumen. Specimens for cytology and bacteriology can be obtained with these brushes. This allows more accurate determination of pulmonary infectious agents. Laser therapy can now be performed through the bronchoscope to burn out endotracheal lesions.

Contraindications

- Patients with hypercapnia and severe shortness of breath who cannot tolerate interruption of high-flow oxygen

Potential complications

- Fever
- Hypoxemia
- Laryngospasm
- Bronchospasm
- Pneumothorax
- Aspiration
- Hemorrhage (after biopsy)

Procedure and patient care

Before

- Explain the procedure to the patient. Allay any fears and allow the patient to verbalize any concerns.
- Obtain informed consent for this procedure.
- Keep the patient NPO for 4 to 8 hours before the test to reduce the risk of aspiration.
- Instruct the patient to perform good mouth care to minimize the risk of introducing bacteria into the lungs during the procedure.
- Remove and safely store the patient's dentures, glasses, or contact lenses before administering the preprocedural medications.
- Administer the preprocedural medications as ordered. Atropine is used to prevent vagally induced bradycardia and to minimize secretions. Meperidine is used to sedate the patient and relieve anxiety.
- Reassure the patient that he or she will be able to breathe during this procedure.
- Instruct the patient not to swallow the local anesthetic sprayed into the throat. Provide a basin for expectoration of the lidocaine.

During

- Note the following procedural steps for *fiberoptic bronchoscopy:*
  1. This test is performed by a pulmonary specialist or a surgeon at the bedside or in an appropriately equipped room.

2. The patient's nasopharynx and oropharynx are anesthetized topically with lidocaine spray before the insertion of the bronchoscope.
3. The patient is placed in the sitting or supine position, and the tube is inserted through the nose or mouth and into the pharynx (Figure 5).
4. After the tube passes into the larynx and through the glottis, more lidocaine is sprayed into the trachea to prevent the cough reflex.

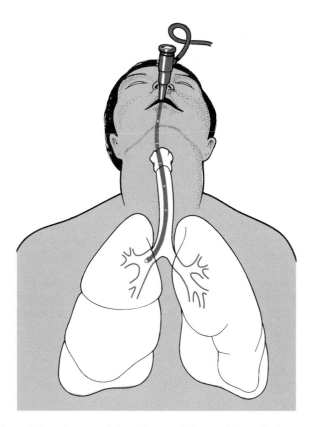

Figure 5 Bronchoscopy. A bronchoscope is inserted through the trachea and into the bronchus.

5. The tube is passed farther, well into the trachea, bronchi, and the first- and second-generation bronchioles, for systematic examination of the bronchial tree.
6. Biopsy specimens and washings are taken if pathology is suspected.
7. If bronchoscopy is performed for pulmonary toilet (removal of mucus), each bronchus is aspirated until clear.

- Note the following procedural steps for *rigid bronchoscopy:*
  1. This test is usually performed in the operating room with the patient under heavy sedation or general anesthesia.
  2. The patient is placed in the supine position with the neck hyperextended.
  3. The tube is inserted through the mouth and larynx and then into the trachea.
- Note that this procedure is performed by a physician in approximately 30 to 45 minutes.
- Tell the patient that because of sedation no discomfort is usually felt.

After

- Instruct the patient not to eat or drink anything until the tracheobronchial anesthesia has worn off and the gag reflex has returned, usually in approximately 2 hours.
- Observe the patient's sputum for hemorrhage if biopsy specimens were removed. A small amount of blood streaking may be expected and is normal for several hours. Large amounts of bleeding can cause a chemical pneumonitis.
- Observe the patient closely for evidence of impaired respiration or laryngospasm. The vocal cords may go into spasms after intubation. Emergency resuscitation equipment should be readily available.
- Inform the patient that postbronchoscopy fever often develops within the first 24 hours.
- If a tumor is suspected, collect a postbronchoscopy sputum sample for a cytology determination.
- Inform the patient that warm saline gargles and lozenges may be helpful if a sore throat develops.

Abnormal findings

Inflammation	Hemorrhage
Strictures	Foreign body
Tuberculosis	Abscess
Cancer	Infection

CA 15-3 tumor marker (Cancer antigen 15-3)

Type of test Blood

Normal findings <22 U/ml

Test explanation and related physiology

The CA 15-3 antigen is a tumor-associated serum marker available for diagnosing and monitoring the treatment of breast cancer. Until now, no other good tumor marker has been available for patients with breast cancer. Carcinoembryonic antigen (CEA, see p. 194), the most widely used tumor marker, is limited by poor sensitivity and specificity for patients with disease. Most recently, the monoclonal antibody technology has permitted the development of CA 15-3 antigen.

CA 15-3 is not as sensitive in the diagnosis of primary breast cancer as other tumor markers are for their respective tumors. That is, CA 15-3 levels are high in only 50% of patients whose presentation is a localized breast cancer or who have a small tumor burden. Eighty percent of patients with metastatic breast cancer, however, do have elevated levels; therefore the usefulness of CA 15-3 as a screening technique in early breast cancers, the most common cancer of women, is quite limited. Benign breast or ovarian disease and other nonbreast malignancies also can cause elevated CA 15-3 levels.

CA 15-3 is useful in monitoring the patient's response to therapy for metastatic breast cancer. A partial or complete response to treatment will be confirmed by declining levels. Likewise, a persistent rise in CA 15-3 levels despite therapy strongly suggests progressive disease.

CA 15-3 levels cannot be used in the surveillance of patients who have had a complete response to breast cancer as a result of surgery, radiation therapy, or chemotherapy. The high sensitivity but lack of specificity noted with this marker often inaccurately suggests recurrent disease when other benign processes exist.

Procedure and patient care

Before

- Explain the procedure to the patient.
- Tell the patient that no fasting is required.

During

- Collect 7 to 10 ml of venous blood in a red-top tube.
- Have the blood sample sent to a central diagnostic laboratory for CA 15-3 determinations. The results are available to the local hospital in 7 to 10 days.

After

- Apply pressure or a pressure dressing to the venipuncture site.
- Observe the venipuncture site for bleeding.

Abnormal finding

▲   **Increased levels**
Metastatic breast cancer

notes

CA 19-9 tumor marker (Cancer antigen 19-9)

Type of test Blood

Normal findings <37 U/ml

Test explanation and related physiology

CA 19-9 antigen is a tumor marker used in diagnosis, evaluation of a patient's response to treatment, and surveillance of patients with pancreatic or hepatobiliary cancer. It is used primarily in the diagnosis of pancreatic carcinoma. For example, in a patient whose presenting symptom is a pancreatic mass or biliary obstruction, greatly elevated CA 19-9 levels would confirm that pancreatic cancer exists. Likewise, patients whose presenting symptoms are ascites, jaundice, and elevated CA 19-9 levels may have a hepatobiliary cancer. CA 19-9 levels, however, may not be elevated in all patients with pancreatic carcinoma. Approximately 70% of patients with pancreatic carcinoma and 65% of patients with hepatobiliary cancer have elevated levels.

CA 19-9 levels are used in the posttreatment surveillance of those who have had pancreatic or hepatobiliary cancers. In the few patients with pancreatic or biliary cancer who have a good response to surgery, chemotherapy, or radiation therapy, a decline in serum levels of CA 19-9 will confirm this response. A rapid rise in CA 19-9 levels may be associated with a recurrent or progressive tumor growth. Mildly elevated levels may exist in patients with gastric cancer, colorectal cancer, or hepatoma, and even in 6% to 7% of patients with nongastrointestinal malignancies. Patients who have pancreatitis, gallstones, cirrhosis, inflammatory bowel disease, or cystic fibrosis also can have minimally elevated levels of CA 19-9.

Because of its lack of sensitivity and specificity, CA 19-9 is not effective in screening for pancreatobiliary tumors in the general population.

Procedure and patient care

Before

- Explain the procedure to the patient.
- Tell the patient that no fasting is required.

During

- Collect 7 to 10 ml of blood in a red-top tube.
- Have the blood sent to a central diagnostic laboratory for CA 19-9 determinations. The results are available to the local hospital in 7 to 10 days.

After

- Apply pressure or a pressure dressing to the venipuncture site.
- Observe the venipuncture site for bleeding.

Abnormal findings

▲ **Increased levels**

Pancreatic carcinoma	Gastric cancer
Hepatobiliary carcinoma	Colorectal cancer
Pancreatitis	Gallstones
Cholecystitis	Cystic fibrosis
Cirrhosis	Lung cancer

notes

CA-125 tumor marker (Cancer antigen-125)

Type of test Blood

Normal findings 0-35 U/ml

Test explanation and related physiology

The detection, extent of disease, and response to treatment of ovarian cancer can be determined by the use of CA-125. This tumor marker has a high degree of sensitivity and specificity for ovarian cancer and has been of great benefit to clinicians. Just as alpha-fetoprotein (AFP) and human chorionic gonadotropin (HCG) are accurate tumor markers for germ cell tumors of the ovary, CA-125 is an extremely accurate marker for epithelial tumors of the ovary. It is elevated in 75% to 80% of women with ovarian cancer.

The CA-125 marker can be used in many ways. It is especially helpful in making the diagnosis of ovarian cancer. For example, CA-125 can be used in women who have abdominal distention, ascites, and a palpable pelvic mass. In these patients, a greatly elevated CA-125 level is strong confirmation that the underlying etiology is an epithelial ovarian malignancy.

The CA-125 serum tumor marker is also used to determine a patient's response to therapy. Serial comparative testing will show a progressive decline in CA-125 levels for patients responding to treatment. Also, CA-125 tumor markers can predict whether or not a second-look (repeat) diagnostic laparotomy will be positive. A second-look laparotomy will detect a residual tumor in 97% of patients whose CA-125 level is greater than 35 U/ml, whereas only 56% of patients with ovarian cancer whose CA-125 level is less than 35 U/ml will have a positive second-look laparotomy. A precipitous fall in CA-125 after two courses of chemotherapy is an accurate predictor of a complete response to chemotherapy.

Finally, CA-125 determinations can be used in posttreatment surveillance of patients with ovarian cancer. In a patient who has had a complete response as a result of radiation therapy, chemotherapy, or surgery, a delayed rise in the CA-125 level may be an early predictor of a recurrent tumor. CA-125 is not an effective screening test for the asymptomatic general public because of its lack of specificity. It is used in a "high-risk" population of women who have a strong family history of ovarian cancer. Elevated levels in the general population indicate that either benign or malignant disease is present in 95% of patients.

Other tumors and benign processes can cause elevated CA-125 levels as well. Diseases that affect the peritoneum, such as cirrhosis, pancreatitis, peritonitis, endometriosis, and pelvic inflammatory disease, can create elevated levels of CA-125. Other malignancies occurring in the female genital tract, pancreas, colon, lung, and breast can also be associated with elevated levels of this protein.

Interfering factors

- The first trimester of pregnancy and normal menstruation may be associated with mild elevations of CA-125 levels.
- Patients with benign peritoneal diseases (e.g., cirrhosis, endometriosis) will have mildly increased levels.

Procedure and patient care

Before
- Explain the procedure to the patient.
- Tell the patient that no fasting or sedation is required.

During
- Collect 7 to 10 ml of blood in a red-top tube.
- Have the blood sent to a central diagnostic laboratory for determination of CA-125 level. The results are available to the local hospital in 3 to 7 days.

After
- Apply pressure or a pressure dressing to the venipuncture site.
- Observe the venipuncture site for bleeding.

Abnormal findings

▲   Increased levels

Malignant disorders	*Benign disorders*
Cancer of the ovary	Cirrhosis
Cancer of the pancreas	Peritonitis
Cancer of the nonovarian female genital tract	Pregnancy
	Endometriosis
Cancer of the breast	Pancreatitis
Cancer of the colon	Pelvic inflammatory disease
Cancer of the lung	
Lymphoma	
Peritoneal carcinomatosis	

calcitonin (Human calcitonin [HCT], Thyrocalcitonin)

Type of test Blood

Normal findings

Basal
  Males: ≤19 pg/ml or ≤19 ng/L (SI units)
  Females: ≤14 pg/ml or ≤14 ng/L (SI units)
Calcium infusion (2.4 mg/kg)
  Males: ≤190 pg/ml or ≤190 ng/L
  Females: ≤130 pg/ml or ≤130 ng/L
Pentagastrin injection (0.5 μg/kg)
  Males: ≤110 pg/ml or ≤110 ng/L
  Females: ≤30 pg/ml or ≤30 ng/L

Test explanation and related physiology

Calcitonin is a hormone secreted by the parafollicular or C cells of the thyroid gland as a response to elevated serum calcium levels. Calcitonin decreases serum calcium levels by inhibiting bone resorption and increasing calcium excretion by the kidneys.

This test is usually indicated to evaluate those with suspected medullary carcinoma of the thyroid. Seventy-five percent of these patients have hypersecretion of calcitonin with normal serum calcium levels. C-cell hyperplasia is also associated with elevated calcitonin levels. Calcitonin is useful in monitoring response to therapy and predicting recurrences of medullary thyroid cancer. It is also useful as a screening test for those with a family history of medullary cancer. Equivocal elevations require testing with IV pentagastrin or calcium to stimulate calcitonin secretion. Pentagastrin stimulation involves an IV infusion over 5 to 10 seconds with blood samples drawn before the injection and at 90 seconds, 2 minutes, and 5 minutes following the infusion. The calcium infusion test can be performed in a variety of ways but is most commonly administered over a 1-minute interval with baseline and 5- and 10-minute postinfusion blood levels.

Elevated levels of this tumor marker also may be seen in people with cancer of the lung, breast, and pancreas. This results from the paraneoplastic syndrome of ectopic production of calcitonin by tumor cells.

Interfering factors

☞ Drugs that may cause *increased* levels include calcium, cholecystokinin, epinephrine, glucagon, pentagastrin, and oral contraceptives.

Procedure and patient care

Before

- Explain the procedure to the patient.
- Tell the patient that an overnight fast is required. Water is permitted.

During

- Collect a venous sample of blood in a heparinized green-top or a chilled red-top tube according to the laboratory's protocol.

After

- Apply pressure or a pressure dressing to the venipuncture site.
- Assess the venipuncture site for bleeding.
- Tell the patient that results may not be available for several days.

Abnormal findings

▲ **Increased levels**

Medullary carcinoma of the thyroid
Oat cell carcinoma of the lung
Breast carcinoma
Pancreatic cancer
Primary hyperparathyroidism
Secondary hyperparathyroidism because of chronic renal failure
Zollinger-Ellison syndrome
Pernicious anemia
Alcoholic cirrhosis
Thyroiditis

notes

calcium, blood (Total/ionized calcium, Ca^{++}, Serum calcium)

Type of test Blood

Normal findings
Adult
  Total: 9.0-10.5 mg/dl or 2.25-2.75 mmol/L (SI units)
  Ionized: 4.5-5.6 mg/dl or 1.05-1.30 mmol/L (SI units)
Elderly: values slightly decreased
Child (total): 8.8-10.8 mg/dl or 2.2-2.7 mmol/L (SI units)
Newborn (total): 9.0-10.6 mg/dl or 2.30-2.65 mmol/L (SI units)
Umbilical cord (total): 9.0-11.5 mg/dl or 2.25-2.88 mmol/L (SI units)

Possible critical values
<6 mg/dl (may lead to tetany)
>14 mg/dl (may lead to coma)

Test explanation and related physiology
The serum calcium test is used to evaluate parathyroid function and calcium metabolism by directly measuring the total amount of calcium in the blood. When the serum calcium level is elevated on at least three separate determinations, the patient is said to have hypercalcemia. About one half of the total calcium exists in the blood in its free (ionized) form, and about one half exists in its protein-bound form (mostly with albumin). The serum calcium level is a measure of both. As a result, when the serum albumin level is low (as in malnourished patients), the serum calcium level will also be low, and vice versa. As a rule of thumb, the total serum calcium level decreases by approximately 0.8 mg for every 1-g decrease in the serum albumin level.

The ionized form of calcium also can be measured by ion-selective electrode techniques or can be calculated from several available formulas. An advantage of measuring the ionized form is that it is unaffected by changes in serum albumin levels. Some physicians consider measurement of ionized calcium more sensitive and reliable than that of total calcium in the detection of primary hyperparathyroidism. Other physicians, however, do not agree. Many laboratories do not have the equipment to perform the ionized calcium assay.

The most common cause of hypercalcemia is hyperparathyroidism. Parathormone (see p. 599) causes elevated calcium levels by increasing gastrointestinal absorption, decreasing urinary excretion, and increasing bone resorption. Malignancy, the second most common cause of hypercalcemia, can cause elevated calcium levels in two main ways. First, tumor metastasis (myeloma, lung, breast, renal cell) to the bone can destroy the bone, causing resorption and pushing calcium into the blood. Second, the cancer (lung, breast, renal cell) can produce a parathyroid hormone–like substance that drives the serum calcium up (ectopic PTH). Excess vitamin D ingestion can increase serum calcium by increasing renal and gastrointestinal absorption. Sarcoidosis, hyperthyroidism, and renal failure can occasionally be associated with elevated calcium levels.

Hypocalcemia occurs in patients with hypoalbuminemia, large blood losses, intestinal malabsorption, renal failure, chronic malnutrition states (alcoholism), rhabdomyolysis, alkalosis, and acute pancreatitis (due to saponification of fat).

Interfering factors

- Vitamin D intoxication may cause *increased* serum calcium levels.
- Excessive ingestion of milk may cause *increased* levels.
- Serum pH can affect calcium values. A decrease in pH causes *increased* calcium levels.
- Prolonged tourniquet time will lower pH and factitiously *increase* calcium levels.
- There is normally a small diurnal variation in calcium, with peak levels occurring around 9 PM.
- Hypoalbuminemia is artifactually associated with *decreased* levels of total calcium.
- Drugs that may cause *increased* levels include calcium salts, hydralazine, lithium, thiazide diuretics, parathyroid hormone (PTH), thyroid hormone, alkaline antacids, Ca salts, ergocalciferol, androgens, and vitamin D.
- Drugs that may cause *decreased* levels include acetazolamide, anticonvulsants, asparaginase, aspirin, calcitonin, cisplatin, corticosteroids, heparin, laxatives, loop diuretics, magnesium salts, diuretics, estrogens, albuterol, and oral contraceptives.

Procedure and patient care

Before
- Explain the procedure to the patient.
- Tell the patient that no fasting is required; however, the se-

rum calcium may be part of a multichemical analysis in
which fasting is required for the other studies.

During

- Collect approximately 7 ml of venous blood in a red-top
  tube. Avoid prolonged tourniquet use.
- List on the laboratory slip any medications that may affect
  test results.

After

- Apply pressure or a pressure dressing to the venipuncture
  site.
- Assess the venipuncture site for bleeding.

Abnormal findings

▲ **Increased levels
(hypercalcemia)**
  Metastatic tumor to the
  bone
  Hyperparathyroidism
  Vitamin D intoxication
  Sarcoidosis
  Milk-alkali syndrome
  Addison's disease
  Paget's disease of bone
  Nonparathyroid PTH–
  producing tumor (e.g.,
  lung or renal carci-
  noma)
  Acromegaly
  Hyperthyroidism

▼ **Decreased values
(hypocalcemia)**
  Hypoparathyroidism
  Renal failure
  Rickets
  Osteomalacia
  Hyperphosphatemia sec-
  ondary to renal failure
  Renal failure
  Vitamin D deficiency
  Malabsorption
  Pancreatitis
  Rhabdomyolysis
  Alkalosis

notes

calcium, urine (Urine calcium, Quantitative calcium)

Type of test Urine (24-hour)

Normal findings Vary with the diet.

Normal diet: 100-300 mg/day or 2.50-7.50 mmol/day (SI units)

Low-calcium diet: 50-150 mg/day or 1.25-3.75 mmol/day (SI units)

Test explanation and related physiology

This quantitative test measures the amount of calcium excreted in the urine within 24 hours. (This test differs from the qualitative Sulkowitch's reagent test, which is rarely performed today.) Excretion of calcium in the urine is increased most commonly in patients with primary hyperparathyroidism, and values are decreased in patients with hypoparathyroidism.

Disagreement exists as to whether the specimen should be collected from the patient who has a normal diet, a normal diet except for milk products, or a controlled diet limited to 100 to 200 mg of calcium. Therefore the reference values vary according to the type of diet.

Interfering factors

✏ Drugs that may *increase* urine calcium levels include antacids, anticonvulsants, carbonic anhydrase inhibitors, diuretics, calcitonin, Ca salts, steroids, mithramycin, and phosphates.

✏ Drugs that may *decrease* urine calcium levels include estrogens, lithium bicarbonates, and oral contraceptives.

Procedure and patient care

Before
- Explain the procedure to the patient.
- Determine the diet regimen recommended by the specific laboratory.
- Give the patient written and oral instructions regarding dietary restrictions.

During
- Begin the 24-hour urine collection after the patient urinates. This is the start time of the collection.
- Discard the first sample.

- Collect all urine passed by the patient during the next 24 hours.
- Post the hours for urine collection in a prominent location.
- Remind the patient to void before defecating so that the urine is not contaminated by feces.
- Instruct the patient not to place toilet paper in the collection container.
- Encourage the patient to drink fluids during the 24 hours, unless this is contraindicated for medical purposes.
- Collect the last specimen as close as possible to the end of the 24 hours.
- Indicate the time the last specimen was collected on the laboratory slip or urine container.
- Store the 24-hour collection in a plastic urine container or an acid-washed glass bottle. Refrigerate the collected urine or keep on ice.
- Note that some laboratories add a preservative to the container to prevent precipitation. Check with the laboratory.
- List on the laboratory slip any medications that may affect test results.

After

- Send the specimen to the laboratory as soon as it is completed.

Abnormal findings

▲ **Increased levels (hypercalciuria)**
Primary hyperparathyroidism
Idiopathic hypercalciuria
Cushing's syndrome
Milk-alkali syndrome
Osteoporosis
Osteolytic bone disease
Renal tubular acidosis
Sarcoidosis
Vitamin D intoxication
Prolonged immobilization

▼ **Decreased values (hypocalciuria)**
Hypoparathyroidism
Vitamin D deficiency
Malabsorption disorder
Renal osteodystrophy

caloric study (Oculovestibular reflex study)

Type of test Electrodiagnostic

Normal findings Nystagmus with irrigation

Test explanation and related physiology

Caloric studies are used to evaluate the vestibular portion of the eighth cranial nerve (CN VIII) by irrigating the external auditory canal with hot or cold water. Normally, stimulation with cold water causes rotary nystagmus (involuntary rapid eye movement) away from the ear being irrigated; hot water induces nystagmus toward the side of the ear being irrigated. If the labyrinth is diseased or the CN VIII is not functioning (e.g., from tumor compression), no nystagmus is induced. This study aids in the differential diagnosis of abnormalities that may occur in the vestibular system, brainstem, or cerebellum. When results are inconclusive, electronystagmography (see p. 349) may be performed.

Contraindications

- Patients with a perforated eardrum
  Cold air may be substituted for the fluid.
- Patients with an acute disease of the labyrinth (e.g., Ménière's syndrome)
  The test can be performed when the acute attack subsides.

Interfering factors

✠ Drugs such as sedatives and antivertigo agents can alter test results.

Procedure and patient care

Before
- Explain the procedure to the patient.
- Hold solid foods before the test to reduce the incidence of vomiting.

During
- Although the exact procedures for caloric studies vary, note the following steps in a typical test:
  1. Before the test, the patient is examined for the presence of nystagmus, postural deviation (Romberg's sign), and past-pointing. This examination provides the baseline values for comparison during the test.

2. The ear canal should be examined and cleaned by a physician before testing to ensure that the water will freely flow to the middle ear area.

3. The ear on the suspected side is irrigated first, because the patient's response may be minimal.

4. After an emesis basin is placed under the ear, the irrigation solution is directed into the external auditory canal until the patient complains of nausea and dizziness, or nystagmus is seen. Usually, this occurs in 20 to 30 seconds.

5. If after 3 minutes no symptoms occur, the irrigation is stopped.

6. The patient is tested again for nystagmus, past-pointing, and Romberg's sign.

7. After approximately 5 minutes, the procedure is repeated on the other side.

- Note that this procedure is usually performed by a physician or technician in approximately 15 minutes.
- Tell the patient that he or she will probably experience nausea and dizziness during the test.

After

- Usually, place the patient on bed rest for approximately 30 to 60 minutes until nausea or vomiting subsides.
- Ensure patient safety related to dizziness.

Abnormal findings

Brainstem inflammation, infarction, or tumor
Cerebellar inflammation, infarction, or tumor
Vestibular or cochlear inflammation or tumor
Acoustic neuroma

notes

carbon dioxide content (CO$_2$ content, CO$_2$ combining power)

Type of test Blood

Normal findings
Adult/elderly: 23-30 mEq/L or 23-30 mmol/L (SI units)
Child: 20-28 mEq/L
Infant: 20-28 mEq/L
Newborn: 13-22 mEq/L

Possible critical values <6 mEq/L

Test explanation and related physiology
The serum CO$_2$ test is usually included with other assessments of electrolytes. This test measures the H$_2$CO$_3$, dissolved CO$_2$, and the bicarbonate ion (HCO$_3^-$) that exists in the serum. Because the amounts of H$_2$CO$_3$ and dissolved CO$_2$ in the blood are so small, CO$_2$ content is a direct measure of HCO$_3^-$ (see p. 147). This anion is second in importance to the chloride ion in electrical neutrality of extracellular and intracellular fluid; its major role is in acid-base balance. Levels of HCO$_3^-$ are regulated by the kidneys. Increases occur with alkalosis, and decreases occur with acidosis.

Interfering factors
- Drugs that may cause *increased* serum CO$_2$ and HCO$_3^-$ levels include aldosterone, barbiturates, bicarbonates, ethacrynic acid, hydrocortisone, loop diuretics, mercurial diuretics, and steroids.
- Drugs that may cause *decreased* levels include methicillin, nitrofurantoin (Furadantin), paraldehyde, phenformin hydrochloride, tetracycline, thiazide diuretics, and triamterene.

Procedure and patient care
Before
- Explain the procedure to the patient.
- Tell the patient that no fasting is required.

During
- Collect approximately 7 to 10 ml of venous blood in a red- or green-top tube.

After
- Apply pressure or a pressure dressing to the venipuncture site.
- Assess the venipuncture site for bleeding.

Abnormal findings

▲ **Increased levels**
Severe diarrhea
Starvation
Severe vomiting
Aldosteronism
Emphysema
Metabolic alkalosis
Gastric suction

▼ **Decreased levels**
Renal failure
Salicylate toxicity
Diabetic ketoacidosis
Metabolic acidosis
Shock

notes

carboxyhemoglobin (COHb, Carbon monoxide)

Type of test Blood

Normal findings

Nonsmoker: <3%
Smoker: ≤12%
Newborn: ≥12%

Possible critical values >20%

20% to 30%: dizziness, headache, disturbances in judgment
30% to 40%: tachycardia, hyperpnea, hypotension, confusion
50% to 60%: coma
>60%: death

Test explanation and related physiology

This test measures the amount of serum COHb, which is formed by the combination of carbon monoxide (CO) and hemoglobin (Hb). CO combines with Hb 200 times more readily than oxygen (O_2) can combine with Hb (oxyhemoglobin). This greater affinity of CO for Hb results in fewer Hb bonds available to combine with O_2 and causes the patient to become hypoxic. CO poisoning is documented by Hb analysis for COHb. A specimen should be drawn as soon as possible after exposure, because CO is rapidly cleared from the Hb by breathing normal air. This test also may be indicated to evaluate patients with complaints of headache, irritability, nausea, vomiting, vertigo, collapse, and coma. Patients exposed to smoke inhalation, exhaust fumes, and fires may be evaluated by this study as well.

Principal sources of CO include tobacco smoke, petroleum and natural gas fuels, automobile exhaust, unvented natural-gas heaters, and defective gas stoves. Continuous exposure to CO can lead to coma and death. The treatment of CO toxicity is administration of high concentrations of O_2.

Procedure and patient care

Before

- Explain the procedure to the patient or the family.
- Obtain the patient history related to any possible source of CO inhalation.
- Assess the patient for signs and symptoms of mild CO toxic-

ity (e.g., headache, weakness, dizziness, malaise, dyspnea) and moderate to severe CO toxicity (e.g., severe headache, bright-red mucous membranes, cherry-red blood). Maintain patient safety precautions if confusion is present.

C

During
- Collect approximately 5 to 10 ml of venous blood in a lavender- or green-top tube.

After
- Apply pressure or a pressure dressing to the venipuncture site.
- Assess the venipuncture site for bleeding.
- Treat the patient as indicated by the physician. Usually, the patient receives high concentrations of O_2.
- Encourage respirations to allow the patient to clear CO from the Hb.

Abnormal finding
Carbon monoxide poisoning

notes

carinoembryonic antigen (CEA)

Type of test Blood

Normal findings <5 ng/ml or 0.0-2.5 μg/L (SI units)

Test explanation and related physiology

The CEA is a protein that normally occurs in fetal gut tissue. By birth, detectable serum levels disappear. In the early 1960s, CEA was found to exist in the bloodstream of adults who had colorectal tumors. Therefore the antigen was thought to be a specific indicator of the presence of colorectal cancer. Subsequently, however, this protein has been found in patients who have a variety of carcinomas (e.g., breast, pancreatic, gastric, hepatobiliary), sarcomas, and even many benign diseases (e.g., ulcerative colitis, diverticulitis, cirrhosis). Chronic smokers also have elevated CEA levels.

Because the CEA level can be elevated in both benign and malignant diseases, it is not considered to be a specific test for colorectal cancer. As a result, CEA is not a reliable screening test for the detection of colorectal cancer in the general population. Its use is limited to determining the prognosis and monitoring the response of tumor to antineoplastic therapy in a patient with cancer. This is especially helpful in patients with breast and gastrointestinal cancers. The CEA level on the initial test is an indicator of tumor burden and prognosis. Smaller and early-staged tumors are likely to have minimal CEA elevations, if not normal CEA levels. A drastic reduction to normal CEA levels is expected with complete eradication of tumor. Therefore this test is used to determine the adequacy of treatment.

This test also is used in the surveillance of patients with cancer. A steadily rising CEA level is occasionally the first sign of tumor recurrence. This makes CEA testing very valuable in the follow-up of patients who have had potentially curative therapy.

It is important to note that many patients with advanced breast or gastrointestinal tumors may not have elevated CEA levels.

Interfering factors

- Smoking
- Benign diseases (e.g., cholecystitis, colitis, diverticulitis)
- Liver diseases (e.g., hepatitis, cirrhosis)

Procedure and patient care

Before

- Explain the procedure to the patient.
- Tell the patient that no fasting is required.

During

- Collect a peripheral blood specimen. The collecting tube varies according to the commercial laboratory. (The two most frequently used laboratories for this test are Abbott Laboratories and Roche Labs.)
- Indicate on the laboratory slip if the patient smokes or has diseases that can affect test results.

After

- Apply pressure or a pressure dressing to the venipuncture site.
- Observe the venipuncture site for bleeding.

Abnormal findings

▲ **Increased levels**

Cancer (gastrointestinal, breast, lung, pancreatic, hepatobiliary)
Inflammation (colitis, cholecystitis, pancreatitis, diverticulitis)

Cirrhosis
Peptic ulcer

notes

cardiac catheterization (Coronary angiography, Angiocardiography, Ventriculography)

Type of test X-ray with contrast dye

Normal findings Normal heart-muscle motion, normal coronary arteries, normal great vessels, and normal intracardiac pressures and volumes

Test explanation and related physiology

Cardiac catheterization is a procedure that allows the heart, great blood vessels, and coronary arteries to be studied. A catheter is passed into the heart through a peripheral vein or artery, depending on whether catheterization of the right or left side of the heart is being performed. Through the catheter, pressures are recorded and radiographic dyes are injected. With the assistance of a computer, cardiac output and other measures of cardiac functions can be determined. Cardiac catheterization is indicated for the following reasons:

1. To identify, locate, and quantitate the severity of atherosclerotic, occlusive coronary artery disease
2. To evaluate the severity of acquired and congenital cardiac valvular or septal defects
3. To determine the presence and the degree of congenital cardiac abnormalities, such as transposition of great vessels, patent ductus arteriosus, and anomalous venous return to the heart
4. To evaluate the success of previous cardiac surgery or balloon angioplasty
5. To evaluate cardiac muscle function
6. To identify and quantify ventricular aneurysms
7. To identify and locate acquired disease of the great vessels, such as atherosclerotic occlusion or aneurysms within the aortic arch
8. To evaluate patients with acute myocardial infarction and to facilitate infusion of thrombolytic agents into the occluded coronary arteries
9. To insert a catheter to monitor right-sided heart pressures, such as pulmonary artery and pulmonary wedge pressures (Table 6 provides pressures and volumes used in cardiac monitoring.)
10. To perform dilation of stenotic coronary arteries (angio-

plasty), to place coronary artery stents, or to perform laser atherectomy

Cardiac catheterization is performed under sterile conditions. In right-sided heart catheterization, usually the subclavian, brachial, or femoral vein is used for vascular access. In left-sided heart catheterization, usually the right femoral artery is cannulated; alternatively, however, the brachial or radial artery may be chosen. As the catheter is placed into the great vessels of the heart chamber, pressures are monitored and recorded. Blood samples for analysis of O_2 content are also obtained. The catheter is advanced with appropriate guidance into the desired position. After pressures are obtained, angiographic visualization of the heart chambers, valves, and coronary arteries is achieved with the injection of radiographic dye.

Transluminal coronary angioplasty is a therapeutic procedure that can be performed during coronary angiography in medical centers where open heart surgery is available. During this procedure, a specific, specially designed balloon catheter is introduced into the coronary arteries and placed across the stenotic area of the coronary artery. This area can then be dilated by controlled inflation of the balloon. The coronary arteriogram is then repeated to document the effects of the forceful dilation of the stenotic area. Coronary arterial stents can be placed at the site of previous stenosis after angioplasty and maintain patency for longer periods of time. Likewise, laser atherectomy of coronary arterial plaques can be performed to more permanently open hard, atheromatous plaques.

Contraindications

- Patients who are unable to cooperate during the test
- Patients who would refuse intervention if an amenable lesion were found
- Patients with an iodine dye allergy who have not received preventive medication for allergy
- Patients who are pregnant, because of radiation exposure to the fetus
- Patients with renal disorders, because iodinated contrast is nephrotoxic
- Patients with a bleeding propensity

Potential complications

- Cardiac arrhythmias (dysrhythmias)
- Perforation of the heart myocardium

TABLE 6 Pressures and volumes used in cardiac monitoring

	Description	Normal values
Pressures		
Routine blood pressure	Routine brachial artery pressure	90-140/60-90 mm Hg
Systolic left ventricular pressure	Peak pressure in the left ventricle during systole	90-140 mm Hg
End-diastolic left ventricular pressure	Pressure in the left ventricle at the end of diastole	4-12 mm Hg
Central venous pressure	Pressure in the superior vena cava	2-14 cm H_2O
Pulmonary wedge pressure	Pressure in the pulmonary venules, an indirect measurement of left atrial pressure and left ventricular end-diastolic pressure	Left atrial: 6-15 mm Hg
Pulmonary artery pressure	Pressure in the pulmonary artery	15-28/5-16 mm Hg
Aortic artery pressure	Same as routine blood pressure	

Volumes

End-diastolic volume (EDV)	Amount of blood present in the left ventricle at the end of diastole	50-90 ml/m^2
End-systolic volume (ESV)	Amount of blood present in the left ventricle at the end of systole	25 ml/m^2
Stroke volume (SV)	Amount of blood ejected from the heart in one contraction (SV = EDV − ESV)	45 ± 12 ml/m^2
Ejection fraction (EF)	Proportion (fraction) of EDV ejected from the left ventricle during systole (EF = SV/EDV)	0.67 ± 0.07
Cardiac output (CO)	Amount of blood ejected by the heart in 1 minute	3-6 L/min
Cardiac index (CI)	Amount of blood ejected by the heart in 1 minute per square meter of body surface area (CI = CO/body surface area)	2.8-4.2 L/min/m^2 for a patient with 1.5 m^2 of body surface area

- Catheter-induced embolic stroke (cerebrovascular accident) or myocardial infarction
- Complications associated with the catheter insertion site, such as arterial thrombosis, embolism, or pseudoaneurysm
- Allergic reactions to iodinated dye
  These vary from flushing, itching, and urticaria to severe, life-threatening anaphylaxis (evidenced by respiratory distress, drop in blood pressure, shock). In the event of anaphylaxis the patient is treated with diphenhydramine (Benadryl), steroids, and epinephrine. Oxygen and endotracheal equipment should be on hand for immediate use.
- Infection at the catheter insertion site
- Pneumothorax following subclavian vein catheterization of the right side of the heart

Procedure and patient care

Before
- Explain the procedure to the patient.
- Obtain written permission from the fully informed patient.
- Allay the patient's fears and anxieties regarding this test. Although this test creates tremendous fear in a patient, it is performed often, and complications are rare.
- Instruct the patient to abstain from oral intake for at least 4 to 8 hours before the test.
- Prepare the catheter insertion site by shaving and scrubbing the skin.
- Determine whether the patient has an iodine dye allergy. If so, Benadryl and steroids should be provided several days before the test if possible. Also, non-ionic iodine contrast dye should be used during the test.
- Mark the patient's peripheral pulses with a pen before catheterization. This will facilitate postcatheterization assessment of the pulses at the affected and nonaffected extremities.
- Provide appropriate precatheterization sedation as ordered by the physician.
- Instruct the patient to void before going to the catheterization laboratory.
- Remove all valuables and dental prostheses before transporting the patient to the catheterization laboratory.
- Obtain IV access for delivery of IV fluids and cardiac drugs if necessary.

During

- Take the patient to the cardiac catheterization lab.
- Note the following procedural steps:
  1. The chosen catheter insertion site is prepared and draped in a sterile manner.
  2. The desired vessel is punctured with a needle.
  3. A wire is placed through the needle and into the catheter.
  4. The angiographic catheter is threaded on top of the wire.
  5. Once the catheter is in the desired location, the appropriate cardiac pressures and volumes are measured.
  6. Cardiac ventriculography is performed with controlled injection of contrast.
  7. Each coronary artery is catheterized. Cardiac angiography is then carried out with a controlled injection of contrast material.
  8. During the injection, x-ray films are rapidly made.
  9. The patient's vital signs must be monitored constantly during this procedure.
  10. If *angioplasty* is performed, the cardiologist appropriately places the catheter and balloon at the stenotic area. Note the following procedural steps:
      a. As the EKG tracing is observed, the balloon is inflated and the stenotic areas are forcefully dilated.
      b. If signs of myocardial ischemia develop, the balloon is immediately deflated.
      c. Usually, inflation of the balloon is continued only for a few seconds.
  11. After obtaining all the required information, the catheter is removed.
- Note that this test is usually performed by a cardiologist in approximately 1 hour.
- Tell the patient that during the injection he or she may experience a severe hot flush. This is uncomfortable but lasts only 10 to 15 seconds.
- Note that some patients have a tendency to cough as the catheter is placed into the pulmonary artery.
- Verbally support the patient as the x-ray films are taken, because the possibly loud noises may frighten the patient.

After

- Monitor the patient's vital signs.
- Apply pressure to the site of vascular access.

- Keep the patient on bed rest for 4 to 8 hours to allow for complete sealing of the arterial puncture.
- Keep the affected extremity extended and immobilized with sandbags to decrease bleeding.
- Assess the puncture site for signs of bleeding, hematoma, or absence of pulse.
- Assess the patient's pulses of both extremities. Compare with preprocedural baseline values.
- Encourage the patient to drink fluids to maintain adequate hydration. Dehydration may be caused by the diuretic action of the dye.
- Evaluate the patient for delayed reaction to the dye (dyspnea, rashes, tachycardia, hives). This usually occurs within the first 2 to 6 hours after the test. Treat with antihistamines or steroids.
- Instruct the patient that the test will be reviewed by the cardiologist and the results will be available in 1 or 2 days.

Abnormal findings

Anatomic variation of the cardiac chambers and great vessels

Coronary artery occlusive disease

Ventricular aneurysm

Ventricular mural thrombi

Intracardiac tumor

Aortic root arteriosclerotic or aneurysmal disease

Anomalies in pulmonary venous return

Acquired or congenital septal defects and valvular abnormalities

Pulmonary emboli

Pulmonary hypertension

notes

cardiac exercise stress testing (Stress testing; Exercise testing; Electrocardiograph [EKG] stress testing, exercise testing)

Type of test Electrodiagnostic

Normal findings Patient able to obtain and maintain maximal heart rate of 85% for predicted age and gender with no cardiac symptoms or EKG change

Test explanation and related physiology

Exercise stress testing is a noninvasive study that provides information about the patient's cardiac function. During stress testing, the EKG, heart rate, and blood pressure are monitored while the patient engages in some type of physical activity (stress). Two methods of stress testing include pedaling a stationary bike and walking on a treadmill. With the stationary bicycle, the pedaling tension is slowly increased to increase the heart rate. With the treadmill test, the speed and grade of incline are increased. The treadmill test is the most frequently used, because it is the most easily standardized and reproducible.

The usual goal of the testing is to increase the heart rate to just below maximal levels or to the "target heart rate." Usually, this target heart rate is 80% to 90% of the maximal heart rate. The test is usually discontinued if the patient reaches that target heart rate or develops any symptoms or EKG changes. The maximal heart rate is determined by a chart that takes into account the patient's age and gender. The normal maximal heart rate for adults varies from 150 to 200 beats/min; patients taking calcium channel blockers and sympathetic blockers have a lower-than-expected maximal heart rate.

Exercise stress testing is based on the principle that occluded arteries will be unable to meet the heart's increased demand for blood during the testing. This may become obvious with symptoms (e.g., chest pain, fatigue, dyspnea, tachycardia, cardiac arrhythmias [dysrhythmias], fall in blood pressure) or EKG changes (e.g., ST-segment variance >1 mm, increasing premature ventricular contractions or other rhythm disturbances). An advantage of stress testing is that these symptoms can be stimulated and identified in a safe environment.

The indications for stress testing are:
1. To evaluate chest pain in a patient suspected of having coronary disease (Occasionally, a person may have signifi-

cant coronary stenosis that is not apparent during normal physical activity. If, however, the pain can be reproduced with exercise, one may infer that coronary occlusion is present.)

2. To determine the limits of safe exercise during a cardiac rehabilitation program or to assist patients with cardiac disease in maintaining good physical fitness
3. To detect labile or exercise-related hypertension
4. To detect intermittent claudication in patients with suspected vascular occlusive disease in the extremities (In this situation, the patient may experience leg muscle cramping while performing the exercise.)
5. To evaluate the effectiveness of treatment in patients who take antianginal or antiarrhythmic medications
6. To evaluate the effectiveness of cardiac intervention (such as bypass grafting or angioplasty)

When exercise testing is not advisable or the patient is unable to exercise to a level adequate to stress the heart, *dipyridamole-thallium scanning* can be substituted for cardiac stress testing. This may be referred to as *chemical stress testing*. Dipyridamole (Persantine) is a coronary vasodilator that simulates the exercise portion of nuclear stress testing. If one coronary artery is significantly occluded, a discrepancy in the coronary blood flow exists and can be visualized on the thallium gamma-detector scanning camera. This discrepancy is accentuated because the dipyridamole-induced vascular dilation steals the blood from the ischemic areas and diverts it to the open, dilated coronary vessels. Caution must be taken, however, because this can precipitate angina or myocardial infarction. This test should be performed only with a cardiologist in attendance. IV aminophylline can reverse the effect of dipyridamole. This scanning technique is usually performed on patients with an orthopedic, arthritic, neurologic, or pulmonary limitation that precludes thallium stress testing.

Another type of chemical testing is called a *dobutamine stress echocardiogram*. This entails administration of progressively greater amounts of dobutamine over 3-minute intervals. An echocardiogram is then performed to detect the induction of cardiac wall motion abnormalities.

A third method of chemical stress testing uses *adenosine*. Uses and indications for adenosine are similar to those of dipyridamole (Persantine), which is described above.

Contraindications

- Patients with unstable angina
- Patients with severe aortic valvular heart disease
- Patients who cannot participate in an exercise program because of their impaired lung or motor function
- Patients who have recently had a myocardial infarction
  In this case, however, limited stress testing can be done.
- Patients with severe congestive heart failure
- Patients who have severe claudication and cannot walk adequately to stress their hearts

Potential complications

- Fatal cardiac arrhythmias
- Severe angina
- Myocardial infarction
- Fainting

Interfering factors

- Heavy meals before testing can divert blood to the gastrointestinal tract.
- Nicotine from smoking can cause coronary artery spasm.
- Medical problems such as left ventricular hypertrophy, hypertension, valvular heart disease (especially of the aortic valve), left bundle-branch block, severe anemia, hypoxemia, and chronic pulmonary disease can affect results.
- ⚕ Drugs that can affect test results include beta-blockers (e.g., propranolol [Inderal]), calcium channel blockers, digoxin, and nitroglycerine.

Procedure and patient care

Before
- Explain the procedure to the patient.
- Instruct the patient to abstain from eating, drinking, and smoking for 4 hours.
- Inform the patient about the risks of the test and obtain informed consent.
- Instruct the patient to bring comfortable clothing and shoes in which to exercise. Slippers are not acceptable.
- Inform the patient if any medications should be discontinued before testing.
- Obtain a pretest EKG.
- Record the patient's vital signs for baseline values.
- Apply and secure appropriate EKG electrodes.

During

- Note that a physician usually is present during stress testing.
- After the patient begins to exercise, adjust the treadmill machine settings to apply increasing levels of stress at specific intervals. It is helpful to encourage and support the patient at each level of increased stress.
- Encourage patients to verbalize any symptoms.
- Note that during the test, the EKG tracing and vital signs are monitored continuously.
- Terminate the test if the patient complains of chest pain, exhaustion, dyspnea, fatigue, or dizziness.
- Note that testing usually takes approximately 45 minutes.
- Inform the patient that the physician in attendance usually interprets the results and will explain them to the patient.

After

- Place the patient in the supine position to rest after the test.
- Monitor the EKG tracing and record vital signs at poststress intervals, until recordings and values return to pretest levels.
- Remove electrodes and paste.

Abnormal findings

Coronary artery occlusive disease

Exercise-related hypertension

Intermittent claudication

Abnormal cardiac rhythms—stress induced

notes

cardiac nuclear scanning (Myocardial scan, Cardiac scan, Nuclear cardiac scanning, Heart scan, Thallium scan, MUGA scan, Isonitrile scan, Sestamibi scan)

Type of test Nuclear scan

Normal findings Normal myocardial ejection fraction and coronary perfusion

Test explanation and related physiology

Cardiac radionuclear scanning is a noninvasive and safe method of recognizing alterations of left ventricular muscle function and coronary artery blood distribution. Many different radiocompound materials can be used, most often technetium-99m pertechnetate, thallium-201, or technetium-99m pyrophosphate. When these compounds are injected intravenously and a radiation detector is placed over the heart, an image of the heart can be recorded and photographed.

In evaluating the patency of the coronary arteries, the characteristic abnormality varies according to the type of radiocompound used. When thallium is used, all normal myocardial cells take up the substance and appear on the photoscan. Ischemic or infarcted cells do not take up the substance and appear as "cold spots," devoid of nuclear material and surrounded by normal cells. Technetium pyrophosphate, however, is taken up only by the ischemic or infarcted cells. Therefore an acute myocardial infarction will show up as a "hot spot" on this type of cardiac photoscan. Technetium Sestamibi (isonitrile) is an even better cardiac imaging agent. Higher-quality images can be obtained on the first pass, providing information similar to angiocardiography. Perfusion images, ventricular function, and gated-pool ejection fractions (GPEFs) can all be obtained with a single injection.

For an evaluation of myocardial function, technetium pertechnetate or technetium-labeled albumin is used to measure the portion of blood ejected from the ventricle. Normally, over 65% of the blood is ejected from the ventricle during systole. Values less than that indicate decreased contractility of the heart caused by ischemia or infarction or by cardiomyopathy. Computers can be synchronized with the electrocardiogram (EKG) during scanning. This computer-assisted *gated* (synchronized) cardiac scan

can allow the myocardial wall to be photographed while in motion. This allows visualization of the myocardium during several cardiac cycles, and contractility of the myocardium can be determined. Furthermore, the amount of blood ejected during systole also can be calculated. This form of determination of ventricular function is called *gated pool imaging* or the *gated pool ejection fraction. Multigated acquisition* (MUGA) *scan* is another name for this test based on the name of the computer machinery originally required. These imaging techniques can provide the same information as radiographic ventriculography, which is performed during cardiac catheterization (see p. 196); however, the nuclear scans are noninvasive and much safer.

Thallium also can be used to assess myocardial ischemia during stress testing (see p. 203). In some cases, no evidence of diminished blood supply to the myocardium is evident during the resting state. When stressed, however, evidence of myocardial ischemia can become quite obvious and is easily detected by *thallium stress testing*. In this form of nuclear cardiac scanning, thallium-201 is injected intravenously during exercise stress testing. The thallium accumulates in the myocardium in direct proportion to the regional myocardial blood flow. The normal myocardium will have much greater thallium activity than the ischemic myocardium. In comparing this stress testing with a resting thallium scan, one can see exercise-induced ischemia. This is called *exercise stress testing with thallium scanning,* or *thallium stress testing.* This test is not only beneficial in detecting coronary occlusive disease, but is also successful in assessing postoperative patency of a coronary bypass graft.

Like thallium, isonitrile (Sestamibi) is also used during stress testing. For this form of nuclear cardiac scanning, Isonitrile is injected and the patient is scanned at rest and at a later time after cardiac stress testing.

Single-photon emission computed tomography (SPECT) has been used to visualize the heart from several different angles. These images are then reconstructed using tomographic techniques, and three-dimensional images of the physiologic cardiac processes are obtained. Areas of myocardial ischemia can be seen with far greater resolution and accurately quantified.

Specific indications for cardiac nuclear scanning include:
1. Screening of adults for past and recent infarction
2. Evaluation of patients with chest pain and uninterpretable or equivocal EKG changes caused by drugs, bundle-branch block, or left ventricular hypertrophy

3. Evaluation of myocardial perfusion before and after coronary artery bypass surgery
4. Quantification and surveillance of myocardial infarction
5. Evaluation of medical and surgical therapy for coronary artery perfusion
6. Evaluation of ventricular function in patients with myocardial disease
7. Evaluation of patients receiving cardiotoxic drugs (e.g., adriamycin chemotherapy)

Contraindications

- Patients who are uncooperative
- Patients who are pregnant, because of fetal exposure to radionuclide material

Interfering factors

- Myocardial trauma
- Recent nuclear scans (e.g., thyroid or bone scan)
- Drugs such as long-acting nitrates

Procedure and patient care

Before

- Explain the procedure to the patient.
- Instruct the patient that a short fasting period may be required.

During

- Take the patient to the nuclear medicine department.
- Note the following procedural steps:
  1. An IV injection of radionuclide material is performed.
  2. Depending on the radionuclide used, scanning is performed 15 minutes to 4 hours later.
  3. A gamma ray detector is placed over the precordium.
  4. The patient is placed in a supine position, then in the lateral position, and then in both the right and left oblique positions.
  5. The gamma-ray scanner records the image of the heart, and a photograph is immediately developed.
  6. For a *thallium exercise stress test,* radioactive thallium is injected during exercise when the patient reaches a maximum heart rate. The patient then lies on a table, and scanning is done. A repeat scan may be done 3 to 4 hours later.
  7. If an *isonitrile stress test* is needed, the patient is injected

and scanned 30 to 60 minutes later for the resting phase. Four hours later, cardiac stress testing is done. After a second injection, scanning is repeated. Milk and a muffin are usually given after each isonitrile injection to facilitate clearing of the radionuclide from the hepatobiliary system.

- Tell the patient that the only discomfort associated with this test is the venipuncture required for injection of the radioisotope.
- Note that myocardial scans are usually performed in less than 30 minutes by a nuclear medicine technician.

After

- Because only tracer doses of radioisotopes are used, note that no precautions need to be taken against radioactive exposure to personnel or family.
- Encourage the patient to drink fluids to aid in the excretion of the radioactive substance.
- Apply pressure or a pressure dressing to the venipuncture site.
- Assess the venipuncture site for bleeding.
- If stress testing was performed, evaluate the patient's vital signs at frequent intervals (as indicated).

Abnormal findings

Coronary artery occlusive disease
Decreased myocardial function associated with ischemia, myocarditis, cardiomyopathy, or congestive heart failure

notes

carotid duplex scanning

Type of test Ultrasound

Normal findings Carotid artery free of plaques and stenosis

Test explanation and related physiology

Carotid duplex scanning is a noninvasive, ultrasound test used on the extracranial carotid artery to detect occlusive disease directly. The duplex concept is based on the ability to define the carotid artery walls within a two-dimensional image and uses a pulse Doppler probe to evaluate flow velocities within the artery. This technique can measure the amplitude and the waveform of the carotid arterial pulse. Furthermore, a two-dimensional image of the carotid artery can be produced. As a result, one can directly visualize possibly stenotic or occluded arteries and the arterial flow disruption.

Procedure and patient care

Before
- Explain the procedure to the patient.
- Tell the patient that no special preparation is required.
- Assure the patient that the study is painless.

During
- Place the patient in the supine position with the head supported to prevent lateral motion.
- Note the following procedural steps:
  1. A water-soluble gel is used to couple the sound from the transducer to the skin surface.
  2. Images of the carotid artery and pulse waveform are obtained.
- Note that this test is performed by an ultrasound technologist in the ultrasound or radiology department in approximately 15 to 30 minutes.
- Tell the patient that no discomfort is associated with this test.

After
- Remove the water-soluble gel from the patient.

Abnormal finding

Carotid artery occlusive disease

ceruloplasmin (Cp)

Type of test Blood

Normal findings
Adults: 23-43 mg/dl
Neonates: 2-13 mg/dl

Test explanation and related physiology

Ceruloplasmin is an alpha$_2$-globulin that binds copper for transport within the circulation after it is absorbed from the gastrointestinal tract. It is an acute-phase reactant that becomes elevated during stress, infection, and pregnancy. However, it rises more slowly than other acute-phase reactants, such as C-reactive protein and erythrocyte sedimentation rate.

Ceruloplasmin is decreased in most instances of Wilson's disease, which is an inherited disorder with inappropriately high unbound copper levels toxic to the body. The copper is deposited in the eye, brain, liver, and kidney. Wilson's disease is fatal unless early treatment is instituted. Because of this, Cp levels are evaluated in teenagers and young adults with hepatitis, cirrhosis, or recurrent neuromuscular incoordination to allow for early detection of Wilson's disease. Early detection is important, because effective therapy is possible in most cases.

Interfering factors

- Values are increased during pregnancy.
- Drugs that may cause *increased* levels include estrogen, birth control pills, tamoxifen, methadone, and phenytoin.

Procedure and patient care

Before
- Explain the procedure to the patient.
- Tell the patient that no fasting is required.

During
- Collect venous blood in a red-top tube.
- Keep the specimen on ice.

After
- Apply pressure or a pressure dressing to the venipuncture site.
- Assess the venipuncture site for bleeding.

- Medical follow-up and genetic counseling are indicated when Wilson's disease is confirmed.

Abnormal findings

▲ **Increased levels**
Pregnancy
Thyrotoxicosis
Cancer
Acute inflammatory reactions (e.g., infection, rheumatoid arthritis)
Biliary cirrhosis
Copper intoxication

▼ **Decreased levels**
Wilson's disease
Normal infants (<6 months)
Nephrotic syndrome
Sprue
Kwashiorkor
Menkes' (kinky-hair) syndrome
Hyperalimentation

notes

cervical mucus test (Fern test)

Type of test Fluid analysis

Normal findings Arborization, or ferning, of cervical mucus during midcycle

Test explanation and related physiology

The cervical mucus can be examined near midcycle and just before menstruation to detect ovulation. Because pregnancy is impossible without ovulation, this study is used in the evaluation of infertility to predict the day of ovulation and to determine whether ovulation occurs.

At ovulation, the cervical mucus is clear, abundant, watery, and elastic. This elasticity, or *spinnbarkheit* (Figure 6), increases at ovulation. Excellent spinnbarkheit occurs when the mucus can be stretched at least 5 to 6 cm.

When the cervical mucus is spread on a clean glass slide and allowed to dry, a pattern of "arborization" or "ferning" occurs. This is caused by the increased levels of salt and water interact-

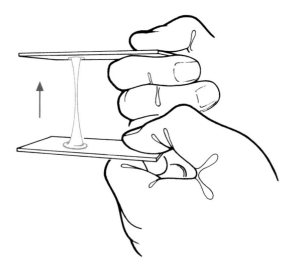

Figure 6 Spinnbarkheit (elasticity) of the cervical mucus increases at ovulation.

ing with the glycoproteins in the mucus during ovulation. This pattern is correlated with estrogen activity and is therefore present in all ovulatory women at midcycle. When the cervical mucus is checked again immediately before menstruation, no ferning is found because of progesterone activity. Therefore, during a normal ovulatory cycle, the ferning of cervical mucus will occur at midcycle and no ferning will occur before menstruation.

Besides its absence in anovulatory premenopausal patients, ferning of the cervical mucus is also absent in postmenopausal, castrated, or normally pregnant women. This is because of the presence of fern-inhibiting progesterone.

Interfering factors

- Slides cleaned with tap water may produce false ferning. The slides used for the mucus must be washed in distilled water.
- Cervical trauma during this procedure may cause blood to mix with the mucus and inhibit ferning.

Procedure and patient care

Before
- Explain the procedure to the patient.
- Tell the patient that no fasting or sedation is required.

During
- Note that this procedure is performed at midcycle to detect estrogen-induced ferning and is repeated approximately 7 days later to detect the progesterone inhibition of ferning.
- Note the following procedural steps:
  1. The patient is placed in the lithotomy position.
  2. A nonlubricated speculum is inserted into the vagina to expose the cervix.
  3. A cotton-tipped applicator is gently inserted into the cervical canal and rotated.
  4. The mucus that adheres to the cotton swab is spread on the clean glass slide and allowed to dry at room temperature. No staining is used.
  5. The dried spread of mucus is examined under the low-power lens of a microscope for the presence of ferning.
- Note that this procedure is performed by a physician in approximately 15 minutes.

- Tell the patient that the only discomfort associated with this study is the insertion of the speculum.

After

- Inform the patient that she is usually given the results immediately after the test.

Abnormal findings

Infertility
Pregnancy

notes

chest tomography (Tomogram, Tomography of the lung)

Type of test X-ray

Normal findings Normal lungs and surrounding structures

Test explanation and related physiology

Tomography is a radiographic examination in which a sequence of x-ray films, each representing a "slice" of the lung at different depths, is taken. Usually, the slices are made 0.5 to 1.0 cm apart throughout the organ being studied. Tomography permits examination of a single layer or plane of tissue that would otherwise be obscured by surrounding tissue on an ordinary film.

For tomography, the x-ray tube and film cassette are rapidly moved in opposite directions while the x-ray film is taken. This technique effectively blurs all the tissue planes except that plane, or slice, being studied.

Tomography is often a helpful adjunct to a routine chest x-ray examination for several reasons:

1. It may reveal properties of a lung lesion (e.g., cavitation, tumor margins) that are normally not seen on chest x-ray films.
2. It provides better visualization of many structures (e.g., the hilus, trachea, mediastinum) that are not clearly seen on a routine chest x-ray film.
3. It may demonstrate many small lesions (e.g., in metastasis) that are not normally seen on a routine chest x-ray film.

Indications for chest tomography have greatly decreased since the advent of computed tomography (CT) of the chest (see p. 269).

Contraindications

- Patients who are pregnant

Interfering factors

- Conditions (e.g., severe pain) that prevent the patient from taking and holding a deep breath

Procedure and patient care

Before

- Explain the procedure to the patient.

- Tell the patient that no fasting is required.
- Instruct the patient to put on an x-ray gown.
- Instruct the patient to remove all metal objects (e.g., necklaces, pins) so that they do not block visualization of part of the chest.
- Tell the patient that he or she will be asked to take a deep breath and hold it while x-ray films are being taken.
- Instruct men to ensure that their testicles are covered, and women to have their ovaries covered, with a lead shield to prevent radiation-induced abnormalities.

During

- Take the nonfasting patient to the radiology department as for a routine chest x-ray film.
- Note the following procedural steps:
  1. With the patient remaining completely still, an x-ray tube is rapidly moved back and forth while the film is rapidly moved in the opposite direction. Excursion of this movement regulates the plane of tissues photographed.
  2. Prone and supine positions may be required.
- Tell the patient that he or she will be unable to detect the fine, synchronized movements of the x-ray tube and film.
- Note that a radiologist performs this test in approximately 15 minutes.
- Tell the patient that no discomfort is associated with chest tomography.

After

- Note that no special care is required following the test.

Abnormal findings

Lung tumor	Bronchiectasis
Tuberculosis	Bronchial occlusion
Lung abscess	Granuloma

notes

chest x-ray (CXR, Chest radiography)

Type of test X-ray

Normal findings Normal lungs and surrounding structures

Test explanation and related physiology

The chest x-ray film is important in the complete evaluation of the pulmonary and cardiac systems. This procedure is often part of the general admission screening workup in adult patients. Much information can be provided by the chest x-ray film. One can identify or follow (by repeated chest x-ray films) the following:

1. Tumors of the lung (primary and metastatic), heart (myxoma), chest wall (soft-tissue sarcomas), and bony thorax (osteogenic sarcoma)
2. Inflammation of the lung (pneumonia), pleura (pleuritis), and pericardium (pericarditis)
3. Fluid accumulation in the pleura (pleural effusion), pericardium (pericardial effusion), and lung (pulmonary edema)
4. Air accumulation in the lung (chronic obstructive pulmonary disease) and pleura (pneumothorax)
5. Fractures of the bones of the thorax or vertebrae
6. Diaphragmatic hernia
7. Heart size, which may vary depending on cardiac function
8. Calcification, which may indicate large-vessel deterioration or old lung granulomas
9. Location of centrally placed intravenous access devices

Most chest x-ray films are taken at a distance of 6 feet, with the patient standing. The sitting or supine position also can be used, but x-ray films taken with the patient in the supine position will not demonstrate fluid levels. A *posteroanterior* (PA) view, with the x-rays passing through the back of the body (posterior) to the front of the body (anterior), is taken first. Then, a *lateral* view, with the x-rays passing through the patient's side, is taken.

Oblique views may be taken with the patient turned at different angles as the x-rays pass through the body. *Lordotic* views provide visualization of the apices (rounded upper portions) of the lungs and are usually used for detection of tuberculosis. *Decubitus* films are taken with the patient in the recumbent lateral position to localize fluid, which becomes dependent within the pleural space (pleural effusion).

Chest x-ray studies are best performed in the radiology department. Studies using a portable x-ray machine may be done at the bedside and are often performed on critically ill patients who cannot leave the nursing unit.

Contraindications

- Patients who are pregnant

Interfering factors

- Conditions (e.g., severe pain) that prevent the patient from taking and holding a deep breath

Procedure and patient care

Before

- Explain the procedure to the patient.
- Tell the patient that no fasting is required.
- Instruct the patient to remove clothing to the waist and to put on an x-ray gown.
- Inform the patient to remove all metal objects (e.g., necklaces, pins) so that they do not block visualization of part of the chest.
- Tell the patient that he or she will be asked to take a deep breath and hold it while the x-ray films are taken.
- Instruct men to ensure that their testicles are covered, and women to have their ovaries covered, with a lead shield to prevent radiation-induced abnormalities.

During

- After the patient is correctly positioned, tell him or her to take a deep breath and hold it until the x-ray films are taken.
- Note that x-ray films are taken by a radiologic technologist in several minutes.
- Inform the patient that no discomfort is associated with chest radiography.

After

- Note that no special care is required following the procedure.

Abnormal findings

Lung tumor
Myxoma
Pneumonia
Pleuritis
Pericarditis
Pleural effusion
Pericardial effusion
Pulmonary edema
Chronic obstructive pulmonary disease

Soft tissue sarcoma
Osteogenic sarcoma
Pneumothorax
Fracture
Diaphragmatic hernia
Atelectasis
Tuberculosis
Lung abscess
Scoliosis
Aortic calcinosis

notes

Chlamydia

Type of test Microscopic examination or blood test

Normal findings

Negative culture
Antibodies: Immunoglobulin test ≤1:640

Test explanation and related physiology

There are many *Chlamydia* species that cause various diseases within the human body. *Chlamydia psittaci* causes respiratory tract infections and occurs with close contact with infected birds. *C. pneumoniae,* another species, causes pneumonia. *C. trachomatis* infection is probably the most frequently occurring sexually transmitted disease in developed countries. Infections of the genitalia are most common, followed by those of the conjunctiva, pharynx, urethra, and rectum. Lymphogranuloma venereum was the first form of venereal disease recognized as a *C. trachomatis* infection; this infection is very common in central Africa. The second serotype of *C. trachomatis* causes the eye disease *trachoma,* which is the most common form of preventable blindness. A third serotype produces genital and urethral infections different from lymphogranuloma. This later type is transmitted by direct contact of the infant with the mother's cervix during vaginal delivery or by direct contact during sexual activity.

Chlamydia infection is thought to be the most prevalent sexually transmitted disease in the United States. This disease is most prevalent in those younger than 20 years, in nulliparas, and in users of nonbarrier contraceptive methods. Also, in those with multiple or recent, new sexual partners, *Chlamydia* is frequently associated with gonorrhea.

Most women colonized with *Chlamydia* are asymptomatic. *Chlamydia* may be associated with cases of pelvic inflammatory disease, particularly in adolescents.

In recognition of the rapidly increasing prevalence of *Chlamydia,* strategies to monitor prevalence, control its spread, and educate the public have been proposed. These strategies include screening all at-risk groups, particularly sexually active adolescents and those with other sexually transmitted disease, for disease. Evaluation of those with signs and symptoms of exposure, as well as potential treatment of all females at high risk for *Chlamydia* disease, has also been proposed.

The *Chlamydia* organism can be detected in many different ways. It seems to be most accurately demonstrated by tissue culture. Although these cultures require a special cell culture line, which takes several days, they are used as the gold standard against which other methods of detection of *Chlamydia* are measured. It is now possible to detect the antigen by direct fluorescent antibody slide staining and enzyme-linked immunosorbent assay (ELISA) technique. These newer techniques are less expensive and more widely available than culture techniques; however, their sensitivity and specificity are lower.

Invasive infection with *C. trachomatis* does produce an immunogenic response. Therefore *Chlamydia* antibodies can be measured using complement fixation, microimmunofluorescence, and ELISA techniques. When a fourfold rise in IgG titer or the presence of specific IgM antibodies is documented, *Chlamydia* disease may be diagnosed.

Interfering factors

- Women presently having their routine menses.
- Patients undergoing antibiotic therapy.

Procedure and patient care

Before

- Explain the procedure to the patient.
- Note that many different methods are used to perform chlamydial tests.

During

- Collect venous blood in a red-top tube.
- Acute and convalescent serum should be drawn 2 to 3 weeks apart.
- A conjunctival smear is obtained by swabbing the eye lesion with a cotton-tipped applicator or scraping with a sterile ophthalmic spatula and smearing on a clean glass slide.
- Sputum cultures (see p. 763) are used to check for *C. psittaci* respiratory infections.
- Note the following procedural steps for *cervical culture:*
  1. The female patient should refrain from douching and bathing in a tub before the cervical culture is performed.
  2. The patient is placed in the lithotomy position.

3. A nonlubricated vaginal speculum is inserted to expose the cervix.
4. The mucus is removed from the squamocolumnar junction of the cervix.
5. A sterile, cotton-tipped swab is inserted into the endocervical canal and moved from side to side for 30 seconds to obtain the culture.
- Note the following procedural steps for *urethral culture:*
  1. The urethral specimen should be obtained from the man before voiding.
  2. A culture is taken by inserting a sterile thin swab gently into the urethra for about 3 to 4 cm.
- Note that these tests are performed by a physician or nurse in several minutes.
- Tell the patient that minimal discomfort is associated with these procedures.

After

- Treat patients who have positive smears with antibiotics.
- Tell affected patients to have their sexual partners examined.

Abnormal findings

Chlamydia infections

notes

chloride, blood (Cl)

Type of test Blood

Normal findings

Adult/elderly: 90-110 mEq/L or 98-106 mmol/L (SI units)
Child: 90-110 mEq/L
Newborn: 96-106 mEq/L
Premature infant: 95-110 mEq/L

Possible critical values <80 or >115 mEq/L

Test explanation and related physiology

Chloride is the major extracellular anion. Its main purpose is to maintain electrical neutrality, mostly as a salt with sodium. It follows sodium losses and accompanies sodium excesses, thus affecting water balance. Chloride also serves as a buffer to assist in acid-base balance. As carbon dioxide increases, bicarbonate moves from the intracellular space to the extracellular space. To maintain electrical neutrality, chloride will shift back into the cell.

Hypochloremia and hyperchloremia rarely occur alone and usually parallel shifts in sodium levels (see p. 754). Signs and symptoms of hypochloremia include hyperexcitability of the nervous system and muscles, shallow breathing, hypotension, and tetany. Signs and symptoms of hyperchloremia include lethargy, weakness, and deep breathing.

Interfering factors

- Drugs that may cause *increased* serum chloride levels include acetazolamide, ammonium chloride, androgens, chlorothiazide, cortisone preparations, estrogens, guanethidine, hydrochlorothiazide, methyldopa, and nonsteroidal antiinflammatory drugs.
- Drugs that may cause *decreased* levels include aldosterone, bicarbonates, corticosteroids, cortisone, hydrocortisone, loop diuretics, thiazide diuretics, and triamterene.

Procedure and patient care

Before

- Explain the procedure to the patient.
- Tell the patient that no fasting is required.

During
- Collect 5 to 10 ml of venous blood in a red- or green-top tube.

After
- Apply pressure or a pressure dressing to the venipuncture site.
- Assess the venipuncture site for bleeding.

Abnormal findings

▲ **Increased levels (hyperchloremia)**
Dehydration
Renal tubular acidosis
Excessive infusion of normal saline
Cushing's syndrome
Eclampsia
Multiple myeloma
Kidney dysfunction
Metabolic acidosis
Hyperventilation
Anemia
Respiratory alkalosis
Hyperparathyroidism

▼ **Decreased levels (hypochloremia)**
Overhydration
Congestive heart failure
Syndrome of inappropriate secretion of antidiuretic hormone
Vomiting
Chronic gastric suction
Chronic respiratory acidosis
Salt-losing nephritis
Addison's disease
Burns
Metabolic alkalosis
Diuretic therapy
Hypokalemia
Aldosteronism
Respiratory acidosis

notes

chloride, urine (Cl)

C

Type of test Urine (24-hour)

Normal findings

Adult/elderly: 110-250 mEq/day or 110-250 mmol/day (SI units)
Child: 15-40 mmol/day
Infant: 2-10 mmol/day

Test explanation and related physiology

Chloride is the major extracellular anion. Its main purpose is to maintain electrical neutrality, mostly as a salt with sodium. It follows sodium losses and accompanies sodium excesses, thus affecting water balance. Chloride also serves as a buffer to assist in acid-base balance. As carbon dioxide increases, bicarbonate moves from the intracellular space to the extracellular space. To maintain electrical neutrality, chloride will shift back into the cell.

A 24-hour urine collection for chloride is useful for evaluating the electrolyte composition of urine and acid-base imbalances.

Interfering factors

- Urine volume and perspiration can affect chloride levels.
- Dietary salt intake affects levels.
- Drugs that may cause *increased* levels include bromides, diuretics, and steroids.

Procedure and patient care

Before

- Explain the procedure to the patient.
- Tell the patient that no special diet is required.

During

- Instruct the patient to begin the 24-hour urine collection after voiding.
- Discard the initial specimen and begin the 24-hour timing at that point.
- Collect all the urine passed during the next 24 hours.
- Show the patient where to store the urine container.
- Keep the specimen on ice or refrigerated during the entire 24 hours.

- Indicate the starting time on the urine container and laboratory slip.
- Post the hours for the urine collection in a prominent location to prevent accidental discarding of the specimen.
- Instruct the patient to void before defecating so that the urine is not contaminated by feces.
- Remind the patient not to put toilet paper in the collection container.
- Encourage the patient to drink fluids during the 24 hours.
- Instruct the patient to collect the last specimen as close as possible to the end of the 24 hours.

After
- Transport the urine specimen promptly to the laboratory.

Abnormal findings

▲ **Increased levels**
Dehydration
Starvation
Salicylate toxicity
Diuretic therapy
Increased salt intake
Salt-losing nephritis

▼ **Decreased levels**
Addison's disease
Malabsorption syndrome
Prolonged gastric suction
  or vomiting
Diarrhea
Congestive heart failure
Emphysema
Pyloric obstruction
Diaphoresis
Reduced salt intake

notes

cholecystography (Oral cholecystogram, Gallbladder series, GB series)

Type of test X-ray with contrast dye

Normal findings
Good visualization of gallbladder
No filling defects
No stones

Test explanation and related physiology
Oral cholecystography provides x-ray visualization of the gall-bladder after the oral ingestion of a radiopaque, iodinated dye that comes in the form of pills. Adequate visualization of the gall-bladder requires concentration of this dye within the gallbladder. The following factors are necessary for adequate dye concentration within the gallbladder:

1. Ingestion of all the dye tablets by the patient.
2. Adequate absorption of the dye from the gastrointestinal tract. Vomiting or diarrhea may preclude this absorption.
3. Abstinence from a meal on the morning of the test. A fatty meal eaten before x-ray films would induce gallbladder emptying of the concentrated dye. No visualization of the gallbladder would occur.
4. Excretion of the dye into the bile. This excretion is inhibited by inadequate hepatocellular function or when the bilirubin level is greater than 2 mg/dl.
5. Patency of the cystic duct. The dye is secreted by the liver through the hepatic duct and enters the gallbladder through the cystic duct. Obstruction of the cystic duct (as found in acute cholecystitis) will prevent the dye from entering the gallbladder.
6. Concentration of the dye within the gallbladder. The mucosa of a chronically inflamed gallbladder is unable to absorb the bile waters and concentrate the dye adequately for visualization.

On x-ray film, the biliary calculi (gallstones) are visualized as radiolucent shadows within a dye-filled gallbladder. Gallbladder polyps and tumors occasionally also can be seen as filling defects.

Occasionally, the gallbladder will not visualize after a single dose of dye tablets is ingested. The test should then be repeated using a double dose. Nonvisualization after a double dose is reliable evidence of chronic cholecystitis as long as none of the previously listed factors necessary for adequate dye concentration have been violated.

The oral cholecystogram is less accurate than the gallbladder ultrasound. It is also more cumbersome to perform. It may take several days to obtain an accurate result. Fasting is required. Gallbladder ultrasonography, however, can be done on an emergency basis; fasting is preferred but not necessary for ultrasonography. When positive, the accuracy of gallbladder ultrasound is unparalleled (see p. 1). Ultrasound has now replaced cholecystography as the primary method of choice in the diagnosis of gallstones.

Contraindications

- Patients who are allergic to iodine dye
  This is a relative contraindication. Most patients who are allergic to iodine dye react only when the dye is administered intravenously.
- Patients who are pregnant
- Patients whose bilirubin is greater than 2 mg/dl
  The dye will not visualize the gallbladder.
- Patients who have another inflammatory process within the abdomen
  The absorption of the orally ingested dye is not adequate for visualization.
- Patients who have diarrhea or vomiting
  They cannot absorb the dye.

Potential complication

- Adverse reaction or allergy to dye
  This rarely occurs, because the dye is not administered intravenously.

Interfering factors

- Barium within the abdomen (usually as a result of an upper GI series or barium enema) will preclude visualization of the gallbladder.
- Vomiting or diarrhea will affect absorption of the radiopaque dye.

Procedure and patient care

Before
- Explain the procedure to the patient.

- Instruct the patient as to the importance of ingesting the appropriate dose of the radiopaque dye.
- Be sure that the serum bilirubin level is less than 1.8 mg/dl.
- Instruct the patient to ingest a low-fat or fat-free meal the evening before testing.
- Assess for iodine dye allergy before administering radiopaque dye. The dye tablets are usually taken 2 hours after the dinner meal. Usually, six 0.5-g iopanoic acid tablets are administered. These are best taken one tablet at a time at 5-minute intervals.
- Inform the radiologist if vomiting or diarrhea occurs after ingestion of the radiopaque dye tablets.
- Instruct the patient to remain NPO except for water after taking the contrast tablets.

During
- Note the following procedural steps:
  1. In the radiology department, several plain x-ray films of the patient's right upper quadrant are taken.
  2. If the patient is to receive a fatty meal, a palatable liquid is ingested.
  3. Repeat x-ray films of the right upper quadrant are performed.
- Note that the x-rays take only a few minutes to perform. They are interpreted by a radiologist, and the results are available later that day.
- Tell the patient that no discomfort is associated with the test.

After
- If the gallbladder does not visualize, note that the patient may be instructed to repeat the procedure with a double dose of radiopaque dye tablets.
- Inform the patient that the radiopaque dye is eventually excreted in the urine. Some patients may report slight dysuria following cholecystography.

Abnormal findings

Gallstones	Cholesterolosis
Gallbladder polyps	Gallbladder cancer
Chronic cholecystitis	Cystic duct obstruction

cholesterol

Type of test Blood

Normal findings Vary with age and testing center
Adult/elderly: <200 mg/dl or <5.20 mmol/L (SI units)
Child: 120-200 mg/dl
Infant: 70-175 mg/dl
Newborn: 53-135 mg/dl

Test explanation and related physiology

Cholesterol is the main lipid associated with arteriosclerotic vascular disease. Cholesterol, however, is required for the production of steroids, bile acids, and cellular membranes. Most of the cholesterol we eat comes from foods of animal origin. The liver metabolizes the cholesterol to its free form, and cholesterol is transported in the bloodstream by lipoproteins. Nearly 75% of the cholesterol is bound to low-density lipoproteins (LDLs), and 25% is bound to high-density lipoproteins (HDLs). Because cholesterol is the main lipid involved in arteriosclerotic disease, high levels of free and bound LDLs are associated with increased risk for arteriosclerotic vascular disease.

Because the liver is required to metabolize ingested cholesterol products, subnormal cholesterol levels are indicative of severe liver diseases. Malnutrition is also associated with low cholesterol levels.

The purpose of cholesterol testing is to identify patients at risk for arteriosclerotic heart disease. Cholesterol testing is usually done as a part of lipid profile testing, which also evaluates lipoproteins (see p. 514) and triglycerides (see p. 819), because, by itself, cholesterol is not a totally accurate predictor of heart disease. There is considerable overlap in what are considered "normal" and "high-risk" levels. Day-to-day cholesterol values in the same individual can vary by 15%. Positional changes can affect these levels. Certain disease states affect cholesterol levels.

Interfering factors

- Pregnancy is usually associated with elevated cholesterol levels.
- Oophorectomy increases levels.

☛ Drugs that may cause *increased* levels include adrenocorticotropic hormone, anabolic steroids, beta-adrenergic blocking
agents, corticosteroids, epinephrine, oral contraceptives,
phenytoin (Dilantin), sulfonamides, thiazide diuretics, cyclo-
sporine, and vitamin D.

☛ Drugs that may cause *decreased* levels include allopurinol,
androgens, bile salt–binding agents, captopril, chlorpropamide, clofibrate, colchicine, colestipol, erythromycin, isoniazid, liothyrinone (Cytomel), lovastatin (Mevacor), monoamine oxidase inhibitors, neomycin (oral), niacin, and nitrates.

Procedure and patient care

Before

- Instruct the patient to fast 12 to 14 hours after eating a low-
fat diet before testing. Only water is permitted.
- Indicate to the patient that dietary intake at least 2 weeks
before testing will affect results.
- Tell the patient that no alcohol should be taken 24 hours
before the test.

During

- Collect 5 to 10 ml of blood in a red-top tube.
- Indicate on the laboratory slip any drugs that may affect
cholesterol levels.

After

- Apply pressure or a pressure dressing to the venipuncture
site.
- Assess the venipuncture site for bleeding.
- Instruct patients with high levels regarding a low-cholesterol
diet, exercise, and appropriate body weight.

Abnormal findings

▲ **Increased levels**
  Hypercholesterolemia
  Hyperlipidemia
  Hypothyroidism
  Uncontrolled diabetes
    mellitus
  Nephrotic syndrome
  Pregnancy
  High-cholesterol diet
  Xanthomatosis
  Hypertension
  Myocardial infarction
  Atherosclerosis
  Biliary cirrhosis
  Stress
  Nephrosis

▼ **Decreased levels**
  Malabsorption
  Malnutrition
  Hyperthyroidism
  Cholesterol-lowering
    medication
  Pernicious anemia
  Hemolytic anemia
  Sepsis
  Stress
  Liver disease
  Acute myocardial infarc-
    tion

notes

cholinesterase (CHS, Pseudocholinesterase, Cholinesterase RBC, Red cell cholinesterase, Acetylcholinesterase)

Type of test Blood

Normal findings

0.5-1.5 mg/dl or 5-15 mg/L (SI units)
7-19 U/ml or 7-19 kU/L (SI units)
(Values vary with laboratory test methods.)

Test explanation and related physiology

Cholinesterases hydrolyze acetylcholine and also other choline esters and thereby regulate nerve impulse transmission at the nerve synapse and neuromuscular junction. Two types of cholinesterases are measured: acetylcholinesterase (true cholinesterase) and pseudocholinesterase. The activity of these enzymes is inhibited by certain insecticides. People with an inherited pseudocholinesterase enzyme deficiency exhibit increased sensitivity to the effects of succinylcholine (a muscle relaxant commonly used during general anesthesia). Succinylcholine is inactivated by pseudocholinesterase.

Declining test results can be used as a sensitive index of exposure to organic phosphate insecticides. This test also can preoperatively identify patients with genetic enzyme alterations in pseudocholinesterase activity. During anesthesia induction, succinylcholine (a blocker of acetylcholine activity) may be used to induce muscle paralysis. Persons with altered amounts of pseudocholinesterase enzyme cannot inactivate succinylcholine; therefore they may experience prolonged muscle paralysis or weakness causing respiratory depression. Serum cholinesterase assay is currently the best screening test for suspected cholinesterase deficiency. Etiologies of deficiencies, besides genetic causes, include chronic liver disease, inorganic phosphate poisoning, malnutrition, and drugs such as atropine and steroids.

Interfering factors

- Pregnancy decreases test values.
- Drugs that may cause *decreased* values include atropine, caffeine, codeine, estrogens, morphine sulfate, neostigmine, oral contraceptives, phenothiazines, theophylline, quinidine, and vitamin K.

Procedure and patient care

Before
- Explain the procedure to the patient.
- Tell the patient that no fasting is required.
- It may be recommended to withhold medications that could alter test results for 12 to 24 hours before the test.

During
- Collect a venous blood sample in a red-top tube.
- Include a listing of all medications taken by the person with the laboratory requisition slip.

After
- Apply pressure or a pressure dressing to the venipuncture site.
- Assess the venipuncture site for bleeding.

Abnormal findings

▼ **Decreased levels**

Poisoning from organic
   phosphate insecticides
Hepatocellular disease

Persons with congenital
   enzyme deficiency
Malnutrition

notes

chorionic villus sampling (CVS, Chorionic villus biopsy [CVB])

C

Type of test Cell analysis

Normal findings No genetic or biochemical disorders

Test explanation and related physiology

The CVS test can be performed between 8 and 12 weeks of gestation for the early detection of genetic and biochemical disorders. Because CVS detects congenital defects early, first-trimester therapeutic abortions can be performed if indicated and desired.

For this study, a sample of chorionic villi is obtained for analysis. The villi in the chorion frondosum are present from 8 to 12 weeks on and are believed to reflect fetal chromosome, enzyme, and DNA content. This permits a much earlier diagnosis of prenatal problems than amniocentesis, which cannot be done before 14 to 16 weeks.

Potential complications

- Accidental abortion
- Infection
- Bleeding
- Fetal limb deformities

Procedure and patient care

Before

- Explain the procedure to the patient.
- Be certain that the physician has obtained a signed consent for the procedure.
- Tell the patient that no food or fluid restrictions are necessary.

During

- Note the following procedural steps:
  1. The patient is placed in the lithotomy position.
  2. A cannula is inserted into the cervix and uterine cavity (Figure 7).
  3. Under ultrasound guidance, the cannula is rotated to the site of the developing placenta.

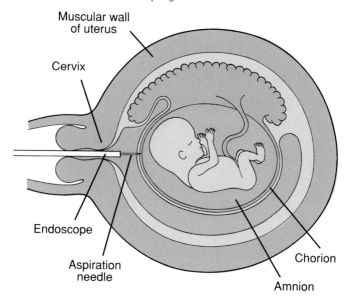

Muscular wall
of uterus

Cervix

Endoscope

Aspiration
needle

Chorion

Amnion

Figure 7 Chorionic villus sampling (CVS). Diagram of an 8-week pregnancy showing endoscopic aspiration of extraplacental villi.

4. A syringe is attached, and suction is applied to obtain several samples of villi.
- Note that this procedure is performed by an obstetrician in approximately 5 minutes.
- Inform the patient that discomfort associated with this test is similar to that of a Pap smear.

After
- Note that some Rh-negative mothers may receive RhoGAM. RhoGAM is given because of the risk of immunization from the fetal blood, which could jeopardize the fetus.
- Monitor the vital signs and check the mother for signs of bleeding.
- Schedule the mother for an ultrasound in 2 to 4 days to affirm the continued viability of the fetus.
- Assess the vaginal area for discharge and drainage; note the color and amount.

- Assess the patient for signs of spontaneous abortion (e.g., cramps, bleeding).
- Inform the patient how she can obtain the results from her physician. Make sure she understands that the results are usually not available for several weeks. (Results may be available much sooner at major medical centers that perform this test.)

Abnormal findings

Genetic and biochemical disorders

notes

chromosome karyotype (Blood chromosome analysis, Chromosome studies, Cytogenetics, Karyotype)

Type of test Blood

Normal findings

Female: 44 autosomes + 2 X chromosomes; karyotype: 46,XX
Male: 44 autosomes + 1 X, 1 Y chromosome; karyotype:
  46,XY

Test explanation and related physiology

This test is used to study an individual's chromosome makeup. The term *karyotyping* refers to the arrangement of cell chromosomes in order from the largest to the smallest to analyze their number and structure. This test involves the determination of chromosome number and structure; variations in either can produce numerous abnormalities. A normal karyotype of chromosomes consists of a pattern of 22 pairs of autosomal chromosomes and a pair of sex chromosomes: XY for the male and XX for the female.

Chromosome karyotyping is useful in evaluating congenital anomalies, mental retardation, growth retardation, delayed puberty, infertility, hypogonadism, primary amenorrhea, ambiguous genitalia, chronic myelogenous leukemia, neoplasm, recurrent miscarriage, prenatal diagnosis in situations of advanced maternal age, Turner's syndrome, Klinefelter's syndrome, Down's syndrome, and other suspected genetic disorders. The products of conception also can be studied to determine the cause of stillbirth or miscarriage.

Procedure and patient care

Before
- Explain the procedure to the patient.
- Determine how the specimen will be collected.
  Obtain preparation guidelines from the laboratory if indicated.
- Many patients are fearful of the test results and require considerable emotional support.

During
- Specimens for chromosome analysis can be obtained from

numerous sources. Leukocytes from a peripheral venipuncture are the most easily and most often used for this study.

- Bone marrow biopsies and surgical specimens also can sometimes be used as sources for analysis.
- During pregnancy, specimens can be collected by amniocentesis (see p. 44) and chorionic villus sampling (see p. 237).
- Fetal tissue or products of conception can be studied, as well, to determine the reason for the loss of the pregnancy.

After

- Aftercare depends on how the specimen was collected.
- Inform the patient that test results are generally not available for several months.
- If the test results show an abnormality, encourage the patient to verbalize his or her feelings. Provide emotional support.

Abnormal findings

Congenital anomalies
Mental retardation
Growth retardation
Delayed puberty
Infertility
Hypogonadism
Primary amenorrhea
Ambiguous genitalia
Chronic myelogenous leukemia

Neoplasm
Recurrent miscarriage
Prenatal diagnosis in situations of advanced maternal age
Turner's syndrome
Klinefelter's syndrome
Down's syndrome

notes

cisternal puncture

Type of test Fluid analysis

Normal findings

Pressure: <200 cm H_2O
Color: clear and colorless
Blood: none
Cells: no red blood cells; <5 lymphocytes/mm^3
Culture and sensitivity: no organisms present
Protein: 15-45 mg/dl cerebrospinal fluid (CSF) (≤70 mg/dl in elderly adults and children)
Glucose: 50-75 mg/dl CSF or 60% to 70% of blood glucose level
Chloride: 700-750 mg/dl
Lactic dehydrogenase (LDH): <2.0-7.2 U/ml
Cytology: no malignant cells
Serology for syphilis: negative
Glutamine: 6-15 mg/dl

Test explanation and related physiology

In certain conditions, a spinal needle may be inserted into the cisterna magna for a cisternal puncture instead of into the subarachnoid space as in a lumbar puncture (see p. 526). This procedure is hazardous because of the proximity of the needle to the brainstem. A cisternal puncture may be indicated in the following conditions:

1. To obtain CSF for examination when it cannot be obtained at the lumbar level (e.g., because of infection, lumbar deformity)
2. To demonstrate a subarachnoid block by performing a cisternal puncture simultaneously with a lumbar puncture
3. For drainage of CSF when a lumbar puncture is contraindicated
4. To introduce contrast material or air for myelography
5. To perform encephalography

With the use of accurate central nervous system imaging (e.g., computed tomography, magnetic resonance imaging), the diagnostic role of this test has greatly diminished.

Contraindications

- Patients with increased intracranial pressure

- Patients with infection near the puncture site
  Meningitis can result from contamination with infected material.
- Patients who have a developmental anomaly at the level of the foramen magnum
- Patients with suspected lesions in the cisterna magna
- Patients who cannot cooperate and remain still during the procedure

Potential complications

- Meningitis
- Herniation of the brain

Procedure and patient care

Before

- Explain the procedure to the patient. Allay the patient's fears and allow time for concerns to be verbalized.
- Obtain consent if required by the institution.
- Inform the patient that his or her head must be kept still during the procedure. Rotation of the neck could cause needle injury to the medulla.
- Tell the patient that no fasting or sedation is usually required.

During

- Note the following procedural steps:
  1. The occipital area at the back of the head is shaved and cleansed with an antiseptic.
  2. The patient is placed on his or her side with a pillow under the head to keep the head and spine aligned. The chin rests on the chest and is held in place by an assistant to prevent rotation.
  3. The needle is inserted approximately 4 to 5 cm between the first cervical vertebra and the rim of the foramen magnum (Figure 8).
  4. The insert (obturator) is removed, and CSF can be seen slowly dripping from the needle.
  5. The needle is then attached to a sterile manometer, and the pressure (opening pressure) is recorded. Before the pressure reading is taken, however, the patient is asked to relax and straighten the legs to reduce the intraabdominal pressure, which causes an increase in CSF pressure.
  6. Three sterile test tubes are filled with 5 to 10 ml of CSF each.

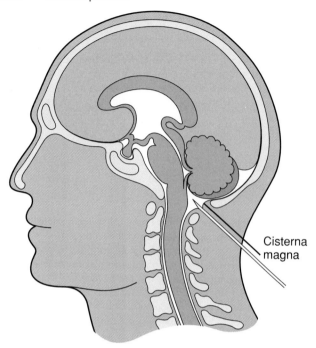

Cisterna
magna

Figure 8 Position of the needle when a cisternal puncture is performed.

7. The pressure (closing pressure) is measured.
- Note that the duration of the procedure is approximately 20 to 60 minutes.
- Tell the patient that this procedure is usually described as painful by most patients.

After
- Apply digital pressure and a bandage to the puncture site.
- Assess the puncture site for drainage of blood or CSF at the puncture site.
- Observe the patient for respiratory complications (e.g., cyanosis, dyspnea, apnea) and irregularities in the heartbeat, which could indicate injury to the medulla.
- Encourage the patient to drink increased amounts of fluid to replace the CSF lost during the procedure.

- Tell the patient that headaches do not usually occur as a result of this procedure.
- Inform the patient that he or she can usually get out of bed in 2 to 3 hours if no problems occur.

Abnormal findings

Subarachnoid block
Brain neoplasm
Spinal cord neoplasm
Cerebral hemorrhage
Meningitis
Encephalitis
Degenerative cord or brain disease
Autoimmune disorder
Hepatic encephalopathy
Coma

Cerebral abscess
Viral or tubercular meningitis
Myelitis
Tumor
Neurosyphilis
Multiple sclerosis
Acute demyelinating polyneuropathy
Subarachnoid bleeding
Reye's syndrome

notes

clostridial toxin assay (*Clostridium difficile,* Antibiotic-associated colitis assay; Pseudomembranous colitis toxic assay)

Type of test Stool

Normal findings Negative (no *Clostridium* toxin identified)

Test explanation and related physiology

Clostridium difficile bacterial infection of the intestine may occur in patients who are immunocompromised or taking broad-spectrum antibiotics (e.g., clindamycin, ampicillin, and cephalosporins). The infection results from depression of the normal flora of the bowel by antibiotics. This increases the amount of *C. difficile* in the intestines. Diarrhea is the common feature and is usually watery and voluminous. Abdominal cramps, fever, and leukocytosis are noted in most patients. Symptoms usually begin 4 to 10 days after the initiation of antibiotic therapy.

The clostridial bacterium releases a toxin that causes necrosis of the colonic epithelium. The detection of this toxin in the stool is therefore diagnostic of clostridial enterocolitis (pseudomembranous colitis). Management of this antibiotic-associated colitis includes immediate cessation of the broad-spectrum antibiotics (if possible), IV replacement of fluid and electrolytes, and institution of metronidazole (Flagyl) or vancomycin (Vancocin) antibiotic therapy.

Procedure and patient care

Before

- Explain the method of stool collection to the patient. Be matter-of-fact to avoid embarrassment to the patient.
- Instruct the patient not to mix urine and toilet paper with the stool specimen.
- Handle the specimen carefully, as though it were capable of causing infection. If the nurse is assisting with the specimen collection, gloves should be worn.

During

- Ask the patient to defecate into a clean container. A rectal swab cannot be used, because it collects inadequate amounts of stool.

- Note that a stool specimen also can be collected by proctoscopy.
- Place the specimen in a closed container and then transport it to the laboratory to prevent deterioration of the toxin.
- If the specimen cannot be processed immediately, refrigerate it.

After

- Maintain enteric isolation precautions on all patients until appropriate therapy is completed.

Abnormal finding

Antibiotic-related pseudomembranous colitis

notes

clot retraction test (Whole-blood clot retraction test)

Type of test Blood

Normal findings
50% to 100% clot retraction in 1-2 hours
Complete retraction within 24 hours

Test explanation and related physiology
The clot retraction test is used to determine if bleeding disorders may be caused by thrombocytopenia (i.e., decreased platelet count), Glanzmann's thrombasthenia (abnormal platelet function), or some other cause of poor platelet function. Clot retraction is prolonged in the first two disorders and is normal in most other causes of platelet dysfunction. Clot retraction is rarely used today because of availability of accurate platelet counts and more accurate methods of determining platelet dysfunction.

If thrombocytopenia exists, the clot retraction will be slower and the clot formation will stay soft and watery. If fibrinolysins are present, no clot retraction will occur. This test is only reliable if the hematocrit and fibrinogen (factor I) concentration (see Table 7, p. 252) are within normal limits.

In addition to thrombocytopenia, poor whole-blood clot retraction occurs in patients with thrombasthenia (abnormal platelets) and Waldenström's macroglobulinemia.

Contraindications
- Patients with low platelet counts
- Patients with hypofibrinogenemia
- Patients taking aspirin

Interfering factors
- Uremia
- Drugs that may alter test results include aspirin and nonsteroidal antiinflammatory agents.

Procedure and patient care
Before
- Explain the procedure to the patient.
- Tell the patient that no fasting is required.

During

- Avoid excessive probing during venipuncture if a coagulation disorder is suspected.
- Collect approximately 5 to 7 ml of venous blood in a red-top tube.
- Avoid hemolysis.
- Indicate on the laboratory slip if the patient is taking aspirin or a nonsteroidal antiinflammatory agent.

After

- Transport the specimen to the laboratory within 1 hour of collection.
- Apply pressure or a pressure dressing to the venipuncture site.
- Assess the venipuncture site for bleeding and bruising.

Abnormal findings

▲ **Increased clot retraction**
Severe anemia
Hypofibrinogenemia

▼ **Decreased or poor clot retraction**
Thrombocytopenia
von Willebrand's disease
Thrombasthenia (abnormal platelets)
Waldenström's macroglobulinemia

notes

coagulating factors concentration (Factor assay, Coagulating factors, Blood-clotting factors)

Type of test Blood

Normal findings 50% to 200% of "normal"

Test explanation and related physiology

The coagulating factors concentration test measures the concentration of specific coagulating factors in the blood. Testing is available to measure the quantity of the following factors:

I (fibrinogen)
II (prothrombin)
V (proaccelerin)
VII (proconvertin stable factor)
VIII (antihemophilic factor)
IX (Christmas factor)
X (Stuart factor)
XI (plasma thromboplastin antecedent)
XII (Hageman factor)

For example, fibrinogen (factor I) is essential to the blood-clotting mechanism, because it is converted to fibrin by the action of thrombin during the coagulation process (Figure 9). Measurement of factor I is often referred to as a *quantitative fibrinogen*. When these factors exist in concentrations below their "minimal hemostatic level," clotting time will be prolonged. These minimal hemostatic levels vary according to the factor involved (Table 7). Common medical conditions associated with decreased factor concentrations are listed in Table 8. It is important to identify the exact factor or factors involved in the coagulating defect so that appropriate blood component replacement can be administered.

Procedure and patient care

Before
- Explain the procedure to the patient.
- Tell the patient that no fasting is required.

During
- Collect approximately 7 to 10 ml of venous blood in a blue-top tube.

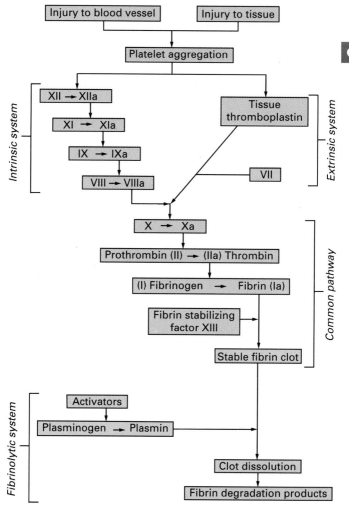

Figure 9 Process of hemostasis and fibrinolysis. Injury to a blood vessel surface or tissue initiates platelet aggregation. The intrinsic or extrinsic system is activated and then activates the common pathway of fibrin formation. Finally, fibrin is physiologically dissolved by the fibrinolytic system.

TABLE 7 Minimum concentration of coagulation factors required for adequate fibrin production

Factor	Minimal hemostatic level (mg/dl)	Blood components*
I	60-100	C, FFP, FWB
II	10-15	P, WB, FFP, FWB
V	5-10	FFP, FWB
VII	5-20	P, WB, FFP, FWB
VIII	30	C, FFP, VIII CONC
IX	30	FFP, FWB
X	8-10	P, WB, FFP, FWB
XI	25	P, WB, FFP, FWB

*Blood components capable of providing specific factor: *C,* cryoprecipitate; *FFP,* fresh frozen plasma; *FWB,* fresh whole blood (<24 hours old); *P,* unfrozen banked plasma; *WB,* banked whole blood; *VIII CONC,* factor VIII concentrate.

TABLE 8 Conditions that may result in coagulation factor deficiency

Condition	Diminished factors
Liver disease	I, II, V, VII, IX, X, XI
Disseminated intravascular coagulation	I, V, VIII
Fibrinolysis	I, V, VIII
Congenital deficiency	I, II, V, VII, VIII, IX, X, XI, XII
Heparin administration	II
Warfarin ingestion	II, VII, IX, X, XI
Autoimmune disease	VIII
Vitamin K deficiency or maldigestion	II, VII, IX, X, XI

After

- Apply pressure or a pressure dressing to the venipuncture site.
- Assess the venipuncture site for bleeding.
- Deliver the blood specimen to the laboratory as soon as possible.

Abnormal findings

Table 8 lists conditions that may result in a coagulation factor deficiency.

notes

colonoscopy

Type of test Endoscopy

Normal findings Normal colon

Test explanation and related physiology

With fiberoptic colonoscopy, the entire colon from anus to cecum can be examined in most patients. As with sigmoidoscopy, benign and malignant neoplasms, polyps, mucosal inflammation, ulceration, and sites of active hemorrhage can be visualized. Diseases such as cancer, polyps, ulcers, and arteriovenous (AV) malformations also can be visualized. Cancers, polyps, and inflammatory bowel diseases can be biopsied through the colonoscope with cable-activated instruments, and sites of active bleeding can be coagulated with the use of laser, electrocoagulation, and injection of sclerosing agents.

This test is recommended for patients who have Hemoccult-positive stools, lower gastrointestinal bleeding, or a change in bowel habits, or are at high risk for colon cancer. The latter group includes patients with a strong personal or family history of colon cancer, polyps, or ulcerative colitis.

Contraindications

- Patients who are uncooperative
  As in all studies that require technical finesse, patient cooperation is essential to successful completion of the test.
- Patients whose medical condition is not stable
  This test requires sedation, which may induce hypotension in the medically unstable patient.
- Patients who are bleeding profusely from the rectum
  The viewing lens will become covered with blood clots, preventing visualization of the lower intestinal tract.
- Patients with a suspected perforation of the colon

Potential complications

- Bowel perforation
- Persistent bleeding from a biopsy site
- Oversedation resulting in respiratory depression

Interfering factors

- Poor bowel preparation
  The stool immediately obstructs the lens and precludes adequate visualization of the colon.

- Active bleeding
  Blood obstructs the lens system and precludes adequate visualization of the colon.

Procedure and patient care

Before

- Explain the procedure to the patient.
- Fully inform the patient as to the risks of the procedure and obtain an informed consent.
- Instruct the patient as to the appropriate bowel preparation. One type is the 2-day bowel preparation, which uses clear liquids for 2 days, along with a strong cathartic such as magnesium citrate and bisacodyl (Dulcolax). On the day of examination, an enema is given. A 1-day preparation using a Colyte bowel preparation has become more widely used. After the patient ingests a gallon of Colyte, enemas are not usually needed. Dulcolax tablets may be taken.
- Avoid an oral bowel preparation in patients with upper gastrointestinal obstruction, suspected acute diverticulitis, or recent bowel resectional surgery.
- Assure patients that they will be appropriately draped to avoid unnecessary embarrassment.
- Administer appropriate preendoscopy sedation, usually meperidine (Demerol) and diazepam (Valium). Often, atropine is ordered to minimize patient secretions.

During

- Note the following procedural steps:
  1. IV access is obtained.
  2. After a rectal examination indicates adequate bowel preparation, the patient is sedated.
  3. The patient is placed in the lateral decubitus position, and the colonoscope is placed into the rectum.
  4. Under direct visualization, the colonoscope is directed to the cecum. Often, a significant amount of manipulation is required to obtain this position.
  5. As in all endoscopy, air is insufflated to distend the bowel for better visualization.
  6. Complete examination of the large bowel is carried out.
  7. Polypectomy, biopsy, and other endoscopic surgery is performed after appropriate visualization.
  8. When the laser or coagulator is used, the air is removed and carbon dioxide is used as an insufflating agent to avoid explosion.

- Note that this test is performed by a physician trained in gastrointestinal endoscopy in approximately 30 to 60 minutes.
- Tell the patient that minimal discomfort is associated with the test.

After
- Explain to patients that air has been insufflated into the bowel. They may experience flatulence or gas pains.
- Examine the abdomen for evidence of colon perforation (abdominal distention and tenderness).
- Assess the patient's vital signs. Watch for a decrease in blood pressure and an increase in pulse as an indication of hemorrhage.
- Inspect the stools for gross blood.
- Notify the physician if the patient develops increased pain or significant gastrointestinal bleeding.
- Allow the patient to eat when fully alert if no evidence of bowel perforation exists.
- Encourage the patient to drink a lot of fluids when intake is allowed. This will make up for the dehydration associated with the bowel preparation.

Abnormal findings

Colon cancer
Colon polyps
Inflammatory bowel disease (e.g., ulcerative or Crohn's colitis)

AV malformations
Hemorrhoids
Ischemic or postinflammatory strictures
Diverticulosis

notes

colposcopy

Type of test Macroscopic examination

Normal findings Normal vagina and cervix

Test explanation and related physiology

Colposcopy provides an in situ macroscopic examination of the vagina and the cervix with a colposcope, which is a macroscope with a light source and a magnifying lens. With this procedure, tiny areas of dysplasia, carcinoma in situ, and invasive cancer that would be missed by the naked eye can be visualized, and biopsy specimens can be obtained. The study is performed on patients with abnormal vaginal epithelial patterns, cervical lesions, or suspicious Pap smear results, and on those exposed to diethylstilbestrol in utero. It may be a sufficient substitute to cone biopsy (removal and examination of a cone of tissue from the cervix) in evaluating the cause of abnormal cervical cytologic findings.

It is important to realize that colposcopy is useful only in identifying a suspicious lesion. Definitive diagnosis requires biopsy of the tissue. One of the major advantages of this procedure is that of directing the biopsy to the area most likely to be truly representative of the lesion. A biopsy performed without colposcopy may not necessarily be representative of the lesion's true pathologic condition, resulting in a significant risk of missing a serious lesion.

The patient will need to have diagnostic conization if:

1. Colposcopy and endocervical curettage do not explain the problem or match the cytologic findings of the Pap smear within one grade.
2. The entire transformation zone is not seen.
3. The lesion extends up the cervical canal beyond the vision of the colposcope.

The need for up to 90% of cone biopsies is eliminated by an experienced colposcopist. Endocervical curettage may routinely accompany colposcopy to detect unknown lesions in the endocervical canal.

Contraindications

- Patients with heavy menstrual flow

Interfering factor
- Failure to cleanse the cervix of foreign materials (e.g., creams, medications) may impair visualization.

Procedure and patient care

Before
- Explain the procedure to the patient.
- Obtain informed consent if required by the institution.

During
- Note the following procedural steps:
  1. The patient is placed in the lithotomy position, and a vaginal speculum is used to expose the vagina and cervix.
  2. After the cervix is sampled for cytologic findings, it is cleansed with a 3% acetic acid solution to remove excess mucus and cellular debris. The acetic acid also accentuates the difference between normal and abnormal epithelial tissues.
  3. The colposcope is focused on the cervix, which is then carefully examined.
  4. Usually, the entire lesion can be outlined, and the most atypical areas selected for biopsy specimen removal.
- Note that colposcopy is performed by a physician in approximately 5 to 10 minutes.
- Tell the patient that some women complain of pressure pains from the vaginal speculum and that momentary discomfort may be felt if biopsy specimens are obtained.

After
- Inform the patient that she may have vaginal bleeding if biopsy specimens were taken. Suggest that she wear a sanitary pad.
- Instruct the patient to abstain from intercourse and not to insert anything (except a tampon) into the vagina until healing of a biopsy is confirmed.
- Inform the patient when and how to obtain the results of this study.

Abnormal findings
Dysplasia

Carcinoma in situ

Invasive cancer

Cervical lesions

complement assay

Type of test Blood

C

Normal findings

Total complement: 75-160 U/ml or 75-160 U/L (SI units)
C3: 55-120 mg/dl or 0.55-1.20 g/L (SI units)
C4: 20-50 mg/dl or 0.20-0.50 g/L (SI units)

Test explanation and related physiology

Serum complements make up a group of globulin proteins that act as enzymes. These enzymes facilitate the immunologic and inflammatory response. The complement system is important for destroying foreign cells and removing foreign materials. Complement increases vascular permeability, allowing antibodies and white blood cells (WBCs) to be delivered to the area of inflammation. Complement also acts to increase chemotaxis (pulling of WBCs to the area of infection), phagocytosis, and immune adherence of the antibody to antigen. These processes are vitally important in the inflammatory response.

The total complement, sometimes labeled CH 50, is made up of nine major components—C1 through C9. Total complement can be measured by the complement fixation test and other hemolytic tests. These tests assess the overall function of the entire complement system. The C3 and C4 components can be quantitated for a more accurate evaluation of the complement system.

Reduced complement levels can be congenital, as in hereditary angioedema, or acquired. Examples of these acquired deficiency diseases include serum sickness, lupus erythematosus, infectious endocarditis, renal transplant rejection, vasculitis, and some forms of glomerulonephritis. In these types of illnesses, the complement components are decreased because of consumption created by the development of the "autoimmune complexes."

Complement components are increased following the onset of various acute or chronic inflammatory diseases or acute tissue damage.

For this test, the blood is mixed with antibody-coated red blood cells (RBCs) of sheep. When complement is present in normal quantities, 50% of the RBCs are lysed. Decreased quantities of complement are associated with lower percentages of sheep RBC lyses.

Usually, specimens for complement assays must be sent out to reference laboratories.

Procedure and patient care

Before
- Explain the procedure to the patient.
- Tell the patient that no fasting or special preparations are required.

During
- Collect 7 to 10 ml of venous blood in a red-top tube.

After
- Apply pressure or a pressure dressing to the venipuncture site.
- Observe the venipuncture site for bleeding.

Abnormal findings

▲ **Increased levels**
Rheumatic fever (acute)
Myocardial infarction (acute)
Ulcerative colitis
Cancer

▼ **Decreased levels**
Cirrhosis
Autoimmune disease (e.g., systemic lupus erythematosus)
Serum sickness (immune complex disease)
Glomerulonephritis
Lupus nephritis
Renal transplant rejection (acute)
Protein malnutrition
Anemia
Malnutrition
Hepatitis
Rheumatoid arthritis
Sjögren's syndrome

notes

complete blood count and differential count (CBC and diff)

C

The CBC and differential count are a series of tests of the peripheral blood that provide a tremendous amount of information about the hematologic system and many other organ systems. They are inexpensively, easily, and rapidly performed as a screening test. The CBC and differential count include automated measurement of the following studies, which are discussed separately:

Red blood cell count (RBC, see p. 694)
Hemoglobin (Hgb, see p. 454)
Hematocrit (Hct, see p. 452)
Red blood cell indices (RBC indices, see p. 697)
    Mean corpuscular volume (MCV)
    Mean corpuscular hemoglobin (MCH)
    Mean corpuscular hemoglobin concentration (MCHC)
White blood cell count (WBC) and differential count (see p. 873)
    Neutrophils (polynucleated cells or "polys," segmented cells or "segs," band cells, stab cells)
    Lymphocytes
    Monocytes
    Eosinophils
    Basophils
Blood smear (see p. 151)
Platelet count (see p. 631)

notes

computed tomography of the abdomen (CAT scan of the abdomen, CT scan of the abdomen)

Type of test X-ray with contrast dye

Normal findings No evidence of abnormality

Test explanation and related physiology

The CT scan of the abdomen is a noninvasive yet very accurate x-ray procedure used to diagnose pathologic conditions such as tumors, cysts, abscesses, inflammation, perforation, bleeding, obstruction, aneurysms, and calculi of the abdominal and retroperitoneal organs. The CT scan image results from passing x-rays through the abdominal organs at many angles. The variation in density of each tissue allows for a variable penetration of the x-rays. Each density is given a numeric value called a *density coefficient,* which is digitally computed into shades of gray. This is then displayed on a television screen as thousands of dots in various shades of gray. The final display appears as an actual photograph of the anatomic area sectioned by x-rays. The image can be enhanced by repeating the CT scan after IV administration of iodine containing contrast dye. These images can be recorded on Polaroid or x-ray film.

Liver tumors, abscesses, trauma, cysts, and anatomic abnormalities can be seen, and pancreatic tumors, pseudocysts, inflammation, calcification, bleeding, and trauma can be detected. The kidneys and urinary outflow tract are well visualized.

Renal tumors and cysts, ureteral obstruction, calculi, and congenital renal and ureteral abnormalities are easily seen with the use of IV contrast injection. Extravasation of urine secondary to trauma or obstruction can also be easily demonstrated. Adrenal tumors and hyperplasia are best diagnosed with this technique. Some radiology literature indicates that the histology of the tumor can be suggested based on the density coefficients shown on the scan.

Although the bowel can be better visualized by an upper GI series, small bowel follow-through, or barium enema, large tumors and perforations of the bowel can be identified with the CT scan, especially when oral contrast is ingested. The spleen can be well visualized for hematoma, laceration, fracture, tumor infiltration, and splenic vein thrombosis with CT scanning. The retroperitoneal lymph nodes can be evaluated. These are usually present, but all nodes with a diameter greater than 2 cm are considered abnormal. The abdominal aorta and its major branches can be evaluated for aneurysmal dilation and intramural thrombi, and the pelvic structures (including the uterus, ovaries, tubes, prostate, and rectum) and musculature can be evaluated for tumors, abscesses, infection, or hypertrophy. Ascites and hemoperitoneum can easily be demonstrated with the CT scan.

Contraindications

- Patients who are allergic to iodinated dye or shellfish
- Patients who are pregnant
- Patients whose vital signs are unstable
- Patients who are very obese, usually over 300 pounds
- Patients who are claustrophobic

Potential complications

- Allergic reaction to iodinated dye
  Allergic reactions vary from flushing, itching, and urticaria to severe, life-threatening anaphylaxis (evidenced by respiratory distress, drop in blood pressure, and/or shock). In the unusual event of anaphylaxis, diphenhydramine (Benadryl), steroids, and epinephrine are added to routine resuscitative efforts. Oxygen and endotracheal equipment should be on hand for immediate use.
- Acute renal failure from dye infusion
  Adequate hydration beforehand may reduce this likelihood.

Interfering factors

  The following can obscure visualization:
- Presence of metallic objects (e.g., hemostasis clips)
- Retained barium from previous studies
- Large amounts of fecal material or gas in the bowel

Procedure and patient care

Before

- Explain the procedure to the patient. The patient's cooperation is necessary, because he or she must lie still during the procedure.
- Obtain informed consent if required by the institution.
- Assess the patient for allergies to iodinated dye or shellfish.
- Inform the radiologist if an allergy to iodinated contrast is suspected. The radiologist may prescribe a Benadryl-and-steroid preparation to be administered before testing. Usu-

ally a hypoallergenic, non-ionic contrast will be used during the test.

- Show the patient a picture of the CT machine. Encourage the patient to verbalize his or her concerns, because some patients may have claustrophobia. Most patients who are mildly claustrophobic can be scanned after appropriate pre-medication with antianxiety drugs.
- Keep the patient NPO for at least 4 hours before the test if oral contrast is to be administered; however, this test can be performed on an emergency basis on patients who have recently eaten.

During

- Note the following procedure for the abdominal CT scan: The patient is taken to the radiology department and placed on the CT scan table. The patient then is placed in an encircling camera (body scanner) that takes pictures of the various levels of the abdomen and pelvis. Any motion will cause blurring and streaking of the final picture. Therefore the patient is asked to remain motionless during x-ray exposure. Television equipment allows for immediate display of the CT scan image, which is then recorded on Polaroid or x-ray film. In a separate room, the technicians manipulate the CT scan table, affecting the level of the abdomen that is scanned. Through audio communication, the patient is instructed to hold his or her breath during x-ray exposure.
- Remember that oral and IV iodinated x-ray contrast dye provides better results for this test. One can accurately differentiate the gastrointestinal organs from the other abdominal organs with oral contrast. Likewise, the vessels and ureters are contrasted with the surrounding structures with use of IV dye.
- Note that this procedure is usually performed by a radiologist in less than 30 minutes. If dye is administered, the procedure time may be doubled, because the CT scan is done both with and without contrast dye.
- Tell the patient that the discomforts associated with this study include lying still on a hard table and the peripheral venipuncture. Mild nausea is a common sensation when contrast dye is used. An emesis basin should be readily available. Some patients may experience a salty taste, flushing, and warmth during the dye injection.

After

- Encourage the patient to drink fluids to avoid dye-induced renal failure and to promote dye excretion.
- Inform the patient that diarrhea may occur after ingestion of the oral contrast.
- Evaluate the patient for delayed reaction to dye (dyspnea, rashes, tachycardia, hives). This may occur 2 to 6 hours after the test. Treat with antihistamines or steroids.

Abnormal findings

Liver: tumor, abscess, bile duct dilation

Pancreas: tumor, pseudocyst, inflammation, bleeding

Spleen: hematoma, fracture, laceration, tumor, venous thrombosis

Gallbladder/biliary system: gallstones, tumor, bile duct dilation

Kidneys: tumor, cyst, ureteral obstruction, calculi, congenital abnormalities

Adrenal: adenoma, cancer, pheochromocytoma, hemorrhage, myelolipoma, hyperplasia

GI tract: perforation, tumor, inflammatory bowel disease, diverticulitis, appendicitis

Uterus, tubes, ovaries: tumor, abscess, infection, hydrosalpinx, cyst, fibroid

Prostate: hypertrophy, tumor

Retroperitoneum: tumor, lymphadenopathy

Abdominal aneurysm

Ascites, hemoperitoneum

Abscess

notes

computed tomography of the brain (CT scan of the brain, Computerized axial transverse tomography [CATT])

Type of test X-ray with contrast dye

Normal findings No evidence of pathologic conditions

Test explanation and related physiology

Computed tomography of the brain consists of a computerized analysis of multiple tomographic x-ray films taken of the brain tissue at successive layers, providing a three-dimensional view of the cranial contents. The CT image provides a view of the head as if one were looking down through its top. The variation in density of each tissue allows for variable penetration of the x-ray beam. An attached computer calculates the amount of x-ray penetration of each tissue and displays this as shades of gray. The image is placed on a television screen and photographed. The final result is a series of actual anatomic pictures of coronal sections of the brain.

The CT scan is used in the differential diagnosis of intracranial neoplasms, cerebral infarctions, ventricular displacement or enlargement, cortical atrophy, cerebral aneurysms, intracranial hemorrhage and hematoma, and arteriovenous (AV) malformation.

Visualization of a neoplasm, previous infarction, or any pathologic process that destroys the blood-brain barrier may be enhanced by IV injection of an iodinated contrast dye. CT scans may be repeated frequently to monitor the progress of any disease or to monitor the healing process. In many cases, CT scanning has eliminated the need for more invasive procedures, such as cerebral arteriography and pneumoencephalography. In many localities, MRI scanning of the brain has replaced the use of CATT scans of the brain.

Contraindications

- Patients who are allergic to iodinated dye or shellfish
- Patients who are claustrophobic
- Patients who are pregnant
- Patients whose vital signs are unstable
- Patients who are very obese, usually over 300 pounds

Potential complications

- Allergic reaction to iodinated dye
  Allergic reactions vary from mild flushing, itching, and urticaria to severe, life-threatening anaphylaxis (evidenced by respiratory distress, drop in blood pressure, shock). In the unusual event of anaphylaxis, diphenhydramine (Benadryl), steroids, and epinephrine are added to routine resuscitation. Oxygen and endotracheal equipment should be on hand for immediate use.
- Acute renal failure from dye infusion
  Adequate hydration beforehand may reduce this likelihood.

Procedure and patient care

Before

- Explain the procedure to the patient. The patient's cooperation is necessary, because he or she must lie still during the procedure.
- Obtain informed consent if required by the institution.
- Show the patient a picture of the CT machine and encourage the patient to verbalize his or her concerns, because some patients may have claustrophobia. Most patients who are mildly claustrophobic can be scanned after appropriate premedication with antianxiety drugs.
- Keep the patient NPO for 4 hours before the study, because contrast dye may cause nausea. It is not usually known before the test if enhanced visualization by dye injection will be indicated. If contrast will not be used, food and fluids may be taken.
- Instruct the patient that wigs, hairpins, clips, or partial dental plates cannot be worn during the procedure, because they hamper visualization of the brain.
- Assess the patient for allergies to iodinated dye or shellfish.
- Inform the radiologist if an allergy to iodinated contrast is suspected. The radiologist may prescribe a Benadryl-and-steroid preparation to be administered before testing. Usually, a hypoallergenic, non-ionic contrast will be used during the test.
- Tell the patient that he or she may hear a "clicking" noise as the scanning machine moves around the head.

During

- Note the following procedure for the brain CT scan:
  The patient lies in the supine position on an examining table with the head resting on a snug-fitting rubber cap within a

water-filled box. The patient's head is enclosed only to the hairline (as in a hair dryer). The face is not covered, and the patient can see out of the machine at all times. Sponges are placed along the side of the head to ensure the patient's head does not move during the study. The scanner passes an x-ray beam through the brain from one side to the other. The machine then rotates 1 degree, and the procedure is repeated at each degree through a 180-degree arc. The machine is then moved, and the entire procedure is repeated through a total of three to seven planes.

- Remember that an iodinated dye will usually then be used. A peripheral IV line is started, and the iodine dye is administered through it. The entire scanning process is repeated.

- Note that this procedure is performed by a radiologist in less than 1 hour. If dye is administered, the procedure time is doubled, because the CT scan is done with and without the contrast dye.

- Tell the patient that the discomforts associated with this study include lying still on a hard table and peripheral venipuncture. Mild nausea is a common sensation when contrast dye is used. An emesis basin should be readily available. Some patients may experience a salty taste, flushing, and warmth during the dye injection.

After

- Encourage the patient to drink fluids, because dye is excreted by the kidneys and causes diuresis.

- Evaluate the patient for delayed reaction to dye (dyspnea, rash, tachycardia, hives). This usually occurs 2 to 6 hours after the test. Treat with antihistamines or steroids.

Abnormal findings

Intracranial neoplasm
Cerebral infarction
Ventricular displacement
Ventricular enlargement
Cortical atrophy
Cerebral aneurysm
Intracranial hemorrhage

Hematoma
AV malformation
Meningioma
Multiple sclerosis
Hydrocephalus
Abscess

notes

computed tomography of the chest (Chest CT scan)

Type of test X-ray with contrast dye

Normal findings No evidence of pathologic conditions

Test explanation and related physiology

Computed tomography of the chest is a noninvasive yet very accurate x-ray procedure for diagnosing and evaluating pathologic conditions, such as tumors, nodules, hematomas, parenchymal coin lesions, cysts, abscesses, pleural effusion, and enlarged lymph nodes affecting the lungs and mediastinum. Tumors, cysts, and fractures of the chest wall and pleura can also be seen. When an IV contrast material is given, vascular structures can be identified, and a diagnosis of aortic or other vascular abnormality can be made. With oral contrast, the esophagus and upper structures can be evaluated for tumor and other conditions. This procedure provides a cross-sectional view of the chest and is especially useful in detecting small differences in tissue densities, demonstrating lesions that cannot be seen with conventional radiology and tomography. The mediastinal structures can be visualized in a manner that cannot be equaled with conventional x-ray and tomographic scans.

The x-ray image results from using a body scanner to pass x-rays through the patient's chest at many different angles. The variation in density of each tissue allows for a variable penetration of the x-rays. Each density is given a numeric value called a *coefficient,* which is digitally computed into shades of gray. This is then displayed on a television screen as thousands of dots in various shades of gray. The final display appears as an actual photograph of the anatomic area sectioned by the x-rays.

Contraindications

- Patients who are pregnant
- Patients who are allergic to iodinated dye or shellfish
- Patients who are claustrophobic
- Patients who are very obese, usually over 300 pounds
- Patients whose vital signs are unstable

Potential complications

- Allergic reaction to iodinated dye
  Allergic reactions may vary from mild flushing, itching, and

urticaria to severe, life-threatening anaphylaxis (evidenced by respiratory distress, drop in blood pressure, shock). In the unusual event of anaphylaxis, diphenhydramine (Benadryl), steroids, and epinephrine are added to routine resuscitation. Oxygen and endotracheal equipment should be on hand for immediate use.

- Acute renal failure from dye infusion
  Adequate hydration beforehand may reduce this likelihood.

Procedure and patient care

Before

- Explain the procedure to the patient. The patient's cooperation is necessary, because he or she must lie still during the procedure.
- Obtain informed consent if required by the institution.
- Assess the patient for allergies to iodinated dye or shellfish.
- Inform the radiologist if an allergy to iodinated contrast is suspected. The radiologist may prescribe a Benadryl-and-steroid preparation to be administered before testing. Usually, a hypoallergenic, non-ionic contrast will be used during the test.
- Show the patient a picture of the CT machine and encourage the patient to verbalize concerns regarding claustrophobia. Most patients who are mildly claustrophobic can tolerate this study after appropriate premedication with antianxiety drugs.
- Keep the patient NPO for 4 hours before the test in the event that contrast dye is administered.

During

- Note the following procedure for the chest CT scan: The patient is taken to the radiology department and asked to remain motionless in a supine position, because any motion will cause blurring and streaking of the final picture. An encircling x-ray camera (body scanner) takes pictures at varying intervals and levels over the chest area. Television equipment allows for immediate display, and the image is recorded on Polaroid or x-ray film. Occasionally, IV dye is administered to enhance the chest image, and the x-ray studies are repeated.
- Note that this procedure is performed by a radiologist in 30 to 45 minutes. If dye is administered, the procedure time

may be doubled, because the CT scan is done with and without contrast dye.

- Tell the patient that the discomforts associated with this study include lying still on a hard table and peripheral venipuncture. Mild nausea is a common sensation when contrast dye is used. An emesis basin should be readily available. Some patients may experience a salty taste, flushing, and warmth during the dye injection.

After

- Encourage patients who received dye injection to increase their fluid intake, because the dye is excreted by the kidneys and causes diuresis.
- Evaluate the patient for delayed reaction to the dye (dyspnea, rashes, tachycardia, hives). This usually occurs 2 to 6 hours after the test. Treat with antihistamines or steroids.

Abnormal findings

Pulmonary tumor
Inflammatory nodules
Granuloma
Cyst
Pleural effusion
Enlarged lymph nodes
Aortic aneurysm
Postpneumonitic scanning

Pneumonitis
Esophageal tumor
Hiatal hernia
Mediastinal tumor (e.g., lymphoma, thymoma)
Primary or metastatic chest wall tumor

notes

computed tomography portogram (CT portogram)

Type of test X-ray with contrast dye

Normal findings No evidence of liver abnormalities

Test explanation and related physiology

A CT scan of the liver (see p. 262) is inaccurate in identifying tumors in the liver smaller than 2 cm. A CT portogram can routinely accurately identify abnormalities in the liver as small as 5 mm. The difference between a CT scan of the liver and a CT portogram is in the manner in which the contrast dye is injected. In a routine CT scan, dye is injected through a peripheral vein. In a CT portogram, dye is injected through a catheter that is placed in the splenic artery. The dye passes through the spleen and into the splenic vein and, subsequently, into the portal vein and its tributaries. Hepatic tumors and cysts, however, do not take up dye. These lesions appear as a filling defect (dark spots) in the liver. Use of this test, therefore, is limited to identification of suspected smaller neoplasms involved in the liver. It is used in cancer patients who are suspected to have liver metastasis. The number and location of these metastatic lesions are best visualized with a CT portogram.

Contraindications

- Patients with allergies to shellfish or iodinated dye
- Patients who are uncooperative or agitated
- Patients who are pregnant
- Patients with renal disorders, because iodinated contrast is nephrotoxic
- Patients with a bleeding propensity
- Patients with unstable cardiac disorders
- Patients who are dehydrated, because they are especially susceptible to dye-induced renal failure

Potential complications

- Allergic reaction to iodinated dye
  These reactions may vary from mild flushing, itching, and urticaria to severe, life-threatening anaphylaxis (evidenced by respiratory distress, drop in blood pressure, and shock). In the unusual event of anaphylaxis, diphenhydramine (Benadryl), steroids, and epinephrine are added to routine

resuscitative efforts. Oxygen and endotracheal equipment should be on hand for immediate use.

- Hemorrhage from the arterial puncture site used for arterial access
- Arterial embolism from dislodgment of an arteriosclerotic plaque
- Soft tissue infection around the puncture site
- Renal failure, especially in elderly patients who are chronically dehydrated or have a mild degree of renal failure
- Pseudoaneurysm development as a result of failure of the puncture site to seal

Procedure and patient care

Before

- Explain the procedure to the patient. Allay any fears and allow the patient to verbalize concerns.
- Ensure that written and informed consent for this procedure is in the patient's chart.
- Assess the possibility of allergies to iodinated dye. Inform the radiologist if an allergy to iodinated contrast is suspected. The radiologist may prescribe Benadryl and a steroid preparation to be administered before the test. Usually, hypoallergenic, non-ionic contrast will be used during the test.
- Determine if the patient has been taking anticoagulants.
- Keep the patient NPO for at least 2 to 4 hours before testing.
- Mark the site of the patient's peripheral pulses with permanent ink before arterial catheterization. This will permit assessment of the peripheral pulses after the procedure.

During

- Note the following preprocedural steps:
  1. The patient may be sedated before being taken to the angiography room, which is usually within the radiology department.
  2. The patient is placed on the x-ray table in the supine position.
  3. If the femoral artery is to be used, the groin is shaved, prepared, and draped in a sterile manner.
  4. The femoral artery is cannulated, and a wire is threaded up that artery and into or near the opening of the splenic artery.

5. A catheter is placed over that wire and into the splenic artery.
6. The patient is transferred to the CT scan unit, which is usually also in the x-ray department.
7. Through the catheter, iodinated contrast material is injected into the splenic artery.
8. CT scan images are taken subsequent to the injection.

- Note that the placement of the arterial catheter takes about 30 minutes and is minimally uncomfortable. This is done by a physician.
- Inform the patient that CT scan imaging takes about 15 minutes and is not uncomfortable. This is done by a technician.

After

- After x-rays are completed, the catheter is removed and a pressure dressing is applied to the puncture site.
- Monitor the patient's vital signs for indications of hemorrhage.
- Assess the peripheral pulse in the extremity used for vascular access and compare it with the preprocedural baseline values.
- Maintain pressure at the puncture site with a 1- to 2-pound sandbag or an IV bag for several hours.
- Keep the patient on bed rest for about 4 to 8 hours following the procedure to allow for complete sealing of the arterial puncture site.
- Evaluate the patient for delayed allergic reaction to the dye (dyspnea, rash, tachycardia, hives). This usually occurs within 2 to 6 hours after the test. Treat the patient as described above.

Abnormal findings

Hepatic tumor
Hepatic cyst
Hepatic hemangioma

notes

contraceptive localization (Intrauterine device [IUD] localization)

Type of test Ultrasound

Normal findings An IUD contraceptive device is located within the endometrial cavity.

Test explanation and related physiology

When a woman is unable to visualize or palpate the string of an IUD, ultrasound is indicated to determine whether the IUD has perforated the uterus, been expulsed, or been incorporated with an intrauterine pregnancy. IUDs have a particular type-specific morphology and can be easily recognized with ultrasound.

If an IUD can be seen on the abdominal x-ray film but cannot be shown to be in the endometrial cavity by ultrasound, one must strongly suspect that the IUD has perforated the uterus.

Interfering factors

- Patients who have had recent GI contrast studies, because barium creates severe distortion of reflective sound waves.
- Patients with air-filled bowel loops, because gas does not transmit sound waves well.
- Failure to fill the bladder, which is often used as a reference point for pelvic sonography.

Procedure and patient care

Before

- Explain the procedure to the patient.
- Give the patient 3 to 4 glasses (200 to 300 ml) of water or other liquid 1 hour before the examination and instruct her not to void until after the procedure is completed. This will allow the bladder to fill and be used as a reference point.
- Tell the patient that no fasting or sedation is required.

During

- Note the following procedural steps:
  1. The patient is taken to the ultrasound room and placed in the supine position on the examination table.
  2. The ultrasonographer, usually a radiologist, applies a greasy, conductive paste to the abdomen to enhance sound transmission and reception.

3. A transducer is passed vertically and horizontally over the skin.
4. Pictures are taken of the sound waves, and a real image is produced.

- Note that this procedure is performed in approximately 20 minutes.
- Inform the patient that no discomfort is associated with this study other than having a full bladder and the urge to void.

After

- Remove the lubricant from the patient's skin.
- Provide an opportunity for the patient to void.

Abnormal findings

Perforation of the uterus
Expulsion of the IUD

Incorporation of the IUD within an intrauterine pregnancy

notes

contraction stress test (CST, Oxytocin challenge test [OCT])

Type of test Manometric

Normal findings Negative

Test explanation and related physiology

The CST, frequently called the *oxytocin challenge test* (OCT), is a relatively noninvasive test of fetoplacental adequacy used in the assessment of high-risk pregnancy. For this study, a temporary stress in the form of uterine contractions is applied to the fetus. The reaction of the fetus to the contractions is assessed by an external fetal heart monitor. Uterine contractions cause transient impediment of placental blood flow. If the placental reserve is adequate, the maternal-fetal oxygen transfer is not significantly compromised during the contractions and the fetal heart rate (FHR) remains normal (a *negative* test). The fetoplacental unit can then be considered adequate for the next 7 days.

If the placental reserve is inadequate, the fetus does not receive enough oxygen during the contraction. This results in intrauterine hypoxia and late deceleration of the FHR. The test is considered to be *positive* if consistent, persistent, late decelerations of the FHR occur with two or more uterine contractions. False-positive results caused by uterine hyperstimulation can occur in 10% to 30% of patients. Thus, positive test results warrant a complete review of other studies (e.g., amniocentesis) before the pregnancy is terminated by delivery.

The test is considered to be *unsatisfactory* if the results cannot be interpreted (e.g., because of hyperstimulation of the uterus, excessive movement of the mother, or deceleration of unknown meaning. In the case of unsatisfactory results, other means of management should be considered.

Two advantages of the CST are that it can be done at any time and that its results are available shortly afterward. Although this test can be performed reliably at 32 weeks of gestation, it usually is done after 34 weeks. CST can induce labor, and a fetus at 34 weeks is more likely to survive an unexpectedly induced delivery than a fetus at 32 weeks. Nonstress testing (see p. 571) of the fetus is the preferred test in almost every instance and can be performed more safely at 32 weeks; it can then be followed 2 weeks later by CST if necessary. The CST may be performed weekly until delivery terminates pregnancy.

The CST can be used clinically in any high-risk pregnancy where fetal well-being is threatened. These include pregnancies marked by diabetes, hypertensive disease of pregnancy (toxemia), intrauterine growth retardation, Rh-factor sensitization, history of stillbirth, postmaturity, or low estriol levels.

Contraindications

- Patients with multiple pregnancy, because the myometrium is under greater tension and is more likely to be stimulated to premature labor
- Patients with a prematurely ruptured membrane, because labor may be stimulated by the CST
- Patients with placenta previa, because vaginal delivery may be induced
- Patients with abruptio placentae, because the placenta may separate from the uterus as a result of the oxytocin-induced uterine contractions
- Patients with a previous hysterotomy, because the strong uterine contractions may cause uterine rupture
- Patients with a previous vertical or classic cesarean section, because the strong uterine contractions may cause uterine rupture (The test can be performed, however, if it is carefully monitored and controlled.)
- Patients with pregnancies of less than 32 weeks, because early delivery may be induced by the procedure

Potential complication

- Premature labor

Interfering factor

- Hypotension may cause false-positive results.

Procedure and patient care

Before
- Explain the procedure to the patient.
- Obtain informed consent for the procedure.
- Teach the patient breathing and relaxation techniques.
- Record the patient's blood pressure and the FHR before the test as baseline values.
- If the CST is performed on an elective basis, the patient may be kept NPO in case labor occurs.

During
- Note the following procedural steps:
  1. After the patient empties her bladder, place her in a semi-Fowler's position and tilted slightly to one side to avoid vena caval compression by the enlarged uterus.
  2. Check her blood pressure every 10 minutes to avoid hypotension, which may cause diminished placental blood flow and a false-positive test result.
  3. Place an external fetal monitor over the patient's abdomen to record the fetal heart tones. Attach an external tokodynamometer to the abdomen at the fundal region to monitor uterine contractions.
  4. Record the output of the fetal heart tones and uterine contractions on a two-channel strip recorder.
  5. Monitor baseline FHR and uterine activity for 20 minutes.
  6. If uterine contractions are detected during this pretest period, withhold oxytocin and monitor the response of the fetal heart tone to spontaneous uterine contractions.
  7. If no spontaneous uterine contractions occur, administer oxytocin (Pitocin) by IV infusion pump.
  8. Increase the rate of oxytocin infusion until the patient is having moderate contractions, then record the FHR pattern.
  9. After the oxytocin infusion is discontinued, continue FHR monitoring for another 30 minutes until the uterine activity has returned to its preoxytocin state. The body metabolizes oxytocin in approximately 20 to 25 minutes.
- Note that the CST is performed safely on an outpatient basis in the labor and delivery unit, where qualified nurses and necessary equipment are available. The test is performed by a nurse with a physician available.
- Note that a new noninvasive method of performing the CST is called the *breast stimulation* or *nipple stimulation technique*. Stimulation of the nipple causes nerve impulses to the hypothalamus that trigger the release of oxytocin into the mother's bloodstream. This causes uterine contractions and may eliminate the need for IV administration of oxytocin. Uterine contractions are usually satisfactory after 15 minutes of nipple stimulation (gentle twisting of the nipples). Advantages of this technique include the ease of performing the test, shorter duration of the study, and elimination of the

need to start, monitor, and stop IV infusions. If sufficient contractions do not result from nipple stimulation, the standard CST procedure is followed.

- Note that the duration of this study is approximately 2 hours.
- Tell the patient that the discomfort associated with the CST may consist of mild labor contractions. Usually, breathing exercises are sufficient to control any discomfort. Administer analgesics if needed.

After
- Monitor the patient's blood pressure and the FHR.
- Discontinue the IV line and assess the site for bleeding.

Abnormal finding
Fetoplacental inadequacy

notes

Coombs' test, direct (Direct antiglobulin test)

Type of test Blood

Normal findings Negative; no agglutination

Test explanation and related physiology

The direct Coombs' test is used to detect autoantibodies against red blood cells (RBCs), which can cause cellular damage, usually to ABO Rh antigens. Many diseases (e.g., erythroblastosis fetalis, lymphomas, lupus erythematosus, mycoplasmal infection, infectious mononucleosis), drugs (e.g., quinidine), and the aftermath of cardiac valvular surgery are associated with the production of these autoantibodies. These antibodies result in hemolytic anemia. Frequently, the production of these autoantibodies against RBCs is not associated with any disease, and the resulting hemolytic anemia is therefore called *idiopathic*.

This test is performed by mixing the patient's RBCs, which are suspected of being covered with autoantibodies against RBCs, with Coombs' serum. Coombs' serum is a solution containing antibodies against human antibodies. If the patient's RBCs are coated with autoantibodies against RBCs, the Coombs' antibodies will react with the autoantibodies on the RBCs and cause agglutination (clumping) of the RBCs. The greater the quantity of antibodies against RBCs, the more clumping occurs. This test is read as *positive* with clumping on a scale of trace to +4. If the RBCs are not coated with autoantibodies against RBCs (immunoglobulins), agglutination will not occur; this is a *negative* test.

When a transfusion with incompatible blood is given, the Coombs' test can detect the patient's antibodies coating the transfused RBCs. The Coombs' test is therefore very helpful in evaluating suspected transfusion reactions.

Interfering factors

- Drugs that may cause false-positive results include ampicillin, captopril, cephalosporins, chlorpromazine (Thorazine), chlorpropamide, hydralazine, indomethacin (Indocin), insulin, isoniazid (INH), levodopa, methyldopa (Aldomet), penicillin, phenytoin (Dilantin), procainamide, quinidine, quinine, rifampin, streptomycin, sulfonamides, and tetracyclines.

Procedure and patient care

Before

- Explain the procedure to the patient.
- Tell the patient that no fasting is required.

During

- Collect approximately 5 to 7 ml of venous blood in a red- or lavender-top tube.
- Use venous blood from the umbilical cord to detect the presence of antibodies in the newborn.
- List on the laboratory slip all medications that the patient has taken in the last few days.

After

- Apply pressure or a pressure dressing to the venipuncture site.
- Assess the venipuncture site for bleeding.

Abnormal findings

Autoimmune hemolytic anemia
Transfusion reaction
Erythroblastosis fetalis
Lymphoma
Lupus erythematosus
Mycoplasmal infection
Infectious mononucleosis

notes

C

Coombs' test, indirect (Blood antibody screening)

Type of test Blood

Normal findings Negative; no agglutination

Test explanation and related physiology

The indirect Coombs' test detects circulating antibodies against RBCs. The major purpose of this test is to determine if the patient has minor serum antibodies (other than the major ABO system) to RBCs that he or she is about to receive by blood transfusion. Therefore this test is the "screening" portion of the "type and screen" routinely performed for blood compatibility testing (crossmatching in the blood bank).

In this test, a small amount of the recipient's serum is added to the donor's RBCs. Then Coombs' serum is added to the mixture. Coombs' serum is a solution containing antibodies against human antibodies. Visible agglutination indicates that the recipient has antibodies to the donor's RBCs. If the recipient has no antibodies against the donor's RBCs, agglutination will not occur; transfusion should then proceed safely and without any transfusion reaction.

Circulating antibodies against RBCs also may occur in an Rh-negative pregnant woman who is carrying an Rh-positive fetus.

Interfering factors

☛ Drugs that may cause false-positive results include antiarrhythmics, antituberculins, cephalosporins, chlorpromazine (Thorazine), insulin, levodopa, methyldopa (Aldomet), penicillins, phenytoin (Dilantin), quinidine, sulfonamides, and tetracyclines.

Procedure and patient care

Before
- Explain the procedure to the patient.
- Tell the patient that no fasting is required.

During
- Collect approximately 7 ml of venous blood in a red-top tube.
- List on the laboratory slip all medications that the patient has taken in the last few days.

After

- Apply pressure or a pressure dressing to the venipuncture site.
- Assess the venipuncture site for bleeding.
- Remember that if this antibody screening test is positive, antibody identification is then done.

Abnormal findings

Incompatible crossmatched blood

Anti-Rh antibodies

Acquired hemolytic anemia

Presence of specific antibody

Erythroblastosis fetalis

notes

cortisol, blood (Hydrocortisone, Serum cortisol)

Type of test Blood

Normal findings

Adult/elderly
  8 AM: 6-28 µg/dl or 170-625 nmol/L (SI units)
  4 PM: 2-12 µg/dl or 80-413 nmol/L (SI units)
Child
  8 AM: 15-25 µg/dl
  4 PM: 5-10 µg/dl
Newborn: 1-24 µg/dl

Test explanation and related physiology

Cortisol is a potent glucocorticoid released from the adrenal cortex in response to stimulation by adrenocorticotropic hormone (ACTH). The best method of evaluating adrenal activity is by directly measuring plasma cortisol levels. Normally, cortisol levels rise and fall during the day; this is called the *diurnal variation*. Cortisol levels are highest around 6 to 8 AM and gradually fall during the day to their lowest point around midnight. Sometimes, the earliest sign of adrenal hyperfunction is the loss of this diurnal variation, even though the cortisol levels are not yet elevated. For example, individuals with Cushing's syndrome often have top-normal plasma cortisol levels in the morning and do not exhibit a decline as the day proceeds. Low levels of plasma cortisol are suggestive of Addison's disease.

For this test, blood is usually collected at 8 AM and again at around 4 PM. One would expect the 4 PM value to be one third to two thirds of the 8 AM value. Normal values may be transposed in individuals who have worked during the night and slept during the day for long periods of time.

Interfering factors

- Physical and emotional stress can artificially elevate cortisol levels.
- Recent radioisotope scans can affect test results.
- Drugs that may cause *increased* levels include estrogen, oral contraceptives, amphetamines, cortisone, and spironolactone (Aldactone).
- Drugs that may cause *decreased* levels include androgens,

aminoglutethimide, betamethasone, danazol, lithium, levodopa, metyrapone, and phenytoin (Dilantin).

Procedure and patient care

Before

- Explain the procedure to the patient to minimize anxiety.
- Assess the patient for signs of physical stress (e.g., infection, acute illness) or emotional stress and report these to the physician.

During

- Collect approximately 7 to 10 ml of venous blood in a red- or green-top tube in the morning after the patient has had a good night's sleep.
- Collect another blood sample at about 4 PM.
- Indicate on the laboratory slip the time of the venipuncture and any drugs that may affect test results.

After

- Apply pressure or a pressure dressing to the venipuncture site.
- Observe the venipuncture site for bleeding.

Abnormal findings

▲ **Increased levels**
Cushing's disease
Adrenal adenoma or car-
cinoma
Ectopic ACTH-
producing tumors
Hyperthyroidism
Obesity
Stress

▼ **Decreased levels**
Addison's disease
Hypopituitarism
Hypothyroidism
Liver disease

notes

cortisol, urine (Hydrocortisone, Urine cortisol)

Type of test Urine (24-hour)

Normal findings

Adult/elderly: 10-100 μg/24 hr or 27-276 nmol/day (SI units)
Adolescent: 5-55 μg/24 hr
Child: 2-27 μg/24 hr

Test explanation and related physiology

Cortisol is a potent glucocorticoid released from the adrenal cortex in response to stimulation by adrenocorticotropic hormone (ACTH). This test is used in the evaluation of adrenocortical function, especially hyperfunction. An elevated cortisol level in a properly collected urine specimen supports the diagnosis of Cushing's syndrome in an unstressed patient.

Interfering factors

- Pregnancy causes increased cortisol levels.
- Recent radioisotope scans can interfere with test results.
- Stress can increase cortisol levels.
- Drugs that may cause *increased* levels include oral contraceptives, danazol, hydrocortisone, and spironolactone (Aldactone).
- Drugs that may cause *decreased* levels include dexamethasone, ethacrynic acid, ketoconazole, and thiazides.

Procedure and patient care

Before

- Explain the procedure to the patient.
- Assess the patient for signs of physical stress (e.g., infection, acute illness) or emotional stress and report these to the physician.

During

- Begin the 24-hour collection after the patient urinates. Discard this specimen.
- Collect all urine passed by the patient during the next 24 hours.
- Post the hours for urine collection in a prominent spot.

- Note that it is not necessary to measure each urine specimen.
- Remind the patient to void before defecating so that the urine is not contaminated by feces.
- Tell the patient not to put toilet paper in the collection container.
- Encourage the patient to drink fluids during the 24 hours unless this is contraindicated for medical purposes.
- Collect the last specimen as close as possible to the end of the 24-hour period. Add this to the collection.
- Place the 24-hour urine collection in a plastic container and keep on ice. Use a preservative.
- Note on the laboratory slip the date and time that the specimen collection began and ended.
- Indicate on the laboratory slip any medications that may affect test results.

After

- Send the specimen to the laboratory promptly.

Abnormal findings

▲ **Increased levels**
Cushing's disease
Adrenal adenoma or carcinoma
Ectopic ACTH-producing tumor
Hyperthyroidism
Obesity
Stress

▼ **Decreased levels**
Addison's disease
Hypopituitarism
Hypothyroidism

notes

C-peptide (Connecting peptide insulin, Insulin C-peptide, Proinsulin C-peptide)

Type of test Blood

Normal findings 0.78-1.89 ng/ml or 0.26-0.62 nmol/L (SI units)

Test explanation and related physiology

C-peptide is formed in the islet of Langerhans of the pancreas during the conversion of proinsulin to insulin and C-peptide. C-peptide is released into the portal vein in a 1:1 ratio with insulin. Because it has a longer half-life than insulin, more C-peptide exists in the peripheral circulation. C-peptide levels correlate with insulin levels in the blood, except in islet cell tumors and possibly in obese patients.

The capacity of the pancreatic beta cells to secrete insulin can be evaluated by measuring insulin or C-peptide. Thus C-peptide is a by-product of *endogenous* insulin synthesis and a marker for endogenous insulin production with or without exogenous insulin injections.

C-peptide is not affected by the presence or absence of insulin antibodies. Therefore residual beta-cell function can be evaluated in the patient with diabetes who is treated with insulin and who may have insulin antibodies. This most often occurs in patients treated with old bovine or pork insulin.

C-peptide values are high in patients with insulinoma. In these patients, C-peptide concentrations parallel the plasma insulin values. This test is also useful in evaluating patients with hypoglycemia and in identifying those patients with factitious hypoglycemia caused by surreptitious injection of insulin. These patients have high circulating levels of insulin and a suppressed C-peptide value, because *exogenous* insulin suppresses *endogenous* insulin release. This suppression does not occur in insulinoma. Normal C-peptide levels occur in diabetics who are in remission. This blood test also can be used to detect the presence of residual tissue in patients who have had a pancreatectomy.

Interfering factors

- Because the majority of C-peptide is degraded in the kidney, renal failure can cause increased levels.

◤ Drugs that may cause *increased* levels of C-peptide include oral hypoglycemic agents (e.g., sulfonylureas).

Procedure and patient care

Before
- Explain the procedure to the patient.
- Instruct the patient to fast for 8 to 10 hours before the test. Only water is permitted.

During
- Collect venous blood in one red-top tube.

After
- Apply pressure or a pressure dressing to the venipuncture site.
- Assess the venipuncture site for bleeding.

Abnormal findings

▲ **Increased levels**
Insulinoma
Renal failure
Pancreas transplant

▼ **Decreased levels**
Factitious hypoglycemia
Radical pancreatectomy
Diabetes mellitus

notes

C-reactive protein test (CRP)

Type of test Blood

Normal findings <0.8 mg/dl

Test explanation and related physiology

C-reactive protein is a nonspecific, acute-phase reactant used to diagnose bacterial infectious disease and inflammatory disorders, such as acute rheumatic fever and rheumatoid arthritis. CRP levels do not consistently rise with viral infections. CRP is an abnormal protein produced primarily by the liver during an acute inflammatory process. A positive test result indicates the presence, but not the cause, of an acute inflammatory reaction. The synthesis of CRP is initiated by antigen-immune complexes, bacteria, fungi, and trauma. CRP is functionally analogous to immunoglobulin G, except that it is not antigen specific. CRP interacts with the complement system.

The CRP test is a more sensitive and rapidly responding indicator than the erythrocyte sedimentation rate (ESR, see p. 363). In an acute inflammatory change, CRP shows an earlier and more intense increase than ESR; with recovery, the disappearance of CRP precedes the return of ESR to normal. The CRP also disappears when the inflammatory process is suppressed by salicylates or steroids.

This test is also useful in evaluating patients with an acute myocardial infarction. The level of CRP correlates with peak levels of the MB isoenzyme of creatine kinase (see p. 293), but CRP peaks occur 1 to 3 days later. Failure of CRP to normalize may indicate ongoing damage to the heart tissue. Levels are not elevated in patients with angina.

This test also may be used postoperatively to detect wound infections. CRP levels increase within 4 to 6 hours after surgery and generally begin to decrease after the third postoperative day. Failure of the levels to fall is an indicator of complications, such as infection or pulmonary infarction.

Interfering factors

- An intrauterine device may cause positive test results because of tissue stress.
- Drugs that may cause *increased* levels include oral contraceptives.

☛ Drugs that may cause *decreased* levels include nonsteroidal antiinflammatories, salicylates, and steroids.

Procedure and patient care

Before

- Explain the procedure to the patient.
- Tell the patient that fasting usually is not required; however, some laboratories require a 4- to 12-hour fast. Water is permitted.

During

- Collect one red-top tube of venous blood.

After

- Apply pressure or a pressure dressing to the venipuncture site.
- Assess the venipuncture site for bleeding.

Abnormal findings

▲ **Increased levels**

Acute rheumatic fever
Rheumatoid arthritis
Acute myocardial infarction
Postoperative wound infection
Pulmonary infarction
Kidney or bone marrow transplant rejection
Malignant disease
Bacterial infection (e.g., tuberculosis)
Crohn's disease
Reiter's syndrome
Vasculitis syndrome
Lupus erythematosus
Tissue necrosis or trauma

notes

creatine phosphokinase (CPK, CP, Creatine kinase [CK])

C

Type of test Blood

Normal findings

Total CPK

Adult/elderly
  Male: 12-70 U/ml or 55-170 U/L (SI units)
  Female: 10-55 U/ml or 30-135 U/L (SI units)
Values are higher after exercise.
Newborn: 68-580 U/L (SI units)

Isoenzymes

CPK-MM: 100%
CPK-MB: 0%
CPK-BB: 0%

Test explanation and related physiology

CPK is found predominantly in the heart muscle, skeletal muscle, and brain. Serum CPK levels are elevated whenever injury occurs to these muscle cells; CPK levels can rise within 6 hours after damage. If damage is not persistent, the levels peak at 18 hours after injury and return to normal in 2 to 3 days.

To test specifically for myocardial muscle injury, electrophoresis is performed to detect the three CPK isoenzymes: CPK-BB (CPK1), CPK-MB (CPK2), and CPK-MM (CPK3). The CPK-MB isoenzyme portion appears to be specific for myocardial cells. CPK-MB levels rise 3 to 6 hours after infarction occurs. If there is no further myocardial damage, the level peaks at 12 to 24 hours and returns to normal 12 to 48 hours after infarction. CPK-MB levels do not usually rise with transient chest pain caused by angina, pulmonary embolism, or congestive heart failure. One can expect to see a rise in CPK-MB in patients with unstable angina, shock, malignant hyperthermia, myopathies, or myocarditis.

A *relative index* can be calculated to determine whether myocardial injury is highly suggestive or indeterminant for myocardial injury. The relative index is a mathematic calculation based on the total CPK value and the CPK-MB value. A CPK-MB value of ≥3.0 ng/ml with a relative index of ≥2.5 is highly suggestive of myocardial injury. If the CPK-MB is >3.0 ng/ml and the relative index is <2.5, the results are indeterminant for myocardial injury.

The CPK-MB isoenzyme level is helpful in both quantifying the degree of myocardial infarction and timing the onset of infarction. With the more frequent use of thrombolytic therapy for myocardial infarction, the CPK-MB isoenzyme is often used to determine appropriateness of thrombolytic therapy. High CPK-MB levels would suggest that significant infarction has already occurred, thereby precluding the benefit of thrombolytic therapy.

Because the CPK-BB isoenzyme is predominantly found in the brain and lung, injury to either of these organs (e.g., cerebrovascular accident, pulmonary infarction) will be associated with elevated levels of this isoenzyme.

The CPK-MM isoenzyme normally comprises almost all of the circulatory total CPK enzymes in healthy people. When the total CPK level is elevated as a result of increases in CPK-MM, there is injury or stress to the skeletal muscle. Examples of this include myopathies, vigorous exercise, multiple IM injections, electroconvulsive therapy, cardioversion, chronic alcoholism, or surgery.

Creatine phosphokinase is the main cardiac enzyme studied in patients with heart disease. Because its blood clearance and metabolism are well-known, its frequent determination can accurately reflect timing, quantity, and resolution of a myocardial infarction. Lactic dehydrogenase (see p. 501) and aspartate aminotransferase (see p. 117) are also important enzymes used to confirm a myocardial infarction.

New blood assays for cardiac markers have promised to rapidly and accurately detect acute myocardial infarction (MI) in the emergency room. One of these new assays is troponin. *Troponin* is a protein complex consisting of three isotypes (T, I, and C). Troponin T and troponin I have the potential to become better diagnostic markers for acute MI than existing enzymes (such as CPK-MB) because these new cardiac isotypes are distinctly different from skeletal isotypes. Monoclonal antibodies to cardiac troponin have been developed that do not cross-react with skeletal muscle forms. At the present time, troponins are mainly used in emergency rooms with a cardiac center where the patient can be monitored for several hours while awaiting test results. Then a decision can be made regarding admission to the cardiac care unit or discharge to home.

Interfering factors

- IM injections can cause elevated CPK levels.
- Strenuous exercise and recent surgery may cause increased levels.
- Early pregnancy may produce decreased levels.
- Drugs that may cause *increased* levels include amphotericin B, ampicillin, some anesthetics, anticoagulants, aspirin, clofibrate, dexamethasone (Decadron), furosemide (Lasix), captopril, colchicine, alcohol, lovastatin, lithium, lidocaine, propranolol, succinylcholine, and morphine.

Procedure and patient care

Before

- Explain the procedure to the patient.
- Discuss with the patient the need and reason for frequent venipuncture in diagnosing myocardial infarction.
- Avoid IM injections in patients with cardiac disease. These injections may falsely elevate the total CPK level.
- Tell the patient that no food or fluid restrictions are necessary.

During

- Collect a venous blood sample in a red-top tube. This is usually done daily for 3 days and then at 1 week.
- Rotate the venipuncture sites.
- Avoid hemolysis.
- Record the time and date of any IM injection.
- Record the exact time and date of venipuncture on each laboratory slip. This aids in the interpretation of the temporal pattern of enzyme elevations.

After

- Apply pressure or a pressure dressing to the venipuncture site.
- Observe the venipuncture site for bleeding.

Abnormal findings

▲ **Increased levels of total CPK**

Acute myocardial infarction

Acute cerebrovascular disease

Electric shock

Convulsions

Muscular dystrophy

Delirium tremens

Chronic alcoholism

Polymyositis

Hypokalemia

Central nervous system trauma

Pulmonary infarction

Dermatomyositis

▲ **Increased levels of CPK-MB isoenzyme**

Acute myocardial infarction

Cardiac aneurysm surgery

Cardiac defibrillation

Malignant hyperthermia

Reye's syndrome

Muscular dystrophy

Cardiac ischemia

Myocarditis

Rhabdomyolysis

▲ **Increased levels of CPK-BB isoenzyme**

Pulmonary infarction

Electroconvulsive therapy

Brain injury

Cerebrovascular accident (stroke)

Shock

Adenocarcinoma

Intestinal ischemia

Pulmonary embolism

Subarachnoid hemorrhage

Seizures

Brain cancer

▲ **Increased levels of CPK-MM isoenzyme**

Muscular dystrophy

Myositis

Delirium tremens

Recent convulsions

Electroconvulsive therapy

Recent surgery

Electromyography

Hypokalemia

Hypothyroidism

IM injections

Crush injuries

Hemophilia

notes

creatinine, blood (Serum creatinine)

Type of test Blood

C

Normal findings
Adult
    Female: 0.5-1.1 mg/dl or 44-97 μmol/L (SI units)
    Male: 0.6-1.2 mg/dl
Elderly: decrease in muscle mass may cause decreased values
Adolescent: 0.5-1.0 mg/dl
Child: 0.3-0.7 mg/dl
Infant: 0.2-0.4 mg/dl
Newborn: 0.3-1.2 mg/dl

Possible critical values >4 mg/dl (indicates serious impairment in renal function)

Test explanation and related physiology

This test measures the amount of creatinine in the blood. Creatinine is a catabolic product of creatine phosphate, which is used in skeletal muscle contraction. The daily production of creatine, and subsequently creatinine, depends on muscle mass, which fluctuates very little. Creatinine, as with blood urea nitrogen (BUN, see p. 837), is excreted entirely by the kidneys and therefore is directly proportional to renal excretory function. Thus, with normal renal excretory function, the serum creatinine level should remain constant and normal. Only renal disorders, such as glomerulonephritis, pyelonephritis, acute tubular necrosis, and urinary obstruction, will cause an abnormal elevation in creatinine. There are slight increases in creatinine levels after meals, especially after ingestion of large quantities of meat. Furthermore, there may be some diurnal variation in creatinine—nadir at 7 AM and peak at 7 PM.

The serum creatinine test, as with the BUN, is used to diagnose impaired renal function. Unlike the BUN, however, the creatinine level is affected very little by hepatic function. The serum creatinine level has much the same significance as the BUN level but tends to rise later. Therefore elevations in creatinine suggest chronicity of the disease process. In general, a doubling of creatinine suggests a 50% reduction in the glomerular filtration rate. The creatinine level is interpreted in conjunction with the BUN. These tests are referred to as *renal function studies*.

Interfering factors

☢ Drugs that may *increase* creatinine values include aminoglycosides (e.g., gentamicin), cimetidine, heavy-metal chemotherapeutic agents (e.g., cisplatin), and other nephrotoxic drugs such as cephalosporins (e.g., cefoxitin).

Procedure and patient care

Before
- Explain the procedure to the patient.
- Tell the patient that no fasting is required.

During
- Collect approximately 5 ml of blood in a red-top tube.
- For pediatric patients, blood is usually drawn from a heel stick.

After
- Apply pressure or a pressure dressing to the venipuncture site.
- Observe the venipuncture site for bleeding.

Abnormal findings

▲ Increased levels
Glomerulonephritis
Pyelonephritis
Acute tubular necrosis
Urinary tract obstruction
Reduced renal blood
flow (e.g., shock, dehydration, congestive heart failure, atherosclerosis)
Diabetes
Nephritis
Rhabdomyolysis
Acromegaly
Gigantism

▼ Decreased levels
Debilitation
Decreased muscle mass
(e.g., muscular dystrophy, myasthenia gravis)

notes

creatinine clearance

Type of test Urine (24-hour); blood

C

Normal findings

Adult (<40 years)
  Male: 90-139 ml/min or 0.87-1.34 ml/sec/m^2
  Female: 80-125 ml/min or 0.77-1.20 ml/sec/m^2
Values decrease 6.5 ml/min/decade of life because of decline
  in glomerular filtration rate (GFR).
Newborn: 40-65 ml/min

Test explanation and related physiology

The creatinine clearance (CC) is a measure of the glomerular filtration rate (GFR; i.e., the number of milliliters of filtrate made by the kidneys per minute). Urine and serum creatinine levels are assessed, and the clearance rate is calculated.

The amount of filtrate made in the kidney depends on the amount of blood present to be filtered and on the ability of the glomeruli to act as a filter. The amount of blood present for filtration is decreased in renal artery atherosclerosis, dehydration, or shock. The ability of the glomeruli to act as a filter is decreased by diseases such as glomerulonephritis, acute tubular necrosis, and most other primary renal diseases. Significant bilateral obstruction to urinary outflow affects glomerular filtration (CC) only after it is long-standing.

When one kidney alone becomes diseased, the opposite kidney, if normal, has the ability to compensate by increasing its filtration rate. Therefore, with unilateral kidney disease or nephrectomy, a decrease in CC is not expected if the other kidney is normal.

Several nonrenal factors may influence CC. With each decade of age, the CC decreases 6.5 ml/min because of a decrease in the GFR. Urine collections are timed, and incomplete collections will falsely decrease CC. Muscle mass varies among people. Decreased muscle mass will give lower CC values. Likewise, ingestion of large meat meals will temporarily increase CC.

The CC test requires a 24-hour urine collection and a serum creatinine level. Creatinine clearance is then computed using the following formula:

$$\text{Creatinine clearance} = \frac{UV}{P}$$

where

U = Number of milligrams per deciliter of creatinine excreted in the urine over 24 hours

V = Volume of urine in milliliters per minute

P = Serum creatinine in milligrams per deciliter

A 24-hour urine collection for creatinine is often measured along with other urine collections to assess the completeness of other 24-hour collections. In patients with normal creatinine, the CC should indicate whether all the urine has been collected for the 24 hours.

Interfering factors

- Exercise may cause increased creatinine values.
- Incomplete urine collection may give a falsely lowered value.
- ✗ Drugs that may cause *increased* levels include aminoglycosides (e.g., gentamicin), cimetidine, heavy-metal chemotherapeutic agents (e.g., cisplatin), and nephrotoxic drugs such as cephalosporins (e.g., cefoxitin).

Procedure and patient care

Before

- Explain the procedure to the patient.
- Tell the patient that no special diet is usually required.
- Note that some laboratories instruct the patient to avoid cooked meat, tea, coffee, or drugs on the day of the test. Check with the laboratory.

During

- Instruct the patient to begin the 24-hour urine collection, after voiding. Discard the initial specimen and start the 24-hour timing as of that point.
- Collect all the urine passed during the next 24 hours.
- Show the patient where to store the urine specimen.
- Keep the specimen on ice or refrigerated during the 24 hours.
- Indicate the starting time on the urine container and laboratory slip.
- Post the hours for the urine collection in a noticeable place to prevent accidental discharge of a specimen.

- Instruct the patient to void before defecating so that urine is not contaminated by feces.
- Remind the patient not to put toilet paper in the collection container.
- Encourage the patient to drink fluids during the 24 hours unless this is contraindicated for medical purposes.
- Instruct the patient to avoid vigorous exercise during the 24 hours, because exercise may cause an increased creatinine clearance.
- Collect the last specimen as close as possible to the end of the 24-hour period. Add this urine to the container.
- Make sure a venous blood sample is drawn in a red-top tube during the 24-hour collection.
- Mark the patient's age, weight, and height on the requisition sheet.

After
- Transport the urine specimen promptly to the laboratory.
- Apply pressure or a pressure dressing to the venipuncture site.
- Observe the venipuncture site for bleeding.

Abnormal findings

▲ **Increased levels**
Exercise
Pregnancy

▼ **Decreased levels**
Impaired kidney function (e.g., renal artery atherosclerosis, glomerulonephritis, acute tubular necrosis)
Conditions causing decreased GFR (congestive heart failure, cirrhosis with ascites, shock, dehydration)

notes

cryoglobulin

Type of test Blood

Normal findings No cryoglobulins detected

Test explanation and related physiology

Cryoglobulins are abnormal globulin protein complexes that exist within the blood of patients with various diseases. These proteins will precipitate reversibly at low temperatures and redissolve with rewarming. These cryoglobulins can precipitate within the blood vessel of the fingers when exposed to cold temperatures. This precipitation causes sludging of the blood within those blood vessels. These patients may have symptoms of purpura, arthralgia, or Raynaud's phenomenon (pain, cyanosis, coldness of the fingers).

These proteins exist in varying degrees depending on the disease entity with which they are associated. Serum levels greater than 5 mg/ml are associated with multiple myeloma, macroglobulinemia, and leukemia. Globulin levels between 1 and 5 mg/ml are associated with rheumatoid arthritis. Levels less than 1 mg/ml can be associated with systemic lupus erythematosus, rheumatoid arthritis, infectious mononucleosis, viral hepatitis, endocarditis, cirrhosis, and glomerulonephritis.

For this test, the blood sample is taken to the chemistry laboratory, where it is refrigerated for 72 hours. After that time the specimen is evaluated for precipitation. If precipitation is identified, it is measured and recorded. The tube is then rewarmed, and the specimen is reexamined for dissolution of that precipitation. If precipitation of the refrigerated specimen is identified and dissolved on rewarming, cryoglobulins are present.

Procedure and patient care

Before

- Explain the procedure to the patient.
- Inform the patient that an 8-hour fast may be required. This will minimize turbidity of the serum caused by ingestion of a recent (especially fatty) meal. Turbidity may make the detection of precipitation rather difficult.

During

- Collect 10 ml of venous blood in a red-top tube that has been prewarmed to body temperature.

After

- Apply pressure or a pressure dressing to the venipuncture site.
- Observe the venipuncture site for bleeding.
- If cryoglobulins are found to be present, warn the patient to avoid cold temperatures and contact with cold objects to minimize Raynaud's symptoms. Tell the patient to wear gloves in cold weather.

Abnormal findings

Multiple myeloma
Leukemia
Macroglobulinemia
Connective tissue disease
  (e.g., lupus erythematosus)

Infectious mononucleosis
Hepatitis
Endocarditis
Lymphoma or other malignancy
Glomerulonephritis

notes

cutaneous immunofluorescence biopsy
(Immunofluorescence skin biopsy, Skin biopsy antibodies, Skin immunohistopathology)

Type of test Microscopic examination of skin tissue

Normal findings Normal skin histology

Test explanation and related physiology

For this study, a skin biopsy is obtained and evaluated by immunofluorescence study. Deposition of human immunoglobulins and complement components is determined by immunofluorescent patterns. This test is useful in detecting immune complexes, complement, and immunoglobulin deposition in systemic and discoid lupus erythematosus, pemphigus, bullous pemphigoid, and dermatitis herpetiformis. This test is also used to confirm the histopathology of skin lesions and to follow the results of treatment.

Procedure and patient care

Before
- Explain the procedure to the patient.
- Obtain an informed consent.

During
- A 4-mm punch biopsy or tissue excision is obtained.

After
- Apply a dry, sterile dressing over the biopsy site.
- Tell the patient that results may not be available for several days.
- Deliver the specimen on ice immediately to the laboratory after the biopsy is taken.

Abnormal findings

Systemic lupus erythematosus
Discoid lupus erythematosus
Pemphigus

Bullous pemphigoid
Dermatitis herpetiformis

notes

cystography (Cystourethrography, Voiding cystography, Voiding cystourethrography)

Type of test X-ray with contrast dye

Normal findings Normal bladder structure and function

Test explanation and related physiology

Filling the bladder with radiopaque contrast material provides visualization of the bladder for radiographic study. Either fluoroscopic or x-ray films demonstrate bladder filling and collapse after emptying. Filling defects or shadows within the bladder indicate primary bladder tumors. Extrinsic compression or distortion of the bladder is seen with pelvic tumor (e.g., rectal, cervical) or hematoma (secondary to pelvic bone fractures). Extravasation of the dye is seen with traumatic rupture, perforation, and fistula of the bladder. Vesicoureteral reflux (abnormal backflow of urine from bladder to ureters), which can cause persistent or recurrent pyelonephritis, also may be demonstrated during cystography. Although the bladder is visualized during an intravenous pyelogram (see p. 487), primary pathologic bladder conditions are best studied by cystography.

Contraindications

- Patients with urethral or bladder infection or injury

Potential complications

- Urinary tract infection
  This may result from catheter placement or the instillation of contaminated contrast material.
- Allergic reaction to iodinated dye
  This rarely occurs, because the dye is not administered intravenously.

Procedure and patient care

Before

- Explain the procedure to the patient.
- Obtain informed consent if required by the institution.
- Give clear liquids for breakfast on the morning of the test.
- Assure the patient that he or she will be draped to prevent unnecessary exposure.
- Insert a Foley catheter if ordered.

During

- Note the following procedural steps:
  1. The patient is taken to the radiology department and placed in a supine or lithotomy position.
  2. Unless the catheter is already present, one is placed.
  3. Through the catheter, approximately 300 ml of air or radiopaque dye (much less for children) is injected into the bladder.
  4. The catheter is clamped.
  5. X-ray films are taken.
  6. If the patient is able to void, the catheter is removed and the patient is asked to urinate while films are taken of the bladder and urethra (voiding cystourethrogram).
- Ensure that males wear a lead shield over the testes to prevent irradiation of the gonads.
- Remember that female patients cannot be shielded without blocking bladder visualization.
- Note that a radiologist performs the study in approximately 15 to 30 minutes.
- Tell the patient that this test is moderately uncomfortable if bladder catheterization is required.

After

- Assess the patient for signs of urinary tract infection.
- Encourage the patient to drink fluids to eliminate the dye and to prevent accumulation of bacteria.

Abnormal findings

Bladder tumor
Pelvic tumor
Hematoma

Bladder trauma
Vesicoureteral reflux

notes

cystometry (Cystometrogram [CMG])

Type of test Manometric

C

Normal findings

Normal sensations of fullness and temperature
Normal pressures and volumes
Maximal cystometric capacity
 Male: 350-750 ml
 Female: 250-550 ml
Intravesical pressure when bladder is empty: usually <40 cm
 H_2O
Detrusor pressure: <10 cm H_2O

Test explanation and related physiology

The purpose of cystometry is to evaluate the motor and sensory function of the bladder when incontinence is present or neurologic bladder dysfunction is suspected. A graphic recording of pressure exerted at varying phases of the filling of the urinary bladder is produced. A pressure/volume relationship of the bladder is made. This urodynamic study assesses the neuromuscular function of the bladder by measuring the efficiency of the detrusor muscle, intravesical pressure and capacity, and the bladder's response to thermal stimulation.

Cystometry can determine whether bladder pathology is caused by neurologic, infectious, or obstructive diseases. Cystometry is indicated to elucidate the causes for frequency and urgency, especially before surgery on the urologic outflow tract. Cystometry is also part of the evaluation for the following: incontinence, persistent residual urine, vesicoureteral reflux, neurologic disorders, sensory disorders, and the effect of certain drugs on bladder function.

Contraindications

- Urinary tract infections because of the possibility of false results and the potential for the spread of infection

Procedure and patient care

Before

- Explain the purpose and the procedure to the patient.
- Tell the patient that no fluid or food restrictions are needed.

- Assure the patient that he or she will be draped to prevent unnecessary exposure.
- Assess the patient for signs and symptoms of urinary tract infection.
- Instruct the patient not to strain while voiding, because the results can be skewed.
- If the patient has a spinal cord injury, transport him or her on a stretcher. The test will then be performed with the patient on the stretcher.

During

- Note the following procedural steps:
    1. Cystometry, usually performed in a urologist's office or a special procedure room, begins with the patient being asked to void.
    2. The amount of time required to initiate voiding and the size, force, and continuity of the urinary stream are recorded. The amount of urine, the time of voiding, and the presence of any straining, hesitancy, or terminal urine dribbling are also recorded.
    3. The patient is placed in a lithotomy or supine position.
    4. A retention catheter is inserted through the urethra and into the bladder.
    5. Residual urine volume is measured and recorded.
    6. Thermal sensation is evaluated by the instillation of approximately 30 ml of room temperature saline solution into the bladder followed by an equal amount of warm water. The patient reports any sensations.
    7. This fluid is withdrawn from the bladder.
    8. The urethral catheter is connected to a cystometer (a tube used to monitor bladder pressure).
    9. Sterile water, normal saline solution, or carbon dioxide gas is slowly introduced into the bladder at a controlled rate, usually with the patient in a sitting position.
    10. Patients are asked to indicate the first urge to void and then when they have the feeling that they must void. The bladder is full at this point.
    11. The pressures and volumes are plotted on a graph.
    12. The patient is asked to void, and the maximal intravesical voiding pressure is recorded.
    13. The bladder is drained for any residual urine.
    14. If no additional studies are to be done, the urethral catheter is removed.

- Throughout the study, ask the patient to report any sensations, such as pain, flushing, sweating, nausea, bladder filling, and an urgency to void.
- Note that certain drugs may be administered during the cystometric examination to distinguish between underactivity of the bladder because of muscle failure and underactivity associated with denervation. Cholinergic drugs (e.g., bethanechol [Urecholine]) may be given to enhance the tone of a flaccid bladder. Anticholinergic drugs (e.g., atropine) may be given to promote relaxation of a hyperactive bladder. If these drugs are to be given, the catheter is left in place. The drugs are given, and the examination is repeated 20 to 30 minutes later using the first test as a control value.
- Note that this test is performed by a urologist in approximately 45 minutes.
- Explain to the patient that the only discomfort is that associated with the urethral catheterization.

After

- Observe the patient for any manifestations of infection (e.g., elevated temperature, chills).
- Examine the urine for hematuria. Notify the physician if the hematuria persists after several voidings.
- Provide a warm sitz bath or tub bath for the patient's comfort if desired.

Abnormal findings

Neurogenic bladder
Bladder obstruction
Bladder infection

Bladder hypertonicity
Diminished bladder capacity

notes

cystoscopy (Endourology)

Type of test Endoscopy

Normal findings Normal structure and function of the urethra, bladder, ureters, and prostate (in males)

Test explanation and related physiology

Cystoscopy provides direct visualization of the urethra and bladder through the transurethral insertion of a cystoscope into the bladder (Figure 10). Cystoscopy is used *diagnostically* to allow:

1. Direct inspection and biopsy of the prostate, bladder, and urethra
2. Collection of a separate urine specimen directly from each kidney by the placement of ureteral catheters

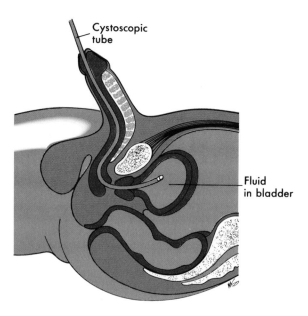

Figure 10 Cystoscopic examination of the male bladder. (From Beare PG, Myers JL: *Principles and practice of adult health nursing,* ed 2, St Louis, 1994, Mosby.)

3. Measurement of bladder capacity and determination of ureteral reflux
4. Identification of bladder and ureteral calculi
5. Placement of ureteral catheters (Figure 11) for retrograde pyelography (see p. 720)
6. Identification of the source of hematuria

Cystoscopy is used *therapeutically* to provide:

1. Resection of small, superficial bladder tumors
2. Removal of foreign bodies and stones
3. Dilation of the urethra and ureters
4. Placement of catheters to drain urine from the renal pelvis
5. Coagulation of bleeding areas

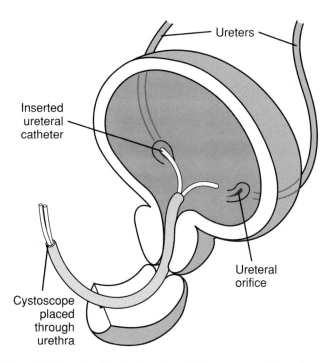

Figure 11 Ureteral catheterization through the cystoscope. Note the ureteral catheter inserted into the right orifice. The left ureteral catheter is ready to be inserted.

6. Implantation of radium seeds into a tumor
7. Resection of hypertrophied or malignant prostate gland overgrowth
8. Placement of ureteral stents for identification of ureters during pelvic surgery

The cystoscope consists primarily of an obturator and a telescope. The obturator is used to insert the cystoscope atraumatically. After the cystoscope is within the bladder, the obturator is removed and the telescope is passed through the cystoscope. The lens and lighting system of the telescope permit adequate visualization of the lower genitourinary tract. Transcopic instruments, such as forceps, scissors, needles, and electrodes, are used when appropriate.

Endourology is an endoscopic procedure that visualizes the bladder and urethra. It is more comprehensive than cystoscopy, because it includes a detailed visualization of the urethra. This test is important in the evaluation of hematuria, chronic infection, suspected stones, and radiographic filling defects. On inspection, the urethra may show inflammation or structural causes of obstruction (e.g., stricture, neoplasia, prostatic hypertrophy). If the obstruction is functional rather than structural (e.g., detrusor–bladder neck dyssynergia), no site of obstruction will be demonstrated by endoscopy.

Potential complications

- Perforation of the bladder
- Sepsis by seeding the bloodstream with bacteria from infected urine
- Hematuria
- Urinary retention

Procedure and patient care

Before

- Explain the procedure to the patient.
- Ensure that an informed consent is obtained.
- If enemas are ordered to clear the bowel, assist the patient as needed and record the results.
- Encourage the patient to drink fluids several hours before the procedure to maintain a continuous flow of urine for collection and to prevent multiplication of bacteria that may be introduced during this technique.
- If the procedure will be done with the patient under local anesthesia, allow a liquid breakfast.

- If the procedure will be performed with the patient under general anesthesia, follow routine precautions. Keep the patient NPO after midnight on the day of the test. Fluids may be given intravenously.
- Administer the preprocedural medications as ordered 1 hour before the study. Sedatives decrease the spasm of the bladder sphincter, decreasing the patient's discomfort.

During

- Note the following procedural steps:
  1. Cystoscopy is usually performed in the operating room but also can be done in the urologist's office.
  2. The patient is placed in the lithotomy position with his or her feet in stirrups.
  3. The external genitalia are cleansed with an antiseptic solution such as povidone-iodine (Betadine).
  4. A local anesthetic is instilled into the urethra if general anesthesia has not been used.
  5. The cystoscope is inserted, and the desired diagnostic or therapeutic studies are performed.
- Instruct the patient to lie very still during the entire procedure to prevent trauma to the urinary tract.
- Tell the patient that he or she will have the desire to void as the cystoscope passes the bladder neck.
- When the procedure is completed, keep the patient on bed rest for a short time.
- Note that if *endourology* is performed, the urethra will also be evaluated.
- Note that this procedure is performed by a urologist in approximately 25 minutes.
- When local anesthesia is used, inform the patient of the associated discomfort (much more than with urethral catheterization).

After

- Instruct the patient not to walk or stand alone immediately after the legs have been removed from the stirrups. The orthostasis that may result from standing erect may cause dizziness and fainting.
- Assess the patient's ability to void for at least 24 hours after the procedure. Urinary retention may be secondary to edema caused by instrumentation.
- Note the urine color. Pink-tinged urine is common. The

presence of bright-red blood or clots should be reported to the physician.

- Monitor the patient for complaints of back pain, bladder spasms, urinary frequency, and burning on urination. Warm sitz baths and mild analgesics may be ordered and given. Sometimes belladonna and opium (B&O) suppositories are given to relieve bladder spasms. Warm, moist heat to the lower abdomen may help to relieve pain and to promote muscle relaxation.
- Encourage increased intake of fluids. A dilute urine decreases dysuria. Fluids also maintain a constant flow of urine to prevent stasis and the accumulation of bacteria in the bladder.
- Check and record the patient's vital signs as ordered. Watch for a decrease in blood pressure and an increase in pulse as an indication of hemorrhage.
- Observe for signs and symptoms of sepsis (elevated temperature, flush, chills, decreased blood pressure, increased pulse).
- Note that antibiotics are occasionally ordered 1 day before and 3 days following the procedure to reduce the incidence of bacteremia that may occur with instrumentation of the urethra and bladder.
- Encourage the patient to use cathartics, especially after cystoscopic surgery. Increases in intraabdominal pressure caused by constipation may initiate severe lower urologic bleeding.

Abnormal findings

Lower urologic tract tumor
Stones in the ureter or bladder
Prostatic hypertrophy
Prostate cancer

Inflammation of the bladder and urethra
Urethral/ureteral stricture
Prostatitis
Vesical neck contracture

notes

cytomegalovirus (CMV)

Type of test Blood

Normal findings No virus isolated

Test explanation and related physiology

CMV is part of the viral family that includes herpes simplex, Epstein-Barr, and varicella-zoster viruses. CMV is widespread and common. Male homosexuals, transplant patients, and AIDS patients are particularly susceptible. Infections are acquired by contact with body secretions or urine. Most patients with acute disease have no or very few (mononucleosis-like) symptoms. Virus culture is the most definitive method of diagnosis. However, a culture cannot differentiate acute infection from chronic, inactive infection. Immunofluorescence, ELISA, and latex agglutination methods reveal much more information about activity of infection.

CMV IgG antibody levels persist for years after infection. Measurement of IgM antibodies, however, indicates a relatively short time of infection (6 to 12 months) and thereby acute or recent infection. There are three different CMV antigens that can be detected immunologically. They are called early, intermediate-early, and late antigens and indicate onset of infection.

Cytomegalovirus is the most common congenital infection. Approximately 10% of infected newborns exhibit permanent damage, usually mental retardation and auditory damage. Fetal infection can cause microcephaly, hydrocephaly, cerebral palsy, mental retardation, or death. No specific therapy is known for this infection. If the diagnosis is established early by viral culture or serology, abortion may be an option. A fourfold increase in CMV titer in paired sera drawn 10 to 14 days apart is usually indicative of an acute infection.

Procedure and patient care

Before

- Explain the procedure to the patient.

During

- For culture specimens, a urine, sputum, or mouth swab is the specimen of choice. Fresh specimens are essential.

- The specimens are cultured in a virus laboratory, which takes about 3 to 7 days.
- For antibody or antigen titer, draw 4 to 7 ml of blood in a gold- or red-top tube.
- Collect a specimen from the mother with suspected acute infection as early as possible.
- Collect the convalescent specimen 2 to 4 weeks later.

After

- Apply pressure or a pressure dressing to the venipuncture site.
- Assess the venipuncture site for bleeding.

Abnormal finding

CMV infection

notes

D-dimer test (Fragment D-dimer, Fibrin degradation fragment)

Type of test Blood

Normal findings

Negative (no D-dimer fragments present)
<250 ng/ml or <250 μg/L (SI units)

Test explanation and related physiology

The fragment D-dimer assesses both thrombin and plasmin activity. D-dimer is a fibrin degradation fragment that is made through fibrinolysis. This assay is a highly specific measurement of the amount of fibrin degradation that occurs. Normal plasma does not have detectable amounts of fragment D-dimer.

This test provides a simple and confirmatory test for disseminated intravascular coagulation (DIC). Positive results of the D-dimer assay correlate with positive results of fibrin degradation products (FDPs) (see p. 394). Although the D-dimer assay is more specific than the FDP assay, it is less sensitive. Therefore combining the FDP and the D-dimer provides a highly sensitive and specific test for recognizing DIC in a patient. Levels increase when a fibrin clot is lysed by thrombolytic therapy. Thrombotic problems such as deep-vein thrombosis, pulmonary embolism, sickle cell anemia, and thrombosis of malignancy are also associated with high D-dimer levels.

Procedure and patient care

Before
- Explain the procedure to the patient.
- Tell the patient that no fasting is required.

During
- Collect a venous blood sample in a blue-top tube.

After
- Apply pressure or a pressure dressing to the venipuncture site.
- Assess the venipuncture site for bleeding. Remember that if the patient is receiving anticoagulants or has coagulopathies, the bleeding time will be increased.

Abnormal findings

▲ **Increased levels**

Fibrinolysis

During thrombolytic or defibrination therapy with tissue plasminogen activator

Deep-vein thrombosis

Pulmonary embolism

Arterial thromboembolism

Disseminated intravascular coagulation

Vaso-occlusive crisis of sickle cell anemia

Pregnancy

Malignancy

Surgery

notes

delta-aminolevulinic acid (Aminolevulinic acid [ALA], Delta-ALA)

D

Type of test Urine (24-hour)

Normal findings 1-7 mg/24 hr or 11.1-57.2 µmol/24 hr (SI units)

Possible critical values >20 mg/24 hr

Test explanation and related physiology

The basic precursor for the porphyrins (see p. 642), delta-ALA, is an enzyme needed for the normal conversion to porphobilinogen during heme synthesis. Impaired conversion, which causes abnormal red blood cell (RBC) formation, occurs in lead intoxication and porphyria. These conditions cause the urine levels of ALA to rise before other chemical or hematologic changes.

Urine levels of ALA are obtained to screen for lead poisoning and to aid in the diagnosis of certain types of genetic deficiencies of porphyrin metabolism. Elevated levels also may be seen in patients with hepatitis and hepatic carcinoma.

Healthy people usually do not have ALA present in their urine. Increased values, however, may be seen in patients taking some medications (e.g., penicillin, barbiturates, griseofulvin).

Interfering factors

✶ Drugs that may cause *increased* ALA levels include penicillin, barbiturates, and griseofulvin.

Procedure and patient care

Before

- Explain the procedure to the patient.

During

- Instruct the patient to begin a 24-hour urine collection after voiding. Discard the initial specimen and start the 24-hour timing at that point.
- Collect all urine passed during the next 24 hours.
- Show the patient where to store the urine container.
- Keep the specimen on ice or refrigerated during the 24 hours.

- Keep the urine in a light-resistant container with a preservative.
- Indicate the starting time on the urine container and on the laboratory slip.
- Post the hours for the urine collection in a noticeable place to prevent accidental discarding of the specimen.
- Instruct the patient to void before defecating so that urine is not contaminated by feces.
- Remind the patient not to put toilet paper in the collection container.
- Encourage the patient to drink fluids during the 24 hours unless this is contraindicated for medical purposes.
- Collect the last specimen as close as possible to the end of the 24-hour period. Add this to the urine collection.
- If the patient has a Foley catheter in place, cover the drainage bag to prevent exposure to light.
- Indicate on the laboratory slip any drugs that may affect test results.

After

- Transport the urine specimen promptly to the laboratory.

Abnormal findings

▲ **Increased levels**

Porphyria   Hepatitis
Lead intoxication   Hepatic carcinoma

notes

---

dexamethasone suppression test (DST, Prolonged/rapid DST, Cortisol suppression test, ACTH suppression test)

D

Type of test Blood; urine (24-hour)

Normal findings

Prolonged method

Expected values (normal)
  Low dose: >50% reduction of plasma cortisol and 17-hydroxycorticosteroid (17-OCHS) levels
  High dose: >50% reduction of plasma cortisol and 17-OCHS levels

Rapid method

  Normal: nearly 0 cortisol levels

Test explanation and related physiology

The DST is an important test for diagnosing adrenal hyperfunction (Cushing's syndrome) and distinguishing its cause. This test is based on pituitary adrenocorticotropic hormone (ACTH) secretion being dependent on the plasma cortisol feedback mechanism. As plasma cortisol levels increase, ACTH secretion is suppressed; as cortisol levels decrease, ACTH secretion is stimulated. Dexamethasone is a synthetic steroid (similar to cortisol) that will suppress ACTH secretion. Under normal circumstances, this results in reduced stimulation to the adrenal glands and, ultimately, a drop of 50% or more in plasma cortisol and 17-OCHS levels. This important feedback system does not function properly in patients with Cushing's syndrome.

In Cushing's syndrome caused by bilateral adrenal hyperplasia (Cushing's disease), the pituitary gland is reset upward and responds only to high plasma levels of cortisone and steroids. In Cushing's syndrome caused by adrenal adenoma or cancer (which acts autonomously), cortisol secretion will continue despite a decrease in ACTH. When Cushing's syndrome is caused by an ectopic ACTH-producing tumor (as in lung cancer), that tumor is also considered autonomous and will continue to secrete ACTH despite high cortisol levels. Again, no decrease occurs in plasma cortisol. Knowledge of the following defects in the normal cortisol-

ACTH feedback system is the basis for understanding the DST:

> Cushing's syndrome caused by:
>> Bilateral adrenal hyperplasia
>>> Low dose: no change
>>> High dose: >50% reduction of plasma cortisol and 17-OCHS levels
>> Adrenal adenoma or carcinoma
>>> Low dose: no change
>>> High dose: no change
>> Ectopic ACTH-producing tumor
>>> Low dose: no change
>>> High dose: no change

The DST also may identify depressed persons likely to respond to electroconvulsive therapy or antidepressants rather than to psychologic or social interventions. ACTH production will not be suppressed after administration of low-dose dexamethasone in these patients.

The *prolonged* DST can be performed over a 6-day period on an outpatient basis. The *rapid* DST is easily and quickly performed and is used primarily as a screening test to diagnose Cushing's syndrome. It is less accurate and less informative than the prolonged DST, but when its results are normal, the diagnosis of Cushing's syndrome can safely be excluded. The ease with which the rapid DST can be performed makes it useful in clinical medicine.

Interfering factors

- Stress can cause ACTH release and obscure interpretation of test results.
- Drugs that can affect test results include barbiturates, estrogens, oral contraceptives, phenytoin (Dilantin), spironolactone (Aldactone), steroids, and tetracyclines.

Procedure and patient care

Before

- Explain the procedure (prolonged or rapid test) to the patient.
- Obtain the patient's weight as a baseline for evaluating side effects of steroids.

During

Prolonged test

- Obtain a baseline 24-hour urine collection for corticosteroids (urine 17-OCHS [see p. 469] or urinary cortisol [see p. 287]).

- Collect blood for determination of baseline plasma cortisol levels (see p. 285) if indicated.
- Collect 24-hour urine specimens daily over a 6-day period. Because 6 continuous days of urine collections are needed, no urine specimens are discarded except for the first voided specimen on day 1, after which the collection begins.
- On day 3, administer a low dose (0.5 mg) of dexamethasone by mouth every 6 hours for a total of 2 mg.
- On day 5, administer a high dose (2.0 mg) of dexamethasone by mouth every 6 hours for a total of 8 mg.
- Administer the dexamethasone with milk or an antacid to prevent gastric irritation.
- Remember that the urine samples for cortisol and 17-OCHS do not need a preservative.
- Note that the creatinine content is measured in all the 24-hour urine collections to demonstrate their accuracy and adequacy.
- Keep the urine specimens refrigerated or on ice during the collection period.

Rapid test
- Give the patient 1 mg of dexamethasone by mouth at 11 PM.
- Administer the dexamethasone with milk or an antacid to prevent gastric irritation.
- If ordered, administer a barbiturate to sedate the patient and to ensure a good night's sleep.
- At 8 AM the next morning, draw blood for determination of the plasma cortisol level before the patient arises.
- If no cortisol suppression occurs after 1 mg of dexamethasone, administer a higher dose (8 mg) to suppress ACTH production. This is referred to as the *overnight 8-mg dexamethasone suppression test.*

After
- Evaluate the patient for evidence of gastric irritation.
- Assess the patient for steroid-induced side effects by monitoring weight, glucose levels, and potassium levels.
- Send specimens to the laboratory promptly.

Abnormal findings

Adrenal hyperfunction (Cushing's syndrome)

Hyperthyroidism
Mental depression

2,3-diphosphoglycerate (2,3-DPG in erythrocytes)

Type of test Blood

Normal findings

12.3 ± 1.87 µmol/g of hemoglobin
4.2 ± 0.64 µmol/ml of erythrocytes
Levels are lower in newborns and even lower in premature infants.

Test explanation and related physiology

This test is used in the evaluation of anemia. 2,3-DPG is a red blood cell (RBC) enzyme that controls oxygen transport from the RBCs to the tissues. Deficiencies of this enzyme result in alterations of the RBC-oxygen dissociation curve that controls release of oxygen to the tissues.

Usually, 2,3-DPG levels increase in response to anemia or hypoxic conditions (e.g., obstructive lung disease, congenital cyanotic heart disease, after vigorous exercise). Increases in 2,3-DPG decrease the oxygen binding of hemoglobin so that increased amounts of oxygen are released to the tissues at lower oxygen tensions. Levels of 2,3-DPG are decreased as a result of inherited genetic defects. This genetic defect parallels sickle cell anemia and hemoglobin C diseases.

Interfering factors

- Levels may be increased after vigorous exercise.
- High altitudes may increase 2,3-DPG levels.
- Banked blood has decreased amounts of 2,3-DPG.
- Acidosis decreases 2,3-DPG levels.

Procedure and patient care

Before
- Explain the procedure to the patient.
- Tell the patient that no fasting is required.

During
- Collect a venous blood sample in a red-top tube.

After
- Apply pressure or a pressure dressing to the venipuncture site.
- Assess the venipuncture site for bleeding.

Abnormal findings

▲ **Increased levels**
  Anemia
  Uremia
  Cirrhosis
  Obstructive lung disease
  Congenital cyanotic heart
    disease
  Hyperthyroidism
  Cystic fibrosis with pul-
    monary involvement
  Chronic renal failure
    (secondary to anemia)

▼ **Decreased levels**
  Polycythemia
  Respiratory distress syn-
    drome
  2,3-DPG disease

D

notes

disseminated intravascular coagulation screening
(DIC screening)

Type of test Refer to specific tests in Table 9.

Normal findings No evidence of DIC

Test explanation and related physiology

This is a group of tests used to detect disseminated intravascular coagulation. Many pathologic conditions can instigate or are associated with DIC. The more common ones include bacterial septicemia, amniotic fluid embolism, retention of a dead fetus, malignant neoplasia, liver cirrhosis, extensive surgery (especially on the liver), postextracorporeal heart bypass, extensive trauma, severe burns, and transfusion reactions.

In DIC, the entire clotting mechanism is triggered inappropriately. This results in significant systemic or localized intravascular formation of fibrin clots. Consequences of this futile clotting are intravascular sludging and excessive bleeding caused by consumption of the platelets and clotting factors that have been

TABLE 9 Disseminated intravascular coagulation screening tests

Test	Positive result
Bleeding time (p. 141)	Prolonged
Platelet count (p. 631)	Decreased
Prothrombin time (p. 678)	Prolonged
Activated partial thrombo-plastin time (p. 601)	Prolonged
Fibrinogen (factor I concentration) (p. 396)	Decreased
Fibrin degradation products (p. 394)	Present
Red blood cell smear (p. 151)	Damaged red blood cells and decreased number of platelets
Euglobulin lysis time (p. 380)	Normal or prolonged
D-dimer (p. 317)	Increased

used in intravascular clotting. The fibrinolytic system is also activated to break down the clot formation and the fibrin involved in the intravascular coagulation. This fibrinolysis results in the formation of fibrin degradation products (FDPs), which, by themselves, act as anticoagulants; these FDPs only serve to enhance the bleeding tendency.

Organ injury can occur as a result of the intravascular clots, which cause microvascular occlusion in various organs. This may cause serious anoxic injury in affected organs. Also, red blood cells (RBCs) passing through partly plugged vessels are injured and subsequently hemolyzed. The result may be ongoing hemolytic anemia. Figure 12 summarizes DIC pathophysiology and effects. Heparin is sometimes used to treat DIC because it inhibits the ongoing futile thrombin formation. This decreases the use of clotting factors and platelets, and bleeding ceases.

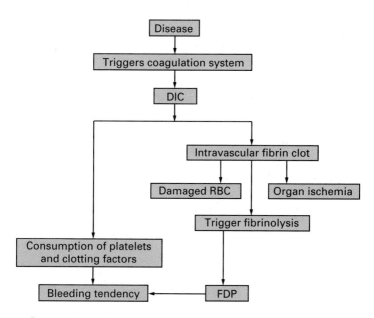

Figure 12 Pathophysiology of disseminated intravascular coagulation *(DIC)*, which may result in bleeding tendency, organ ischemia, and hemolytic anemia. *RBC,* Red blood cell; *FDP,* fibrin degradation product.

When a patient with a bleeding tendency is suspected to have DIC, a series of readily performed laboratory tests should be performed (Table 9). With these tests, the hematologist can make the appropriate diagnosis confidently. All these tests are discussed separately.

notes

Doppler studies

Type of test Ultrasound

Normal findings

Venous

A normal Doppler venous signal with spontaneous respiration
Normal venous system without evidence of occlusion

Arterial

Normal arterial Doppler signal with systolic and diastolic components
No reduction in blood pressure in excess of 20 mm Hg compared with the normal extremity
A normal ankle-to-brachial arterial blood pressure index of 0.85 or greater
No evidence of arterial occlusion

Test explanation and related physiology

Doppler studies are used to identify occlusion of the veins or arteries. *Venous* patency is demonstrated through Doppler ultrasound by detecting moving red blood cells (RBCs) within the vein. The Doppler transducer directs an ultrasound beam at the vein. Moving RBCs reflect the beam back to the transducer, which then transforms the flow velocity into a "swishing" noise augmented by an audio speaker. If the vein is occluded, no swishing sounds are detected.

With *arterial* Doppler studies, one can identify and locate peripheral arteriosclerotic occlusive disease of the extremities. By slowly deflating blood pressure cuffs placed on the calf and ankle, the systolic pressure in the various arteries of the extremities can be accurately measured by detecting the first evidence of blood flow with the Doppler transducer. The extremely sensitive Doppler ultrasound detector can recognize the "swishing" sound of even the most minimal blood flow. Normally, there is a minimal drop in systolic blood pressure from the arteries of the arms to those of the legs. If the drop in blood pressure exceeds 20 mm Hg, occlusive disease is believed to exist immediately proximal to the area tested.

Interfering factors

- Venous or arterial occlusive disease proximal to the site of testing
- Cigarette smoking, because nicotine can cause constriction of the peripheral arteries and alter the results

Procedure and patient care

Before

- Explain the procedure to the patient.
- Inform the patient that this is a painless procedure.
- Remove all clothing from the extremity to be examined.
- Instruct the patient to abstain from cigarette smoking for at least 30 minutes before the test.

During

- Note the following procedural steps:

Venous Doppler studies
1. A conductive gel is applied to the skin overlying the venous system of the extremity in multiple areas.
2. Usually, for the lower extremity, the deep venous system is identified in the ankle, calf, thigh, and groin.
3. The characteristic "swishing" sound of the Doppler indicates a patent venous system. Failure to detect this signal indicates venous occlusion.
4. Usually, both the superficial and venous systems are evaluated.

Arterial Doppler studies
1. These are performed with the use of blood pressure cuffs, which are placed around the thigh, calf, and ankle.
2. A conductive paste is applied to the skin overlying the artery distal to the cuffs.
3. The proximal cuff is inflated to a level above systolic blood pressure in the normal extremity.
4. The Doppler ultrasound transducer is placed immediately distal to the inflated cuff.
5. The pressure in the cuff is slowly released.
6. The highest pressure at which blood flow is detected by the characteristic "swishing" Doppler signal is recorded as the blood pressure of that artery.
7. The test is repeated at each successive level.
8. When the ankle pressure is divided by the arm (brachial artery) pressure, this is known as the *AB index*. If the AB

index is less than 0.85, significant arterial occlusive disease exists within the extremity.

- Note that these studies are usually performed in the vascular laboratory or radiology department and take approximately 30 minutes.

After

- Encourage the patient to verbalize his or her fears in terms of test results.
- Remove the transducer gel from the extremity.
- Inform the patient that the physician must interpret the studies and that results will be available in a few hours.

Abnormal findings

Venous occlusion, secondary to thrombosis or thrombo-phlebitis
Small or large vessel arterial occlusive disease

Spastic arterial disease (e.g., Raynaud's phenomenon)
Small vessel arterial occlusive disease (as in diabetes)
Embolic arterial occlusion

notes

echocardiography (Cardiac echo, Heart sonogram, Transthoracic echocardiography [TTE])

Type of test Ultrasound

Normal findings

Normal position, size, and movement of the cardiac valves and heart muscle wall

Normal directional flow of blood within the heart chambers

Test explanation and related physiology

Echocardiography is a noninvasive ultrasound procedure used to evaluate the structure and function of the heart. In diagnostic ultrasonography, a harmless, high-frequency sound wave emitted from a transducer penetrates the heart. Sound waves are bounced off the heart structures and reflected back to the transducer as a series of echoes. These echoes are amplified and displayed on an oscilloscope. Tracings also can be recorded on moving graph paper or on videotape. The study usually includes M-mode recordings, two-dimensional recordings, and a Doppler study.

M-mode echocardiography is a linear tracing of the motion of the heart structures over time. This allows the various cardiac structures to be located and studied regarding their movement during a cardiac cycle.

Two-dimensional echocardiography angles a beam within one sector of the heart. This produces a picture of the spatial anatomic relationships within the heart.

A recent addition has been *color Doppler echocardiography*. This test detects the pattern of the blood flow and measures changes in velocity of blood flow within the heart and great vessels. These variations in blood flow and velocity alter the ultrasound frequency. By assigning computerized weighted numbers to these altered frequencies, one is able to map and determine origins of velocity changes and blood turbulence. Turbulent blood or altered velocity and direction of blood flow can then be identified by changes in color. This is seen in a photograph. In most Doppler ultrasound, color flow imaging, blue and red represent the direction of a given stream of blood; the various hues from dull to bright represent varying blood velocities. The most useful application of the color flow imaging is in determining the direction and turbulence of blood flow across regurgitant or narrowed valves. Doppler color flow imaging also may be helpful in assessing proper functioning of prosthetic valves.

Echocardiography, in general, is used in the diagnosis of a pericardial effusion, valvular heart disease (e.g., mitral valve prolapse, stenosis, regurgitation), subaortic stenosis, myocardial wall abnormalities (e.g., cardiomyopathy), infarction, and aneurysm. Cardiac tumors (e.g., myxomas) are easily diagnosed with ultrasound. Atrial and ventricular septal defects and other congenital heart diseases are also recognized by ultrasound. Finally, postinfarction mural thrombi are readily apparent with this testing.

It is now possible to perform echocardiography via the esophagus using a probe mounted on an endoscope. This is referred to as *transesophageal echocardiography*, TEE (see p. 815).

Contraindications

- Patients who are uncooperative

Interfering factors

- Chronic obstructive pulmonary disease (COPD)
  Patients who have severe COPD have a significant amount of air and space between the heart and the chest cavity. Air space does not conduct ultrasound waves well.
- Obesity
  In obese patients, the space between the heart and the transducer is greatly enlarged; therefore accuracy of the test is decreased.

Procedure and patient care

Before

- Assure the patient that this is a painless study.
- Complete the request for the echocardiogram, including the pertinent patient history.

During

- Note the following procedural steps:
  1. The patient is placed in the supine position.
  2. Electrocardiographic (EKG) leads are placed (see p. 335).
  3. A gel, which allows better transmission of sound waves, is placed on the chest wall immediately under the transducer.
  4. Ultrasound is directed to the heart, and appropriate tracings are obtained.

- Note that this procedure usually takes approximately 45 minutes and is performed by an ultrasound technician in a darkened room within the cardiac laboratory or radiology department.
- Tell the patient that no discomfort is associated with this study but that the transmission gel is usually cooler than body temperature.

After

- Remove the gel from the patient's chest wall.
- Inform the patient that the physician must interpret the study and that the results will be available in a few hours.

Abnormal findings

Valvular stenosis
Valvular regurgitation
Mitral valve prolapse
Pericardial effusion
Ventricular or atrial mural thrombi

Myxoma
Poor ventricular muscle motion
Septal defects

notes

electrocardiography (Electrocardiogram [ECG, EKG])

Type of test Electrodiagnostic

Normal findings Normal heart rate (60-100 beats/min), rhythm, and wave deflections

E

Test explanation and related physiology

The EKG is a graphic representation of the electrical impulses that the heart generates during the cardiac cycle. These electrical impulses are conducted to the body's surface, where they are detected by electrodes placed on the patient's limbs and chest. The monitoring electrodes detect the electrical activity of the heart from a variety of spatial perspectives. The EKG lead system is composed of several electrodes that are placed on each of the four extremities and at varying sites on the chest. Each combination of electrodes is called a *lead*.

A *12-lead EKG* provides a comprehensive view of the flow of the heart's electrical currents in two different planes. There are six limb leads (combination of electrodes on the extremities) and six chest leads (corresponding to six sites on the chest). Leads I, II, and III are considered the *standard* limb leads. Lead I records the difference in electrical potential between the left arm (LA) and the right arm (RA). Lead II records the electrical potential between the RA and the left leg (LL). Lead III reflects the difference between the LA and the LL. The right leg (RL) electrode is an inactive ground in all leads. There are three *augmented* limb leads: aV_R, aV_L, and aV_F (*a*, augmented; *V*, vector [unipolar]; *R*, right arm; *L*, left arm; *F*, left foot or leg). The augmented leads measure the electrode potential between the center of the heart and the right arm (aV_R), the left arm (aV_L), and the left leg (aV_F). The six standard chest, or *precordial*, leads (V_1, V_2, V_3, V_4, V_5, V_6) are recorded by placing electrodes at six different positions on the chest, surrounding the heart.

The EKG is recorded on special paper with a graphic background of horizontal and vertical lines for rapid measurement of time intervals (*X* coordinate) and voltages (*Y* coordinate). Time duration is measured by vertical lines 1 mm apart, each representing 0.04 second. Voltage is measured by horizontal lines 1 mm apart. Five 1-mm squares equal 0.5 mV.

The normal EKG pattern is composed of waves arbitrarily designated by the letters *P*, *Q*, *R*, *S*, and *T*. The Q, R, and S waves are grouped together and described as the QRS complex. The significance of the waves and time intervals is as follows (Figure 13):

P wave. This represents atrial electrical depolarization associated with atrial contraction. It represents electrical activity associated with the spread of the original impulse from the sinoatrial (SA) node through the atria. If the P waves are absent or altered, the cardiac impulse originates outside the SA node.

PR interval. This represents the time required for the impulse to travel from the SA node to the atrioventricular (AV) node. If this interval is prolonged, a conduction delay exists in the AV node (e.g., a first-degree heart block). If the PR interval is shortened, the impulse must have reached the ventricle through a "shortcut" (as in Wolff-Parkinson-White syndrome).

QRS complex. This represents ventricular electrical depolarization associated with ventricular contraction. This complex consists of an initial downward (negative) deflection (Q wave), a large upward (positive) deflection (R wave), and a small downward deflection (S wave). A widened QRS complex indicates abnormal or prolonged ventricular depolarization time (as in a bundle-branch block).

ST segment. This represents the period between the completion of depolarization and the beginning of repolarization of the ventricular muscle. This segment may be elevated or depressed in transient muscle ischemia (e.g., angina) or in muscle injury (as in the early stages of myocardial infarction).

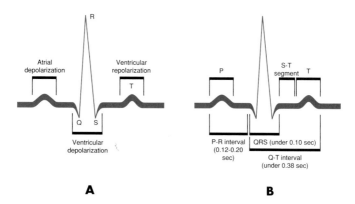

A   **B**

Figure 13 A, Normal EKG deflections during depolarization and repolarization of the atrium and ventricles. **B,** Principal EKG intervals between P, QRS, and T waves.

T wave. This represents ventricular repolarization (i.e., return to neutral electrical activity).

Through the analysis of these waveforms and time intervals, valuable information about the heart may be obtained. The EKG is used primarily to identify abnormal heart rhythms (arrhythmias, or dysrhythmias) and to diagnose acute myocardial infarction, conduction defects, and ventricular hypertrophy. It is important to note that the EKG may be normal, even in the presence of heart disease, if the heart disorder does not affect the electrical activity of the heart.

For some patients at high risk for malignant ventricular dysrhythmias, a *signal-averaged EKG (SAEKG)* can be performed. This test averages several hundred QRS waveforms to detect late potentials that are likely to lead to ventricular dysrhythmias. SAEKGs have been a useful precursor to electrophysiologic studies (see p. 351) because they can identify patients with unexplained syncope who may have ventricular tachycardias induced by the electrophysiologic study. SAEKGs can be performed by the bedside in 15 to 20 minutes and must be ordered separately from a standard EKG.

Interfering factors

- Inaccurate placement of the electrodes
- Electrolyte imbalances
- Poor contact between the skin and the electrodes
- Movement or muscle twitching during the test
- ▼ Drugs that can affect results include digitalis, quinidine, and barbiturates

Procedure and patient care

Before

- Explain the procedure to the patient.
- Tell the patient that no food or fluid restriction is necessary.
- Assure the patient that the flow of electric current is *from* the patient. He or she will feel nothing during this procedure.
- Expose only the patient's chest and arms. Keep the abdomen and thighs adequately covered.

During

- Note the following procedural steps:
  1. The skin areas designated for electrode placement are prepared by using alcohol swabs or sandpaper to remove

skin oil or debris. Sometimes the skin is shaved if the patient has a large amount of hair.

2. Electrode paste is applied to ensure electrical conduction between the skin and the electrodes.

3. The four limb leads are usually held in place by straps that encircle the extremity. Newer machines have clamps that can easily be opened and applied to the extremity.

4. Many cardiologists recommend that arm electrodes be placed on the upper arm, because fewer muscle tremors are detected there.

5. The chest leads are applied either one at a time, three at a time, or six at a time, depending on the type of EKG machine.

   These leads are positioned as follows:

   V_1: in the fourth intercostal space (4ICS) at the right sternal border

   V_2: in 4ICS at the left sternal border

   V_3: midway between V_2 and V_4

   V_4: in 5ICS at the midclavicular line

   V_5: at the left anterior axillary line at the level of V_4 horizontally

   V_6: at the left midaxillary line on the level of V_4 horizontally

- List medications the patient is taking on the EKG request form.
- Note that cardiac technicians, nurses, or physicians perform this procedure in less than 5 minutes at the bedside or in the cardiology clinic.
- Tell the patient that although this procedure carries no discomfort, he or she must lie still in the supine position without talking while the EKG is recorded.

After

- Remove the electrodes from the patient's skin and wipe off the electrode gel.
- Indicate on the EKG strip or request slip if the patient was experiencing chest pain during the study. The pain may be correlated to an arrhythmia on the EKG.

Abnormal findings

Arrhythmia (dysrhythmia)
Acute myocardial infarction
Conduction defects
Ventricular hypertrophy
Wolff-Parkinson-White syndrome

Conduction system disease
Myocardial ischemia
Hypertrophy of the heart
Pulmonary infarction
Electrolyte imbalance
Pericarditis

E

notes

electroencephalography (Electroencephalogram [EEG])

Type of test Electrodiagnostic

Normal findings Normal frequency, amplitude, and characteristics of brain waves

Test explanation and related physiology

The EEG is a graphic recording of the electrical activity of the brain. EEG electrodes are placed on the scalp over multiple areas of the brain to detect and record electrical impulses within the brain. This study is invaluable in the investigation of epileptic states, where the focus of seizure activity is characterized by rapid, spiking waves seen on the graph. Patients with cerebral lesions (e.g., tumors, infarctions) will have abnormally slow EEG waves depending on the size and location of the lesion. Because this study determines the overall activity of the brain, it can be used to evaluate trauma and drug intoxication and also to determine cerebral death in comatose patients.

The EEG also can be used to monitor cerebral blood flow during surgical procedures. For example, during carotid endarterectomy, the carotid vessel must be temporarily occluded. When this surgery is performed with the patient under general anesthesia, the EEG can be used for the early detection of cerebral tissue ischemia, which would indicate that continued carotid occlusion will result in a cerebrovascular accident (stroke) syndrome. Temporary shunting of the blood during the surgery is then required.

Interfering factors

- Fasting may cause hypoglycemia, which could modify the EEG pattern.
- Drinks containing caffeine (e.g., coffee, tea, cocoa, cola) interfere with the test results.
- Body and eye movements during the test can cause changes in the brain wave patterns.
- Drugs that may affect test results include sedatives.

Procedure and patient care

Before

- Explain the procedure to the patient.
- Assure the patient that this test cannot "read the mind" or detect senility.

- Assure the patient that the flow of electrical activity is *from* the patient. He or she will not feel anything during the test.
- Instruct the patient to wash his or her hair the night before the test. No oils, sprays, or lotion should be used.
- Check if the physician wants to discontinue any medications before the study. (Anticonvulsants should be taken unless contraindicated by the physician.)
- Instruct the patient if sleeping time should be shortened the night before the test. Adults may not be allowed to sleep more than 4 or 5 hours, and children not more than 5 to 7 hours, if a sleep EEG will be done.
- Do *not* administer any sedatives or hypnotics before the test, because they will cause abnormal waves on the EEG.
- Inform the patient not to fast before the study. Fasting may cause hypoglycemia, which could alter test results.
- Instruct the patient not to drink any coffee, tea, cocoa, or cola on the morning of the test because of their stimulating effect.
- Tell the patient that he or she needs to remain still during the test. Any movement, including opening the eyes, will create interference and alter the EEG recording.

During
- Note the following procedural steps:
  1. The EEG is usually performed in a specially constructed room that is shielded from outside disturbances.
  2. The patient is placed in a supine position on a bed or reclining on a chair.
  3. Sixteen or more electrodes are applied to the scalp with electrode paste in a uniform pattern over both sides of the head, covering the prefrontal, frontal, temporal, parietal, and occipital areas.
  4. One electrode may be applied to each earlobe for grounding.
  5. After the electrodes are applied, the patient is instructed to lie still with his or her eyes closed.
  6. The technician continuously observes the patient during the EEG recording for any movements that could alter results.
  7. Approximately every 5 minutes, the recording is interrupted to permit the client to move if desired.

- In addition to the resting EEG, note that the following *activating procedures* can be performed:
  1. The patient is *hyperventilated* (asked to breathe deeply 20 times a minute for 3 minutes) to induce alkalosis and cerebral vasoconstriction, which can activate abnormalities.
  2. *Photostimulation* is performed by flashing a light over the patient's face with the eyes opened or closed. Photostimulated seizure activity may be seen on the EEG.
  3. A *sleep EEG* may be performed to aid in the detection of some abnormal brain waves that are seen only if the patient is sleeping (e.g., frontal lobe epilepsy). The sleep EEG is performed after orally administering methyprylon (Noludar) or chloral hydrate (Noctec). A recording is performed while the patient is falling asleep, while the patient is asleep, and while the patient is waking.
- Note that this study is performed by an EEG technician in approximately 45 minutes to 2 hours.
- Tell the patient that no discomfort is associated with this study, other than possibly missing sleep.

After

- Help the patient to remove the electrode paste. The paste may be removed with acetone or witch hazel.
- Instruct the patient to shampoo the hair.
- Ensure safety precautions until the effects of any sedatives have worn off. Keep the bed's siderails up.
- Tell the patient that one who has had a sleep EEG should not drive home alone.

Abnormal findings

Seizure disorders (e.g., epilepsy)
Brain tumor
Brain abscess
Head injury
Cerebral death
Encephalitis
Intracranial hemorrhage
Cerebral infarct
Narcolepsy
Alzheimer's disease

notes

electromyography (EMG)

Type of test Electrodiagnostic

Normal findings No evidence of neuromuscular abnormalities

Test explanation and related physiology

By placing a recording electrode into a skeletal muscle, one can monitor the electrical activity of a skeletal muscle in a way very similar to electrocardiography. The electrical activity is displayed on an oscilloscope as an electrical waveform. An audio-electrical amplifier can be added to the system so that both the appearance and sound of the electrical potentials can be analyzed and compared simultaneously. EMG is used to detect primary muscular disorders along with muscular abnormalities caused by other system diseases (e.g., nerve dysfunction, sarcoidosis, paraneoplastic syndrome).

Spontaneous muscle movement, such as fibrillation and fasciculation, can be detected during EMG. When seen, these waves indicate injury or disease of the nerve innervating that muscle or spastic myotonic muscle disease. Reduced amplitude size of the electrical waveform is indicative of a primary muscle disorder (e.g., polymyositis, muscular dystrophies, various myopathies). A progressive decrease in amplitude of the electrical waveform is a classic sign of myasthenia gravis. A decrease in the number of muscle fibers able to contract is seen with peripheral nerve damage. This study is usually done in conjunction with nerve conduction studies (see p. 346) and also may be called *electromyoneurography.*

Contraindications

- Patients receiving anticoagulant therapy
- Patients with extensive skin infection

Potential complication

- Rarely, hematoma at the needle insertion site

Interfering factors

- Edema, hemorrhage, or thick subcutaneous fat can interfere with test results.
- Patients with excessive pain may have false results.

Procedure and patient care

Before

- Explain the procedure to the patient. Allay any fears and allow the patient to express concerns.
- Obtain informed consent if required by the institution.
- Tell the patient that fasting is not usually required; however, some facilities may restrict stimulants (coffee, tea, cocoa, cola, cigarettes) for 2 to 3 hours before the test.
- If serum enzyme tests (e.g., AST [SGOT], CPK, LDH) are ordered, the specimen should be drawn before EMG or 5 to 10 days after the test, because the EMG may cause misleading elevations of these enzymes.
- Premedication or sedation is usually avoided because of the need for patient cooperation.

During

- Note the following procedural steps:
  1. This study is usually done in an EMG laboratory.
  2. The patient's position depends on the muscle being studied.
  3. A needle that acts as a recording electrode is inserted into the muscle being examined.
  4. A reference electrode is placed nearby on the skin surface.
  5. The patient is asked to keep the muscle at rest.
  6. The oscilloscope display is viewed for any evidence of spontaneous electrical activity, such as fasciculation or fibrillation.
  7. The patient is asked to contract the muscle slowly and progressively.
  8. The electrical waves produced are examined for their number, form, and amplitude.
- Note that the EMG is performed by a physical therapist, physiatrist, or neurologist in approximately 20 minutes.
- Tell the patient that this test is moderately uncomfortable. Slight pain may occur with the insertion of the needle electrode.

After

- Observe the needle site for hematoma or inflammation.
- Provide pain medication if needed.

Abnormal findings

Polymyositis
Muscular dystrophy
Multiple sclerosis
Myopathy
Amyotrophic lateral sclerosis
Muscle denervation
Muscular abnormalities
  caused by diseases of other
  systems (e.g., nerve dysfunc-
  tion, sarcoidosis, paraneo-
  plastic syndrome)

Traumatic injury
Myasthenia gravis
Guillain-Barré syndrome
Diabetic neuropathy
Anterior poliomyelitis

E

notes

electroneurography (ENG, Nerve conduction studies)

Type of test Electrodiagnostic

Normal findings

No evidence of peripheral nerve injury or disease
(Conduction velocity is usually decreased in the elderly.)

Test explanation and related physiology

Electroneurography, or nerve conduction studies, allow for
the detection and location of peripheral nerve injury or disease.
By initiating an electrical impulse at one site (proximal) of a nerve
and recording the time required for that impulse to travel to a
second site (distal) of the same nerve, the conduction velocity
of any impulse in that nerve can be determined. This study is
usually done in conjunction with electromyography (see p. 343)
and also may be called *electromyoneurography*.

The normal value for conduction velocity varies from one
nerve to another. Individual variation also exists. It is always best
to compare the conduction velocity of the suspected side with
the contralateral nerve conduction velocity. In general, a range
of normal conduction velocity will be approximately 50 to 60
m/sec.

Traumatic transection or contusion of a nerve will usually
cause maximal slowing of conduction velocity in the affected side
as compared with the normal side. Neuropathies, both local and
generalized, also will cause a slowing of conduction velocity. A
velocity greater than normal does not indicate a pathologic condition.

Because conduction velocity requires contraction of a muscle
as an indication of an impulse arriving at the recording electrode,
primary muscular disorders may cause a falsely slow nerve conduction velocity. This "muscular" variable is eliminated if one
evaluates the suspected pathologic muscle group before performing nerve conduction studies. This evaluation can be done by
measuring distal latency (i.e., the time required for stimulation
of the distal end of the nerve to cause muscular contraction).
The nerve conduction study is then performed normally by
stimulating the proximal portion of the nerve bundle. Conduction velocity is determined by the following equation:

$$\text{Conduction velocity (in meters per second)} = \frac{\text{Distance (in meters)}}{\text{Total latency} - \text{Distal latency}}$$

Interfering factor

- Patients in severe pain may have false results.

Procedure and patient care

Before

- Explain the procedure to the patient. Allay any fears and allow the patient to express concerns.
- Obtain informed consent if required by the institution.
- Tell the patient that no fasting or sedation is usually required.

During

- Note the following procedural steps:
    1. This test can be performed in a nerve conduction laboratory or at the patient's bedside.
    2. The patient's position depends on the area of suspected peripheral nerve injury or disease.
    3. A recording electrode is placed on the skin overlying a muscle innervated solely by the relevant nerve.
    4. A reference electrode is placed nearby.
    5. All skin-to-electrode connections are ensured by using electrical paste.
    6. The nerve is stimulated by a shock-emitting device at an adjacent location.
    7. The time between nerve impulse and muscular contraction (distal latency) is measured in milliseconds on an EMG machine.
    8. The nerve is similarly stimulated at a location proximal to the area of suspected injury or disease.
    9. The time required for the impulse to travel from the site of initiation to muscle contraction (total latency) is recorded in milliseconds.
    10. The distance between the site of stimulation and the recording electrode is measured in centimeters.
    11. Conduction velocity is converted to meters per second and is computed as in the previous equation.
- Note that this test takes approximately 15 minutes and is performed by a physiatrist or a neurologist.

- Tell the patient that this test is uncomfortable in that a mild shock is required for nerve impulse stimulation.

After
- Remove the electrode gel from the patient's skin.

Abnormal findings

Peripheral nerve injury or disease

Myasthenia gravis

Muscular dystrophy

Tumor

Guillain-Barré syndrome

Carpal tunnel syndrome

Diabetic neuropathy

notes

electronystagmography

Type of test Electrodiagnostic

Normal findings

Normal nystagmus response
Normal oculovestibular reflex

Test explanation and related physiology

Electronystagmography is used to evaluate nystagmus (involuntary rapid eye movement) and the muscles controlling eye movement. By measuring changes in the electrical field around the eye, this study can make a permanent recording of eye movement at rest and in response to various stimuli. It delineates the presence or absence of nystagmus, which is caused by the initiation of the oculovestibular reflex. Nystagmus should occur when initiated by visual or caloric (see p. 188) stimuli. If nystagmus does not occur with stimulation, the cerebral cortex (temporal lobe), auditory nerve, or brainstem is abnormal. Tumors, infection, ischemia, and degeneration can cause such abnormalities. This test is used in the differential diagnosis of lesions in the vestibular system, brainstem, and cerebellum. It also may help evaluate unilateral hearing loss and vertigo. Unilateral hearing loss may be due to middle ear problems or nerve injury. If the patient experiences nystagmus with stimulation, the auditory nerve is working and hearing loss can be blamed on the middle ear.

Contraindications

- Patients with perforated eardrums, who should not have water irrigation
- Patients with pacemakers

Interfering factors

- Blinking of the eyes can alter test results.
- ✘ Drugs that can alter results include sedatives, stimulants, and antivertigo agents.

Procedure and patient care

Before

- Explain the procedure to the patient.
- Instruct the patient not to apply facial makeup before the test, because electrodes will be taped to the skin around the eyes.

- Hold solid food before the test to reduce the likelihood of vomiting.
- Instruct the patient not to drink caffeine or alcoholic beverages for approximately 24 to 48 hours (as ordered) before the test.
- Check with the physician regarding withholding any medications that could interfere with the test results.

During

- Note the following procedural steps:
  1. This procedure is usually performed in a darkened room with the patient seated or lying down on an examining table.
  2. If there is any wax in the ear, it is removed.
  3. Electrodes are taped to the skin around the eyes.
  4. Various procedures are used to stimulate nystagmus, such as pendulum tracking, changing head position, changing gaze position, and caloric tests (see p. 188).
  5. Several recordings are made with the patient at rest and to demonstrate patient response to various procedures (e.g., blowing air into the ear, irrigating the ear with water).
  6. Nystagmus response is compared with the expected ranges, and the results are recorded as normal, borderline, or abnormal.
- Note that this procedure is performed by a physician or audiologist in approximately 1 hour.
- Tell the patient that nausea and vomiting may occur during the test.

After

- Consider prescribing bed rest until nausea, vertigo, or weakness subsides.

Abnormal findings

Brainstem lesions

Vestibular system lesions

Cerebellum lesions

Congenital disorder

Demyelinating disease

notes

electrophysiologic study (EPS, Cardiac mapping)

Type of test Electrodiagnostic

Normal findings Normal conduction intervals, refractive periods, and recovery times

Test explanation and related physiology

In this invasive procedure, electrode catheters are fluoroscopically placed through a peripheral vein and into the right atrium and/or ventricle. With close cardiac monitoring, the electrode catheters are used to pace the heart and potentially induce arrhythmias (dysrhythmias). Defects in the heart conduction system can then be identified; arrhythmias that are otherwise unapparent also can be induced, identified, and treated. The effectiveness of the antiarrhythmic drugs (e.g., lidocaine, phenytoin, quinidine) can be assessed by determining the electrical threshold required to induce arrhythmias.

Contraindications

- Patients who are uncooperative
- Patients with acute myocardial infarction

Potential complications

- Cardiac arrhythmias (dysrhythmias) leading to ventricular tachycardia or fibrillation
- Perforation of the myocardium
- Catheter-induced embolic cerebrovascular accident (stroke) or myocardial infarction
- Peripheral vascular problems
- Hemorrhage
- Phlebitis at the venipuncture site

Interfering factors

✔ Drugs that may interfere with test results include analgesics, sedatives, and tranquilizers.

Procedure and patient care

Before

- Instruct the patient to fast for 6 to 8 hours before the procedure. Usually, fluids are permitted until 3 hours before the test.
- Obtain an informed consent from the patient.

- Encourage the patient to verbalize any fears regarding this test.
- Shave and prepare the catheter insertion site.
- Collect a blood sample for potassium or drug levels, if indicated.
- Obtain peripheral IV access for the administration of drugs.

During
- Note the following procedural steps:
  1. After being transported to the cardiac catheterization laboratory, the patient has electrocardiographic (EKG) leads attached.
  2. The catheter insertion site, usually the femoral vein, is prepared and draped in a sterile manner.
  3. Under fluoroscopic guidance, the catheter is passed to the atrium and ventricle.
  4. Baseline surface intracardiac EKGs are recorded.
  5. Various parts of the cardiac electroconduction system are stimulated by atrial or ventricular pacing.
  6. Mapping of the electroconduction system and its defects is performed.
  7. Arrhythmias (dysrhythmias) are identified.
  8. Drugs may be administered to assess their efficacy in preventing EPS-induced arrhythmias.
- Note that this procedure is performed by a cardiologist within a darkened cardiac catheterization laboratory in approximately 1 to 4 hours.
- Tell the patient that he or she may experience palpitations, light-headedness, or dizziness when arrhythmias are induced. Report these sensations to the physician. For most patients, this is an anxiety-producing experience.
- Inform the patient that discomfort from catheter insertion is minimal.

After
- Keep the patient on bed rest for approximately 6 to 8 hours.
- Evaluate the venous access site for swelling and bleeding.
- Monitor the patient's vital signs for at least 2 to 4 hours for hypotension and arrhythmias (dysrhythmias). Additional monitoring is especially important for certain medications that the patient received during the test. For example, if the patient received quinidine, he or she should be monitored for hypotension and abdominal cramping.

- Continue cardiac monitoring to identify arrhythmias. Transfer arrangements to a monitored unit may be necessary.
- Cover the area with sterile dressings if the electrical catheter is left in place for subsequent studies.

Abnormal findings

Electroconduction defects

Cardiac arrhythmia (dysrhythmia)

Sinoatrial node defects (e.g., sick sinus syndrome)

Atrioventricular node defects and heart blocks

notes

endometrial biopsy

Type of test Microscopic examination of tissue

Normal findings
No pathologic conditions
Presence of a "secretory-type" endometrium 3 to 5 days before normal menses

Test explanation and related physiology
An endometrial biopsy can determine whether ovulation has occurred. A biopsy specimen taken 3 to 5 days before normal menses should demonstrate a "secretory-type" endometrium on histologic examination if ovulation and corpus luteum formation have occurred. If not, only a preovulatory "proliferative-type" endometrium will be seen.

Occasionally, an endometrial biopsy is performed to indicate estrogen's effect in patients with suspected ovarian dysfunction or absence. Similarly, adequate circulating progesterone levels can be determined by identifying secretory endometrium. Another major use of endometrial biopsy is to diagnose endometrial cancer, tuberculosis, polyps, or inflammatory conditions and to evaluate uterine bleeding.

Contraindications
- Patients with infections (e.g., trichomonal, candidal, or suspected gonococcal) of the cervix or vagina
- Patients in whom the cervix cannot be visualized (e.g., because of abnormal position or previous surgery)

Potential complications
- Perforation of the uterus
- Uterine bleeding
- Interference with early pregnancy
- Infection

Procedure and patient care
Before
- Explain the procedure to the patient.
- Ensure that written and informed consent for this procedure is obtained from the patient.

- Tell the patient that no fasting or sedation is usually required.

During

- Note the following procedural steps:
  1. The patient is placed in the lithotomy position, and a pelvic examination is performed to determine the position of the uterus.
  2. The cervix is exposed and cleansed.
  3. A biopsy instrument is inserted into the uterus, and specimens are obtained from the anterior, posterior, and lateral walls.
  4. The specimens are placed in a solution containing 10% formalin solution and sent to the pathologist for histologic examination.
- Note that this procedure is performed by an obstetrician/gynecologist in approximately 10 to 30 minutes.
- Tell the patient that this procedure may cause momentary discomfort (menstrual-type cramping).

After

- Assess the patient's vital signs at regular intervals for the next 48 hours. Any temperature elevation should be reported to the physician, because this procedure may activate pelvic inflammatory disease.
- Advise the patient to wear a pad, because some vaginal bleeding is to be expected. Instruct the patient to call her physician if excessive bleeding (requiring more than one pad per hour) occurs.
- Inform the patient that douching and intercourse are not permitted for 72 hours after the biopsy specimen removal.
- Instruct the patient to rest during the next 24 hours and to avoid heavy lifting to prevent uterine hemorrhage.

Abnormal findings

Anovulation
Tumor
Tuberculosis

Polyps
Inflammatory condition

notes

endoscopic retrograde cholangiopancreatography
(ERCP, ERCP of the biliary and pancreatic ducts)

Type of test Endoscopy

Normal findings

Normal size of biliary and pancreatic ducts

No obstruction or filling defects within the biliary or pancreatic ducts

Test explanation and related physiology

With the use of a fiberoptic endoscope, ERCP provides radiographic visualization of the bile and pancreatic ducts. This is especially useful in patients with jaundice. If a partial or total obstruction of those ducts exists, characteristics of the obstructing lesion can be demonstrated. Stones, benign strictures, cysts, ampullary stenosis, anatomic variations, and malignant tumors can be identified. Only ERCP and percutaneous transhepatic cholangiography (PTHC) can provide direct visualization of the biliary and pancreatic ducts. PTHC (see p. 613) is an invasive procedure with significant morbidity; ERCP is associated with much less morbidity but must be performed by an experienced endoscopist.

In contrast to an oral cholecystogram or an IV cholangiogram, which does not visualize the biliary tree when high levels of bilirubin are present, the biliary ducts of jaundiced patients can be visualized by ERCP. As a result, this test is extremely important in the evaluation of patients with jaundice.

Incision of the papillary muscle in the ampulla of Vater can be performed through the scope at the time of ERCP. This incision widens the distal common duct so that common bile duct gallstones can be removed. Stents can be placed through strictured bile ducts with the use of ERCP, and the bile of jaundiced patients can be internally drained. Pieces of tissue and brushings of the common bile duct can be obtained by ERCP for pathologic review.

Contraindications

- Patients who are uncooperative
  Cannulation of the ampulla of Vater requires that the patient lie very still.
- Patients whose ampulla of Vater is not accessible endoscopically because of previous upper gastrointestinal surgery (e.g.,

gastrectomy patients whose duodenum containing the ampulla is surgically separated from the stomach)
- Patients with esophageal diverticula
  The scope can fall into a diverticulum and perforate its wall.
- Patients with known acute pancreatitis

Potential complications
- Perforation of the esophagus, stomach, or duodenum
- Gram-negative sepsis
  This results from introducing bacteria through the biliary system and into the blood. Usually, this occurs in patients who have obstructive jaundice.
- Pancreatitis
  This results from pressure of the dye injection.
- Aspiration of gastric contents into the lungs
- Respiratory arrest as a result of oversedation

Interfering factor
- Barium within the abdomen as a result of a previous upper GI series or barium enema x-ray studies precludes adequate visualization of the biliary and pancreatic ducts.

Procedure and patient care

Before
- Explain the procedure to the patient.
- Obtain informed consent from the patient.
- Inform the patient that breathing will not be compromised by the insertion of the endoscope.
- Keep the patient NPO as of midnight the day of the test.
- Administer appropriate premedication (e.g., midazolam [Versed] and atropine) if ordered.

During
- Note the following procedural steps:
  1. A flat plate of the abdomen is taken to ensure that any barium from previous studies will not obscure visualization of the bile duct.
  2. The patient is placed in the supine position or on the left side.
  3. The patient is usually sedated with a narcotic and a sedative/hypnotic.
  4. The pharynx is sprayed with a local anesthetic (lidocaine [Xylocaine]) to inactivate the gag reflex and to lessen the discomfort caused by the passage of the scope.

5. A side-viewing fiberoptic duodenoscope is inserted through the oral pharynx and passed through the esophagus, stomach, and into the duodenum (Figure 14).
6. Glucagon is often administered intravenously to minimize the spasm of the duodenum and to improve visualization of the ampulla of Vater.
7. Through the accessory lumen within the scope, a small catheter is passed through the ampulla and into the common bile or pancreatic ducts.
8. Radiographic dye is injected, and x-ray films are taken.

- Note that the test usually takes approximately 1 hour and is performed by a physician trained in endoscopy. The x-ray films are interpreted by the radiologist.
- Tell the patient that no discomfort is associated with the dye

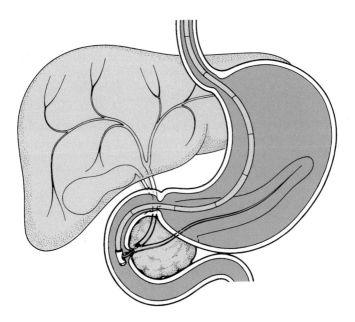

Figure 14 Endoscopic retrograde cholangiopancreatography (ERCP). The fiberoptic scope is passed into the duodenum. Note the small catheter being advanced into the biliary duct.

injection but that minimal gagging may occur during the initial introduction of the scope into the oral pharynx.

After

- Do *not* allow the patient to eat or drink until the gag reflex returns.
- Observe the patient closely for development of abdominal pain, nausea, and vomiting. This may herald the onset of ERCP-induced pancreatitis.
- Observe safety precautions until the effects of the sedatives have worn off.
- Monitor the patient for signs of respiratory depression. Medication (e.g., naloxone [Narcan]) should be available to counteract serious respiratory depression. Resuscitative equipment should also be present.
- Assess the patient for signs and symptoms of septicemia, which may indicate the onset of ERCP-induced cholangitis.
- Inform the patient that he or she may be hoarse and have a sore throat for several days. Drinking cool fluids and gargling will help to relieve some of this soreness.

Abnormal findings

Tumor, strictures, or gallstones of the common bile duct

Sclerosing cholangitis

Biliary sclerosis

Cysts of the common bile duct

Tumor, strictures, inflammation, or pseudocyst of the pancreatic duct

Anatomic biliary or pancreatic duct variations

notes

Epstein-Barr virus titer (EBV)

Type of test Blood

Normal findings

Titers ≤1:10 are nondiagnostic.

Titers of 1:10 to 1:60 indicate infection at some undetermined time.

Titers of 1:320 or greater suggest active infection.

Fourfold increase in titer in paired sera drawn 10 to 14 days apart is usually indicative of an acute infection.

Test explanation and related physiology

EBV infects 80% of the U.S. population. Once infection occurs, the virus becomes dormant but can be reactivated later. EBV infection can produce infectious mononucleosis (IM). In Africa, EBV has been associated with Burkitt's lymphoma. In China, EBV infection has been associated with nasopharyngeal carcinoma. Mononucleosis is seen most often in children, adolescents, and young adults. Clinical features include those of acute fatigue, fever, sore throat, lymphadenopathy, and splenomegaly. Laboratory findings of lymphocytosis, atypical lymphocytes, and the development of transient serum heterophil antibodies are found in patients with acute EBV infection. Most patients with infectious mononucleosis recover uneventfully and return to normal activity within 4 to 6 weeks.

After recovery from primary EBV infection, a lifelong, latent EBV-carrier status is established. In the last several years, specific immunologic tests to identify EBV activity indicate that latent EBV can reactivate and become associated with a constellation of chronic signs and symptoms resembling infectious mononucleosis. Clinical manifestations of chronic EBV are variable and include nonspecific symptoms, such as profound fatigue, pharyngitis, myalgia, arthralgia, low-grade fever, headache, paresthesia, and loss of abstract thinking.

Serologic tests are the only way to make the diagnosis of EBV. The heterophil agglutination slide test (monospot test) is explained on p. 562. Other, more specific immunologic tests indicate more precisely the timing of the infection (Table 10). The viral capsid antigen-antibodies (VCAs) can be IgG or IgM. The

TABLE 10 Serologic studies and the timing of infections

Serologic study	Appears/ disappears	Clinical significance
Mono spot heterophil	5 days/2 weeks	Acute or convalescent infection
VCA-IgM	7 days/3 months	Acute or convalescent infection
VCA-IgG	7 days/exists for life	Acute, convalescent, or old infection
EBNA-IgG	3 weeks/exists for life	Old infection
EA-D	7 days/2 weeks	Acute or convalescent infection

EBV nuclear antigen (EBNA) is located in the nuclei of the infected lymphocyte. Another EBV antigen is called the early antigen (EA). There are two EA antigens. One is spread diffusely about the cytoplasm of the infected cell (EA-D), and the other is restricted to only one area of the cytoplasm (EA-R). The EA-D is commonly found in nasopharyngeal cancer. The EA-R is commonly found in Burkitt's lymphoma.

The interpretation of EBV antibody tests is based on the following assumptions:

1. Once the person becomes infected with EBV, the anti-VCA antibodies appear first.
2. Anti-EA (EA-D or EA-R) antibodies appear next or are present with anti-VCA antibodies early in the course of illness. An anti-EA antibody titer greater than 80 in a patient 2 years after acute infectious mononucleosis indicates chronic EBV syndrome.
3. As the patient recovers, anti-VCA and anti-EA antibodies decrease and anti-EBNA antibodies appear. Anti-EBNA antibody persists for life and reflects a past infection.
4. After the patient is well, anti-VCA and anti-EBNA antibodies are always present but at lower ranges. Occasionally, anti-EA antibody also may be present after the patient recovers.

Procedure and patient care

Before
- Explain the procedure to the patient.
- Tell the patient that no fasting or special preparation is required.

During
- Collect 5 to 10 ml of venous blood in a red-top tube.
- Record the day of onset of illness on the laboratory slip.
- Obtain serum samples as soon as possible after the onset of the illness.
- Obtain a second blood specimen 14 to 21 days later.

After
- Apply pressure or a pressure dressing to the venipuncture site.
- Observe the venipuncture site for bleeding.

Abnormal findings

Infectious mononucleosis
Chronic fatigue syndrome
Chronic EBV carrier state

Burkitt's lymphoma
Nasopharyngeal cancer

notes

erythrocyte sedimentation rate (ESR, Sed rate test)

Type of test Blood

Normal findings

Westergren method

Male: up to 15 mm/hr
Female: up to 20 mm/hr
Child: up to 10 mm/hr
Newborn: 0-2 mm/hr

Test explanation and related physiology

The ESR is a nonspecific test used to detect inflammatory, neoplastic, infectious, and necrotic processes. Because the ESR is nonspecific, it is not diagnostic for any particular organ disease or injury. The test is performed by measuring the distance (in millimeters) that red blood cells (RBCs) descend (or settle) in normal saline in 1 hour. Because these pathologic conditions increase the protein content of plasma, RBCs have a tendency to stack up on one another, increasing their weight and causing them to descend faster. Therefore, in these diseases, the ESR will be increased.

The test can be used to detect disease that is otherwise not suspected. Many physicians use the ESR test in this way for routine patient evaluation for vague symptoms. Other physicians regard this test as so nonspecific that it is useless as a routine study. The ESR test occasionally can be helpful in differentiating disease entities or complaints: for example, in the patient with chest pain, the ESR will be increased with myocardial infarction but will be normal with angina.

The ESR is a fairly reliable indicator of the course of disease and therefore can be used to monitor disease therapy, especially for inflammatory autoimmune diseases. In general, as the disease worsens, the ESR increases; as the disease improves, the ESR decreases. If the results of the ESR are equivocal or inconsistent with the clinical impressions, the C-reactive protein test (see p. 291) is often performed.

Interfering factors

- Artificially low results can occur when the collected specimen is allowed to stand longer than 3 hours before the testing.

- Pregnancy (second and third trimester) can cause elevated levels.
- Menstruation can cause elevated levels.
- Drugs that may cause *increased* ESR levels include dextran, methyldopa (Aldomet), oral contraceptives, penicillamine, procainamide, theophylline, and vitamin A.
- Drugs that may cause *decreased* levels include aspirin, cortisone, and quinine.

Procedure and patient care

Before

- Explain the procedure to the patient.
- Hold medications that may affect test results if indicated.

During

- Collect approximately 5 to 10 ml of venous blood in a lavender-top tube.

After

- Transport the specimen immediately to the laboratory.
- Apply pressure or a pressure dressing to the venipuncture site.
- Assess the venipuncture site for bleeding.

Abnormal findings

▲ **Increased levels**
Toxemia
Syphilis
Nephritis
Multiple myeloma
Bacterial infection
Acute pelvic inflammatory disease
Pneumonia
Rheumatoid arthritis
Rheumatic fever
Acute myocardial infarction
Hyperfibrinogenemia
Systemic lupus erythematosus
Severe anemia
Hodgkin's disease
Carcinoma

▼ **Decreased levels**
Congestive heart failure
Sickle cell anemia
Hypofibrinogenemia
Polycythemia vera
Infectious mononcleosis
Degenerative arthritis
Angina pectoris

esophageal function studies (Esophageal manometry, Esophageal motility studies)

E

Type of test Manometric

Normal findings

Lower esophageal sphincter pressure: 10-20 mm Hg
Swallowing pattern: normal peristaltic waves
Acid reflux: negative
Acid clearing: <10 swallows
Bernstein test: negative

Test explanation and related physiology

Esophageal function studies include the following:
1. Determination of the *lower esophageal sphincter (LES) pressure* (manometry).
2. Graphic recording of esophageal swallowing waves, or *swallowing pattern* (manometry).
3. Detection of reflux of gastric acid back into the esophagus (acid reflux).
4. Detection of the ability of the esophagus to clear acid (acid clearing).
5. An attempt to reproduce symptoms of heartburn (Bernstein test).

Manometry studies

Two manometry studies are used in assessing esophageal function: (1) measurement of LES pressure and (2) graphic recording of swallowing waves (motility). The LES is a sphincter muscle that acts as a valve to prevent reflux of gastric acid into the esophagus. Free reflux of gastric acid occurs when the sphincter pressures are low. An example of such a disorder in adults is gastroesophageal reflux; in children, it is called chalasia (incompetent or relaxed LES).

With increased sphincter pressure, as found in patients with achalasia (failure of the LES to relax normally with swallowing), and with diffuse esophageal spasms, food cannot pass from the esophagus into the stomach. Increased LES pressures are noted on manometry. In achalasia, few if any swallowing waves are detected. In contrast, diffuse esophageal spasm is characterized by strong, frequent, asynchronous, and nonpropulsive waves.

Acid reflux with pH probe

Acid reflux is the primary component of gastroesophageal reflux. Patients with an incompetent LES will regurgitate gastric acid into the esophagus. This will then cause a drop in pH testing done by the pH probe.

Acid clearing

Patients with normal esophageal function can completely clear hydrochloric acid from the esophagus in less than 10 swallows. Patients with decreased esophageal motility (frequently caused by severe esophagitis) require a greater number of swallows to clear the acid.

Bernstein test (acid perfusion)

The Bernstein test is simply an attempt to reproduce the symptoms of gastroesophageal reflux. If the patient suffers pain with the instillation of hydrochloric acid into the esophagus, the test is positive and proves the patient's symptoms are caused by reflux esophagitis. If the patient has no discomfort, a cause other than esophageal reflux must be sought to explain the patient's discomfort.

Contraindications

- Patients who cannot cooperate
- Patients who are medically unstable

Potential complication

- Aspiration of gastric contents

Interfering factors

- Eating shortly before the test may affect results.
- Drugs such as sedatives can alter test results.

Procedure and patient care

Before

- Explain the procedure to the patient.
- Instruct the patient not to eat or drink anything for at least 8 hours before the test.
- Allay any fears and allow the patient to verbalize concerns. Be sensitive to the patient's fears about choking during the procedure.

During

- Note the following procedural steps:
  1. Esophageal studies are usually performed in the endoscopy laboratory.

2. The fasting, unsedated patient is asked to swallow two or three very tiny tubes. The tubes are equipped so that pressure measurements can be taken at 5-cm intervals (Figure 15).

3. The outer ends of the tubes are attached to a pressure transducer.

4. All tubes are passed into the stomach; then three tubes are slowly pulled back into the esophagus. A rapid and extreme increase in the pressure readings indicates the high-pressure zone of the LES.

5. The LES pressure is recorded.

6. With all tubes in the esophagus, the patient is asked to swallow. Motility wave patterns are recorded.

7. The pH indicator probe is placed in the esophagus.

8. The patient's stomach is filled with approximately 100 ml of 0.1-N hydrochloric acid. A decrease in the pH of the esophageal pH probe indicates gastroesophageal reflux.

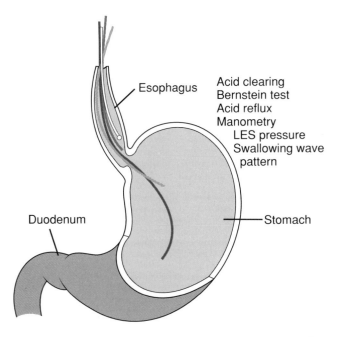

Figure 15 Esophageal function studies demonstrating placement of manometry tubes and a pH probe within the esophagus.

9. Hydrochloric acid is instilled into the esophagus, and the patient is asked to swallow. The number of swallows is counted to determine acid clearing. More than 10 swallows to clear the acid (as determined by the pH probe) indicates decreased esophageal motility.

10. Finally, 0.1-N hydrochloric acid and saline solution are alternately instilled into the esophagus for the Bernstein test. The patient is not told which solution is being infused. If the patient volunteers symptoms of discomfort while the acid is running, the test is considered positive. If no discomfort is recognized, the test is negative.

- Note that these tests are performed by an esophageal technician in approximately 30 minutes.
- Inform the patient that the test results are interpreted by a physician and are available in a few hours.
- Tell the patient that except for some initial gagging when swallowing the tubes, these tests are not uncomfortable.

After

- Inform the patient that it is not unusual to have a mild sore throat after placement of the tubes.

Abnormal findings

Presbyesophagus
Diffuse esophageal spasm
Chalasia

Achalasia
Gastroesophageal reflux
Reflux esophagitis

notes

esophagogastroduodenoscopy (EGD, Upper gastrointestinal [UGI] endoscopy, Gastroscopy)

E

Type of test Endoscopy

Normal findings Normal esophagus, stomach, and duodenum

Test explanation and related physiology

Endoscopy enables direct visualization of the upper gastrointestinal (GI) tract by means of a long, flexible, fiberoptic-lighted scope. The esophagus, stomach, and duodenum are examined for tumors, varices, mucosal inflammations, hiatal hernias, polyps, ulcers, and obstructions. The endoscope has one to three channels. The first channel is used for viewing, the second for insufflation of air and aspiration of fluid, and the third for passing cable-activated instruments to perform a biopsy of suspected pathologic tissue. Probes also can be passed through the third channel to allow for coagulation or injection of sclerosing agents to areas of active GI bleeding. A laser beam can pass through the endoscope to perform endoscopic surgery (e.g., obliteration of tumors or polyps, control of bleeding), and the fiberoptics of endoscopy are so refined that video images and "still pictures" can be taken.

With endoscopy, one can not only evaluate the esophagus, stomach, and duodenum, but with the use of an extralong fiberoptic endoscope, one can also visualize and perform a biopsy of tissue in the upper small intestinal tract. This procedure is referred to as *enteroscopy*. Abnormalities of the small intestine, such as arteriovenous (AV) malformations, tumors, enteropathies (e.g., celiac disease), and ulcerations, can be diagnosed with enteroscopy. Besides being much more sensitive and specific than an upper GI series in diagnosing diseases of the esophagus, stomach, and duodenum, EGD also can be used therapeutically. An experienced endoscopist often can control active GI bleeding by electrocoagulation, laser coagulation, or the injection of sclerosing agents such as alcohol. Also, with the endoscope, benign and malignant strictures can be dilated to reestablish patency of the upper GI tract. Biliary stents and a percutaneous gastrostomy can be placed with the use of EGD. The role of endoscopic surgery is expanding in light of its dramatic success and minimal morbidity.

Contraindications

- Patients who cannot cooperate fully
  As in all studies that require technical finesse, patient cooperation is essential for successful, safe, and accurate test completion.
- Patients with severe upper GI bleeding
  The viewing lens will become covered with blood clots, preventing adequate visualization. If the stomach can be lavaged and aspirated to clear the blood clots, however, EGD can be performed.
- Patients with esophageal diverticula
  The scope can easily fall into the diverticulum and perforate the wall of the esophagus.
- Patients with suspected perforation
  The perforation can be worsened by the insufflation of pressurized air into the GI tract.
- Patients who have had recent GI surgery
  The anastomosis may not be able to withstand the pressure of the required air insufflation. This may lead to anastomotic disruption.

Potential complications

- Perforation of the esophagus, stomach, and duodenum
- Bleeding from a biopsy site
- Pulmonary aspiration of gastric contents
- Oversedation from the medication administered during the test
- Hypotension induced by the sedative medication
  Usually, however, the patient already has some significant element of hypovolemia or dehydration.
- Local IV phlebitic reaction to the injection of sclerosing sedative medication

Interfering factors

- Food in the stomach
- Excessive GI bleeding

Procedure and patient care

Before

- Explain the procedure to the patient.
- Obtain informed consent if required by the institution.
- Instruct the patient to abstain from eating as of midnight the day of the test.

- Reassure the patient that this test is not painful. Tell the patient that the throat will be anesthetized with a spray to depress the gag reflex.
- Encourage the patient to verbalize fears. Provide support.
- Remove the patient's dentures and eyewear before testing.
- Remind the patient that he or she will not be able to speak during the test but that respiration will not be affected.
- Instruct the patient not to bite down on the endoscope.
- Instruct the patient as to appropriate oral hygiene, because the tube will be passed through the mouth.

During
- Note the following procedural steps:
  1. The patient is placed on the endoscopy table in the left lateral decubitus position.
  2. The throat is topically anesthetized with viscous lidocaine (Xylocaine) or another anesthetic spray. This is to decrease the gag reflex caused by passage of the endoscope.
  3. The patient is usually sedated. This minimizes anxiety and allows the patient to experience a "light" sleep.
  4. The endoscope is gently passed through the mouth and finally into the esophagus; once in the esophagus, visualization can be performed.
  5. Air is insufflated to distend the upper GI tract for adequate visualization.
  6. The esophagus, stomach, and duodenum are evaluated.
  7. During *enteroscopy,* the upper small bowel is visualized and a biopsy is performed if needed.
  8. Biopsy or any endoscopic surgery is performed with direct visualization.
  9. At the completion of direct inspection and surgery, the excess air and GI secretions are aspirated through the scope.
- Note that the test is performed in the endoscopy laboratory by a physician trained in GI endoscopy and takes approximately 20 to 30 minutes.
- Tell the patient that the test is mildly uncomfortable.

After
- Inform the patient that he or she may have hoarseness or a sore throat after the test.
- Withhold any fluids until the patient is completely alert and the swallowing reflex returns to normal, usually 2 to 4 hours.

- Observe the patient's vital signs. Evaluate the patient for bleeding, fever, abdominal pain, dyspnea, or dysphagia.
- Inform the patient that he or she may experience some post-endoscopic bloating, belching, and flatulence.
- Observe safety precautions until the effects of the sedatives have worn off.
- Inform the patient that the sedation may cause some retrograde and antegrade amnesia for a few hours.

Abnormal findings

Tumor (benign or malignant) of the esophagus, stomach, or duodenum

Esophageal diverticula

Hiatal hernia

Esophagitis, gastritis, duodenitis

Gastroesophageal varices

Peptic ulcer

Peptic stricture and subsequent scarring

Extrinsic compression by a cyst or tumor outside the upper GI tract

Source of upper GI bleeding

notes

estriol excretion (Estrogen fractions)

Type of test Urine (24-hour); blood

Normal findings Rising estriol levels, indicating normal fetal growth

E

Possible critical values Values 40% below the average of two previous values demand immediate evaluation of fetal well-being.

Test explanation and related physiology

Serial urine and blood studies for estriol excretion provide an objective means of assessing placental function and fetal normality in high-risk pregnancies. Excretion of estriol (the largest form of estrogen, which exists in the blood and urine) increases around the eighth week of gestation and continues to rise until shortly before delivery. Estriol is produced in the placenta from estrogen precursors, which are made in the fetal adrenal gland and liver; the measurement of excreted estriol is an important index of fetal well-being. Rising values indicate an adequately functioning fetoplacental unit. Decreasing values suggest fetoplacental deterioration (failing pregnancy, dysmaturity, preeclampsia/eclampsia, complicated diabetes mellitus, encephaly, fetal death) and require prompt reassessment of the pregnancy. If the estriol levels fall, early delivery of the fetus may be indicated.

Serial studies usually begin at approximately 28 to 30 weeks of gestation and are then repeated weekly. The frequency of these estriol determinations can be increased as needed to evaluate a high-risk pregnancy. Collection may be done daily. Although the first collection is the baseline value, all collection results are compared with previous ones, because decreasing values suggest fetal deterioration. Some physicians suggest using an average of three previous values as a control value.

Estriol excretion studies can be done using 24-hour urine tests or blood studies. Because urinary creatinine excretion is relatively constant, its determination can be used to assess the adequacy of the 24-hour urine collection for estriol. A serially increasing estriol/creatinine ratio is a favorable sign in pregnancy. Plasma estriol determinations also can be used to evaluate the fetoplacental unit. These studies can conveniently and rapidly assess the quantity of free estriol in the plasma by radioimmunoassay. The plasma collected by venipuncture is an accurate reflection of the current status of the placenta and fetus. The advantage of the plasma estriol determination is that it is more easily obtained than a 24-hour urine specimen and less affected by medications.

Unfortunately, only severe placental distress will decrease urinary estriol sufficiently to reliably predict fetoplacental stress. Furthermore, plasma and urinary estriol levels are normally associated with significant daily variation, which may confuse serial results. Maternal illnesses such as hypertension, preeclampsia, anemia, and impaired renal function can also factitiously decrease urinary estriol levels. Because these problems create a high number of false-positive and false-negative findings, most clinicians now use nonstress fetal monitoring (see p. 571) to indicate fetal-placental health.

Interfering factors

- Recent administration of radioisotopes may alter test results.
- Glycosuria and urinary tract infections can increase urine estriol levels.
- Drugs that may *elevate* levels include adrenocorticosteroids, ampicillin, estrogen-containing drugs, phenothiazines, and tetracyclines.
- Drugs that may *decrease* levels include clomiphene.

Procedure and patient care

Before

- Explain the procedure to the patient.
- If the patient is going to collect the 24-hour urine specimen at home, give her the collection bottle (with a preservative) and instruct her to keep the urine refrigerated.
- Tell the patient that no food or fluid restrictions are needed.

During

Blood

- Collect approximately 5 ml of venous blood in a red-top tube.

24-hour urine

- Instruct the patient to begin the 24-hour urine collection after voiding. Discard the initial specimen and start the 24-hour timing at that point.
- Collect all urine passed during the next 24 hours. Make sure the patient knows where to store the urine container.
- Keep the specimen on ice or refrigerated during the 24-hour collection period.

- Indicate the starting time on the urine container and laboratory slip.
- Post the hours for the urine collection in a prominent place to prevent accidental discarding of the specimen.
- Instruct the patient to void before defecating so that the urine is not contaminated by feces.
- Remind the patient not to put toilet paper in the collection container.
- Encourage the patient to drink fluids during the 24 hours.
- Collect the last specimen as close as possible to the end of the 24-hour period. Add this urine to the collection.
- List any drugs that may affect test results on the laboratory slip.

After

- Apply pressure or a pressure dressing to the venipuncture site.
- Observe the venipuncture site for bleeding.
- Transport the 24-hour urine specimen promptly to the laboratory.
- Inform the patient how and when to obtain the results of this study.

Abnormal findings

▲ **Increased levels**
Ovarian tumor
Testicular tumor
Adrenal tumor
Multiple pregnancy
Urinary tract infection
Glucosuria

▼ **Decreased levels**
Failing pregnancy
Fetal distress
Dysmaturity
Preeclampsia/eclampsia
Complicated diabetes mellitus
Anencephaly
Congenital anomaly
Fetal death
Turner's syndrome
Hypopituitarism
Adrenogenital syndrome
Stein-Leventhal syndrome
Anorexia nervosa
Menopause
Placental insufficiency
Rh isoimmunization

estrogen receptor assay (ER assay, ERA, Estradiol receptor)

Type of test Microscopic examination

Normal findings

Negative: ≤10 fmol/mg of protein
Positive: >10 fmol/mg of protein

Test explanation and related physiology

The ER assay is useful in determining the prognosis and treatment of breast cancer. The assay is used to determine whether a tumor is likely to respond to endocrine therapy or to removal of the ovaries or adrenal gland. Tumors with a positive ER assay are more than twice as likely to respond to endocrine therapy than an ER-negative tumor. Hormone receptor assays should be done on all primary or recurrent breast carcinomas. Levels tend to be higher in postmenopausal women than in premenopausal women. In general, ER-positive tumors have a better prognosis than ER-negative tumors. ER status is now being evaluated on other gynecologic tumors, but its exact role in these patients has yet to be defined.

Slightly over 50% of patients with breast carcinoma who are ER-positive respond to endocrine therapy (e.g., tamoxifen, estrogens, androgens, oophorectomy, adrenalectomy). The response is greater when the progesterone receptors (see p. 662) are also positive. Patients whose breast cancers lack these hormone receptors (are ER negative) have a much lower chance of tumor response to hormone therapy and may not be candidates for this form of treatment.

Specimens are obtained by the pathologist from surgical specimens. One gram of tissue is required. More recently, an ER assay can be performed by immunohistochemical methods on fixed, paraffin-embedded tissue or microscope slides. With these newer methods, much less tissue is required.

Interfering factors

- Delay in tissue fixation may cause deterioration of receptor proteins and produce lower values.
- Hormones should be discontinued before breast biopsy is performed. Antiestrogen preparations (e.g., tamoxifen [Nol-

vadex]) during the past 2 months may cause false-negative ER assays.

✔ Exogenous hormones that are taken for contraceptive purposes or menopausal estrogens may produce lower receptor values.

Procedure and patient care

Before

- Explain the procedure to the patient.
- Before biopsy, a gynecologic history is obtained, including menopausal status and exogenous hormone use.

During

- The surgeon obtains tumor tissue.
- This tissue is placed on ice and immediately transferred to the pathology department.
- Part of the tissue is used for routine histology, and at least 1 g is frozen.
- The frozen specimen is sent (in dry ice) to a central laboratory for ER analysis.
- If immunohistochemical methods of ER assays are used, the specimen is fixed as soon as it arrives at the lab.

After

- Results are usually available in 2 weeks.

Abnormal findings

Nonapplicable

notes

ethanol (Ethyl alcohol, Blood alcohol, Blood EtOH)

Type of test Blood; urine; gastric; breath

Normal findings None

Possible critical values >300 mg/dl

Test explanation and related physiology

Ethanol depresses the central nervous system and may lead to coma and death. This test is usually performed to evaluate alcohol-impaired driving or overdose. Proper collection, handling, and storage of the blood alcohol are important for medicolegal cases involving sobriety. The blood test is the specimen of choice. Blood is taken from a peripheral vein in living patients and from the aorta in cadavers. Ethanol also can be detected in the urine, in gastric contents, or by breath analyzer.

Blood alcohol levels between 50 to 100 mg/dl (0.05% to 0.10% weight/volume) are considered legal intoxication. At this level, flushing, slowing of reflexes, and impaired visual activity are noted. Depression of the central nervous system occurs with levels over 100 mg/dl, and fatalities are reported with levels over 400 mg/dl.

Interfering factors

- Elevated blood ketones (as with diabetic ketoacidosis) can cause false elevation of blood and breath test results.

Procedure and patient care

Before

- Explain the procedure to the patient.
- Follow the institution's protocol if the specimen will be used for legal purposes.

During

- Use a povidone-iodine wipe instead of an alcohol wipe for cleansing the venipuncture site.
- Collect a venous blood sample in a gray- or red-top tube according to the agency's protocol.
- If a gastric or urine specimen is indicated, approximately 20 to 50 ml of fluid is necessary.
- Breath analyzers are taken at the end of expiration after a deep inspiration.

After

- Apply pressure or a pressure dressing to the venipuncture site.
- Assess the venipuncture site for bleeding.
- Follow the agency's protocol regarding specimen collection.
- The exact time of specimen collection should be indicated. Also, in some instances, signatures of the collector and a witness may be needed for legal evidence.

Abnormal finding

Alcohol overdose

notes

euglobulin lysis time (Euglobulin clot lysis, Fibrinolysis/euglobulin lysis)

Type of test Blood

Normal findings 90 minutes to 6 hours

Possible critical values <1 hour, indicating excessive fibrinolytic activity (danger of bleeding)

Test explanation and related physiology

The euglobulin lysis test is used to evaluate systemic fibrinolysis. The fibrinolytic system normally breaks down small fibrin deposits. When this system is abnormally overactive, as in primary fibrinolysis, any fibrin clot that is formed will be dissolved immediately, resulting in a bleeding tendency. This system is only minimally overactive in disseminated intravascular coagulation (DIC, secondary fibrinolysis).

The euglobulin lysis time is a measure of the activity of this fibrinolytic system. Fibrin formed in the euglobulin fraction of plasma is normally very rapidly dissolved by plasmin (fibrinolysin). The time measured from clot formation to clot lysis is referred to as the *euglobulin lysis time*. In primary fibrinolysis (caused by streptokinase administration, cancer of the prostate, shock, or other conditions), the euglobulin lysis time is rapid (short). In DIC, the euglobulin lysis time is usually normal; however, if all the plasmin has been consumed, the time may be prolonged (see Figure 9, p. 251).

This is one of the best tests to differentiate primary fibrinolysis from DIC. This differentiation is important in considering appropriate therapy for the patient with a bleeding tendency. Epsilon-aminocaproic acid may be required to treat primary fibrinolysis; heparin may be indicated for DIC.

This test also may be used to monitor streptokinase or urokinase therapy in patients with acute myocardial infarction.

Interfering factors

- Vigorous exercise, increasing age, and hyperventilation may cause increased fibrinolysis.
- Postmenopausal women and normal newborns may have decreased fibrinolysis.
- Decreased fibrinogen levels may result in a falsely shortened

lysis time because of the reduced amount of fibrin to be lysed.

- Patients who are obese may have decreased fibrinolysis.
- Drugs that may cause *increased* fibrinolysis include steroids and adrenocorticotropic hormone.

Procedure and patient care

Before

- Explain the procedure to the patient.
- Instruct the patient not to exercise before the blood sample is collected.
- Tell the patient that no fasting is required.

During

- Collect approximately 5 ml of blood in a blue-top tube.
- Avoid excessive agitation of the blood sample.
- Deliver the blood specimen to the laboratory immediately on ice.

After

- Apply pressure or a pressure dressing to the venipuncture site.
- Assess the venipuncture site for bleeding.

Abnormal findings

▲ **Increased fibrinolysis (shortened lysis time)**

Incompatible blood transfusion

Cirrhosis

Thrombocytopenia purpura

Leukemia

Obstetric complications (e.g., antepartum hemorrhage, septic abortion, hydatidiform mole, amniotic embolism)

Primary fibrinolysis (e.g., caused by streptokinase or urokinase administration, cancer of the prostate, shock)

Prostatic cancer

Shock

Extensive vascular trauma or surgery

▼ **Decreased fibrinolysis (increased lysis time)**

Prematurity

Diabetes

evoked potential studies (EP studies, Evoked brain potentials, Evoked responses, Visual-evoked potentials, Auditory brainstem-evoked potentials, Somatosensory-evoked responses)

Type of test Electrodiagnostic

Normal findings No neural conduction delay

Test explanation and related physiology

EP studies focus on changes and responses in brain waves that are evoked from stimulation of a sensory pathway. The study of EPs grew out of early work with the electroencephalogram (EEG) (see p. 340). Although the EEG measures "spontaneous" brain electrical activity, the sensory EP study measures minute voltage changes produced in response to a specific stimulus, such as a light pattern, a click, or a shock. In contrast to the EEG, which records signals that reach amplitudes of up to 50 to 100 μV, EP signals are usually less than 5 μV. Because of this, they can only be detected with an averaging computer. The computer averages out (or cancels) unwanted random waves to sum the evoked response that occurs at a specific time after a given stimulus.

Clinical abnormalities are usually detected by an increase in *latency,* which refers to the delay between the stimulus and the wave response. Latency depends on factors such as body size, position of the body where the stimulus is applied, conduction velocity of axons in the neural pathways, number of synapses in the system, location of nerve generators of EP components (brainstem or cortex), and presence of central nervous system pathology. Conduction delays indicate damage to the nerve fibers of the sensory system being evaluated. EPs are divided by sensory modality into visual, auditory, and somatosensory responses.

Visual-evoked responses (VERs) are usually stimulated by a strobe light flash, reversible checkerboard pattern, or retinal stimuli. A visual stimulus to the eye causes an electrical response in the occipital area that can be recorded with electrodes placed along the vertex and on the occipital lobes. Ninety percent of patients with multiple sclerosis show abnormal latencies in VERs, a phenomenon attributed to demyelination of nerve fibers. In addition to patients with multiple sclerosis, those with other neurologic disorders (e.g., Parkinson's disease) show an abnormal latency with VERs. The degree of latency seems to correlate with the disease severity. Abnormal results also may be seen in patients with lesions of the optic nerve, optic tract, visual center, and eye. Absence of binocularity, which is a neurologic developmental disorder in infants, can be detected and evaluated by VERs. This test also can be used during eye surgery to provide a warning of possible damage to the optic nerve.

Auditory brainstem-evoked potentials (ABEPs) are usually stimulated by clicking sounds to evaluate the central auditory pathways of the brainstem. Either ear can be evoked to detect lesions in the brainstem that involve the auditory pathway without affecting hearing. One of the most successful applications of ABEPs has been screening low-birth-weight newborns for auditory disorders. This enables infants with poor hearing to be fitted with corrective devices as soon as possible before learning to speak. ABEPs also have great therapeutic implications in the early detection of posterior fossa tumors.

Somatosensory-evoked responses (SERs) are usually stimulated by sensory stimulus to an area of the body. The time is then measured for the current of the stimulus to travel along the nerve to the cortex of the brain. SERs are used to evaluate patients with spinal cord injuries, to monitor spinal cord functioning during surgery and treatment of diseases (e.g., multiple sclerosis), to evaluate the location and extent of areas of brain dysfunction after head injury, and to pinpoint tumors at an early stage.

One of the main benefits of EPs is their objectivity, because voluntary patient response is not needed. This makes EPs useful with nonverbal and uncooperative patients. This objectivity permits the distinction of organic from psychogenic problems. This is invaluable in settling lawsuits concerning workmen's compensation insurance. The projected future of EPs will aid in diagnosing and monitoring mental disorders and child learning disabilities and in detecting adult mental disorders (e.g., alcoholic brain damage).

Procedure and patient care

Before

- Explain the procedure to the patient.
- Instruct the patient to shampoo his or her hair before the test.
- Tell the patient that no fasting or sedation is required.

During

- Note that the position of the electrode depends on the type of EP study to be done:
    1. For *VERs,* electrodes are placed on the scalp along the vertex and the cortex lobes. Stimulation occurs by using a strobe light, checkerboard pattern, or retinal stimuli.
    2. *ABEPs* are stimulated with clicking noises or tone bursts delivered via earphones. The responses are detected by scalp electrodes placed along the vertex and on each earlobe.
    3. *SERs* are stimulated using electrical stimuli applied to nerves at the wrist (medial nerve) or the knee (peroneal nerve). The response is detected by electrodes placed over the sensory cortex of the opposite hemisphere on the scalp.
- Note that this study is performed by a physician in less than 30 minutes.
- Tell the patient that little discomfort is associated with this study.

After

- Remove the gel used for the adherence of the electrodes.

Abnormal findings

Multiple sclerosis
Parkinson's disease
Tumor
Absence of binocularity
Auditory disorder
Spinal cord injury

Spinal cord dysfunction
Optic tract lesions
Eye lesions
Visual field defects
Cerebrovascular accident
  (stroke)

notes

fecal fat (Fat absorption, Quantitative stool fat determination)

Type of test Stool

Normal findings
Fat: 5 g/24 hr
Retention coefficient: ≥95%

Test explanation and related physiology
The fecal fat test measures the fat content in the stool. The total output of fecal fat per 24 hours in a 3-day stool collection provides the most reliable measurement.

Children with cystic fibrosis have mucous plugs that obstruct the pancreatic ducts. The pancreatic enzymes (amylase, lipase, trypsin, and chymotrypsin) cannot be expelled into the duodenum and are therefore either completely absent or present only in diminished quantities within the gastrointestinal tract. Lipase and bicarbonate are lipolytic, and without them fat is not digested for absorption. This results in impaired fat absorption (malabsorption). These patients have large, greasy, and foul-smelling stools; this is known as *steatorrhea*.

Although reliable, analysis of fecal fat is not specific to cystic fibrosis. Any condition that may cause malabsorption (e.g., sprue, Crohn's disease, Whipple's disease) or maldigestion (e.g., bile duct obstruction, pancreatic duct obstruction secondary to tumor or gallstones) is also associated with increased fecal fat. Short-gut syndrome is also associated with high fecal fat output.

Interfering factors
▼ Drugs that may alter test results include enemas and laxatives, especially mineral oil.

Procedure and patient care
Before
- Explain the procedure to the patient.
- Give the patient instructions regarding the appropriate diet (a diet diary may be requested by the laboratory):
  1. For adults, usually 100 g of fat per day is suggested for 3 days before and throughout the collection period.
  2. Children, and especially infants, cannot ingest 100 g of fat. Therefore, a *fat retention coefficient* is determined by

measuring the difference between ingested fat and fecal fat and then expressing that difference (the amount of fat retained) as a percentage of the ingested fat:

$$\frac{\text{Ingested fat} - \text{Fecal fat}}{\text{Ingested fat}} \times 100\% = \text{Fat coefficient}$$

- Note that the fat retention coefficient in normal children and adults is 95% or greater. A low value indicates steatorrhea.
- Instruct the patient to defecate in a dry, clean container. Occasionally, a tongue blade is required to transfer the stool to the specimen container.
- Tell the patient not to urinate in the stool container.
- Inform the patient that even diarrheal stools should be collected.
- Instruct the patient that toilet paper should not be placed in the stool container.
- Tell the patient not to take any laxatives or enemas during this test, because they will interfere with intestinal motility and alter test results.

During

- Collect each stool specimen and send immediately to the laboratory during the 24- to 72-hour testing period.
- Label each specimen and include the time and date of collection.
- If the specimen is collected at home, give the patient a large stool container to keep in the freezer.

After

- Inform the patient that a normal diet can be resumed.

Abnormal findings

▲ Increased levels

Cystic fibrosis

Malabsorption secondary to sprue, celiac disease, Whipple's disease, Crohn's disease (regional enteritis), or radiation enteritis

Maldigestion secondary to obstruction of the pancreatobiliary tree (e.g., cancer, stricture, gallstones)

Short-gut syndrome secondary to surgical resection, surgical bypass, or congenital anomaly

ferritin

Type of test Blood

Normal findings

Male: 12-300 ng/ml or 12-300 µg/L (SI units)
Female: 10-150 ng/ml or 10-150 µg/L (SI units)
Children
    Newborn: 25-200 ng/ml
    1 month: 200-600 ng/ml
    2-5 months: 50-200 ng/ml
    6 months-15 years: 7-142 ng/ml

Test explanation and related physiology

The serum ferritin study is a good indicator of available iron stores. Ferritin, the major iron storage protein, is normally present in the serum in concentrations directly related to iron storage. In normal patients, 1 ng/ml of serum ferritin corresponds to approximately 8 mg of stored iron. Ferritin levels in adult men and postmenopausal women are generally significantly higher than in younger adult females. Decreases are associated with iron deficiency anemia and are also seen in patients with severe protein depletion. Increased levels are a sign of iron excess, as seen in hemochromatosis, hemosiderosis, megaloblastic anemia, hemolytic anemia, recent blood transfusion, and certain liver disorders.

A limitation of this study is that ferritin levels also can be elevated in conditions not reflecting iron stores (e.g., acute inflammatory diseases, infections, metastatic cancer, lymphomas). If iron deficiency were to occur in patients with these diseases, it would not be recognized because the levels of ferritin would be factitiously elevated by the concurring disease.

When combined with the serum iron level and total iron-binding capacity (TIBC, see p. 492), this test is useful in differentiating and classifying anemias. For example, in patients with iron deficiency anemia, the ferritin, iron, and saturation levels are low, whereas the TIBC and transferrin levels are high. Ferritin levels are normal or high in patients with thalassemia.

Interfering factors

- Recent transfusions and recent ingestion of a meal containing a high iron content may cause elevated ferritin levels.

- Hemolytic diseases may be associated with an artificially high iron content.
- Disorders of excessive iron storage (e.g., hemochromatosis, hemosiderosis) are associated with high ferritin levels.
- Menstruating women may have decreased ferritin levels.
- Drugs that may *increase* ferritin levels include iron preparations.

Procedure and patient care

Before
- Explain the procedure to the patient.
- Tell the patient that no fasting is required.

During
- Collect approximately 5 to 7 ml of venous blood in a red-top tube.

After
- Apply pressure or a pressure dressing to the venipuncture site.
- Assess the venipuncture site for bleeding.

Abnormal findings

▲ **Increased levels**
Hemochromatosis
Hemosiderosis
Megaloblastic anemia
Hemolytic anemia
Alcoholic/inflammatory
  hepatocellular disease
Inflammatory disease
Hodgkin's disease
Breast cancer

▼ **Decreased levels**
Iron deficiency anemia
Severe protein deficiency
Hemodialysis

notes

fetal scalp blood pH

Type of test Blood

Normal findings

pH: 7.25-7.35
O_2 saturation: 30% to 50%
Po_2: 18-22 mm Hg
Pco_2: 40-50 mm Hg
Base excess: 0 to -10 mEq/L

Test explanation and related physiology

Measurement of fetal scalp blood pH provides valuable information on fetal acid-base status. This screening test is useful clinically for diagnosing fetal distress.

Although the oxygen partial pressure (Po_2), carbon dioxide partial pressure (Pco_2), and bicarbonate ion concentration can be measured with the fetal scalp blood sample, the pH is the most useful clinically. The pH normally ranges from 7.25 to 7.35 during labor; a mild decline within the normal range is noted with contractions and as labor progresses.

Fetal hypoxia causes anaerobic glycolysis, resulting in excess production of lactic acid. This causes an increase in hydrogen ion concentration (acidosis) and a decrease in pH. Acidosis reflects the effect of hypoxia on cellular metabolism. A high correlation exists between low pH levels and low Apgar scores.

Contraindications

- Patients with premature membrane rupture
- Patients with active cervical infection (e.g., gonorrhea)

Potential complications

- Continued bleeding from the puncture site
- Hematoma
- Ecchymosis
- Infection

Procedure and patient care

Before

- Explain the procedure to the patient.
- Obtain informed consent for this procedure.
- Tell the patient that no fasting or sedation is required.

During

- Note the following procedural steps:
  1. Amnioscopy is performed with the mother in the lithotomy position.
  2. The cervix is dilated, and the endoscope (amnioscope) is introduced into the cervical canal.
  3. The fetal scalp is cleansed with an antiseptic and dried with a sterile cotton ball.
  4. A small amount of petroleum jelly is applied to the fetal scalp to cause droplets of fetal blood to bead.
  5. After the skin on the scalp is pierced with a small metal blade, beaded droplets of blood are collected in long, heparinized capillary tubes.
  6. The tube is sealed with wax and placed on ice to retard cellular respiration, which can alter the pH.
  7. The physician performing the procedure applies firm pressure to the puncture site to retard bleeding.
  8. Scalp blood sampling can be repeated as necessary.
- Note that this study is performed by a physician in approximately 10 to 15 minutes.
- Tell the patient that she may be uncomfortable during the cervical dilation.

After

- Inform the patient that she may have vaginal discomfort and menstrual-type cramping.

After delivery

- Assess the newborn and identify and document the puncture site(s).
- Cleanse the fetal scalp puncture site with an antiseptic solution and apply an antibiotic ointment.

Abnormal finding

Fetal distress

notes

fetoscopy

Type of test Endoscopy

Normal findings No fetal distress

Test explanation and related physiology

Fetoscopy is an endoscopic procedure that allows direct visualization of the fetus via the insertion of a tiny, telescope-like instrument through the abdominal wall and into the uterine cavity (Figure 16). Direct visualization may lead to diagnosis of a

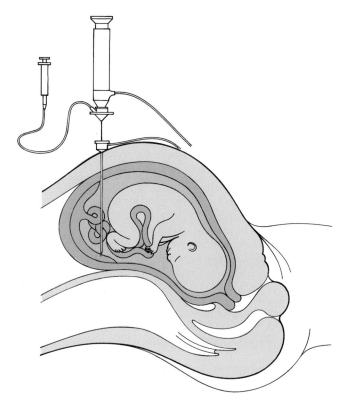

Figure 16 Fetoscopy for fetal blood sampling.

severe malformation, such as a neural tube defect. During the procedure, fetal blood samples to detect congenital blood disorders (e.g., hemophilia, sickle cell anemia) can be drawn from a blood vessel in the umbilical cord for biochemical analysis. Fetal skin biopsies also can be done to detect primary skin disorders.

Fetoscopy is performed at approximately 18 weeks of gestation. At this time, the vessels of the placental surface are of adequate size and the fetal parts are readily identifiable. A therapeutic abortion would not be as hazardous at this time as it would be if it were done later in the pregnancy.

Potential complications

- Spontaneous abortion
- Premature delivery
- Amniotic fluid leak
- Intrauterine fetal death
- Amnionitis

Procedure and patient care

Before

- Explain the procedure to the patient.
- Obtain informed consent for this procedure.
- Assess the fetal heart rate (FHR) before the test to serve as a baseline value.
- Administer meperidine (Demerol) if ordered before the test, because it crosses the placenta and quiets the fetus. This prevents excessive fetal movement, which would make the procedure more difficult.

During

- Note the following procedural steps:
  1. The woman is placed in the supine position on an examining table.
  2. The abdominal wall is anesthetized locally.
  3. Ultrasonography is performed to locate the fetus and the placenta.
  4. The endoscope is inserted.
  5. Biopsies and blood samples may be obtained.
- Note that this procedure is performed by a physician in 1 to 2 hours.
- Tell the patient that the only discomfort associated with this study is the injection of the local anesthetic.

After

- Assess the FHR and compare with the baseline value to detect any side effects related to the procedure.
- Monitor the mother and fetus carefully for alterations in blood pressure, pulse, uterine activity, fetal activity, vaginal bleeding, and loss of amniotic fluid.
- Administer RhoGAM to mothers who are Rh negative unless the fetal blood is found to be Rh negative.
- Note that a repeat ultrasound is usually performed the day after the procedure to confirm the adequacy of the amniotic fluid and fetal viability.
- Instruct the mother to avoid strenuous activity for 1 to 2 weeks following the procedure and to report any pain, bleeding, amniotic fluid loss, or fever.
- At times, if ordered, administer antibiotics prophylactically after the test to prevent amnionitis.

Abnormal findings

Developmental defects (e.g., neural tube defects)
Congenital blood disorders (e.g., hemophilia, sickle cell anemia)
Primary skin disorders

notes

fibrin degradation products (FDPs, Fibrin split products [FSPs], Fibrin breakdown products)

Type of test Blood

Normal findings <10 μg/ml or dilution <1:20

Possible critical values >40 μg/ml

Test explanation and related physiology

Measurement of FDPs provides a direct indication of the activity of the fibrinolytic system. When plasma acts to dissolve fibrin blood clots, FDPs (X, D, E, and Y) are formed. These degradation products, which have an anticoagulant effect and inhibit clotting, can be measured. When present in large amounts, they indicate increased fibrinolysis, as occurs in disseminated intravascular coagulation (DIC) and primary fibrinolytic disorders. This test is one of the DIC screening tests.

Interfering factors

- Traumatic venipunctures may alter test results.
- Drugs that may cause *increased* levels include barbiturates, heparin, streptokinase, and urokinase.

Procedure and patient care

Before
- Explain the procedure to the patient.
- Tell the patient that no fasting is required.

During
- Draw the sample before initiating heparin therapy.
- Collect a venous blood sample (usually only 2 ml) in a small, blue-top tube or in the colored tube designated by the laboratory.
- Avoid excessive agitation of the blood sample.
- Note that it is best to place the blood on ice and take it immediately to the hematology laboratory.
- List on the laboratory slip any drugs that may cause elevated levels.

After
- Apply pressure or a pressure dressing to the venipuncture site.
- Assess the venipuncture site for bleeding.

Abnormal findings

▲ **Increased levels**

Liver disease
Congenital heart disease
Leukemia
Thromboembolic state
Transplant rejection
Renal disease
Obstetric complications
  (e.g., preeclampsia, ab-
  ruptio placentae, intra-
  uterine fetal death)

Following massive blood
  transfusion
Disseminated intravascular
  coagulation
Hypoxia
Portacaval shunt
Infection
Burns
Septicemia
Following cardiopulmonary
  pump surgery

F

notes

fibrinogen (Factor I, Quantitative fibrinogen)

Type of test Blood

Normal findings
Adult: 200-400 mg/dl or 2.0-4.0 g/L (SI units)
Newborn: 125-300 mg/dl

Possible critical values <100 mg/dl

Test explanation and related physiology

Fibrinogen (factor I) is primarily used to aid in the diagnosis of suspected bleeding disorders. Fibrinogen is essential to the blood-clotting mechanism. It is converted to fibrin by action of thrombin during the coagulation process (see Figure 9, p. 251). Fibrinogen, which is produced by the liver, is also an acute-phase protein reactant. It rises sharply during instances of tissue inflammation or tissue necrosis. High levels also may be a useful predictor for increased risk of coronary artery or cerebrovascular disease. Reduced levels can be seen in patients with liver disease, malnourished states, large transfusions, and consumptive coagulopathies (e.g., disseminated intravascular coagulation).

Interfering factors

- Blood transfusions within the past month may affect test results.
- Drugs that may cause *increased* levels include estrogens and oral contraceptives.
- Drugs that may cause *decreased* levels include anabolic steroids, androgens, asparaginase, phenobarbital, streptokinase, urokinase, and valproic acid.

Procedure and patient care

Before
- Explain the procedure to the patient.
- Tell the patient that no fasting is required.

During
- Collect one tube of venous blood in a blue-top tube.

After
- Apply pressure or a pressure dressing to the venipuncture site.
- Assess the venipuncture site for bleeding.

Abnormal findings

▲ **Increased levels**
Rheumatoid arthritis
Hepatitis
Acute infection
Menstruation
Pregnancy (late)
Multiple myeloma
Glomerulonephritis
Pneumonia

▼ **Decreased levels**
Congenital afibrinogen-
emia
Disseminated intravascu-
lar coagulation
Fibrinolysis
Severe liver disease
Advanced carcinoma
Coagulation factor (fi-
brinogen) deficiency
Eclampsia
Recent trauma

F

notes

fibrinogen uptake test with ^{125}I (Fibrinogen uptake test [FUT], Radioactive fibrinogen scanning)

Type of test Nuclear scan

Normal findings No area of increased radionuclide uptake within the venous system of the lower extremity

Test explanation and related physiology

The iodine-125 fibrinogen uptake test (^{125}I FUT) is a noninvasive radionuclear study used to identify thrombi in the veins of the lower extremities. When thrombi form, large amounts of fibrinogen are present at the site of clot formation. Fibrinogen is an important hemostatic factor (factor I) (see Figure 9, p. 251). When fibrinogen is tagged with ^{125}I and given intravenously, it can be detected by a gamma ray detector. At areas where clot formation is occurring (e.g., venous thromboses), the ^{125}I count will be greatly increased. The test is approximately 80% to 90% accurate in the diagnosis of deep-vein thrombophlebitis.

Although clinicians previously thought the test could recognize only clots being formed, it is now known that the ^{125}I FUT can detect established clots. This test is also useful in the early detection of subclinical deep-vein thrombosis. Therefore, immobilized patients at great risk for deep-vein thrombophlebitis can be identified early. However, the ^{125}I FUT has several disadvantages:

1. This test cannot detect deep-vein thrombosis in the proximal thigh. Normally, high quantities of fibrinogen exist in that area, and the background counts are too high to detect minimal degrees of increased uptake.
2. It is necessary to wait at least 24 hours between administering ^{125}I and detecting increased fibrinogen uptake. This is a major disadvantage when one needs to know immediately if thrombosis exists.
3. Because the fibrinogen used in this test is obtained from donated blood, the inherent risks of blood transfusion exist.

Initially, this test was used to evaluate medicosurgical or obstetric patients at high risk for the formation of deep-vein thrombosis. These patients were studied over 1 to 2 weeks to detect extremely early deep-vein thrombosis. Patients can be studied daily for 7 to 14 days after administration of ^{125}I.

Contraindications

- Patients for whom the diagnosis of deep-vein thrombosis is needed in less than 24 hours
- Patients with ongoing inflammation in the leg (e.g., superficial phlebitis, cellulitis, active arthritis)
  Fibrinogen exists in increased levels at these areas and will give a false-positive result.
- Patients with lymphedema, because the fibrinogen level is high in the extremities
- Patients who are allergic to iodine or shellfish
  A steroid-and-diphenhydramine (Benadryl) preparation may be used for these patients.

Interfering factors

- Other areas of inflammation within the suspected extremity
- Lymphedema

Procedure and patient care

Before

- Explain the procedure to the patient.
- Determine whether the patient is allergic to iodine or shellfish.
- Assess the patient's extremity for signs of inflammation or lymphedema.
- Tell the patient that no fasting or sedation is required.

During

- Note the following procedural steps:
  1. The patient is transferred to the nuclear medicine department, where ^{125}I fibrinogen is administered.
  2. The extremity is marked in multiple areas for subsequent examination.
  3. Countered readings are obtained 10 minutes after ^{125}I administration over the premarked sites.
  4. The patient is returned to his or her room.
  5. Twenty-four hours later, either at the patient's bedside or on return to the nuclear medicine department, the Geiger-like detector is placed over the previously marked areas for counter readings.
  6. The amount of ^{125}I identified at the premarked sites is recorded and compared with the amount present in the opposite leg or in the precordium.

7. If the amount of ^{125}I detected at any area is 15 times greater than normal extremity, heart, or baseline preinjection levels, the test is considered positive for deep-vein thrombosis.

- To avoid uptake of ^{125}I by the thyroid gland, provide Lugol's solution or potassium iodine, if ordered, for the patient before and during the scanning procedure.
- Note that a nuclear medicine technologist performs this procedure in less than 1 hour daily.
- Tell the patient that no discomfort is associated with this test other than the fibrinogen injection.

After
- Caution all nursing mothers to refrain from breastfeeding for 24 to 48 hours after injection of ^{125}I.

Abnormal finding

Deep-vein thrombophlebitis

notes

folic acid (Folate)

Type of test Blood

Normal findings 5-20 µg/ml or 14-34 mmol/L (SI units)

Test explanation and related physiology

Folic acid, one of the B vitamins, is necessary for normal function of red and white blood cells (RBCs, WBCs) and for the adequate synthesis of certain purines and pyrimidines, which are precursors for deoxyribonucleic acid (DNA). As with vitamin B_{12} (see p. 727), folate depends on normal function of the intestinal mucosa.

Folic acid blood levels are performed to evaluate hemolytic disorders and to detect anemia caused by folic acid deficiency (in which the RBCs are abnormally large, causing a megaloblastic anemia). These RBCs have a shortened life span and impaired oxygen-carrying capacity.

The main causes of folic acid deficiency include dietary deficiency, malabsorption syndrome, pregnancy, and certain anticonvulsant drugs. Decreased folic acid levels are seen in patients with folic acid deficiency anemia (megaloblastic anemia), hemolytic anemia, malnutrition, malabsorption syndrome, malignancy, liver disease, sprue, and celiac disease. Some drugs (e.g., anticonvulsants, antimalarials, alcohol, aminopterin, and methotrexate) are folic acid antagonists and interfere with nucleic acid synthesis.

Elevated levels of folic acid may be seen in patients with pernicious anemia. The folic acid test may be done in conjunction with tests for vitamin B_{12} levels (see p. 727). This test for folate is often done in the workup for alcoholic patients to assess the patient's nutritional status.

Interfering factors

☛ Drugs that may cause *decreased* folic acid levels include alcohol, aminopterin, aminosalicylic acid (PAS), ampicillin, antimalarials, chloramphenicol, erythromycin, estrogens, methotrexate, oral contraceptives, penicillin, phenobarbital, phenytoin, and tetracyclines.

Procedure and patient care

Before

- Explain the procedure to the patient.

- Tell the patient that no fasting is usually required. (However, some laboratories prefer an 8-hour fast.)
- Instruct the patient not to consume alcoholic beverages before the test.
- Draw the specimen before starting folate therapy.

During

- Collect approximately 7 to 10 ml of venous blood in a red-top tube.
- Avoid hemolysis.
- Indicate on the laboratory slip any medications that may affect test results.

After

- Apply pressure or a pressure dressing to the venipuncture site.
- Assess the venipuncture site for bleeding.
- Transport the blood immediately to the laboratory after collection.

Abnormal findings

▲ **Increased levels**
Pernicious anemia
Vegetarianism

▼ **Decreased levels**
Folic acid deficiency anemia
Hemolytic anemia
Malnutrition
Malabsorption syndrome (e.g., sprue, celiac disease)
Malignancy
Liver disease
Pregnancy
Alcoholism
Anorexia nervosa

notes

gallbladder nuclear scanning (Hepatobiliary scintigraphy, Hepatobiliary imaging, Biliary tract radionuclide scan, Cholescintigraphy, DISIDA scanning, HIDA scanning, IDA gallbladder scanning)

Type of test Nuclear scan

Normal findings Gallbladder, common bile duct, and duodenum visualize within 60 minutes after radionuclide injection. (This confirms patency of the cystic and common bile ducts.)

G

Test explanation and related physiology

Through the use of iminodiacetic acid analogues (IDAs) labeled with technetium-99m (^{99m}Tc), the biliary tract can be evaluated in a safe, accurate, and noninvasive manner. These radionuclide compounds are extracted by the liver and excreted into the bile. Cholescintigraphy is valuable in evaluating patients for suspected gallbladder disease. The primary use of this study is to diagnose acute cholecystitis in patients who have acute right upper quadrant abdominal pain. Failure to visualize the gallbladder 60 to 120 minutes after injection of the radionuclide dye is virtually diagnostic of an obstruction of the cystic duct, which occurs in the pathophysiology of acute cholecystitis. Delayed filling of the gallbladder is associated with chronic or acalculus cholecystitis. This procedure is also helpful in diagnosing biliary duct obstructions.

This procedure is superior to oral cholecystography, IV cholangiography, ultrasonography, and CT of the gallbladder in the detection of cholecystitis. Also, with cholescintigraphy, gallbladder function can be numerically determined by calculating the capability of the gallbladder to eject its contents. It is believed that an ejection fraction below 35% indicates primary gallbladder disease. Occasionally, morphine sulfate is given intravenously. The morphine causes increased ampullary contraction. Not only can this reproduce the patient's symptoms of biliary colic, but it also serves to force the bile containing the radionuclide into the gallbladder. The scan time can therefore be decreased with the use of morphine.

Contraindication

- Pregnancy, because of the risk of fetal damage

Interfering factor

- If the patient has not eaten for more than 24 hours, the radionuclide may not fill the gallbladder. This would produce a false-positive result.

Procedure and patient care

Before

- Explain the procedure to the patient.
- Assure the patient that he or she will not be exposed to large amounts of radioactivity.
- Instruct the patient to fast for at least 2 hours before the test. This fasting is preferable but not mandatory.

During

- Note the following procedural steps:
  1. After IV administration of a ^{99m}Tc-labeled IDA analogue (e.g., DISIDA, PIPIDA, HIDA), the right upper quadrant of the abdomen is scanned.
  2. Serial images are obtained over 1 hour.
  3. Subsequent images can be obtained at 15- to 30-minute intervals.
  4. If the gallbladder, common bile duct, or duodenum is not visualized within 60 minutes after injection, delayed images are obtained up to 4 hours later.
  5. Images are recorded on Polaroid or x-ray film.
  6. When an ejection fraction is to be determined, the patient is given a fatty meal or cholecystokinin to evaluate emptying of the gallbladder. The gallbladder is continually scanned to measure the percentage of isotope ejected.
- Note that a radiologist performs this study in 1 to 4 hours in the nuclear medicine department.
- Tell the patient that the only discomfort associated with this procedure is the IV injection of radionuclide.

After

- Obtain a meal for the patient if indicated.

Abnormal findings

Acute cholecystitis
Chronic cholecystitis
Acalculus cholecystitis

Common bile duct obstruction secondary to gallstones, tumor, or stricture

gallium scan

Type of test Nuclear scan

Normal findings

Diffuse, low level of gallium uptake, especially in the liver and spleen

No increased gallium uptake within the body

Test explanation and related physiology

A gallium scan of the total body is usually performed 24, 48, and 72 hours after an IV injection of radioactive gallium. Gallium is a radionuclide that is concentrated by areas of inflammation and infection, by abscesses, and by benign and malignant tumors. Not all types of tumors, however, will concentrate gallium. Lymphomas are particularly gallium avid. Other tumors that can be detected by a gallium scan include sarcomas, hepatomas, and carcinomas of the gastrointestinal tract, kidney, uterus, stomach, and testicle.

This test is useful in detecting metastatic tumor, especially lymphoma, even when other diagnostic imaging tests are normal. The gallium scan also is useful in demonstrating a source of infection in patients with a fever of unknown origin. Unfortunately, this test is not specific enough to differentiate among tumor, infection, inflammation, or abscess.

Some organs (liver, spleen, bone, colon) normally retain gallium. Therefore a normal total-body gallium scan study would demonstrate some uptake in these organs, but this uptake is much less concentrated than in pathologic areas (e.g., tumor, inflammation).

Contraindication

- Pregnancy, because of the risk of fetal damage

Procedure and patient care

Before

- Explain the procedure to the patient.
- Usually, administer a cathartic or enema to the patient to minimize increased gallium uptake within the bowel.

During

- Note the following procedural steps:
  1. The unsedated patient is injected with gallium.

2. A total-body scan may be performed 4 to 6 hours later by slowly passing a radionuclide detector over the body.
3. The images provided by the detector are recorded on Polaroid or x-ray film.
4. Additional scans are usually taken 24, 48, and 72 hours later.
5. During the scanning process, the patient is positioned in the supine, prone, and lateral positions.

- Note that a nuclear medicine technologist performs each scan in approximately 30 to 60 minutes. Repeated scanning, however, is required. Repeated injections are not necessary.
- Inform the patient that test results are interpreted by a physician trained in nuclear medicine and are usually available 72 hours after the injection.
- Tell the patient that no pain or discomfort is associated with this procedure other than the IV injection. However, it occasionally can be uncomfortable to lie still on a hard table for the duration required.

After

- Assure the patient that only tracer doses of radioisotopes have been used and that no precautions against radioactive exposure to others are necessary.

Abnormal findings

Tumor
Infection

Noninfectious inflammation
Abscess

notes

gamma-glutamyl transpeptidase (GGTP, γ-GTP, gamma-glutamyl transferase [GGT])

Type of test Blood

Normal findings
Male and female over age 45: 8-38 U/L
Female under age 45: 5-27 U/L
Elderly: slightly higher than adult level
Child: similar to adult level
Newborn: 5 times higher than adult level

G

Test explanation and related physiology

The biliary enzyme GGTP participates in the transfer of amino acids and peptides across the cellular membrane and possibly participates in glutathione metabolism. Highest concentrations of this enzyme are found in the liver cells, biliary tract, kidney, spleen, heart, intestine, brain, and prostate gland. This test is used to detect liver cell dysfunction, and it very accurately reveals evidence of cholestasis. As with leucine aminopeptidase and 5′-nucleotidase, the elevation of GGTP generally parallels that of alkaline phosphatase; however, GGTP is more sensitive. Also, as with 5′-nucleotidase and leucine aminopeptidase, GGTP is not increased in bone diseases as is alkaline phosphatase. A normal GGTP level with an elevated alkaline phosphatase level would imply skeletal disease. An elevated GGTP and elevated alkaline phosphatase level would imply hepatic disease.

Another important clinical aspect of GGTP is that it can detect heavy alcohol ingestion. This enzyme rises rapidly even after a small intake of alcohol. It is therefore very useful in the evaluation of alcoholic patients. GGTP is elevated in approximately 75% of these patients.

Why this enzyme is elevated 4 to 10 days after an acute myocardial infarction is not clear. It may represent the associated hepatic insult.

Interfering factors

- Values may be decreased in late pregnancy.
- Drugs that may cause *increased* GGTP levels include alcohol, phenytoin (Dilantin), and phenobarbital.
- Drugs that may cause *decreased* levels include clofibrate and oral contraceptives.

Procedure and patient care

Before
- Explain the procedure to the patient.
- Tell the patient that an 8-hour fast is recommended. Only water is permitted.

During
- Collect approximately 7 to 10 ml of venous blood in a red-top tube.
- Indicate on the laboratory slip any medications the patient is taking that may affect test results.

After
- Apply pressure or a pressure dressing to the venipuncture site.
- Assess the venipuncture site for bleeding. Patients with liver dysfunction often have prolonged clotting times.

Abnormal findings

▲ Increased levels
Hepatitis
Cirrhosis
Hepatic necrosis
Hepatic ischemia
Myocardial infarction (4-10 days after)
Congestive heart failure
Hepatic tumor
Hepatotoxic drugs
Cholestasis
Alcohol ingestion
Jaundice
Pancreatitis

notes

gastric analysis (Tube gastric analysis, Tubeless gastric analysis, Diagnex Blue test)

Type of test Fluid analysis

Normal findings

Tube gastric analysis
    Basal acid output: 2-5 mEq/hr
    Maximal acid output: 10-20 mEq/hr
Tubeless gastric analysis: detectable dye in urine

G

Test explanation and related physiology

With gastric analysis, the contents of the stomach are aspirated to determine the amount of acid produced by the parietal cells within the stomach lining during the resting or basal state (basal acid output [BAO]) and during the stimulated state (maximal acid output [MAO]). This information is useful in the following clinical settings:

1. To differentiate causes of hypergastrinemia. Patients who have high gastrin levels because of antacid ingestion, previous antipeptic surgery, or atrophic gastritis will have reduced values of BAO and MAO. Patients who have high gastrin levels resulting from Zollinger-Ellison (ZE) syndrome or G-cell hyperplasia will have elevated levels of BAO and MAO.

2. To determine whether a gastric ulcer is benign or malignant. Because a benign peptic ulcer requires the presence of acid, ulcerations that occur in the absence of acid (as determined by gastric analysis) will usually be malignant. Differentiation between benign and malignant, however, can be better determined by biopsy directed by esophagogastroduodenoscopy (see p. 369).

3. To determine the presence of ZE syndrome. In this disease, a pancreatic islet cell tumor secretes high levels of gastrin, which constantly and maximally stimulates the stomach to secrete acid. Therefore the stomach is always in the stimulated state and never in the resting state. This causes the value of the BAO to approach that of the MAO. The BAO/MAO ratio would then be greater than 0.6 in ZE syndrome. Because of the development of direct measurement of serum gastrin levels, however, gastric analysis is no longer used for this purpose.

4. To determine the efficacy of medical or surgical antiulcer therapy. To be therapeutic, medical or surgical treatment of peptic ulcer disease must substantially decrease the acid output of the stomach. Baseline values are determined by a pretreatment gastric analysis. The study is repeated during treatment. Effective therapy is indicated by a 50% reduction in the quantity of acid produced. This last indication is probably the only present use for gastric analysis.

Contraindications

- Patients with carcinoid syndrome

Potential complications

- Because histamine is the most frequently used drug to stimulate gastric acid, patients with congestive heart failure, carcinoid syndrome, or hypertension may have their conditions exacerbated.

Interfering factors

- Surgical vagotomy may alter test results.
- Smoking stimulates secretion of the gastric cells.
- Food or fluid alters gastric acid secretion.
- ✸ Drugs that may *increase* gastric acid secretion include adrenergic blockers, caffeine, calcium salts, cholinergics, corticosteroids, ethanol, and reserpine.
- ✸ Drugs that may *decrease* gastric acid secretion include antacids, anticholinergics, H_2-blocking agents (e.g., Tagamet, Pepcid, Zantac), and tricyclic antidepressants.

Procedure and patient care

Before

- Explain the procedure to the patient. Most patients are very apprehensive about this study.
- Instruct the patient to keep NPO after midnight on the day of the test.
- Instruct the patient to abstain from anticholinergic medications, which may inhibit the stimulating action of the histamine.
- Instruct the patient to abstain from smoking, which stimulates gastric acid secretion.

During

- Note the following procedural steps:

Tube gastric analysis

1. To assess the gastric acid secretion reliably, a nasogastric (NG) tube must be inserted into the dependent portion of the stomach.

2. A syringe is attached to the tube while initial gastric acid is aspirated and discarded.

3. Four subsequent samples are aspirated at 15-minute intervals. These are marked as BAO. The BAO is determined by multiplying the number of milliequivalents in the highest basal sample by four. Then histamine, 0.04 mg/kg body weight, is administered subcutaneously to the patient. (Occasionally, betazole hydrochloride is administered.)

4. Eight subsequent specimens are taken at 15-minute intervals. These are the MAO specimens. The MAO is determined by multiplying the number of milliequivalents of the highest measurement by 4.

Tubeless gastric analysis

1. In this type of test, which uses Diagnex Blue (Diagnex Blue test), the patient is asked to ingest a gastric stimulant (e.g., a tablet of caffeine).

2. A resin dye, such as Diagnex Blue, is then ingested. If the gastric contents contain hydrochloric acid (HCl), the stomach acid displaces the dye from the Diagnex resin.

3. The dye is absorbed by the bowel and excreted in the urine in approximately 2 hours. The urine will be changed to a blue color. The absence of a blue color in the urine usually indicates the absence of HCl in the stomach.

- Note that the gastric analysis is usually performed by a nurse or physician in approximately 3 hours. It can be performed in a laboratory or at the patient's bedside.

- Tell the patient that except for the initial gagging usually associated with insertion of the NG tube, this test is not uncomfortable. (No NG tube insertion is needed for the tubeless test.)

After

- Observe the patient for side effects of the histamine injection. They may include uterine, intestinal, or bronchial spasm.

- Observe the patient for capillary dilation, which may be evidenced by increased pulse rate and mildly decreased blood pressure.

- If the tubeless gastric analysis uses Diagnex, inform the patient that the urine may stay blue or blue-green for several days.

Abnormal findings

Zollinger-Ellison syndrome

Peptic ulceration

Inadequate therapeutic effect from surgical vagotomy

Inadequate therapeutic antipeptic ulcer medication

Pernicious anemia

notes

gastric emptying scan

Type of test Nuclear scan

Normal findings
No delay in gastric emptying
Gastric emptying complete in 90 minutes

Test explanation and related physiology
   This study involves having the patient ingest a solid or liquid
"test meal" containing a radionuclide such as technetium (Tc).
The stomach is then scanned until gastric emptying is complete.
This study is used to assess the stomach's ability to empty solids
or liquids and to evaluate disorders that may cause a delay in
gastric emptying, such as obstruction (caused by peptic ulcers
or gastric malignancies) and gastroparesis. This scan is also useful in determining the patency of a gastrointestinal (GI) anastomosis.

Contraindications
- Patients who are pregnant or lactating

Procedure and patient care
Before
- Explain the procedure to the patient.
- Assure the patient that no pain is associated with this study.
- Inform the patient that only a small dose of nuclear material
  is ingested. Reassure the patient that this is a safe dose.
- Instruct the patient to keep NPO after midnight on the day
  of the test.

During
- Note the following procedural steps:
  1. In the nuclear medicine department, the patient is asked
     to ingest a test meal. In the *solid-emptying* study, the pa-
     tient eats a cooked egg white containing Tc. In the
     liquid-emptying study, the patient drinks orange juice
     containing Tc.
  2. After ingestion of the test meal, the patient lies supine
     under a gamma ray detector camera that records images
     until gastric emptying has been complete. This may take
     several hours.

- Note that this procedure lasts approximately 90 minutes, depending on the gastric emptying time.
- Inform the patient that the test is interpreted by a nuclear medicine physician and that results are available the same day.
- Remind the patient that no discomfort is associated with the test.

After

- Assure the patient that he or she has ingested only a small amount of nuclear material. No radiation precautions need to be taken against the patient or his or her bodily secretions.

Abnormal findings

Gastric obstruction caused by gastric ulcer or cancer
Nonfunctioning GI anastomosis
Gastroparesis caused by diabetes or neuropathy

notes

gastrin

Type of test Blood

Normal findings

<200 pg/ml or <200 ng/L (SI units)
Levels are higher in elderly patients.

Test explanation and related physiology

Gastrin is a hormone produced by the G cells located in the distal part of the stomach (antrum). Gastrin is a potent stimulator of gastric acid. In normal gastric physiology, an alkaline environment (created by food or antacids) stimulates the release of gastrin. Gastrin then stimulates the parietal cells of the stomach to secrete gastric acid. The pH environment in the stomach is thereby reduced. By negative feedback, this low-pH environment suppresses further gastrin secretion.

Zollinger-Ellison (ZE) syndrome (gastrin-producing pancreatic tumor) and G-cell hyperplasia (overfunctioning of G cells in the distal stomach) are associated with high serum gastrin levels. Patients with these tumors have aggressive peptic ulcer disease. Unlike the patient with routine peptic ulcers, the patient with ZE syndrome or G-cell hyperplasia has a high incidence of complicated and recurrent peptic ulcers. It is important to identify this latter group of patients to institute more appropriate, aggressive medical and surgical therapy. The serum gastrin level will be normal in the patient with routine peptic ulcer and greatly elevated in patients with ZE syndrome or G-cell hyperplasia.

It is important to note, however, that patients who are taking antacid peptic ulcer medicines, have had peptic ulcer surgery, or have atrophic gastritis will have a high serum gastrin level. However, levels usually are not as high as in patients with ZE syndrome or G-cell hyperplasia.

Not all patients with ZE syndrome exhibit increased levels of serum gastrin. Some may have "top" normal gastrin levels, which makes these patients difficult to differentiate from patients with routine peptic ulcer disease. ZE syndrome or G-cell hyperplasia can be diagnosed in these "top" normal patients by gastrin stimulation tests using calcium or secretin. Patients with these diseases will have greatly increased serum gastrin levels associated with the infusion of these drugs.

Interfering factors

- Peptic ulcer surgery
  This creates a persistent alkaline environment, which is the strongest stimulant to gastrin.
- Ingestion of high-protein food can result in an increase in serum gastrin two to five times the normal level.
- ☒ Diabetic patients taking insulin may have falsely elevated levels.
- ☒ Drugs that may *increase* serum gastrin levels include antacids, H_2-blocking agents (e.g., Tagamet, Zantac), and hydrogen pump inhibitors (e.g., Prilosec).
- ☒ Drugs that may *decrease* levels include anticholinergics and tricyclic antidepressants.

Procedure and patient care

Before

- Explain the procedure to the patient.
- Usually, instruct the patient to fast for 12 hours. Water is permitted.
- Tell the patient to avoid alcohol for at least 24 hours.

During

- Collect approximately 5 to 7 ml of venous blood in a red-top tube.
- For the *calcium infusion test,* administer calcium gluconate intravenously for 3 hours. A preinfusion serum gastrin level is then compared with specimens taken every 30 minutes for 4 hours.
- For the *secretin test,* administer secretin intravenously. Preinjection and postinjection serum gastrin levels are taken at 15-minute intervals for 1 hour after injection.
- Indicate on the laboratory slip any drugs that may affect test results.

After

- Apply pressure or a pressure dressing to the venipuncture site.
- Observe the venipuncture site for bleeding.

Abnormal findings

▲ **Increased levels**

ZE syndrome	Pernicious anemia
G-cell hyperplasia	Atrophic gastritis

gastroesophageal reflux scan (GE reflux scan, Aspiration scan)

Type of test   Nuclear scan

Normal findings   No evidence of gastroesophageal reflux

Test explanation and related physiology

GE reflux scans are used to evaluate patients with symptoms of heartburn, regurgitation, vomiting, and dysphagia. Also, these scans are used to evaluate the medical or surgical treatment of patients with GE reflux. Finally, *aspiration scans* may be used to detect aspiration of gastric contents into the lungs.

Contraindications

- Patients who cannot tolerate abdominal compression
- Patients who are pregnant or lactating

Procedure and patient care

Before

- Explain the procedure to the patient.
- Assure the patient that no pain is associated with this test.
- Instruct the patient to eat a full meal just before the study.

During

- Note the following procedural steps:

GE reflux scan

1. The patient is placed in the supine position and asked to swallow a tracer cocktail (e.g., orange juice, diluted hydrochloric acid, and technetium-99m-labeled colloid).
2. Images are taken of the patient over the esophageal area.
3. The patient is asked to assume other positions to determine whether GE reflux occurs and, if so, in what position.
4. A large abdominal binder that contains an air-inflatable cuff is placed on the patient's abdomen. This is insufflated to increase abdominal pressure.
5. Images are again taken over the esophageal area to determine if any GE reflux occurs.

Aspiration scans

1. These scans may be performed by adding a radionuclide to the patient's evening meal and keeping the patient in the supine position until the next morning.

2. Images are made over the lung fields to detect esophago-tracheal aspiration of the tracer.
- In infants being evaluated for chalasia, note that the tracer is added to the feeding or formula. Nuclear tracer films are then taken over the next hour, with delayed films as needed.
- Note that this procedure is performed in the nuclear medicine department in approximately 30 minutes.
- Remind the patient that no discomfort is associated with this test.

After

- Assure the patient that he or she has ingested only a small dose of nuclear material. No radiation precautions need to be taken against the patient or his or her bodily secretions.

Abnormal findings

Gastroesophageal reflux
Pulmonary aspiration

notes

gastrointestinal bleeding scan (Abdominal scintigraphy, GI scintigraphy)

Type of test   Nuclear scan

Normal findings   No collection of radionuclide in GI tract

Test explanation and related physiology

The GI bleeding scan is a test used to localize the site of bleeding in patients who are having GI hemorrhage. The scan also can be used in patients who have intraabdominal hemorrhage from an unknown source. Localization of the source of GI bleeding can be quite difficult. When surgery is required under these circumstances, it is difficult, cumbersome, and prolonged. The surgeon may have extreme difficulty finding the source of bleeding.

Endoscopy has proved to be extremely useful in determining the source of intestinal bleeding; however, endoscopy is not helpful if the source is within the small intestine or the colon. Although colonoscopy allows excellent visualization of the colon when it is cleared out, it is extremely difficult to see when acute, active intestinal bleeding is occurring. Arteriography can determine the site of bleeding, but the rate of bleeding must exceed 0.5 ml/min for detection. Also, GI bleeding can be intermittent, and the arteriogram could be falsely negative.

A GI scintigram is much more sensitive in locating the site of GI bleeding; however, it is not very specific in pinpointing the site of bleeding. Usually, when positive, the exact source of bleeding cannot be localized any more accurately than indicating the affected quadrant of the abdomen (e.g., right upper, left lower). This test is usually performed by injecting sulfur colloid labeled with technetium-99m (^{99m}Tc) or ^{99m}Tc-labeled red blood cells (RBCs) into the patient. If the patient is bleeding at a rate in excess of 0.05 ml/min, pooling of the radionuclide will ultimately be detected in the abnormal segment of the intestine. Few false-positive results occur. The test will only localize the bleeding; it will not indicate the exact pathologic condition causing the bleeding. With this test result, if surgery is required, the surgeon is directed to the abnormal area and hopefully can detect and resect the pathologic bleeding source.

Contraindications

- Patients who are pregnant or lactating
- Medically unstable patients whose stay in the nuclear medicine department may be risky

Interfering factor

- Barium within the GI tract may mask a small source of bleeding.

Procedure and patient care

Before

- Explain the procedure to the patient.
- Assess the patient's vital signs to ensure that they are stable for the patient's transfer to and from the nuclear medicine department.
- Accompany the patient to the nuclear medicine department if vital signs are questionably stable.
- Assure the patient that only a small amount of nuclear material will be administered.
- Instruct the patient to notify the nuclear medicine technologist if he or she has a bowel movement during the test. Blood in the GI tract can act as a cathartic.
- Inform the patient that no pretest preparation is required.
- Inform the nuclear medicine technologist to notify the nurse of all bloody bowel movements that occur while the patient is in the nuclear medicine department.

During

- Note the following procedural steps:
  1. Ten millicuries of freshly prepared ^{99m}Tc-labeled sulfur colloid is administered intravenously to the patient. If ^{99m}Tc-labeled RBCs are to be used, 3 to 5 ml of the patient's own blood is combined with the ^{99m}Tc and reinjected into the patient.
  2. Immediately after administration of the radionuclide, the patient is placed under a scintillation camera.
  3. Multiple images of the abdomen are obtained at short intervals (5 to 15 minutes). Scintigrams are recorded on Polaroid or x-ray film.
  4. Detection of radionuclide in the abdomen indicates the site of bleeding. If no bleeding sites are noted in the first hour, the scan is repeated at hourly intervals for as long as 24 hours.

- Note that areas of the bowel hidden by the liver or spleen may not be adequately evaluated by this procedure. Also, the rectum cannot be easily evaluated, because other pelvic structures (e.g., the bladder) obstruct the view. If the initial study is negative and subsequent films give evidence of active bleeding, a repeat scan may be performed.
- Note that this test is usually performed in approximately 20 to 30 minutes by a technologist in the nuclear medicine department.
- Tell the patient that the only discomfort associated with this study is the injection of the radioisotope.

After

- Reevaluate the patient's vital signs on return to the nursing unit.
- Assure the patient that only tracer doses of radioisotopes have been used and that no precautions against radioactive exposure to others are necessary.

Abnormal findings

Ulcer
Angiodysplasia
Diverticulosis

Tumor
Polyps
Inflammatory bowel disease

notes

glucagon

Type of test Blood

Normal findings 30-210 pg/ml or 30-210 ng/L (SI units)

Test explanation and related physiology

Glucagon is a hormone secreted by the alpha cells of the pancreatic islets of Langerhans. Glucagon is secreted in response to hypoglycemia and increases the blood glucose by breaking down glycogen to glucose by inhibiting passage of glucose into the cell and by encouraging efflux of glucose from the cell. Elevated glucagon levels may indicate the diagnosis of a *glucagonoma* (i.e., an alpha islet cell neoplasm).

With a glucagon deficiency, serum levels are low. Arginine is a potent stimulator of glucagon. If the glucagon levels fail to rise even with arginine infusion, the diagnosis of glucagon deficiency is confirmed. In patients with diabetes, glucagon secretion does not decrease following ingestion of a carbohydrate meal, but with arginine infusion, great increases in glucagon occur.

Because glucagon is thought to be metabolized by the kidneys, renal failure or rejection of a transplanted kidney may result in increased serum glucagon levels and create significant hypoglycemia.

Interfering factors

- Test results may be invalidated if a patient has undergone a radioactive scan within the previous 48 hours.
- Levels may be elevated after prolonged fasting or moderate to severe exercise.
- ✴ Drugs that may cause *increased* levels include some amino acids (e.g., arginine), danazol, glucocorticoids, gastrin, insulin, and nifedipine.
- ✴ Drugs that may cause *decreased* levels include atenolol, propranolol, and secretin.

Procedure and patient care

Before

- Explain the procedure to the patient.
- Tell the patient that fasting is necessary for 10 to 12 hours before the test. Only water is permitted.

During

- Collect a venous blood sample in a lavender-top tube.

After

- Apply pressure or a pressure dressing to the venipuncture site.
- Assess the venipuncture site for bleeding.
- Place the specimen on ice and send it immediately to the laboratory.

Abnormal findings

▲ **Increased levels**
  Glucagonoma
  Diabetes mellitus
  Chronic renal failure
  Severe stress
  Acromegaly
  Cirrhosis
  Acute pancreatitis
  Pheochromocytoma

▼ **Decreased levels**
  Idiopathic glucagon deficiency
  Chronic pancreatitis
  Postpancreatectomy

G

notes

glucose, blood (Blood sugar, Fasting blood sugar [FBS])

Type of test Blood

Normal findings
Cord: 45-96 mg/dl or 2.5-5.3 mmol/L (SI units)
Premature infant: 20-60 mg/dl or 1.1-3.3 mmol/L
Neonate: 30-60 mg/dl or 1.7-3.3 mmol/L
Infant: 40-90 mg/dl or 2.2-5.0 mmol/L
Child <2 years: 60-100 mg/dl or 3.3-5.5 mmol/L
Child >2 years to adult: 70-105 mg/dl or 3.9-5.8 mmol/L
Elderly: increase in normal range after age 50 years

Possible critical values
Adult male: <50 and >400 mg/dl
Adult female: <40 and >400 mg/dl
Infant: <40 mg/dl
Newborn: <30 and >300 mg/dl

Test explanation and related physiology
The serum glucose test is helpful in diagnosing many metabolic diseases. Serum glucose levels must be evaluated according to the time of day they are performed. For example, a glucose level of 135 mg/dl may be abnormal if the patient is in the fasting state, but this level would be within normal limits if the patient had eaten a meal within the last hour.

In general, true glucose elevations indicate diabetes mellitus; however, one must be aware of many other possible causes of hyperglycemia. Similarly, hypoglycemia has many causes. The most common cause is inadvertent insulin overdose in patients with brittle diabetes.

Glucose determinations must be performed frequently in new diabetic patients to monitor closely the insulin dosage to be administered. Finger stick blood glucose determinations are often performed before meals and at bedtime. Results are compared with a sliding-scale insulin chart ordered by the physician to provide coverage with SQ regular insulin.

Interfering factors
- Many forms of stress (e.g., trauma, general anesthesia, cerebrovascular accident, myocardial infarction) can cause increased serum glucose levels.

- Caffeine may cause *increased* levels.
- ✠ Drugs that may cause *increased* levels include antidepressants (tricyclics), beta-adrenergic blocking agents, corticosteroids, dextrose IV infusion, dextrothyroxine, diazoxide, diuretics, epinephrine, estrogens, glucagon, isoniazid, lithium, phenothiazines, phenytoin, salicylates (acute toxicity), and triamterene.
- ✠ Drugs that may cause *decreased* levels include acetaminophen, alcohol, anabolic steroids, clofibrate, disopyramide, gemfibrozil, insulin, monoamine oxidase inhibitors, pentamidine, propranolol, tolazamide, and tolbutamide.

G

Procedure and patient care

Before

- Explain the procedure to the patient.
- For FBS, keep the patient fasting at least 8 hours. Water is permitted.
- To prevent starvation, which may artificially raise the glucose levels, the patient should not fast longer than 16 hours.
- Withhold insulin or oral hypoglycemics until after blood is obtained.

During

- Collect approximately 7 ml of venous blood in a red- or gray-top tube.
- Glucose levels can also be evaluated by performing a finger stick and using either a visually read or a reflectance meter. The advantage of the *visually read* test is that it does not require an expensive machine. However, the patient must be able to visually interpret the color of the reagent strip. Using *reflectance meters* (e.g., Glucometer, Accu Check bG, Stat Tek) improves the accuracy of the blood glucose determination. However, this method is more complex because it requires machine calibration and control testing.

After

- Apply pressure or a pressure dressing to the venipuncture site.
- Observe the venipuncture site for bleeding.
- Be certain that the patient receives a meal after fasting blood work.

Abstract findings

▲ **Increased levels
(hyperglycemia)**

Diabetes mellitus
Acute stress response
Cushing's disease
Pheochromocytoma
Hyperparathyroidism
Adenoma of the pancreas
Pancreatitis
Diuretic therapy
Corticosteroid therapy
Acromegaly

▼ **Decreased levels
(hypoglycemia)**

Insulinoma
Hypothyroidism
Hypopituitarism
Addison's disease
Extensive liver disease

notes

glucose, postprandial (2-hour postprandial glucose [2-hour PPG], 2-hour postprandial blood sugar, 1-hour glucose screen for gestational diabetes mellitus)

Type of test Blood

Normal findings

2-hour PPG

0-50 years: <140 mg/dl or <7.8 mmol/L (SI units)
50-60 years: <150 mg/dl
60 years and older: <160 mg/dl

1-hour glucose screen for gestational diabetes
<140 mg/dl

Test explanation and related physiology

The 2-hour PPG test is a measurement of the amount of glucose in the patient's blood 2 hours after a meal (postprandial) is ingested. For this study, a meal acts as a glucose challenge to the body's metabolism. In normal patients, insulin is secreted immediately after a meal in response to the elevated blood glucose level, causing the level to return to the premeal range within 2 hours. In patients with diabetes, the glucose level usually is still elevated 2 hours after the meal. The PPG is an easily performed screening test for diabetes mellitus. If the results are abnormal, a glucose tolerance test (see p. 433) may be performed to confirm the diagnosis.

The 1-hour glucose screen is used to detect gestational diabetes mellitus (GDM), which is the most common medical complication of pregnancy. Gestational diabetes is carbohydrate intolerance first recognized during pregnancy. GDM affects 3% to 8% of pregnant women, with up to half of these women developing overt diabetes later in life. The detection and treatment of GDM may reduce the risk for several adverse perinatal outcomes (such as excessive fetal growth and birth trauma, fetal death, or neonatal morbidity).

Screening for GDM is performed with a 50-g oral glucose load followed by a glucose level determination 1 hour later. Screening is done between weeks 24 and 28 of gestation. However, patients with risk factors, such as a previous history of GDM, may benefit from earlier screening. Patients whose serum glucose level equals or exceeds 140 mg/dl should be evaluated by a 3-hour glucose tolerance test (GTT) (see p. 433).

Interfering factors

- Smoking during the testing period may increase the blood glucose level.
- Stress can increase glucose levels.

Procedure and patient care

Before

- Explain the procedure to the patient.
- For the *2-hour PPG*, instruct the patient to eat the entire meal (with at least 75 g of carbohydrates) and then not to eat anything else until the blood is drawn.
- For the *1-hour glucose screen for GDM*, give the fasting or nonfasting patient a 50-g oral glucose load.
- Instruct the patient not to smoke during the testing.
- Inform the patient that he or she should rest during the 1- or 2-hour interval.

During

- Collect approximately 7 ml of blood in a red- or gray-top tube 1 or 2 hours after the patient has eaten the test meal.

After

Apply pressure or a pressure dressing to the venipuncture site. Observe the venipuncture site for bleeding.

Abnormal findings

▲ **Increased levels**
Diabetes mellitus
Gestational diabetes mellitus
Cushing's syndrome
Acromegaly
Malnutrition
Hyperthyroidism
Pheochromocytoma

▼ **Decreased levels**
Addison's disease
Steatorrhea
Islet cell adenoma
Anterior pituitary insufficiency

notes

glucose, urine (Urine sugar, Urine glucose)

Type of test Urine

Normal findings
Random specimen: Negative
24-hour specimen: <0.5 g/day or <2.78 mmol/day (SI units)

Test explanation and related physiology

A qualitative glucose test is usually part of a routine urinalysis. This screening test for the presence of glucose within the urine may indicate the likelihood of diabetes mellitus. This diagnosis must be confirmed by other tests (e.g., glucose tolerance test, glycosylated hemoglobin test). Urine glucose tests are also used to monitor the effectiveness of diabetes therapy; however, this is largely supplanted today by finger stick determinations of blood glucose levels.

In patients with diabetes whose conditions are not well controlled with hypoglycemic agents, blood glucose levels can become very high. High glucose levels also can be produced artificially by IV administration of dextrose-containing fluids. When the blood glucose level exceeds 180 mg/dl (the renal threshold), glucose begins to spill over into the urine (glycosuria). As the blood glucose level increases further, the amount of glucose spilling into the urine also increases.

Interfering factors

- Drugs that may cause false-positive tests with Clinitest but not with Clinistix or Tes-Tape include acetylsalicylic acid, aminosalicylic acid, ascorbic acid, cephalothin, chloral hydrate, nitrofurantoin, streptomycin, and sulfonamides.
- Drugs that may cause false-negative tests include ascorbic acid (Clinistix, Tes-Tape), levodopa (Clinistix), and phenazopyridine (Clinistix, Tes-Tape).
- Drugs that may cause *increased* urine glucose levels include aminosalicylic acid, cephalosporins, chloral hydrate, chloramphenicol, dextrothyroxine, diazoxide, diuretics (loop and thiazide), estrogens, glucose infusions, isoniazid, levodopa, lithium, nafcillin, nalidixic acid, and nicotinic acid (large doses).

Procedure and patient care

Before

- Explain the procedure to the patient.
- Read the directions on the bottle or container of the reagent strips.
- Check the expiration date on the bottle before use.
- Inform the patient that urine tests for glucose may be performed at specified times during the day, generally before meals and at bedtime, and that test results may be used to determine insulin requirements.

During

- Because accuracy is necessary, collect a "fresh" urine specimen. The stagnant urine that has been in the bladder for several hours will not accurately reflect the serum glucose level at testing.
- Preferably, obtain a *double-voided specimen:*
  1. Collect a urine specimen 30 to 40 minutes before the time the urine specimen is actually needed.
  2. Discard this first specimen.
  3. Give the patient glass of water to drink.
  4. At the required time obtain a second specimen, which is tested for glucose.
- Inform the patient that testing for glucose can be easily performed using enzyme tests such as Clinistix, Diastix, or Tes-Tape.
- Remember that urine glucose also can be determined using the Clinitest method (a copper-reducing approach).
- If a 24-hour specimen is required, refrigerate the urine during the collection period.

After

- Record the urine glucose results on the patient's chart.

Abnormal findings

▲   **Increased levels**

Diabetes mellitus	Infection
Cushing's syndrome	Drug therapy
Severe stress (e.g., trauma, surgery)	Pregnancy
	Low renal threshold

glucose-6-phosphate dehydrogenase (G-6-PD screen)

Type of test Blood

Normal findings Negative (screening test) or 8.0-8.6 U/g of hemoglobin

Test explanation and related physiology

Glucose-6-phosphate dehydrogenase is an enzyme used in glucose metabolism. In the red blood cell, a G-6-PD deficiency causes precipitation of hemoglobin and cellular membrane changes. This may result in hemolysis of variable severity. This disease is a sex-linked, recessive trait carried on the X chromosome. Affected males inherit this abnormal gene from their mothers, who are usually asymptomatic. Hemolytic episodes in these individuals may be triggered by drugs (e.g., sulfonamides, nitrofurantoin, phenacetin, antipyretics, primaquine), infections, acidosis, stress, or certain foods (e.g., fava beans). The two common types of G-6-PD deficiency are Mediterranean, affecting Sephardic Jews, and type A, affecting the black population. This test is used to diagnose G-6-PD deficiency in suspected individuals.

Interfering factors

✠ Drugs that may cause *increased* G-6-PD levels include antipyretics, ascorbic acid, aspirin, nitrofurantoin (Furadantin), phenacetin, primaquine, quinidine, sulfonamides, thiazide diuretics, tolbutamide (Orinase), and vitamin K.

Procedure and patient care

Before
- Explain the procedure to the patient.
- Tell the patient that no fasting is required.

During
- Collect approximately 5 ml of venous blood in a lavender- or green-top tube.
- Avoid hemolysis.

After
- Apply pressure or a pressure dressing to the venipuncture site.
- Assess the venipuncture site for bleeding.

- If the test indicates a G-6-PD deficiency, give the patient a
list of drugs that may precipitate hemolysis. Instruct patients
with the Mediterranean type of this disease not to eat fava
beans. Teach patients to read labels on any over-the-counter
drugs for the presence of agents (e.g., aspirin, phenacetin)
that may cause hemolytic anemia.

Abnormal findings

▲ **Increased levels**
Pernicious anemia
Myocardial infarction
Hepatic coma
Hyperthyroidism
Chronic blood loss
Megaloblastic anemia

▼ **Decreased levels**
G-6-PD deficiency
Hemolytic anemia
Infection
Septicemia
Diabetic acidosis

notes

glucose tolerance test (GTT, Oral glucose tolerance test [OGTT])

Type of test Blood; urine

Normal findings

Serum test

Fasting: 70-115 mg/dl or <6.4 mmol/L (SI units)
30 minutes: <200 mg/dl or <11.1 mmol/L
1 hour: <200 mg/dl or <11.1 mmol/L
2 hours: <140 mg/dl or <7.8 mmol/L
3 hours: 70-115 mg/dl or <6.4 mmol/L
4 hours: 70-115 mg/dl or <6.4 mmol/L

Urine test

Negative

Test explanation and related physiology

In the GTT, the patient's ability to tolerate a standard oral glucose load is evaluated by obtaining serum and urine specimens for glucose level determinations before glucose administration and then at 30 minutes, 1 hour, 2 hours, 3 hours, and sometimes 4 hours after the administration. Patients with an appropriate insulin response are able to tolerate the dose quite easily, with only a minimal and transient rise in serum glucose levels within 1 hour after ingestion. In normal patients, glucose will not spill over into the urine.

Patients with diabetes, who have a deficiency of active insulin, will not be able to tolerate this load. As a result, their serum glucose levels will be greatly elevated from 1 to 5 hours (Figure 17). Also, glucose can be detected in their urine.

Gestational diabetes also can be diagnosed by the GTT. Generally, the diagnosis of diabetes can be made if two or more of the results exceed the following:

Fasting: 105 mg/dl
1 hour: 190 mg/dl
2 hours: 165 mg/dl
3 hours: 145 mg/dl

Occasionally, a patient is unable to tolerate the oral glucose load (e.g., patients with prior gastrectomy, short-bowel syndrome, or malabsorption). In these instances, an *intravenous glucose tolerance test* (IV-GTT) can be performed by administering

G

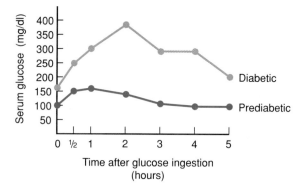

Figure 17 Glucose tolerance test curve for a diabetic patient and a prediabetic patient.

the glucose load intravenously. The values for the IV-GTT differ slightly from those of the oral GTT because the IV glucose is absorbed faster.

Glucose intolerance also may exist in patients with Cushing's syndrome, pheochromocytoma, aldosteronism, myxedema, chronic renal failure, cirrhosis, and acromegaly.

Contraindications

- Patients with serious concurrent infections or endocrine disorders, because glucose intolerance will be observed even though these patients may not be diabetic

Potential complications

- Dizziness, tremors, anxiety, sweating, euphoria, or fainting during testing
  If these symptoms occur, a blood specimen is obtained. If the glucose level is too high, the test may need to be stopped and insulin administered.

Interfering factors

- Smoking during the testing period stimulates glucose because of the nicotine.
- Stress (e.g., from surgery, infection) can increase glucose levels.
- Exercise during the testing can affect glucose levels.
- Drugs that may cause glucose intolerance include antihyper-

tensives, antiinflammatory drugs, aspirin, beta-blockers, furosemide, nicotine, oral contraceptives, psychiatric drugs, steroids, and thiazide diuretics.

Procedure and patient care

Before

- Explain the procedure to the patient.
- Educate the patient about the importance of having adequate food intake with adequate carbohydrates for at least 3 days before the test.
- Instruct the patient to fast for 12 hours before the test.
- Instruct the patient to discontinue drugs that could interfere with the test results.
- Give the patient written instructions explaining the pretest dietary requirement.
- Obtain the patient's weight to determine the appropriate glucose loading dose.

During

- Obtain fasting blood and urine specimens.
- Administer the oral glucose solution, usually a 75- to 100-g carbohydrate load.
- Give pediatric patients a carbohydrate load of 1.75 g/kg body weight, up to a maximum of 75 g.
- Instruct the patient to ingest the entire glucose load.
- Tell the patient that he or she cannot eat anything until the test is completed. However, encourage the patient to drink water. No other liquids should be taken.
- Inform the patient that tobacco, coffee, and tea are not allowed, because they cause physiologic stimulation.
- Collect approximately 5 ml of venous blood in a gray-top tube at 30 minutes and at hourly periods. Apply pressure or a pressure dressing to the sites.
- Collect urine specimens at hourly periods.
- Mark on the tubes the time that the specimens are collected.
- Assess the patient for reactions such as dizziness, sweating, weakness, and giddiness. (These are usually transient.)
- For the IV-GTT, administer the glucose load intravenously over 3 to 4 minutes.
- Indicate on the laboratory slip any drugs that may affect test results.

After

- Send all specimens promptly to the laboratory.
- Allow the patient to eat and drink normally.
- Administer insulin or oral hypoglycemics if ordered.
- Assess the venipuncture sites for bleeding.

Abnormal findings

Diabetes mellitus
Gestational diabetes
Cushing's syndrome
Pancreatic cancer
Somogyi response to hypogly-
  cemia

Pheochromocytoma
Aldosteronism
Myxedema
Chronic renal failure
Cirrhosis
Acromegaly

notes

glycosylated hemoglobin (GHb, GHB, Glycohemoglobin, Hemoglobin [Hb] A$_{1c}$, Diabetic control index)

Type of test Blood

Normal findings Vary with laboratory method employed

Adult/elderly: 4% to 8%
Child: 1.8% to 4.0%
Good diabetic control: 7%
Fair diabetic control: 10%
Poor diabetic control: 13% to 20%

G

Test explanation and related physiology

The GHb test provides an accurate long-term index of the patient's average blood glucose level by measuring the patient's glycohemoglobin, or GHb. Glycohemoglobin is a minor hemoglobin (with A$_1$ components). These A$_1$ components (hemoglobin A$_{1a}$, A$_{1b}$, and A$_{1c}$), which make up approximately 4% to 8% of the total hemoglobin, are glycosylated (i.e., they have glucose attached to them). Hb A$_{1c}$ is usually measured. (If Hb A$_1$ is measured, its value is always 2.4% higher than that of the A$_{1c}$ component.)

As the red blood cell (RBC) circulates, it combines some of its hemoglobin with some of the glucose in the bloodstream to form glycohemoglobin. This glycosylation is irreversible. The amount of GHb depends on the amount of glucose available in the bloodstream over the RBC's 120-day life span. Because old RBCs are constantly being destroyed and new ones are constantly being formed, determination of the GHb value reflects the average blood sugar level for the 100- to 120-day period *before* the test. The more glucose the RBC was exposed to, the greater the GHb percentage. One important advantage of this test is that the sample can be drawn at any time, because it is not affected by short-term variations (e.g., food intake, exercise, stress, hypoglycemic agents, patient cooperation).

The GHb test is particularly beneficial for:
1. Evaluating the success of diabetic treatment
2. Comparing and contrasting the success of past and new forms of diabetic therapy
3. Determining the duration of hyperglycemia in patients with newly diagnosed diabetes

4. Providing a sensitive estimate of glucose imbalance in patients with mild diabetes
5. Individualizing diabetic control regimens
6. Providing a feeling of reward for many patients when the test shows achievement of good diabetic control

Interfering factors

- Low values may occur with sickle cell anemia, with chronic renal failure, and in pregnancy.
- Falsely elevated values occur when the RBC life span is lengthened (as in thalassemia).

Procedure and patient care

Before

- Explain the procedure to the patient.
- Tell the patient that fasting is not indicated.

During

- Collect approximately 5 ml of venous blood in a gray- or lavender-top tube.

After

- Apply pressure or a pressure dressing to the venipuncture site.
- Assess the venipuncture site for bleeding.

Abnormal findings

▲ **Increased levels**
Newly diagnosed diabetic patient
Poorly controlled diabetic patient
Hyperglycemia
Chronic renal failure
Pregnancy
Splenectomy
Iron deficiency anemia
Hemodialysis

▼ **Decreased levels**
Hemolytic anemia (caused by increased erythrocyte turnover)

notes

gonorrhea culture

Type of test Microscopic examination

Normal findings No evidence of *Neisseria gonorrhoeae*

Test explanation and related physiology

Cultures for gonococcal infections are performed on men and women with suspected gonorrhea. If the culture is positive, sexual partners should be evaluated and treated. Cervical cultures are usually done for women; urethral cultures are done for men. Rectal and throat cultures are performed in persons who have engaged in anal and oral intercourse. Because rectal gonorrhea accompanies genital gonorrhea in a high percentage of women, rectal cultures may be recommended in all women with suspected gonorrhea. Performing a culture for gonorrhea is also part of the prenatal workup. If the culture is positive, treatment during pregnancy can prevent possible fetal complications (e.g., ophthalmia neonatorum) and maternal complications. Rectal and orogastric cultures should be done on the neonates of infected mothers.

Gram stains of smears or bacterial cultures should be taken before a patient begins antibiotic therapy. Bacterial cultures use a special medium such as Thayer-Martin, designed for the cultivation of *N. gonorrhoeae*.

Interfering factors

- *N. gonorrhoeae* is very sensitive to lubricants and disinfectants.
- Menses may alter test results.
- Female douching within 24 hours of a cervical culture makes fewer organisms available for culture.
- Male voiding within 1 hour of a urethral culture washes secretions out of the urethra.
- Fecal material may contaminate an anal culture.

Procedure and patient care

Before

- Explain the purpose and procedure to the patient. Use a matter-of-fact, nonjudgmental approach.
- Tell the patient that no fasting or sedation is required.

During
- Obtain cultures as follows:

Cervical culture
1. The female patient is told to refrain from douching and tub bathing before the cervical culture.
2. The patient is placed in the lithotomy position, and a non-lubricated vaginal speculum is inserted to expose the cervix.
3. Cervical mucus is removed with a cotton ball held in a ring forceps.
4. A sterile cotton-tipped swab is inserted into the endocervical canal and moved from side to side to obtain the culture.

Anal canal culture
1. An anal culture of the female or male patient is taken by inserting a sterile, cotton-tipped swab approximately 1 inch into the anal canal.
2. If stool contaminates the swab, a repeat swab is taken.

Urethral culture
1. The urethral specimen should be obtained from the male patient before voiding. Voiding within 1 hour of collection washes secretions out of the urethra, making fewer organisms available for culture.
2. A culture is taken by inserting a sterile swab gently into the anterior urethra.
3. It is advisable to place the male patient in the supine position to prevent falling if vasovagal syncope occurs during introduction of the cotton swab or wire loop into the urethra.
4. The patient is observed for hypotension, bradycardia, pallor, sweating, nausea, and weakness.

Oropharyngeal culture
1. This culture should be obtained in male and female patients who have engaged in oral intercourse.
2. A throat culture is best obtained by depressing the patient's tongue with a wooden tongue blade and touching the posterior wall of the throat with a sterile cotton-tipped swab.

- Note that gonorrheal cultures are obtained by a physician or nurse in several minutes.
- Tell the patient that little discomfort is associated with these procedures.

After

- Place the swabs in a Thayer-Martin medium and roll them from side to side.
- Label and send the culture bottle to the microbiology laboratory.
- Transport the specimen to the laboratory as soon as possible. Handle all specimens as though they were capable of transmitting disease.
- Do not refrigerate the specimen.
- Mark the laboratory slip with the collection time, date, source of specimen, patient's age, current antibiotic therapy, and clinical diagnosis.
- Advise the patient to avoid intercourse and all sexual contact until test results are available.
- If the culture results are positive, tell the patient to receive treatment and to have sexual partners evaluated.
- Note that repeat cultures should be taken after completion of treatment to evaluate therapy.

Abnormal finding

Gonorrhea

notes

growth hormone (GH, Human growth hormone [HGH], Somatotropin hormone [SH])

Type of test Blood

Normal findings

Men: <5 ng/ml or <5 µg/L (SI units)
Women: <10 ng/ml or <10 µg/L
Children: 0-10 ng/ml or 0-10 µg/L
Newborn: 10-40 ng/ml or 10-40 µg/L

Test explanation and related physiology

Growth hormone, or somatotropin, is secreted by the anterior pituitary gland and plays a central role in modulating growth from birth until the end of puberty. In the total absence of growth hormone, linear growth occurs at one half to one third of the normal rate. Growth hormone also plays a role in the control of body anabolism throughout life by increasing protein synthesis, increasing the breakdown of fatty acids in adipose tissue, and increasing the blood glucose level.

If growth hormone secretion is insufficient during childhood, limited growth and dwarfism may result. Also, delay in sexual maturity may be a result in adolescents with reduced growth hormone levels. Conversely, overproduction of growth hormone during childhood results in gigantism, with the person reaching nearly 7 to 8 feet in height. An excess of growth hormone during adulthood results in acromegaly, which is characterized by an increase in bone thickness and width but no increase in height.

Growth hormone tests are used to confirm hypopituitarism or hyperpituitarism. Because growth hormone secretion is episodic, random measurements are not adequate determinants of growth hormone deficiency. Screening for insulin-like growth factor (IGF-1) or somatomedin C (see p. 759) provides a more accurate reflection of the mean plasma concentration of growth hormone. A growth hormone stimulation test (see p. 445) can be performed to evaluate the body's ability to produce growth hormone.

Interfering factors

- Random measurements of growth hormone are not adequate determinants of growth hormone deficiency, because hormone secretion is episodic.

- A radioactive scan performed within the week before the test may affect test results, because levels are determined by radioimmunoassay.
- Growth hormone secretion is increased by stress, exercise, and low blood glucose levels.
- Drugs that may cause *increased* levels include amphetamines, arginine, dopamine, estrogens, glucagon, histamine, insulin, levodopa, methyldopa, and nicotinic acid.
- Drugs that may cause *decreased* levels include corticosteroids and phenothiazines.

Procedure and patient care

G

Before
- Explain the procedure to the patient.
- The patient should not be emotionally or physically stressed, because this can increase growth hormone levels.
- It is preferred that the patients be fasting and well rested. Water is permitted.

During
- Collect one red-top tube of venous blood.
- Because approximately two thirds of the total production of growth hormone occurs during sleep, growth hormone secretion also can be measured during hospitalization by obtaining blood samples while the patient is sleeping.

After
- Apply pressure or a pressure dressing to the venipuncture site.
- Assess the venipuncture site for bleeding.
- Indicate the patient's fasting status and the time the blood is collected on the laboratory slip. Include the patient's recent activity (e.g., sleeping, walking, eating).
- Send the blood to the laboratory immediately after collection, because the half-life of growth hormone is only 20 to 25 minutes.

Abnormal findings

▲ **Increased levels**
Gigantism
Acromegaly
Diabetes mellitus
Anorexia nervosa
Stress
Major surgery
Hypoglycemia
Starvation
Deep-sleep state
Exercise

▼ **Decreased levels**
Pituitary insufficiency
Dwarfism
Hyperglycemia
Failure to thrive
Growth hormone deficiency

notes

growth hormone stimulation test (GH provocation test, Insulin tolerance test [ITT], Arginine test)

Type of test Blood

Normal findings Growth hormone levels >10 ng/ml or 10 μg/L (SI units)

Test explanation and related physiology

Because growth hormone (see p. 442) secretion is episodic, random measurements of plasma growth hormone are not adequate tests of growth hormone deficiency. To diagnose growth hormone deficiency, growth hormone stimulation tests are indicated. One of the most reliable growth hormone stimulators is insulin-induced hypoglycemia, in which the blood glucose declines to less than 40 mg/dl. Other growth hormone stimulants include vigorous exercise and drugs such as arginine, glucagon, levodopa, and clonidine. For children, a double-stimulated test is usually performed using an arginine infusion followed by insulin-induced hypoglycemia. Arginine is an amino acid that stimulates growth hormone secretion; hypoglycemia also stimulates growth hormone secretion. A growth hormone concentration over 10 μg/L after stimulation effectively excludes growth hormone deficiencies.

Contraindications

- Patients with epilepsy
- Patients with cerebrovascular disease
- Patients with myocardial infarction
- Patients with low basal plasma cortisol levels

Interfering factor

- A radioactive scan performed within 1 week before the test may affect test results.

Procedure and patient care

Before

- Explain the procedure very carefully to the patient and, if appropriate, to the parents.
- Instruct the patient to remain NPO after midnight on the morning of the test. Water is permitted.

During

- Note the following procedural steps:
  1. A heparin lock IV line is inserted for the administration of medications and the withdrawal of frequent blood samples.
  2. Baseline blood levels are obtained for growth hormone, glucose, and cortisol.
  3. Venous samples for growth hormone are obtained at 0, 60, and 90 minutes after injection of arginine and/or insulin.
  4. Blood glucose levels are monitored at 15- to 30-minute intervals with the glucometer. The blood sugar should drop to less than 40 mg/dl for effective measurement of growth hormone reserve.
- Monitor the patient for signs of hypoglycemia, postural hypotension, somnolence, diaphoresis, and nervousness. Ice chips are often given during the test for patient comfort.
- This procedure is usually performed by a nurse with a physician in proximity.
- This test takes approximately 2 hours to perform.
- Tell the patient that the minor discomfort associated with this test results from the insertion of the IV line and the hypoglycemic response induced by the insulin injection.
- Growth hormone also can be stimulated by vigorous exercise. This entails running or stair-climbing for 20 minutes. Blood samples of growth hormone are obtained at 0, 20, and 40 minutes.

After

- Observe the venipuncture site for bleeding.
- Inform the patient and family that results may not be available for approximately 7 days. Many laboratories only run growth hormone tests once per week.
- After the test, the patient receives cookies and punch or an IV glucose infusion.
- Send the blood to the laboratory immediately after collection, because the half-life of growth hormone is only 20 to 25 minutes.

Abnormal finding

Growth hormone deficiency

Ham's test (Acid serum test for paroxysmal nocturnal hemoglobinuria [PNH])

Type of test Blood

Normal findings 10% to 50% hemolysis of red blood cells

Test explanation and related physiology

Ham's test is used to identify paroxysmal nocturnal hemoglobinuria (PNH), which is an acquired bone marrow stem cell defect. In these patients, intravascular hemolysis intermittently occurs during sleep. The etiology is not known. The abnormal red blood cells (RBCs) have a membrane defect that creates complement-antibody complexes on the RBC membrane. When these complexes are present, the cell is very sensitive to hemolysis. Hemolysis can be especially provoked by exposing these RBCs to a mild fall in serum pH.

Ham's test is performed by incubating the suspected patient's RBCs with fresh autologous or ABO-compatible homologous serum adjusted to a pH of 6.5 using dilute hydrochloric acid. The amount of hemolysis is then quantified photometrically. A positive test is when 10% to 80% hemolysis of RBCs is observed.

Contraindications

- Patients with recent blood transfusions

Procedure and patient care

Before

- Explain the procedure to the patient.
- Tell the patient that no fasting is required.

During

- Collect approximately 5 to 7 ml of venous blood in a lavender-top tube.
- Indicate if the patient has had a recent blood transfusion.

After

- Apply pressure or a pressure dressing to the venipuncture site.
- Assess the venous puncture site for bleeding.

Abnormal findings

▲   Increased levels
PNH
Type II congenital dyserythropoietic anemia

haptoglobin

Type of test Blood

Normal findings
Adult: 100-150 mg/dl or 16-31 µmol/L (SI units)
Newborn: 0-10 mg/dl

Possible critical values <40 mg/dl

Test explanation and related physiology

The serum haptoglobin test is used to detect intravascular destruction (hemolysis) of red blood cells (RBCs). Haptoglobins are glycoproteins produced by the liver. These haptoglobins are powerful, free hemoglobin-binding proteins. In hemolytic anemias associated with the hemolysis of RBCs, the released hemoglobin is quickly bound to haptoglobin and the new complex is quickly catabolized. This causes a greatly decreased amount of free haptoglobin in the serum; this decrease cannot be quickly compensated for by normal liver production. As a result, the patient demonstrates a transient, reduced level of haptoglobin in the serum.

Haptoglobins are also decreased in patients with primary liver disease not associated with hemolytic anemias. This occurs because the diseased liver is unable to produce these glycoproteins. Hematoma can reduce haptoglobin levels by the absorption of hemoglobin into the blood and binding with haptoglobin.

Elevated haptoglobin concentrations are found in many inflammatory diseases and therefore can be used as a nonspecific "acute-phase" protein in much the same way as a sedimentation rate test (see p. 363). That is, levels of haptoglobin increase with severe infection, inflammation, tissue destruction, acute myocardial infarction, burns, and some cancers.

Interfering factors

- Ongoing infection can cause falsely elevated test results.
- ✠ Drugs that may cause *increased* haptoglobin levels include androgens and steroids.
- ✠ Drugs that may cause *decreased* levels include chlorpromazine, diphenhydramine, indomethacin, isoniazid, nitrofurantoin, oral contraceptives, quinidine, and streptomycin.

Procedure and patient care

Before
- Explain the procedure to the patient.
- Tell the patient that no fasting is required.

During
- Collect at least 2 ml of venous blood in a red-top tube.
- Avoid hemolysis, which may alter test results.

After
- Apply pressure or a pressure dressing to the venipuncture site.
- Assess the venipuncture site for bleeding.

Abnormal findings

▲ **Increased levels**
  Collagen disease
  Infection
  Tissue destruction
  Biliary obstruction
  Nephritis
  Pyelonephritis
  Ulcerative colitis
  Peptic ulcer
  Myocardial infarction
  Acute rheumatic disease
  Neoplasia

▼ **Decreased levels**
  Hemolytic anemia
  Transfusion reactions
  Prostatic heart valves
  Systemic lupus erythema-
    tosus
  Primary liver disease not
    associated with hemo-
    lytic anemia
  Erythroblastosis fetalis
  Hematoma
  Tissue hemorrhage
  Chronic liver disease

notes

***Helicobacter pylori* antibodies test** (*Campylobacter pylori*, Anti–*Helicobacter pylori* immunoglobulin G [IgG] antibody, *Campylobacter*-like organism [CLO] test)

Type of test   Blood, microscopic examination of antral or duodenal biopsy specimen, breath test

Normal findings   Not present

Test explanation and related physiology

Helicobacter pylori, a bacteria that can be found in the mucus covering the gastric mucosa, has been recognized as a risk factor for gastric diseases, such as duodenal ulcers or chronic gastritis. This bacillus may also be a possible cause of gastric carcinoma. Gastric colonization by this organism has been reported in about 90% to 95% of patients with a duodenal ulcer, in 60% to 70% of patients with a gastric ulcer, and in about 20% to 25% of patients with gastric cancer.

Approximately 10% of healthy persons under age 30 have gastric colonization with *H. pylori*. Gastric colonization increases with age, with people over 60 having rates similar to their ages. Most patients with gastric colonization by *H. pylori* remain asymptomatic and never develop ulceration.

Interfering factors

- *H. pylori* can be transmitted by endoscopy procedures.

Procedure and patient care

Before

- Explain the procedure to the patient.
- Tell the patient that no fasting is required for the blood test.
- If a biopsy or culture will be obtained by endoscopy, see discussion of esophagogastroduodenoscopy (EGD) (p. 369).

During

- Collect a venous blood sample according to the protocol of the laboratory performing the test.
- A gastric or duodenal biopsy can be obtained by endoscopy. Keep the specimen moist by the addition of approximately 5 ml of sterile saline.
- The *breath test* depends on the ability of *H. pylori* to break down urea into carbon dioxide and ammonia via its enzyme, urease. For this method of testing, a dose of radioactive ^{14}C

or nonradioactive ^{13}C urea is given by mouth. The isotopic CO_2 concentration is determined by breath collection.

After

- Apply pressure or a pressure dressing to the venipuncture site.
- Assess the venipuncture site for bleeding.
- If endoscopy was used to obtain a culture, see procedure for EGD (p. 369). The specimen should be transported to the laboratory within 30 minutes after collection.

Abnormal findings

▲   **Increased levels**

Acute and chronic gastri- Gastric ulcer
  tis Gastric carcinoma
Duodenal ulcer

notes

hematocrit (Hct, Packed red blood cell volume, Packed cell volume [PCV])

Type of test Blood

Normal findings

Male: 42% to 52% or 0.42-0.52 volume fraction (SI units)
Female: 37% to 47% or 0.37-0.47 volume fraction (SI units)
   (pregnancy: >33%)
Elderly: values may be slightly decreased
Child: 31% to 43%
Infant: 30% to 40%
Newborn: 44% to 64%

Possible critical values <15%

Test explanation and related physiology

The Hct is a measure of the percentage of red blood cells (RBCs) in the total blood volume. It is routinely performed as part of a complete blood count (CBC). Therefore the Hct closely reflects the hemoglobin (Hgb) and RBC values. The Hct in percentage points usually is approximately three times the Hgb concentration in grams per deciliter when RBCs are of normal size and contain normal amounts of Hgb. Normal values also vary according to gender and age. Abnormal values indicate the same pathologic states as abnormal RBC counts and Hgb concentrations (see pp. 694 and 454).

Interfering factors

- Abnormalities in RBC size may alter Hct values.
- Extremely elevated white blood cell counts may affect values.
- Hemodilution and dehydration may affect the Hct level.
- Pregnancy usually causes slightly decreased values because of hemodilution.
- Living in high altitudes causes increased values.
- Values may not be reliable immediately after hemorrhage.
- ✴ Drugs that may cause *decreased* levels include chloramphenicol and penicillin.

Procedure and patient care

Before

- Explain the procedure to the patient.
- Tell the patient that no fasting is required.

During
- Collect approximately 5 to 7 ml of venous blood in a lavender-top tube; however, only 0.5 ml is required when using capillary tubes.
- Avoid hemolysis.

After
- Apply pressure or a pressure dressing to the venipuncture site.
- Assess the venipuncture site for bleeding.

Abnormal findings

▲ **Increased levels**
Congenital heart disease
Polycythemia vera
Severe dehydration
Shock
Erythrocytosis
Severe diarrhea
Eclampsia
Trauma
Surgery
Burns
Dehydration

▼ **Decreased levels**
Anemia
Hyperthyroidism
Cirrhosis
Hemolytic reaction
Hemorrhage
Dietary deficiency
Bone marrow failure
Hodgkin's disease
Organ failure
Normal pregnancy
Rheumatoid arthritis
Multiple myeloma
Malnutrition
Leukemia

notes

hemoglobin (Hb, Hgb)

Type of test Blood

Normal findings
Male: 14-18 g/dl or 8.7-11.2 mmol/L (SI units)
Female: 12-16 g/dl or 7.4-9.9 mmol/L
    (pregnancy: >11 g/dl)
Elderly: values are slightly decreased
Child: 11-16 g/dl
Infant: 10-15 g/dl
Newborn: 14-24 g/dl

Possible critical values <5.0 g/dl

Test explanation and related physiology

The Hgb concentration is a measure of the total amount of Hgb in the peripheral blood. The test is normally performed as part of a complete blood count (CBC). Hgb serves as a vehicle for oxygen and carbon dioxide transport. As with the red blood cell (RBC) count, normal values vary according to gender and age. The clinical implications of this test closely parallel those of the RBC count (see p. 694). In addition, however, changes in plasma volume are more accurately reflected by the Hgb concentration. Dilutional overhydration decreases the concentration, whereas dehydration tends to cause an artificially high value. Slight decreases in the values of Hgb and the hematocrit during pregnancy reflect the expanded blood volume; the number of cells is actually increased during pregnancy.

Interfering factors

- Slight Hgb decreases normally occur during pregnancy because of the expanded blood volume.
- Living in high-altitude areas causes high Hgb values.
- ✔ Drugs that may cause *increased* levels include gentamicin and methyldopa (Aldomet).
- ✔ Drugs that may cause *decreased* levels include antibiotics, antineoplastic drugs, aspirin, indomethacin (Indocin), rifampin, and sulfonamides.

Procedure and patient care

Before

- Explain the procedure to the patient.
- Tell the patient that no fasting is required.

During

- Collect approximately 5 to 7 ml of venous blood in a lavender-top tube.
- Avoid hemolysis.
- List on the laboratory slip any drugs that may affect test results.

After

- Apply pressure or a pressure dressing to the venipuncture site.
- Observe the venipuncture site for bleeding.

Abnormal findings

▲   **Increased levels**

Congenital heart disease
Polycythemia vera
Hemoconcentration of the blood
Chronic obstructive pulmonary disease
Congestive heart failure
High altitudes
Severe burns
Dehydration

▼   **Decreased levels**

Anemia
Severe hemorrhage
Hemolysis
Hodgkin's disease
Hemoglobinopathies
Cancer
Nutritional deficiency
Lymphoma
Systemic lupus erythematosus
Sarcoidosis
Kidney disease
Chronic hemorrhage
Splenomegaly
Sickle cell anemia

notes

hemoglobin electrophoresis (Hgb electrophoresis)

Type of test Blood

Normal findings

Adult/elderly

Hgb A_1: 95% to 98%
Hgb A_2: 2% to 3%
Hgb F: 0.8% to 2%
Hgb S: 0%
Hgb C: 0%

Children: Hgb F

Newborn: 50% to 80%
6 months: 8%
>6 months: 1% to 2%

Test explanation and related physiology

Hgb electrophoresis is a test that enables abnormal forms of Hgb (hemoglobinopathies) to be detected. Although many different Hgb variations have been described, the more common types are A_1, A_2, F, S, and C. Each major Hgb type is electrically charged to varying degrees. When placed in an electromagnetic field, the Hgb variants migrate at different rates and therefore spread apart from each other; each band can be quantitated as a percentage of the total Hgb.

The form Hgb A_1 constitutes the major component of Hgb in the normal red blood cell (RBC). Hgb A_2 is only a minor component (2% to 3%) of the normal Hgb total. Hgb F is the major Hgb in the fetus but exists in only minimal quantities in the normal adult. Levels of Hgb F greater than 2% in patients over 3 years of age are considered abnormal. Hgb F is able to transport oxygen when only small amounts of oxygen are available (as in fetal life). In patients requiring compensation for prolonged chronic hypoxia (as in congenital cardiac abnormalities), Hgb F may be found in increased levels to assist in the transport of the available oxygen.

Hgb S is an abnormal form of Hgb associated with sickle cell anemia, which occurs predominantly in American blacks. Hgb S is a relatively insoluble variant. When little oxygen is available, it assumes a crescent (sickle) shape that greatly distorts the RBC morphology. Vascular sludging is a consequence of the localized sickling and may lead to organ infarction.

The Hgb C variant is another that exists in American blacks. RBCs containing Hgb C have a decreased life span and are more readily lysed than normal RBCs. Mild to severe hemolytic anemia may result.

The Hgb contents of the common hemoglobinopathies, as determined by electrophoresis, are as follows:

Sickle cell disease (homozygous SS)
Hgb S: 80% to 100%
Hgb A_1: 0%
Hgb A_2: 2% to 3%
Hgb F: <2%

Sickle cell trait (heterozygous SA)
Hgb S: 20% to 40%
Hgb A_1: 60% to 80%
Hgb A_2: 2% to 3%
Hgb F: 2%

Hemoglobin C disease (homozygous)
Hgb C: 90% to 100%
Hgb A_1: 0%
Hgb A_2: 2% to 3%
Hgb F: 2%

Hemoglobin H disease
Hgb A_1: 65% to 90%
Hgb A_2: 2% to 3%
Hgb H: 5% to 30%

Thalassemia major (homozygous)
Hgb A_1: 5% to 20%
Hgb A_2: 2% to 3%
Hgb F: 65% to 100%

Thalassemia minor (heterozygous)
Hgb A_1: 50% to 85%
Hgb A_2: 4% to 6%
Hgb F: 1% to 3%

Interfering factor

- Blood transfusions within the previous 12 weeks may alter test results.

Procedure and patient care

Before

- Explain the procedure to the patient.
- Tell the patient that no fasting is required.

During

- Collect approximately 7 ml of venous blood in a lavender-top tube.

After

- Apply pressure or a pressure dressing to the venipuncture site.
- Assess the venipuncture site for bleeding.

Abnormal findings

Sickle cell disease   Hemoglobin H disease
Sickle cell trait   Thalassemia major
Hemoglobin C disease   Thalassemia minor

notes

hepatitis virus studies (Hepatitis-associated antigen [HAA], Australian antigen)

Type of test Blood

Normal findings Negative

Test explanation and related physiology

Hepatitis is an inflammation of the liver caused by a virus. Three common viruses are now recognized to cause this disease: hepatitis A, hepatitis B, and hepatitis non-A, non-B (also called hepatitis C virus).

Hepatitis A virus (HAV) was originally called *infectious hepatitis*. It has a short incubation period of 2 to 6 weeks. HAV is excreted in the stool and transmitted via the oral-fecal route. Although tests are not yet available to detect HAV antigen, two types of antibodies to HAV can be detected.

The first type of antibody to HAV is immunoglobulin (Ig) M antibody (HAV-Ab/IgM), which appears approximately 3 to 4 weeks after exposure or just before hepatocellular enzyme elevations occur. These IgM levels usually return to normal in approximately 8 weeks.

The second type of antibody is IgG (HAV-Ab/IgG), which appears approximately 2 weeks after the beginning of the IgM increase and slowly returns to normal levels. The IgG enzyme can remain detectable for more than 10 years after the infection. If the IgM antibody is elevated in the absence of the IgG antibody, acute hepatitis is suspected. If, however, IgG is elevated in the absence of IgM elevation, this indicates the convalescent or chronic stage of HAV viral infection.

Hepatitis B virus (HBV) is commonly known as *serum hepatitis*. It has a long incubation period of 5 weeks to 6 months. HBV is most frequently transmitted by blood transfusion; however, it also can be contracted via exposure to other body fluids. HBV may cause a severe and unrelenting form of hepatitis ending in liver failure and death. Its incidence is increased among blood transfusion recipients, male homosexuals, dialysis patients, transplant patients, IV drug abusers, and patients with leukemia or lymphoma.

The HBV, also called the *Dane particle,* is made up of an inner core surrounded by an outer capsule. The outer capsule contains the hepatitis B surface antigen (HBsAg), formerly called

H

Australian antigen. The inner core contains HBV core antigen (HBcAg). The hepatitis B e-antigen (HBeAg) is also found within the core. Antibodies to these antigens are called *HBsAb, HBcAb,* and *HBeAb.* The tests used to detect these antigens and antibodies are as follows (Table 11):

1. *Hepatitis B surface antigen* (HBsAg). This is the most frequently and easily performed test for hepatitis B, and this is the first test to become abnormal. HBsAg rises before the onset of clinical symptoms, peaks during the first week of symptoms, and returns to normal by the time jaundice subsides. HBsAg generally indicates active infection by HBV. If the level of this antigen persists in the blood, the patient is considered to be a carrier.

2. *Hepatitis B surface antibody* (HBsAb). This antibody appears approximately 4 weeks after the disappearance of the surface antigen and signifies the end of the acute infection phase. HBsAb also signifies immunity to subsequent infection. Concentrated forms of this agent constitute the hyperimmunoglobulin given to patients who have come in contact with HBV-infected patients (e.g., contact by an inadvertent needle prick from a needle previously used on a patient with HBV infection). HBsAb is the antibody that denotes immunity after administration of hepatitis B vaccine.

TABLE 11 Hepatitis testing

Hepatitis test	Appears/disappears	Clinical significance
HBsAg	2-6 weeks/1-3 months	Active infection, carrier state
HBsAb	2-6 weeks/life	Convalescent, denotes immunity to HBV
HBcAb	2 weeks/3-6 months	Past infection, chronic hepatitis
HBeAg	3-5 days/2-4 weeks	Acute infection, denotes infectivity
HBeAb	1-4 weeks/4-6 years	Convalescent, denotes decreased infectivity

3. *Hepatitis B core antigen* (HBcAg). No tests are currently available to detect this antigen.

4. *Hepatitis B core antibody* (HBcAb). This antibody appears approximately 1 month after infection with HBsAg and declines (although remains elevated) over several years. HBcAb is also present in patients with chronic hepatitis. The HBcAb level is elevated during the time lag between the disappearance of HBsAg and the appearance of HBsAb. This interval is called the *core window*. During the core window, HBcAb is the only detectable marker of a recent hepatitis infection.

5. *Hepatitis B e-antigen* (HBeAg). This antigen is generally not used for diagnostic purposes but rather as an index of infectivity. The presence of HBeAg correlates with early and active disease, as well as with high infectivity in acute HBV infection. The persistent presence of HBeAg in the blood predicts the development of chronic HBV infection.

6. *Hepatitis B e-antibody* (HBeAb). This antibody indicates that an acute phase of HBV infection is over, or almost over, and that the chance of infectivity is greatly reduced.

Non-A, non-B hepatitis, also called *hepatitis C,* is transmitted in a manner similar to HBV. The incubation period is 2 to 12 weeks after exposure. The clinical manifestations of the illness parallel HBV. Most patients with hepatitis caused by blood transfusion have the non-A, non-B type. A hepatitis non-A, non-B viral titer to detect HCV IgG antibodies is now available to detect these infections; however, no vaccine protection exists against this form of hepatitis.

Procedure and patient care

Before
- Explain the procedure to the patient.
- Tell the patient that no fasting is required.

During
- Collect approximately 5 to 7 ml of venous blood in a red-top tube.
- Note that most of the testing for hepatitis is done by radioimmunoassay. Usually, a hepatitis profile that includes several HBV antigens and antibodies is performed.

After

- Apply pressure or a pressure dressing to the venipuncture site.
- Assess the venipuncture site for bleeding.
- Handle the specimen as if it were capable of transmitting hepatitis.
- Immediately discard the needle in the appropriate receptacle.
- Send the specimen promptly to the laboratory.

Abnormal findings

▲ **Increased levels**

Hepatitis A
Hepatitis B
Non-A, non-B hepatitis

Chronic carrier state, hepatitis B
Chronic hepatitis B

notes

herpes genitalis (Herpesvirus type 2, Herpes simplex virus type 2 [HSV 2])

Type of test Microscopic examination

Normal findings No virus present

Test explanation and related physiology

Herpes simplex virus can be classified as either type 1 or type 2. Type 1 is primarily responsible for oral lesions; HSV 2 is a sexually transmitted viral infection of the urogenital tract. Vesicular lesions may occur on the penis, scrotum, vulva, perineum, perianal region, vagina, or cervix. Because most infants become infected if they pass through a birth canal containing HSV, determining its presence at delivery is necessary. Congenital infections may result in problems such as microcephaly, chorioretinitis, and mental retardation in the newborn. Disseminated neonatal herpesvirus infections carry a high incidence of infant mortality. A vaginal delivery is possible if no virus is present, and birth by cesarean section is needed if HSV is present. Viral testing can be performed on males or females to determine the risk of sexual transmission.

Culture is still the gold standard for HSV detection. Blood tests are available for detection of HSV 1 and HSV 2 antigen. Unfortunately, the accuracy is not high enough to be used routinely. Their advantage is that results can be available in a day. Serologic tests for antibodies at present are cumbersome because they require repeated blood tests during the acute and convalescent phases of the acute episode.

Procedure and patient care

Before
- Explain the procedure to the patient.
- Tell the female patient to refrain from douching and tub bathing before the cervical culture is performed.
- Obtain the urethral specimen from the male patient before voiding.

During
- Obtain cultures as follows:

Urethral culture
1. A culture is taken by inserting a sterile swab gently into the anterior urethra or genital skin lesion of the male patient.

2. It is advisable to place the male patient in the supine position to prevent falling if vasovagal syncope occurs during introduction of the cotton swab or wire loop into the urethra.

3. The patient is observed for hypotension, bradycardia, pallor, sweating, nausea, and weakness.

Cervical culture

1. The female patient is placed in the lithotomy position, and a vaginal speculum is inserted.

2. Cervical mucus is removed with a cotton ball.

3. A sterile cotton-tipped swab is inserted into the endocervical canal and moved from side to side to obtain the culture. If a genital lesion is present, swabs from that area will be more sensitive in indicating infection.

- For pregnant women with herpes genitalis, note that the cervix is cultured weekly for the herpesvirus beginning 4 to 6 weeks before the due date. Vaginal delivery is possible if the following criteria are met:

1. The two most recent cultures are negative.

2. The woman is not experiencing any symptoms.

3. No lesions are visible on inspection of the vagina and vulva.

4. Throughout pregnancy, the woman has not had more than one positive culture, during which she was symptom free.

After

- Inform the patient how to obtain the test results.

Abnormal finding

Herpesvirus infection

notes

HLA-B27 antigen (Human lymphocyte antigen B27)

Type of test Blood

Normal findings Negative

Test explanation and related physiology

The HLA antigens are the major histocompatibility (tissue compatibility) antigens important in tissue recognition. These antigens are under direct genetic control and share a locus on the chromosome. Many HLA antigens exist, but HLA-B27 has the most clinical relevance. This antigen is often found in patients with ankylosing spondylitis and Reiter's syndrome. HLA-B27 is used to detect and confirm these diagnoses. HLA-B27 is found in 5% to 7% of normal patients, but approximately 80% to 90% of patients with ankylosing spondylitis or Reiter's syndrome have HLA-B27.

For this test, lymphocytes from the patient are extracted and incubated with anti-HLA-B27 cytotoxic antibody. If the patient has HLA-B27 antigen, a complex will be formed on the cell surface. Serum complement is then added to the mixture, killing the lymphocyte and recognizing the titer of HLA-B27.

Procedure and patient care

Before
- Explain the procedure to the patient.
- Tell the patient that no fasting or special preparation is required.

During
- Collect at least 10 ml of venous blood in a heparinized solution.

After
- Apply pressure or a pressure dressing to the venipuncture site.
- Assess the venipuncture site for bleeding.

Abnormal findings

▲ Increased levels
Ankylosing spondylitis
Reiter's syndrome

Holter monitoring (Ambulatory monitoring, Ambulatory electrocardiography, Event recorder)

Type of test Electrodiagnostic

Normal findings Normal sinus rhythm

Test explanation and related physiology

Holter monitoring is a continuous recording of the electrical activity of the heart. This can be performed for periods up to 48 hours. With this technique, an electrocardiogram (EKG) is recorded continuously on magnetic tape during unrestricted activity, rest, and sleep. The Holter monitor is equipped with a clock that permits accurate time monitoring on the EKG tape. The patient is asked to carry a diary and record daily activities, as well as any cardiac symptoms that may develop during the period of monitoring.

Most units in present use are equipped with an "event marker." This is a button the patient can push when symptoms such as chest pain, syncope, or palpitations are experienced. This type of monitor is referred to as an *event recorder*. Many recorders store the rhythm immediately preceding activation of the recorder. Stored information can be transmitted by telephone to a recording station.

The Holter monitor is used primarily to identify suspected cardiac rhythm disturbances and to correlate these disturbances with symptoms such as dizziness, syncope, palpitations, or chest pain. The monitor is also used to assess pacemaker function and the effectiveness of antiarrhythmic medications.

After completion of the determined time period, usually 24 to 72 hours, the Holter monitor is removed from the patient and the record tape is played back at high speeds. The EKG tracing is usually interpreted by computer, which can detect any significant abnormality that occurred during the testing. A report then can be generated as to the frequency and severity of abnormal cardiac events, especially in relation to the patient's symptoms.

Contraindications

- Patients who are unable to cooperate with maintaining the lead placement from the monitor to the body
- Patients who are unable to maintain an accurate diary of significant activities or events

Interfering factor
- Interruption in the electrode contact with the skin

Procedure and patient care

Before
- Explain the procedure to the patient.
- Instruct the patient about care of the Holter monitor.
- Inform the patient about the necessity of ensuring good contact between the electrodes and the skin.
- Teach the patient how to maintain an accurate diary. Stress the need to record significant symptoms.
- Instruct the patient to note in the diary if any interruption in Holter monitoring occurs.
- Assure the patient that the electrical flow is coming *from* the patient and that he or she will not experience any electrical stimulation from the machine.
- Instruct the patient not to bathe during the period of cardiac monitoring.
- Tell the patient to minimize the use of electrical devices (e.g., electric toothbrushes, shavers), which may cause artificial changes in the EKG tracing.

During
- Prepare the sites for electrode placement with alcohol. (This is usually done in the cardiology department by a technologist.)
- Securely place the gel and electrodes at the appropriate sites. Usually, the chest and abdomen are the most appropriate locations for limb-lead electrode placement. The precordial leads also may be placed.
- Usually, do not use the extremities for electrode placement to minimize alterations in tracing that occur with normal physical activity.
- Encourage the patient to call if he or she has any difficulties.

After
- Gently remove the tape and other paraphernalia securing the electrodes.
- Wipe the patient clean of electrode gel.
- Inform the patient that the Holter monitoring interpretation will be available in a few days.

Abnormal finding
Cardiac arrhythmia (dysrhythmia)

human T-cell lymphotrophic (HTLV) I/II antibody

Type of test Blood

Normal findings Negative

Test explanation and related physiology

Several forms of HTLV, a human retrovirus, affect humans. HTLV-I is associated with adult T-cell leukemia. HTLV-II is associated with adult hairy-cell leukemia. Humans can be infected with these viruses, however, and not develop any malignancy. The human immunodeficiency viruses (HIVs), which are known to be the cause of acquired immunodeficiency syndrome (AIDS), are also retroviruses; however, HTLV infection is not associated with AIDS. HTLV transmission is similar, however, to HIV transmission (e.g., body fluid contamination, intravenous drug use, sexual contact, and so on).

Also, HTLV-I has been associated with neurologic disorders such as tropical spastic paraparesis. Again, positive serum values of this antibody are not necessarily associated with disease.

Procedure and patient care

Before
- Explain the procedure to the patient.
- Tell the patient that no fasting is required.

During
- Collect approximately 7 ml of venous blood in a red-top tube.

After
- Apply pressure or a pressure dressing to the venipuncture site.
- Assess the venipuncture site for bleeding.

Abnormal findings

Acute HTLV infection
Adult T-cell leukemia

Hairy-cell leukemia
Tropical spastic paraparesis

notes

17-hydroxycorticosteroids (17-OCHS)

Type of test Urine (24-hour)

Normal findings

Male

<8 years: <1.5 mg/24 hr
<12 years: <4.5 mg/24 hr
Adult: 4.5-10.0 mg/24 hr
Elderly: values lower than for adult

Female

<8 years: <1.5 mg/24 hr
<12 years: <4.5 mg/24 hr
Adult: 2.5-10.0 mg/24 hr
Elderly: values lower than for adult

H

Test explanation and related physiology

This urine study is used to assess adrenocortical function by measuring the cortisol metabolites (17-OCHS) in a 24-hour urine collection. Because the excretion of cortisol metabolites follows a diurnal variation, a 24-hour collection is necessary. Elevated levels of 17-OCHS are seen in patients with hyperfunctioning of the adrenal gland (Cushing's syndrome) whether this condition is caused by a pituitary or adrenal tumor, bilateral adrenal hyperplasia, or ectopic tumors producing adrenocorticotropic hormone (ACTH). Low levels of 17-OCHS are seen in patients who have a hypofunctioning adrenal gland (Addison's disease) as a result of destruction of the adrenals (by hemorrhage, infarction, metastatic tumor, or autoimmunity), surgical removal of an adrenal gland without appropriate steroid replacement, congenital enzyme deficiency, hypopituitarism, or adrenal suppression after prolonged exogenous steroid ingestion.

Testing the urine for this hormone metabolite is only an indirect measure of adrenal function. Urine and plasma levels of cortisol (see pp. 287 and 285) provide a much more accurate measurement of adrenal function.

Interfering factors

- Emotional and physical stress (e.g., infection) and licorice ingestion may cause increased adrenal activity.
- Drugs that may cause *increased* 17-OCHS levels include ac-

etazolamide, chloral hydrate, chlorpromazine, colchicine, erythromycin, meprobamate, paraldehyde, quinidine, quinine, and spironolactone.

▪ Drugs that may cause *decreased* levels include estrogens, oral contraceptives, phenothiazines, and reserpine.

Procedure and patient care

Before

- Explain the procedure to the patient.
- Note that drugs are usually withheld several days before the urine collection. Check with the physician and laboratory for specific guidelines.
- Assess the patient for signs of stress and report these to the physician.

During

- Do not administer to the patient any drugs that may interfere with test results.
- Begin the 24-hour urine collection after the patient urinates. Discard this urine and note this as the start time of the test.
- Collect all urine passed by the patient during the next 24 hours.
- Post the hours for the urine collection in a prominent spot.
- Note that it is not necessary to measure each urine specimen.
- Tell the patient to void before defecating so that the urine is not contaminated by feces.
- Inform the patient that toilet paper should not be placed in the collection container.
- Encourage the patient to drink fluids during the 24 hours, unless this is contraindicated for medical purposes.
- Collect the last specimen as close as possible to the end of the 24-hour collection. Add this to the container.
- Keep the urine specimen refrigerated or on ice during the entire collection.

After

- Send the urine to the chemistry laboratory as soon as the test is completed.
- List on the laboratory slip any medications the patient may be taking that can affect test results.

Abnormal findings

▲ **Increased levels**

Cushing's syndrome
Pituitary tumor
Adrenal tumor
Bilateral adrenal hyperplasia
Ectopic adrenocorticotropic hormone–producing tumor
Acromegaly
Thyrotoxicosis
Severe hypertension
Stress

▼ **Decreased levels**

Addison's disease
Adrenal infarction
Adrenal hemorrhage
Surgical removal of the adrenals
Congenital enzyme deficiency
Adrenal suppression from steroid therapy
Hypopituitarism
Hypothyroidism
Adrenogenital syndrome

notes

H

5-hydroxyindoleacetic acid (5-HIAA)

Type of test Urine (24-hour)

Normal findings

2-6 mg/24 hr or 10.4-31.2 μmol/day (SI units)
Female levels lower than male levels

Test explanation and related physiology

Quantitative analysis of urine levels of 5-HIAA is used to detect and to follow the clinical course of patients with carcinoid
tumors. Carcinoid tumors are serotonin-secreting tumors that
may grow in the appendix, intestine, lung, or any tissue derived
from the neuroectoderm. These tumors contain *argentaffin-
staining (enteroendocrine) cells*, which produce serotonin and
other powerful neurohormones that are metabolized by the liver
to 5-HIAA and excreted in the urine. These powerful neurohormones are responsible for the clinical presentation of carcinoid
syndrome (bronchospasm, flushing, diarrhea). This test is used
not only to identify patients with carcinoid tumor but also to
reevaluate those with known tumor by using serial levels of urinary 5-HIAA. Rising levels of 5-HIAA indicate progression of
tumor; falling levels of 5-HIAA indicate a therapeutic response
of the tumor to antineoplastic therapy.

Interfering factors

- Bananas, plantain, pineapple, kiwi fruit, walnuts, plums, pe-
  cans, and avocados can factitiously elevate 5-HIAA levels.
- Drugs that may cause *increased* 5-HIAA levels include acet-
  anilid, acetophenetidin (phenacetin), glyceryl guaiacolate
  (guaifenesin [Robitussin]), methocarbamol, acetaminophen,
  and reserpine.
- Drugs that may cause *decreased* levels include chlorpromazine, ethyl alcohol, heparin, imipramine (Tofranil), isoniazid
  (INH), levodopa, MAO inhibitors, methenamine, methyldopa (Aldomet), phenothiazines, promethazine (Phenergan),
  aspirin, and tricyclic antidepressants.

Procedure and patient care

Before

- Explain the procedure to the patient.
- Instruct the patient to refrain from eating foods containing

serotonin (e.g., plums, pineapples, bananas, eggplant, tomatoes, avocados, walnuts) for several days (usually 3) before and during testing.

During

- To begin the 24-hour urine collection, discard the patient's initial specimen and start the timing at that point.
- Collect all urine passed during the next 24 hours.
- Show the patient where to store the urine specimen.
- Keep the specimen on ice or in a refrigerator during the 24-hour collection. A preservative is needed to keep the specimen at an appropriate pH.
- Post the hours for urine collection in a noticeable place to prevent accidental discarding of the specimen.
- Instruct the patient to void before defecating so that urine is not contaminated by stool.
- Tell the patient not to put toilet paper in the urine container.
- Collect the last specimen as close as possible to the end of the 24-hour collection. Add this urine to the container.

After

- Send the urine specimen to the laboratory promptly.
- List on the laboratory slip any medications that may affect the test results.

Abnormal finding

▲   **Increased levels**
    Carcinoid tumor

notes

hysterosalpingography (Uterotubography, Uterosalingography, Hysterogram)

Type of test X-ray with contrast dye

Normal findings
Patent fallopian tubes
No defects in uterine cavity

Test explanation and related physiology

In hysterosalpingography, the uterine cavity and fallopian tubes are visualized radiographically after the injection of contrast material through the cervix. Uterine tumors, intrauterine adhesions, and developmental anomalies can be seen. Tubal obstruction caused by internal scarring, tumor, or kinking also can be detected. A possible therapeutic effect of this test is that passage of dye through the tubes may clear mucous plugs, straighten kinked tubes, or break up adhesions. This test also may be used to document adequacy of surgical tubal ligation.

Contraindications

- Patients with infections of the vagina, cervix, or fallopian tubes, because there is risk of extending the infection
- Patients with uterine bleeding, because contrast material may enter the open blood vessels
- Patients with suspected pregnancy, because contrast material might induce abortion

Potential complications

- Infection of the endometrium (endometritis)
- Infection of the fallopian tubes (salpingitis)
- Uterine perforation
- Allergic reaction to iodinated dye or shellfish
  This rarely occurs, because the dye is not administered intravenously.

Interfering factors

- Fecal material or gas in the bowel may obscure visualization.
- Tubal spasm or excessive traction may cause the appearance of a stricture in normal fallopian tubes.
- Excessive traction may displace adhesions, making tubes appear normal.

Procedure and patient care

Before

- Explain the procedure to the patient. Ask the patient when she had her last menstrual period. If pregnancy is suspected, the test is not performed.
- Obtain informed consent if required by the institution.
- Assess the patient for allergy to iodine dye or shellfish. Report positive findings to the radiologist. (Allergic reactions in this study are rare, because the dye is not administered intravenously.)
- Instruct the patient to take laxatives the night before the test, if ordered.
- Administer enemas or suppositories on the morning of the test, if ordered.
- Administer sedatives (e.g., diazepam [Valium]) or antispasmodics, if ordered, before the test.
- Tell the patient that no food or fluid restrictions are needed.

During

- Note the following procedural steps:
  1. A plain x-ray film of the abdomen is often taken before the test to ensure that the preparation adequately eliminated gastrointestinal gas or feces.
  2. After voiding, the patient is placed on the fluoroscopy table in the lithotomy position.
  3. A speculum is inserted into the vagina, and the cervix is visualized and cleansed.
  4. Contrast material is injected during fluoroscopy, and x-ray films are taken.
  5. More dye is injected so that the entire upper genital tract (uterus and tubes) can be filled.
  6. This test can be considered to be satisfactorily performed only if the uterus and the tubes are distended to their maximal capacity or fluid flows through the fallopian tubes.
- Note that this procedure is performed by a physician in approximately 15 to 30 minutes.
- Tell the patient that she may feel occasional, transient menstrual-type cramping and that she may have shoulder pain caused by subphrenic irritation from the dye as it leaks into the peritoneal cavity.

After

- Inform the patient that a vaginal discharge (sometimes bloody) may be present for 1 to 2 days after the test. A perineal pad should be worn.
- Evaluate the patient for delayed reaction to dye (dyspnea, rash, tachycardia, hives). If this occurs, treat with antihistamines or steroids.
- Inform the patient that cramping and dizziness may occur following this study.
- Evaluate the patient for signs and symptoms of infection (e.g., fever, increased pulse rate, pain). Instruct the patient to call her physician and report these symptoms if they occur.

Abnormal findings

Uterine tumor (e.g., leiomyoma, cancer)
Internal scarring
Kinking secondary to adhesions
Extrauterine pregnancy
Uterine fistula

Developmental anomaly (e.g., uterus bicornis)
Intrauterine adhesions
Tumor of the fallopian tubes
Fallopian tube occlusion

notes

hysteroscopy

Type of test Endoscopy

Normal findings Normal structure and function of the uterus

Test explanation and related physiology

Hysteroscopy is an endoscopic procedure that provides direct visualization of the uterine cavity by inserting a hysteroscope (a thin, telescope-like instrument) through the vagina and cervix and into the uterus. Hysteroscopy can be used to evaluate and diagnose many abnormalities of the uterus, such as abnormal uterine bleeding, infertility, repeated miscarriages, uterine adhesions (Asherman's syndrome), polyps, fibroids, and displaced intrauterine devices (IUDs).

In addition to diagnosing and evaluating uterine problems, hysteroscopy can also correct uterine problems. For example, uterine adhesions and small fibroids can be removed through the hysteroscope, thus avoiding open abdominal surgery. Hysteroscopy can also be used to perform endometrial ablation, which destroys the uterine lining in order to treat some cases of heavy uterine bleeding.

The hysteroscope can be used with many other instruments. For example, it may be done before a dilation and curettage (D&C) or concurrently with a laparoscopy. Hysteroscopy may also confirm the results of other tests, such as hysterosalpingography (see p. 474).

Contraindications

- Patients with pelvic inflammatory disease (PID)
- Patients with vaginal discharge

Potential complications

- Uterine perforation
- Infection

Procedure and patient care

Before

- Explain the procedure to the patient.
- Obtain informed consent for this procedure.
- Schedule the procedure after menstrual bleeding has ceased and before ovulation. This allows better visualization of the

inside of the uterus and avoids damage to a newly formed pregnancy.

- Inform the patient that hysteroscopy may be performed with local, regional, or general anesthesia. If general anesthesia will be given, the patient should be NPO for at least 8 hours before the test. This test may also be performed without anesthesia.
- Tell the patient to void before the procedure because a distended bladder can be more easily perforated.

During

- Note the following procedural steps:
  1. Hysteroscopy may be performed in the operating room or in the doctor's office. Local, regional, general, or no anesthesia may be used. (The type of anesthesia depends on other procedures that may be done at the same time.)
  2. The patient is placed in the lithotomy position. The vaginal area is cleansed with an antiseptic solution.
  3. The cervix may be dilated before this procedure.
  4. The hysteroscope is inserted through the vagina and cervix and into the uterus.
  5. A liquid or gas is released through the hysteroscope to expand the uterus for better visualization.
  6. If minor surgery will be performed, small instruments will be inserted through the hysteroscope.
  7. For more detailed or complicated procedures, a laparoscope may be used (see p. 506) to concurrently view the outside of the uterus.
  8. After the desired procedure is performed, the hysteroscope is removed.
- Note that hysteroscopy is performed by a physician in approximately 30 minutes.
- Inform the patient who will be having general or regional anesthesia that she will not experience any discomfort. Tell the patient receiving local anesthesia that she may feel some cramping during the procedure.

After

- Tell the patient that it is normal to have slight vaginal bleeding and cramps for a day or two after the procedure.
- Inform the patient that signs of fever, severe abdominal pain, or heavy vaginal discharge or bleeding should be reported to her physician.
- If the patient has any discomfort from the gas inserted dur-

ing the hysteroscopy or laparoscopy, assure her that this usually lasts less than 24 hours.

Abnormal findings

Uterine bleeding
Uterine fibroids
Asherman's syndrome
Septate uterus

Uterine polyps
Uterine cancer
Displaced IUD

notes

H

immunoglobulin electrophoresis (Gamma globulin electrophoresis)

Type of test   Blood

Normal findings

IgG: 565-1765 mg/dl
IgA: 85-385 mg/dl
IgM: 55-375 mg/dl
IgD and IgE: minimal

Test explanation and related physiology

Protein within the blood is made up of albumin and globulin. Several types of globulin exist, one of which is gamma globulin. Antibodies are made up of gamma globulin protein and are called *immunoglobulins*. There are many classes of immunoglobulins (antibodies). Immunoglobulin G (IgG) constitutes approximately 75% of the serum immunoglobulins; therefore it constitutes the majority of circulating blood antibodies. IgA constitutes approximately 15% of the immunoglobulins within the body and is present primarily in the secretions of the gastrointestinal tract, in saliva, and in tears. IgM is an immunoglobulin primarily responsible for ABO blood grouping and rheumatoid factor. IgE often mediates an allergic response and is measured to detect allergic diseases. IgD, which constitutes the smallest portion of the immunoglobulins, is rarely evaluated or detected.

Serum electrophoresis is used to detect diseases of hypersensitivity, immune deficiencies, autoimmune diseases, chronic infections, multiple myeloma, chronic viral infections, and intrauterine fetal infections. For this test, the serum is placed on a slide containing agar gel, and an electric current is passed through this gel. Immunoglobulins are separated out and electrophoresed according to the quantity and difference in electrical charge. Specific antisera are placed alongside the slide to identify the specific type of immunoglobulin present.

Interfering factors

☛ Drugs that may cause *increased* immunoglobulin levels include therapeutic gamma globulin, hydralazine, isoniazid (INH), phenytoin (Dilantin), procainamide, and tetanus toxoid and antitoxin.

Procedure and patient care

Before

- Explain the procedure to the patient.
- Tell the patient that no fasting or special preparation is required.

During

- Collect 7 to 10 ml of venous blood in a red-top tube.
- Indicate on the laboratory slip if the patient has received any vaccinations or immunizations within the past 6 months. Also, list any drugs that may affect test results.

After

- Apply pressure or a pressure dressing to the venipuncture site.
- Observe the venipuncture site for bleeding.

Abnormal findings

▲ **Increased IgG levels**
Chronic infection
Hyperimmunization
Severe malnutrition
Sarcoidosis
Rheumatic fever
Liver disease
IgG multiple myeloma
Rheumatoid arthritis

▲ **Increased IgE levels**
Allergy (e.g., hay fever, asthma, anaphylaxis)

▲ **Increased IgA levels**
Cirrhosis
Rheumatic fever
Inflammatory bowel disease
Alcoholism
Chronic infection
Carcinoma, especially involving the GI or hepatobiliary tract

▼ **Decreased IgG levels**
Agammaglobulinemia
Lymphoid hyperplasia
Amyloidosis
Congenital IgG deficiency
Preeclampsia
Leukemia

▼ **Decreased IgE levels**
Agammaglobulinemia

▼ **Decreased IgA levels**
Agammaglobulinemia
Malignancy
Use of lymphopenic drugs (e.g., chemotherapy, steroids)
Protein-losing gastroenteropathies (e.g., inflammatory bowel disease)

▲ **Increased IgM levels**
Macroglobulinemia
Rheumatoid arthritis
Brucellosis
Lymphosarcoma
Other autoimmune disease
Viral infection (e.g., infectious mononucleosis)
Malaria
Fungal infection

▼ **Decreased IgM levels**
Agammaglobulinemia
Lymphoid hyperplasia
Leukemia
Amyloidosis

notes

insulin antibody test (Anti-insulin antibody)

Type of test   Blood

Normal findings   No antibody detected for bovine or porcine insulin

Test explanation and related physiology

Insulin antibodies appear in nearly all patients with diabetes treated with exogenous (bovine or porcine) insulin. These antibodies develop from impurities in animal insulin. The most common type of anti-insulin antibody is immunoglobulin (Ig) G, but IgA, IgM, IgD, and IgE also have been reported. Most of these insulin antibodies do not cause clinical problems, but they may complicate most insulin assays (see p. 485). IgM may cause insulin resistance. Insulin allergy may result from IgE antibodies to insulin.

These insulin antibodies are also found in patients with factitious hypoglycemia from surreptitious administration of insulin. In these cases, C-peptide (see p. 289) studies may be indicated to determine whether hypoglycemia is caused by insulin abuse, because C-peptide is not found in commercial insulin preparations. Occasionally, the glucose tolerance of a patient with diabetes will deteriorate because of the development of anti-insulin antibodies. These antibodies neutralize the insulin, and greater doses may be required.

Interfering factor

- Radioactive scans within 7 days before the test may interfere with the test result.

Procedure and patient care

Before

- Explain the procedure to the patient.
- Tell the patient that no fasting is required.

During

- Collect a venous blood sample in a red-top tube.

After

- Apply pressure or a pressure dressing to the venipuncture site.
- Assess the venipuncture site for bleeding.

Abnormal findings

▲ **Increased levels**
Insulin resistance
Allergies to insulin
Factitious hypoglycemia

notes

insulin assay

Type of test Blood

Normal findings

5-24 µU/ml or 36-179 pmol/L (SI units)
Newborn: 3-20 µU/ml

Possible critical values >30 µU/ml

Test explanation and related physiology

The hormone insulin can be measured successfully by radio-immunoassay in most larger laboratories. Insulin regulates blood glucose levels by facilitating the movement of glucose out of the bloodstream and into the cells. Insulin secretion is primarily reactive to the blood glucose level. Normally, as the blood glucose level increases, the insulin level also increases; as the glucose level decreases, insulin release stops. This test is used to diagnose insulinoma and to evaluate abnormal lipid and carbohydrate metabolism.

Some investigators believe that measuring the ratio of the blood sugar and insulin levels on the same specimen obtained during the oral glucose tolerance test (GTT, see p. 433) is more reliable than measuring insulin levels alone. Compared with the oral GTT, the insulin assay can show characteristic curves in certain situations. For example, patients with juvenile diabetes have low fasting insulin and display flat GTT insulin curves because of little or no increase in insulin levels. Patients who are mildly diabetic have normal fasting insulin levels and display GTT curves with a delayed rise. Most patients being treated with insulin for diabetes develop anti-insulin antibodies (see p. 483) within a few months. These antibodies can interfere with insulin radioimmunoassay results by competing with the insulin antibodies used in the insulin assay. After the patient fasts 12 to 14 hours, the insulin/glucose ratio should be less than 0.3. Patients with insulinoma have ratios greater than this. To increase the sensitivity and specificity for insulinoma, Turner and others have proposed amended insulin/glucose ratios using variable mathematic "fudge" factors. The Turner amended ratio of over 50 suggests insulinoma.

Interfering factors

- Food intake and obesity may cause increased insulin levels.
- Recent administration of radioisotopes may affect test results.
- Drugs that may cause *increased* insulin levels include corticosteroids, levodopa, and oral contraceptives.

Procedure and patient care

Before

- Explain the procedure to the patient.
- Keep the patient NPO for 8 hours.

During

- Collect approximately 5 ml of venous blood in a red-top tube and pack it in ice.
- Avoid hemolysis.
- If the serum insulin level will be measured during the GTT, collect the blood sample before oral ingestion of the glucose load and often, at designated intervals, after glucose ingestion.

After

- Apply pressure or a pressure dressing to the venipuncture site.
- Observe the venipuncture site for bleeding.
- Transport the specimen immediately to the laboratory.

Abnormal findings

▲ **Increased levels**
Insulinoma
Cushing's syndrome
Acromegaly
Obesity

▼ **Decreased levels**
Diabetes

notes

intravenous pyelography (IVP, Excretory urography [EUG], Intravenous urography [IUG, IVU])

Type of test X-ray with contrast dye

Normal findings

Normal size, shape, and position of the kidneys, renal pelvis, ureters, and bladder

Normal kidney excretory function as evidenced by the length of time for passage of contrast material through the kidneys

Test explanation and related physiology

IVP is an x-ray study that uses radiopaque contrast material to visualize the kidneys, renal pelvis, ureters, and bladder. The dye is injected intravenously, filtered out at the kidney by the glomeruli, and then passed through the renal tubules. X-ray films taken at set intervals over the next 30 minutes will show passage of the dye material through the kidneys and ureters and into the bladder.

If the artery leading to one of the kidneys is blocked, the dye cannot enter that part of the renal system and that kidney or portion thereof will not be visualized. If the artery is partially blocked, the length of time required for the appearance of the contrast material will be prolonged.

With primary glomerular disease (e.g., glomerulonephritis), the glomerular filtrate is reduced, which causes a reduction in the quantity of dye filtered. Therefore it requires more time for enough dye to enter the kidney filtrate and allow for renal opacification. As a result, kidney visualization is delayed. This provides an estimate of renal function.

Defects in dye filling of the kidney can indicate renal tumors or cysts. Often, intrinsic tumors, stones, extrinsic tumors, and scarring can partially or completely obstruct the flow of dye through the collecting system (pelvis, ureters, bladder). If the obstruction has been of sufficient duration, the collecting system proximal to the obstruction will be dilated (hydronephrosis). Retroperitoneal and pelvic tumors, aneurysms, and enlarged lymph nodes also can produce extrinsic compression and distortions of the opacified collecting system.

IVP is also used to assess the effect of trauma on the urinary system. Renal hematomas distort the renal contour. Renal artery laceration is suggested by nonopacification of one kidney. Laceration of the kidneys, pelvis, ureters, or bladder often causes urine leaks, which are identified by dye extravasation from the urinary system.

IVP is also used to assess a patient for congenital absence or malposition of the kidneys. Horseshoe kidneys (connection of the two kidneys), double ureters, and pelvic kidneys are typical congenital abnormalities.

Nephrotomography provides radiographic visualization of the kidney using tomographic technique following the IV injection of a radiopaque dye. Tomography is a radiographic technique by which a sequence of x-ray films, each representing a visual "slice" through the organ, is taken. Tomography permits examination of a single layer or plane of the organ that would otherwise be obscured by the surrounding structures. Nephrotomography permits visualization of different planes of the kidney to differentiate solid renal and adrenal tumors from benign renal cysts.

Contraindications

- Patients who are allergic to shellfish or iodinated dyes and who have not received premedication with prednisone and diphenhydramine (Benadryl)
- Patients who are severely dehydrated, because this can cause renal shutdown and failure
  Geriatric patients are particularly vulnerable.
- Patients with renal insufficiency, as evidenced by a blood urea nitrogen (BUN) value greater than 40 mg/dl, because the iodinated nephrotoxic dye can worsen kidney function
- Patients with multiple myeloma, because the iodinated nephrotoxic dye can worsen renal function

Potential complications

- Allergic reaction to iodinated dye
  Allergic reactions vary from mild flushing, itching, and urticaria to severe, life-threatening anaphylaxis (evidenced by respiratory distress, drop in blood pressure, or shock). In the unusual event of anaphylaxis, the patient may be treated with diphenhydramine (Benadryl), steroids, and epinephrine. Oxygen and endotracheal equipment should be on hand for immediate use.
- Infiltration of contrast dye
  This is avoided by ensuring the patency of the IV line. In the event of infiltration, a local injection of hyaluronidase

may be given to hasten the absorption of iodine and the resolution of the reaction.
- Renal failure
  This occurs most often in elderly patients who are chronically dehydrated before the dye injection.

Interfering factors

- Fecal material, gas, or barium in the bowel may obscure visualization of the renal system.
- Abnormal renal function studies may prevent adequate visualization of the urinary tract.
- Retained barium from previous studies may obscure visualization. Studies using barium (e.g., barium enema) should be scheduled *after* an IVP.

Procedure and patient care

Before
- Explain the procedure to the patient. Inform the patient that several x-ray films will be taken over 30 minutes.
- Obtain informed consent if required by the institution.
- Check the patient for allergies to iodinated dye and shellfish.
- Inform the radiologist if an allergy to iodine is suspected. The radiologist may prescribe a Benadryl-and-steroid preparation to be administered before the test. Usually, a hypoallergenic, nonionic contrast will be used during the test.
- Give the patient a laxative (e.g., castor oil) or a cathartic, as ordered, the evening before the test.
- Inform the patient of the required food and fluid restrictions. Some institutions prefer abstinence from solid foods for 8 hours before testing. Some allow a clear-liquid breakfast on the test day.
- Ensure adequate hydration for the patient (IV or oral) before and after the test to avoid dye-induced renal failure.
- Note that pediatric patients will have decreased fasting times, as ordered on an individual basis.
- Note that elderly and debilitated patients should have fasting times indicated specifically for them.
- Note that patients receiving high rates of IV fluids may have infusion rates decreased for several hours before the study to increase the concentration of the dye within the urinary system.
- Assess the patient's BUN and creatinine levels. Abnormal

renal function could deteriorate as a result of the dye injection.

- Schedule any barium studies *after* completion of the IVP.
- Give the patient an enema or suppository on the morning of the study, if ordered.

During

- Note the following procedural steps:
  1. The patient is taken to the radiology department and placed in the supine position.
  2. A plain film of the abdomen (KUB) is taken to ensure that no residual stool obscures visualization of the renal system. This also screens for calculi in the renal collecting system.
  3. Skin testing for iodine allergy is often done.
  4. A peripheral IV line is started (if not in place), and a contrast dye (e.g., Hypaque, Renografin) is given.
  5. X-ray films are taken at specific times, usually at 1, 5, 10, 15, 20, and 30 minutes, and sometimes longer, to follow the course of the dye from the cortex of the kidney to the bladder.
  6. Tomography may be performed to identify a mass.
  7. The patient is taken to the bathroom and asked to void.
  8. A postvoiding film is taken to visualize the empty bladder.
- Note that occasionally it is necessary to partially occlude the ureters temporarily to obtain a better film of the collecting system in the upper part of the ureters. This is done by compressing the abdomen with an inflatable rubber tube, which is wrapped tightly around the abdomen slightly below the umbilicus.
- For *nephrotomography,* note that the x-ray tube and film cassette are rapidly moved in opposite directions while the x-ray film is taken. This technique effectively blurs all tissue planes except that plane or "slice" being studied.
- Note that this test is performed by a radiologist in approximately 45 minutes.
- Inform the patient that the dye injection often causes a transitory flushing of the face, a feeling of warmth, a salty taste in the mouth, or even transient nausea. Initial IV needle placement and lying on a hard x-ray table are the only other discomforts associated with IVP.

After

- Assess the patient's urinary output. A decreased output may be an indication of renal failure.
- Evaluate the patient for delayed reaction to dye (e.g., dyspnea, rashes, tachycardia, hives). This usually occurs within the first 2 to 6 hours after the test. Treat with antihistamines or steroids.
- Encourage the patient to drink fluids to counteract fluid depletion caused by the test preparation.
- Evaluate elderly and debilitated patients for weakness because of the combination of fasting and catharsis necessary for test preparation. Instruct these patients to ambulate only with assistance.
- Maintain the patient on adequate oral or IV hydration for several hours after the IVP.

Abnormal findings

Pyelonephritis

Glomerulonephritis

Kidney tumor (benign or malignant)

Renal hematoma, laceration

Tumor of the collecting system

Bladder tumor

Absence of a kidney

Renal or ureteral calculi

Hydronephrosis

Prostate enlargement (male)

Congenital abnormality

Extrinsic compression of the collecting system (e.g., caused by tumor, aneurysm)

Trauma to the kidneys, ureters, or bladder

notes

iron level and total iron-binding capacity (Fe and TIBC, Transferrin saturation, Transferrin)

Type of test Blood

Normal findings
Iron: 60-190 μg/dl or 13-31 μmol/L (SI units)
TIBC: 25-420 μg/dl or 45-73 μmol/L (SI units)
Transferrin: 200-400 μg/dl
Transferrin saturation: 30% to 40%

Test explanation and related physiology
Abnormal levels of iron and TIBC are characteristic of many diseases, including iron deficiency anemia. Most of the iron in the body is found in the hemoglobin of the red blood cells (RBCs). Iron, supplied by the diet, is absorbed in the small intestine and transported to the plasma. There the iron is bound to a globulin protein called *transferrin* and carried to the bone marrow for incorporation into hemoglobin. The serum iron determination is a measurement of the quantity of iron bound to transferrin. In many laboratories TIBC is not performed; transferrin is directly measured. The TIBC is a direct, quantitative measurement of transferrin. The percentage of saturation is calculated by dividing the serum iron level by the TIBC:

$$\text{Transferrin saturation (\%)} = \frac{\text{Serum iron level}}{\text{TIBC}} \times 100\%$$

The normal value for transferrin saturation is 30% to 40%. Calculation of transferrin saturation is helpful in determining the cause of abnormal iron and TIBC levels. (See also test for ferritin, p. 387.)

Iron deficiency anemia has many causes, including:
1. Insufficient iron intake
2. Inadequate gut absorption
3. Increased requirements (as in growing children and late pregnancy)
4. Loss of blood (as in menstruation, bleeding peptic ulcer, and colon neoplasm)

Iron deficiency results in a decreased production of hemoglobin, which in turn results in a small, pale (microcytic, hypochromic) RBC. A decreased serum iron level, elevated TIBC, and low transferrin saturation value are characteristic of iron deficiency anemia. A decrease in the mean corpuscular volume and mean corpuscular hemoglobin concentration (MCV, MCHC; see p. 697) is also found.

Chronic illness (e.g., infections, neoplasia, cirrhosis) is characterized by a low serum iron level, decreased TIBC, and normal transferrin saturation. Pregnancy is marked by high levels of protein, including transferrin. Because iron requirements are high, it is not unusual to find low serum iron levels, high TIBC, and a low percentage of transferrin saturation in late pregnancy.

Increased intake or absorption of iron (as in hemochromatosis) leads to elevated iron levels. In such cases, the TIBC is unchanged; as a result, the percentage of transferrin saturation is very high. Excess iron is usually deposited in the brain, liver, and heart and causes severe dysfunction of these organs. Massive blood transfusions also may cause elevated serum iron levels.

Because serum iron levels may vary significantly during the day, the blood specimen should be drawn in the morning, especially when the results are used to monitor iron replacement therapy. The patient should refrain from eating for approximately 12 hours to avoid artificially high iron measurements caused by eating food with a high iron content. Blood transfusions also will greatly increase the iron level, although only transiently, and should be avoided before serum iron level determinations.

On the other hand, TIBC varies minimally according to intake. The TIBC is more of a reflection of liver function (transferrin is produced by the liver) and nutrition than of iron metabolism. TIBC values often are used to monitor the course of patients receiving hyperalimentation.

Contraindications

- Patients with hemolytic diseases, because they may have an artificially high iron content

Interfering factors

- Recent blood transfusions may affect test results.
- Recent ingestion of a meal containing high iron content may affect test results.
- Hemolytic diseases may be associated with an artificially high iron content.
- ☛ Drugs that may cause *increased iron* levels include chloramphenicol, dextran, estrogens, ethanol, iron preparations, methyldopa, and oral contraceptives.

☙ Drugs that may cause *decreased iron* levels include adreno-corticotropic hormone (ACTH), cholestyramine, chloramphenicol, colchicine, deferoxamine, methicillin, and testosterone.
☙ Drugs that may cause *increased TIBC* levels include fluorides and oral contraceptives.
☙ Drugs that may cause *decreased TIBC* levels include ACTH and chloramphenicol.

Procedure and patient care

Before

- Explain the procedure to the patient.
- Keep the patient fasting for 12 hours before the blood test. Water is permitted.
- Assess the patient for a history of recent blood transfusion and recent meals high in iron content. Both may affect test results.

During

- Collect approximately 5 to 7 ml of venous blood in a red-top tube. The specimen should always be obtained using a 20-gauge or larger needle.
- Avoid hemolysis, because the iron contained in the RBC will pour out into the serum and cause artificially high iron levels.
- Indicate on the laboratory slip any drugs that may affect test results.

After

- Apply pressure or a pressure dressing to the venipuncture site.
- Assess the venipuncture site for bleeding.

Abnormal findings

▲ **Increased serum iron levels**

Hemosiderosis
Hemochromatosis
Hemolytic anemia
Hepatitis
Hepatic necrosis
Lead toxicity
Iron poisoning

▼ **Decreased serum iron levels**

Insufficient dietary iron
Chronic blood loss
Inadequate absorption of iron
Pregnancy (late)
Iron deficiency anemia
Neoplasia
Chronic gastrointestinal blood loss
Chronic hematuria
Chronic heavy physiologic or pathologic menstruation

▲ **Increased TIBC levels**

Oral contraceptives
Pregnancy (late)
Polycythemia vera
Iron deficiency anemia

▼ **Decreased TIBC levels**

Hypoproteinemia
Inflammatory diseases
Cirrhosis
Hemolytic anemia
Pernicious anemia
Sickle cell anemia

notes

17-ketosteroids (17-KS)

Type of test   Urine (24-hour)

Normal findings

Male: 7-25 mg/24 hr or 24-88 μmol/day (SI units)
Female: 4-15 mg/24 hr or 14-52 μmol/day (SI units)
Elderly: values decrease with age
Child
  Under 12 years: <5 mg/24 hr
  12-15 years: 5-12 mg/24 hr

Test explanation and related physiology

This urine test is used to measure adrenocortical function by measuring 17-KS in the urine. 17-KS are metabolites of the non-testosterone androgenic sex hormones that are secreted from the adrenal cortex and the testes. The principal 17-ketosteroid is dehydroepiandrosterone (DHEA). In men, approximately one third of the hormone metabolites come from the testes and two thirds come from the adrenal cortex; in women and children, almost all the excreted hormones (androgens) are derived from the adrenal cortex. Therefore this test is very useful in diagnosing adrenocortical dysfunction. Elevated 17-KS levels are frequently seen in patients with congenital adrenal hyperplasia and testosterone tumors of the adrenal glands. These diseases frequently cause virilization syndromes. Testicular tumors rarely cause elevations in 17-KS. Low levels of 17-KS have little clinical significance.

Interfering factors

- Stress may increase adrenal activity.
- Drugs that may cause *increased* 17-KS levels include antibiotics, chloramphenicol, chlorpromazine, dexamethasone, meprobamate, phenothiazines, quinidine, secobarbital, and spironolactone (Aldactone).
- Drugs that may cause *decreased* levels include estrogen, oral contraceptives, probenecid, promazine, reserpine, salicylates (prolonged use), and thiazide diuretics.

Procedure and patient care

Before

- Explain the procedure to the patient.
- Withhold all drugs (with physician approval) for several days beforehand.
- Assess the patient for signs of stress and report these to the physician.

During

- Begin the 24-hour urine collection after the patient urinates; discard this specimen.
- Collect all urine passed by the patient during the next 24 hours.
- Post the hours for the urine collection in a prominent spot.
- Remember that it is not necessary to measure each urine specimen.
- Tell the patient to void before defecating so that the urine is not contaminated by feces.
- Inform the patient that toilet paper should not be placed in the collection container.
- Encourage the patient to drink fluids during the 24 hours, unless this is contraindicated for medical purposes.
- Remember that the urine collection needs a preservative.
- Refrigerate the urine throughout the collection.
- Collect the last specimen as close as possible to the end of the 24-hour period. Add this to the urine collection.

After

- Indicate on the laboratory slip the start and end times of the specimen collection.
- List on the laboratory slip any medications that may affect test results.
- Send the specimen to the laboratory as soon as the test is completed.

K

Abnormal findings

▲ **Increased levels**

Congenital adrenal hyperplasia

Pregnancy

Adrenocorticotropic hormone administration

Cushing's syndrome

Testosterone- or estrogen-secreting tumors of the adrenals, ovaries, or testes

Severe stress or infection

Hyperpituitarism

Ovarian neoplasia

▼ **Decreased levels**

Addison's disease

Hypogonadism

Hypopituitarism

Myxedema

Severe debilitating disease

Nephrosis

Gout

Castration

Thyrotoxicosis

notes

kidney, ureter, and bladder x-ray study (KUB)

Type of test X-ray

Normal findings

No evidence of calculi
Normal gastrointestinal (GI) gas pattern

Test explanation and related physiology

The KUB is a *flat plate,* or simple x-ray film, of the abdomen.
It is often referred to as a *plain film,* or *scout film,* of the abdomen. The KUB is similar to the supine view on an *obstruction series* (see p. 575) and can be performed to demonstrate the size, shape, location, and malformations of the kidneys and bladder. The KUB can also be used to identify calculi in these organs and in the ureters. This is often one of the first studies done to diagnose other intraabdominal diseases, such as intestinal obstruction, soft tissue masses, and a ruptured viscus. The KUB is useful in detecting abnormal accumulations of gas within the GI tract and finding ascites. This study involves no contrast medium and poses no risk to the patient.

Contraindications

- Patients who are pregnant

Interfering factor

- Retained barium from previous studies can obscure visualization.

Procedure and patient care

Before

- Explain the procedure to the patient.
- Tell the patient that no fasting or sedation is required.
- Schedule this study before any barium studies.
- Ensure that the male patient has a lead sheet over his testicles to prevent their irradiation.
- Note that the female ovaries cannot be shielded because of their proximity to the kidneys, ureters, and bladder.

During

- Note that in the radiology department the patient is placed in the supine position with the arms extended overhead. X-ray films are taken of the patient's abdomen.

K

- Note that the KUB is performed by a radiologic technologist in a few minutes and is interpreted by a radiologist.
- Inform the patient that results are available in approximately 1 hour.
- Tell the patient that no discomfort is associated with this study.

After

- Schedule intravenous pyelography or GI studies after completion of the KUB.

Abnormal findings

Malformations
Calculi
Abnormal accumulation of
  gas
Ascites

Intestinal obstruction
Soft tissue masses
Ruptured viscus

notes

lactic dehydrogenase (LDH)

Type of test Blood

Normal findings

Adult/elderly: 45-90 U/L (30° C), 115-225 IU/L, or 0.4-1.7 µmol/L (SI units)

Isoenzymes in adult/elderly values

LDH-1: 17% to 27%
LDH-2: 27% to 37%
LDH-3: 18% to 25%
LDH-4: 3% to 8%
LDH-5: 0% to 5%

Child: 60-170 U/L (30° C)
Infant: 100-250 U/L
Newborn: 160-450 U/L

Test explanation and related physiology

The enzyme LDH is found in many body tissues, especially the heart, liver, kidneys, skeletal muscle, brain, red blood cells, and lungs. The serum LDH level rises within 24 to 72 hours after a myocardial infarction (MI), peaks in 3 to 4 days, and returns to normal in approximately 14 days. This makes the serum LDH level especially useful for a delayed diagnosis of patients with MI (e.g., where the patient reports having had severe chest pain 4 days earlier). Because LDH is widely distributed through the body, the total LDH level is not a specific indicator of myocardial disease. LDH, as with creatine phosphokinase (CPK, see p. 293), is more useful diagnostically when fractionated into isoenzymes. Five LDH isoenzymes, called LDH-1 through LDH-5, may be separated by electrophoresis. Isoenzyme LDH-1 comes mainly from the heart and blood vessels; LDH-2 comes primarily from the reticuloendothelial system; LDH-3 comes from the lungs and other tissues; LDH-4 comes from the kidney, placenta, and pancreas; and LDH-5 comes mainly from the liver and striated muscle. Normally, serum levels of LDH-2 are higher than those of the other four isoenzymes. Diseases affecting the specific organ will cause elevations of total LDH and the specific LDH isoenzyme. LDH is also measured in abnormal body fluid collections such as in pleural effusions. If the pleural LDH/serum LDH ratio is greater than 0.6, the effusion is said to be an exudate.

In patients with MI, the LDH-1 level is a more sensitive and specific indicator of MI than the total LDH level. Its sensitivity is over 95%. LDH-1 activity greater than LDH-2 activity strongly supports the diagnosis of MI. This is referred to as a *flipped* LDH, because the normal LDH-1/LDH-2 ratio of less than 1 is reversed. In an acute MI, the flipped LDH ratio usually appears in 12 to 24 hours and is present within 48 hours in approximately 80% of patients. When LDH-2 is greater than LDH-1 (a normal LDH-1/LDH-2 ratio), it is considered reliable evidence against MI. The patient with chest pain may have had an ischemic episode or only minimal heart damage. Other diseases (e.g., pulmonary infarction, hemolysis, congestive heart failure) that cause an increase in LDH levels may obscure the enzyme diagnosis of MI unless isoenzyme levels are determined.

Some laboratories measure only the LDH-1 level. An elevated LDH level with greater than 40% LDH-1 is considered diagnostic of myocardial damage.

Interfering factors

- Hemolysis of blood will cause false-positive LDH levels.
- Drugs that may cause *increased* LDH levels include alcohol, anesthetics, aspirin, clofibrate, fluorides, mithramycin, narcotics, and procainamide.
- Drugs that may cause *decreased* levels include ascorbic acid.

Procedure and patient care

Before
- Explain the procedure to the patient.
- Tell the patient that no fasting is required.
- Inform the patient if he or she will be receiving frequent venipuncture for the evaluation of an MI.

During
- Collect approximately 7 to 10 ml of venous blood in a red-top tube.
- Because many diseases cause an increased LDH level, identify disease conditions on the laboratory slip.
- Record the data and time when blood was drawn on the laboratory slip for an accurate evaluation of the temporal pattern of enzyme elevations.

After
- Apply pressure or a pressure dressing to the venipuncture site.
- Assess the venipuncture site for bleeding.

Abnormal findings

▲ **Increased values**

Myocardial infarction
Pulmonary disease (e.g., infarction)
Hepatic disease (e.g., hepatitis)
Red blood cell disease (e.g., hemolytic anemia)
Skeletal muscle disease and injury
Renal parenchymal disease (e.g., infarction)
Intestinal ischemia and infarction
Cerebrovascular accident
Neoplastic states
Infectious mononucleosis
Heat stroke
Pancreatitis
Collagen disease
Fracture
Muscular dystrophy
Shock
Hypotension

notes

L

lactose tolerance test

Type of test Blood

Normal findings Adult/elderly: rise in plasma glucose levels >20 mg/dl

Test explanation and related physiology

This test is performed to detect lactose intolerance. Lactose is a dissaccharide typically found in dairy products; during digestion, lactose is broken down into glucose and galactose by the intestinal enzyme lactase. Because lactose-intolerant patients have an absence of lactase, lactose digestion will not occur. Thus the small bowel is flooded with a high lactose load. Bacterial metabolism of the lactose occurs within the intestine. This creates a strong cathartic effect. Symptoms of lactose intolerance include abdominal cramping, flatus, abdominal bloating, and diarrhea.

In this test, the patient is provided a lactose load. If lactase is not present in sufficient quantities, lactose is not metabolized to glucose and galactose. Plasma levels of glucose do not rise as expected. Therefore, lower-than-expected serum glucose levels suggest intestinal lactase deficiency.

While all adults have some degree of lactase reduction, severe lactose intolerance occurs in patients with inflammatory bowel disease, short-gut syndrome, and other malabsorption syndromes.

Interfering factors

- Enterogenous steatorrhea
- Strenuous exercise
- Smoking, which may increase blood glucose levels

Procedure and patient care

Before

- Explain the procedure to the patient. Inform the patient that four blood samples will be needed.
- Instruct the patient to fast 8 hours before testing.
- Instruct the patient to avoid strenuous exercise for 8 hours before testing. This may factitiously affect the blood glucose level.
- Inform the patient that smoking is prohibited before testing. This may falsely increase the blood glucose level.

During

- Obtain 5 to 7 ml of venous blood in a gray-top tube from the fasting patient.
- Provide a specified dose of lactose for the patient. Usually, dilute 100 g of lactose with 200 ml of water for ingestion in adults.
- Note that pediatric doses of lactose are based on weight.
- Collect three more blood samples at 30, 60, and 120 minutes after the ingestion of lactose.
- Tell the patient that the only discomfort is the venipuncture; however, patients with lactase deficiency will have the symptoms previously described.

After

- Apply pressure or a pressure dressing to the venipuncture site.
- Observe the venipuncture site for bleeding.
- Note that patients with abnormal test results may receive a monosaccharide tolerance test (e.g., glucose or galactose tolerance test).

Abnormal findings

▼ **Decreased levels**

Lactase insufficiency

Enterogenous diarrhea

notes

laparoscopy (Pelvic endoscopy, Gynecologic video laparoscopy)

Type of test Endoscopy

Normal findings Normal-appearing female reproductive organs

Test explanation and related physiology

During a laparoscopy, the abdominal organs can be visualized by inserting a fiberoptic scope through the abdominal wall and into the peritoneum. Usually, a television camera is applied to the scope, and the scope's view is seen on color monitors. This is particularly helpful in diagnosing abdominal and pelvic adhesions, ovarian tumors and cysts, and other tubal and uterine causes of infertility. Also, endometriosis, ectopic pregnancy, ruptured ovarian cyst, and salpingitis can be detected during an evaluation for pelvic pain. This procedure is also used to stage carcinomas. Surgical procedures (e.g., cholecystectomy, appendectomy, hernia repair, tubal ligation, oophorectomy, hiatal hernia repair, bowel resection, and many more) can easily be performed with the laparoscope.

Contraindications

- Patients with local peritonitis, because laparoscopy may spread the infection throughout the abdominal cavity
- Patients who have had multiple surgical procedures, because adhesions may have formed between the viscera and the abdominal wall
- Patients with suspected intraabdominal hemorrhage, because visualization through the scope will be obscured by the blood

Potential complications

- Perforation of the bowel, with spilling of intestinal contents into the peritoneum
- Hemorrhage
- Acidosis from carbon dioxide inflation of the abdominal cavity

Interfering factors

- Adhesions or extreme obesity may obstruct the field of vision.

Procedure and patient care

Before

- Explain the procedure to the patient.
- Ensure that an informed consent for this procedure is obtained.
- If enemas are ordered to clear the bowel, assist the patient as needed and record the results.
- Because the procedure is usually performed with the patient under general anesthesia, follow the routine general anesthesia precautions.
- Shave and prepare the patient's abdomen as ordered.
- Keep the patient NPO after midnight on the day of the test. IV fluids may be given.
- Instruct the patient to void before going to the operating room, because a distended bladder can be easily penetrated.

During

- Note the following procedural steps:
  1. Pelvic endoscopy is usually performed in the operating room. The patient is placed in a modified lithotomy or Trendelenburg position so that the intestines move away from the pelvis, permitting better visualization of the pelvic organs.
  2. After the abdominal skin is cleansed, a blunt-tipped needle is inserted through a small incision in the subumbilical area and into the peritoneal cavity.
  3. The peritoneal cavity is filled with approximately 3 to 4 L of carbon dioxide to separate the abdominal wall from the intraabdominal viscera, enhancing visualization of pelvic and abdominal structures.
  4. A laparoscope is inserted through a cannula to examine the abdomen (Figure 18).
  5. After the desired procedure is completed, the laparoscope is removed and the carbon dioxide is allowed to escape.
  6. The incision(s) is closed with a few skin stitches and covered with an adhesive bandage.
- Note that laparoscopy is performed by a surgeon.
- Inform the patient who will be under general anesthesia that she will feel no discomfort. Most patients will have mild incisional pain later, however, and also may complain of shoulder or subcostal discomfort from pneumoperitoneum.

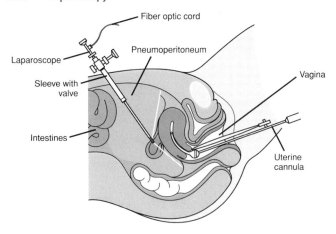

Figure 18 Gynecologic laparoscopy.

After

- Assess the patient frequently for signs of bleeding (increased pulse rate, decreased blood pressure), perforated viscus (abdominal tenderness, guarding, decreased bowel sounds), and acidosis (increased respiratory rate). Report any significant findings to the physician.
- If the patient has shoulder or subcostal discomfort from pneumoperitoneum, assure her that this usually lasts only 24 hours. Minor analgesics usually relieve this discomfort.

Abnormal findings

Pelvic adhesions	Cancer
Ovarian tumor	Uterine fibroids
Ovarian cyst	Abscess
Endometriosis	Infection
Ectopic pregnancy	Ascites
Ruptured ovarian cyst	Liver nodules
Salpingitis	Portal hypertension
Pelvic inflammatory disease	Other abdominal organ pathology

Legionnaires' disease antibody test

Type of test Blood

Normal findings No *Legionella* antibody titer

Test explanation and related physiology

Legionnaires' disease was originally described as a fulminating pneumonia caused by *Legionella pneumophila*. Nearly half of the clinical cases have been caused by serogroup type 1. The diagnosis can be made by culturing this organism from a suspected infected fluid such as blood, sputum, or pleural fluid. The most common method, however, is to detect the antibody directed against the Legionnaires' bacterium in the patient's blood. The indirect fluorescent antibody assay method is used.

A diagnosis of Legionnaires' disease can be made when a single antibody titer is 1:256 or greater. Another way to make the diagnosis is to perform the antibody test 1 and 3 weeks after the onset of symptoms. A fourfold rise in titer between the acute (1 week) and the convalescent (3 week) phases of at least 1:128 is diagnostic.

Procedure and patient care

Before
- Explain the procedure to the patient.
- Tell the patient that no fasting is required.

During
- Collect approximately 5 to 7 ml of blood in a red-top tube.

After
- Apply pressure or a pressure dressing to the venipuncture site.
- Observe the venipuncture site for bleeding.

Abnormal finding

▲ **Increased levels**
   Legionnaires' disease

leucine aminopeptidase (LAP)

Type of test   Blood; urine (24-hour)

Normal findings

Blood
   Male: 80-200 U/ml
   Female: 75-185 U/ml
Urine: 2-18 U/24 hr

Test explanation and related physiology

Produced exclusively by the liver, LAP, is used in diagnosing liver disorders and in the differential diagnosis of increased levels of alkaline phosphatase (ALP, see p. 36). LAP levels tend to parallel ALP levels in hepatic disease. LAP is a sensitive indicator of cholestasis; however, unlike ALP, LAP remains normal in bone disease. LAP can be detected in both the blood and the urine. Patients with elevated serum LAP levels will always show elevations in urine levels. When the urine LAP level is elevated, however, the blood level may have already returned to normal.

Interfering factors

- Pregnancy may cause increased values.
- Drugs that may cause *increased* LAP levels include estrogens and progesterones.

Procedure and patient care

Before
- Explain the procedure to the patient.
- Tell the patient that no fasting is required.

During
- Collect approximately 7 to 10 ml of venous blood in a red-top tube.
- If a urine sample is needed, follow the procedure for a 24-hour urine collection (see p. 374).
- Indicate on the laboratory slip any medications the patient is taking that may affect test results.

After
- Apply pressure or a pressure dressing to the venipuncture site.

- Assess the venipuncture site for bleeding. Patients with liver dysfunction often have prolonged clotting times.

Abnormal findings

▲ **Increased levels**

Hepatitis
Cirrhosis
Hepatic necrosis
Hepatic ischemia

Hepatic tumor
Hepatotoxic drugs
Cholestasis
Gallstones

notes

lipase

Type of test Blood

Normal findings 0-110 units/L or 0-417 U/L (SI units) (values are method dependent)

Test explanation and related physiology

The most common cause of an elevated serum lipase level is acute pancreatitis. Lipase is an enzyme secreted by the pancreas into the duodenum to break down triglycerides into fatty acids. As with amylase (see p. 51), lipase appears in the bloodstream following damage to the pancreatic acinar cells. Because lipase was thought to be produced only in the pancreas, elevated serum levels were considered to be specific to pathologic pancreatic conditions. Other conditions can be associated with elevated lipase levels. Because lipase is excreted through the kidneys, elevated lipase levels are often found in patients with renal failure. Intestinal infarction or obstruction also can be associated with lipase elevation. However, the lipase elevations are less than 3 times the upper limit of normal, as compared with pancreatitis, where they are often 5 to 10 times normal values.

In acute pancreatitis, elevated lipase levels usually parallel serum amylase levels. The lipase levels usually rise 24 to 48 hours after the onset of pancreatitis, however, and remain elevated for 5 to 7 days. Thus they peak later and remain elevated longer than the serum amylase levels. Therefore serum lipase levels are more useful in the late diagnosis of acute pancreatitis. Lipase levels are less useful in more chronic pancreatic diseases (e.g., chronic pancreatitis, pancreatic carcinoma).

Interfering factors

▮ Drugs that may cause *increased* lipase levels include bethanechol, cholinergics, codeine, indomethacin, meperidine, methacholine, and morphine.

▮ Drugs that may cause *decreased* levels include calcium ions.

Procedure and patient care

Before

- Explain the procedure to the patient.
- Instruct the patient to remain NPO, except for water, for 8 to 12 hours before the test.

During

- Collect 5 to 7 ml of venous blood in a red-top tube.
- Indicate on the laboratory slip drugs that may affect test results.

After

- Apply pressure or a pressure dressing to the venipuncture site.
- Observe the venipuncture site for bleeding.

Abnormal findings

Acute pancreatitis
Chronic relapsing pancreatitis
Acute cholecystitis

Renal failure
Intestinal obstruction
Intestinal infarction

notes

L

lipoproteins (High-density lipoprotein [HDL], Low-density lipoprotein [LDL], Very-low-density lipoprotein [VLDL])

Type of test Blood

Normal findings

HDL
  Male: >45 mg/dl or >0.75 mmol/L (SI units)
  Female: >55 mg/dl or >0.91 mmol/L (SI units)
LDL: 60-180 mg/dl or <3.37 mmol/L (SI units)
VLDL: 25% to 50%

Test explanation and related physiology

Lipoproteins are proteins in the blood whose main purpose is to transport cholesterol, triglycerides, and other fats. With the use of electrophoresis, these lipoproteins can be grouped into chylomicrons, which are primarily triglycerides; LDLs, which are primarily cholesterol; VLDLs, which are mainly triglycerides; and HDLs, which are predominantly protein.

HDLs are carriers of cholesterol. It is suspected that the purpose of HDLs is to remove the cholesterol from the peripheral tissues and to transport this to the liver for excretion. Also, HDLs may have a protective effect by preventing cellular uptake of cholesterol and lipids. These potential actions may be the source of the protective cardiovascular characteristics associated with HDLs within the blood. The HDL/total cholesterol ratio should be at least 1:5, with 1:3 being ideal.

LDLs are also cholesterol rich. Cholesterol carried by LDLs can be deposited into the peripheral tissues and is associated with an increased risk of arteriosclerotic heart and peripheral vascular disease. Therefore, high levels of LDL are atherogenic. The LDL level should be less than 160 mg/dl in persons with coronary artery disease and less than 180 mg/dl in those without disease.

VLDLs, although carrying a small amount of cholesterol, are the predominant carriers of blood triglycerides. To a lesser degree, VLDLs are also associated with an increased risk of arteriosclerotic occlusive disease.

The HDL, LDL, and VLDL levels are a part of a lipid profile test that also evaluates cholesterol (see p. 232) and triglycerides (see p. 819). The lipoprotein test is used to assess the risk of coronary artery disease. High levels of the "protective" HDL are associated with a decreased risk of coronary disease, whereas high levels of LDL and VLDL are associated with an increased risk of coronary occlusive disease.

Levels of HDL are increased in patients who engage in frequent physical activity or who use moderate doses of alcohol. On the other hand, LDL and VLDL are known to be increased in patients who have poor dietary habits associated with an increased intake of animal fats and snack foods. Genetic makeup, however, is probably the most important determinant of lipoprotein level.

The VLDL value is usually expressed as a percentage of total cholesterol. Levels in excess of 25% to 50% are associated with increased risk of coronary disease. The LDL is derived by subtracting the HDL plus one fifth of the triglycerides from the total cholesterol:

$$\text{LDL} = \text{Total cholesterol} - (\text{HDL} + \text{Triglycerides}/5)$$

There are other formulas for deriving LDL, which may account for different sets of normal values. (See also test for apolipoprotein, p. 95.)

Interfering factors

- Smoking and alcohol ingestion decrease HDL levels.
- Binge eating can alter lipoprotein values.
- Exercise can raise HDL levels.
- ✔ Drugs that may cause *increased* lipoprotein levels include aspirin, oral contraceptives, phenothiazines, steroids, and sulfonamides.

Procedure and patient care

Before

- Instruct the patient to fast for 12 to 14 hours before testing. Only water is permitted.
- Inform the patient that dietary indiscretion within the previous few weeks may influence lipoprotein levels.

During

- Collect 5 to 10 ml of venous blood in a red-top tube.
- Indicate on the laboratory slip any drugs that may affect test results.

After

- Apply pressure or a pressure dressing to the venipuncture site.

- Observe the venipuncture site for bleeding.
- Instruct patients with high lipoprotein levels regarding diet, exercise, and appropriate body weight.

Abnormal findings

▲ **Increased HDL levels**
Liver disease

▲ **Increased LDL and VLDL levels**
Hyperlipidemia
Increased ingestion of fatty foods and animal fats
Increased risk of arterio-sclerotic heart disease

▼ **Decreased HDL levels**
Increased risk of arterio-sclerotic heart disease

▼ **Decreased LDL and VLDL levels**
Malnutrition
Malabsorption

notes

liver biopsy

Type of test Microscopic examination of tissue

Normal findings Normal liver histology

Test explanation and related physiology

Liver biopsy is a safe, simple, and valuable method of diagnosing pathologic liver conditions. For this study, a specially designed needle is inserted through the abdominal wall and into the liver. A piece of liver tissue is removed for microscopic examination. Percutaneous liver biopsy is used in the diagnosis of various liver disorders, such as cirrhosis, hepatitis, drug reaction, granuloma, and tumor. Biopsy is indicated for:

1. Patients with unexplained hepatomegaly
2. Patients with persistently elevated liver enzymes
3. Patients with suspected primary or metastatic tumor, as determined by other studies
4. Patients with unexplained jaundice
5. Patients with suspected hepatitis
6. Patient with suspected infiltrative diseases (e.g., sarcoidosis, amyloidosis)

The biopsy may be performed by a "blind" stick or may be directed with the use of a computed tomography (CT) or magnetic resonance imaging (MRI) scan. Directed scans are used if there is a specific area of the liver that is suspicious and from which tissue must be obtained (e.g., a metastatic tumor). The "blind" stick is used if the liver is diffusely involved.

Contraindications

- Uncooperative patients who cannot remain still and hold their breath during sustained exhalation
- Patients with impaired hemostasis
- Patients with anemia who could not tolerate major blood loss associated with inadvertent puncture of an intrahepatic blood vessel
- Patients with infections in the right pleural space or right upper quadrant, because the biopsy may spread the infection
- Patients with obstructive jaundice
  In these patients, bile within the ducts is under pressure and may subsequently leak into the abdominal cavity after needle penetration.

- Patients with a hemangioma
  This is a very vascular tumor, and bleeding after a biopsy may be severe.

Potential complications

- Hemorrhage caused by inadvertent puncture of a blood vessel within the liver
- Chemical peritonitis caused by inadvertent puncture of a bile duct, with subsequent leakage of bile into the abdominal cavity
- Pneumothorax (collapsed lung) caused by improper placement of the biopsy needle into the adjacent chest cavity

Procedure and patient care

Before

- Explain the procedure to the patient. Many patients are apprehensive about this procedure.
- Obtain an informed consent.
- Ensure that all coagulation tests are normal.
- Instruct the patient to keep NPO after midnight on the day of the test.
- Administer any sedative medications as ordered.

During

- Note the following procedural steps:
  1. The patient is placed in the supine or left lateral position.
  2. The skin area used for puncture is anesthetized locally.
  3. The patient is asked to exhale and hold the exhalation. This causes the liver to descend and reduces the possibility of a pneumothorax. Frequently, the patient practices exhalation two or three times before insertion of the needle.
  4. During the patient's sustained exhalation, the physician rapidly introduces the biopsy needle into the liver and obtains liver tissue.
     a. Several types of needles are available.
     b. Occasionally, the biopsy needle is inserted under CT guidance. This is especially useful when tissue from a specific area of the liver is needed.
  5. The needle is withdrawn from the liver.
- Note that this test is performed by a physician in approximately 15 minutes.
- Inform the patient that he or she may have minor discom-

fort during injection of the local anesthetic and during needle insertion.

After

- Place the tissue sample into a specimen bottle containing formalin and send it to the pathology department.
- Apply a small dressing over the needle insertion site.
- Place the patient on his or her right side for approximately 1 to 2 hours. In this position, the liver capsule is compressed against the chest wall, thereby decreasing the risk of hemorrhage or bile leak.
- Assess the patient's vital signs frequently for evidence of hemorrhage (increased pulse, decreased blood pressure) and peritonitis (increased temperature).

Abnormal findings

Benign tumor
Malignant tumor (primary or metastatic)
Abscess
Cyst

Hepatitis
Infiltrative diseases (e.g., amyloidosis, hemochromatosis, cirrhosis)

notes

liver/spleen scanning (Liver scanning)

Type of test Nuclear scan

Normal findings Normal size, shape, and position of the liver and spleen

Test explanation and related physiology

This radionuclide procedure is used to outline and detect structural changes of the liver and spleen. A radionuclide, usually technetium sulfur-labeled albumin colloid, is administered intravenously. Later, a gamma ray detector is placed over the right upper and left upper quadrants of the patient's abdomen. This records the distribution of the radioactive particles of the liver and spleen. Images are obtained and recorded on Polaroid or x-ray film.

Because the scan can only demonstrate filling defects greater than 2 cm in diameter, false-negative results may occur in patients with space-occupying lesions (e.g., tumors, cysts, granulomas, abscesses) smaller than 2 cm. The scan may be incorrectly interpreted as positive for filling defects in patients with cirrhosis because of the distortion of the patient's liver parenchyma. The liver scan can detect tumors, cysts, granulomas, abscesses, and diffuse infiltrative processes affecting the liver (e.g., amyloidosis, sarcoidosis).

Splenic hematomas, abscesses, cysts, tumors, and infiltrate processes such as granulomas also can be detected.

Contraindications

- Patients who are pregnant or lactating, because of risk of damage to the fetus or infant.

Interfering factor

- Barium in the GI tract overlying the liver or spleen will produce defects on the scan that may be mistaken for masses.

Procedure and patient care

Before

- Explain the procedure to the patient.
- Tell the patient that no fasting or premedication is required.
- Assure the patient that he or she will not be exposed to large

amounts of radiation, because only tracer doses of isotopes are used.

During

- Note the following procedural steps:
  1. The patient is taken to the nuclear medicine department, where the radionuclide is administered intravenously. (For inpatients, a nuclear medicine technologist may administer the radionuclide at the bedside.)
  2. Thirty minutes after injection, a gamma ray detector is placed over the right upper quadrant of the patient's abdomen.
  3. The patient is placed in supine, lateral, and prone positions so that all surfaces of the liver can be visualized.
  4. The radionuclide image is recorded on Polaroid or x-ray film.
- Note that this procedure is performed by a trained technologist in approximately 1 hour. A physician trained in nuclear medicine interprets the results.
- Tell the patient that the only discomfort associated with this procedure is the IV injection of the radionuclide.

After

- Because only tracer doses of radioisotopes are used, inform the patient that no precautions need to be taken by others against radiation exposure.

Abnormal findings

Tumor of the liver or spleen
Abscess of the liver or spleen
Hematoma of the liver or spleen
Infiltrative processes (e.g., sarcoidosis, amyloidosis, or granuloma of the liver or spleen)

Hepatic or splenic cyst
Tuberculosis
Cirrhosis
Portal hypertension

notes

long-acting thyroid stimulator (LATS, Thyroid-stimulating immunoglobulin [TSIG])

Type of test Blood

Normal findings Negative

Test explanation and related physiology

The LATS antibody is an IgG immunoglobulin directed against the thyroid cell plasma membrane. LATS mimics the action of thyroid-stimulating hormone (TSH). LATS stimulates the thyroid gland to produce and secrete excessive amounts of thyroid hormone. This inhibits TSH secretion through the normal feedback mechanism. LATS can be found in about half of the patients with Graves' disease. It also can be found in some patients with Hashimoto's thyroiditis and in some patients with hyperparathyroidism. LATS is found most frequently in patients with Graves' disease associated with exophthalmos and/or pretibial edema. Its effect on the thyroid is long lasting, and titers do not decrease until nearly 1 year after successful treatment of the thyroid disease. Because LATS crosses the placenta, it may be found in neonates whose mothers have Graves' disease.

Interfering factor

- Recent administration of radioactive iodine may affect test results.

Procedure and patient care

Before

- Explain the procedure to the patient.
- Tell the patient that no fasting or special preparation is required.

During

- Collect approximately 5 ml of venous blood in a red-top tube.
- Notify the laboratory if the patient has received radioactive iodine in the preceding 2 days.
- Handle the blood sample gently. Hemolysis may interfere with interpretation of test results.

After

- Apply pressure or a pressure dressing to the venipuncture site.
- Observe the venipuncture site for bleeding.

Abnormal findings

▲ **Increased levels**
   Hyperthyroidism
   Malignant exophthalmos
   Graves' disease

notes

long bones x-ray

Type of test X-ray

Normal findings No evidence of fracture, tumor, infection, or congenital abnormalities

Test explanation and related physiology

X-ray films of the long bones are usually taken when the patient has complaints about a particular body area. Fractures or tumors are readily detected by x-ray studies. In patients who have a severe or chronic infection overlying a bone, an x-ray film may detect the infection involving that bone (osteomyelitis). X-ray studies of the long bones also can detect joint destruction and bone spurring as a result of persistent arthritis. Growth patterns can be followed by serial x-ray studies of a long bone, usually the wrists and hands. Healing of a fracture also can be documented and followed. X-ray films of the joints reveal the presence of joint effusions and soft tissue swelling as well.

Procedure and patient care

Before
- Explain the procedure to the patient.
- Carefully handle any injured parts of the patient's body.
- Instruct the patient that he or she will need to keep the extremity still while the x-ray film is being taken. This can sometimes be difficult, especially when the patient has severe pain associated with a recent injury.
- Shield the patient's testes, ovaries, or pregnant abdomen to avoid exposure from scattered radiation.
- Tell the patient that no fasting or sedation is required.

During
- Note that in the x-ray department, the patient is asked to place the involved extremity in several positions. An x-ray film is taken of each position.
- Note that this test is routinely performed by a radiologic technologist within several minutes.
- Tell the patient that no discomfort is associated with this test, except possibly from moving the extremity.

After
- Administer an analgesic for relief of pain if indicated.

Abnormal findings

Fractures
Tumors
Infection
Osteomyelitis

Joint destruction
Bone spurring
Abnormal growth pattern
Joint effusion
Arthritis

notes

L

lumbar puncture and cerebrospinal fluid examination (LP and CSF examination, Spinal tap, Spinal puncture, Cerebrospinal fluid analysis)

Type of test Fluid analysis

Normal findings

Pressure: less than 200 cm H_2O
Color: clear and colorless
Blood: none
Cells: no red blood cells; <5 lymphocytes/mm^3
Culture and sensitivity: no organisms present
Protein: 15-45 mg/dl CSF (up to 70 mg/dl in elderly adults and children)
Protein electrophoresis
    Prealbumin: 2% to 7%
    Albumin: 56% to 76%
    Alpha$_1$ globulin: 2% to 7%
    Alpha$_2$ globulin: 4% to 12%
    Beta globulin: 8% to 18%
    Gamma globulin: 3% to 12%
    Oligoclonal bands: none
    IgG: 0.0-4.5 mg/dl
Glucose: 50-75 mg/dl CSF or 60% to 70% of blood glucose level
Chloride: 700-750 mg/dl
Lactic dehydrogenase (LDH): <2.0-7.2 U/ml
Lactic acid: 10-25 mg/dl
Cytology: no malignant cells
Serology for syphilis: negative
Glutamine: 6-15 mg/dl

Test explanation and related physiology

By placing a needle in the subarachnoid space of the spinal column, one can measure the pressure of that space and obtain CSF for examination. The examination may assist in the diagnosis of primary or metastatic brain or spinal cord neoplasm, cerebral hemorrhage, meningitis, encephalitis, degenerative brain disease, autoimmune diseases involving the central nervous system, neurosyphilis, and demyelinating disorders (e.g., multiple sclerosis, acute demyelinating polyneuropathy).

Lumbar puncture may be used therapeutically to inject thera-peutic or diagnostic agents and to administer spinal anesthetics. Examination of the CSF includes evaluation for the presence of blood, bacteria, and malignant cells, along with quantitation of the amount of glucose and protein present. Color is noted, and various other tests such as a serologic test for syphilis (see p. 776), are performed.

Pressure

By attaching a sterile manometer to the needle used in LP, the pressure within the subarachnoid space can be measured. A pressure above 200 cm H_2O is considered abnormal. Because the subarachnoid space surrounding the brain is freely connected to the subarachnoid space of the spinal cord, any increase in in-tracranial pressure will be directly reflected as an increase at the lumbar site. Tumors, hydrocephalus, and intracranial bleeding can cause increased intracranial and spinal pressure. When this normal connection is suspected to be obstructed by tumor or postinfection scarring, a *Queckenstedt-Stookey test* is performed (see Procedure and Patient Care).

Color

Normal CSF is clear and colorless. A cloudy appearance may indicate an increase in the white blood cell (WBC) count or pro-tein. Normally, CSF contains no blood. A red tinge to the CSF indicates the presence of blood. Blood may be present because of subarachnoid bleeding or because the needle used in the LP has inadvertently penetrated a blood vessel. These causes of the bleeding must be differentiated. With a traumatic puncture, the blood within the CSF will clot. No clotting occurs in a patient with subarachnoid hemorrhage. Also, with a traumatic tap, the fluid clears toward the end of the procedure as successive CSF samples are obtained. This clearing does not occur with a sub-arachnoid hemorrhage.

Blood

Blood within the CSF indicates cerebral hemorrhage into the subarachnoid space or a traumatic tap as just described above.

Cells

The number of red blood cells is merely an indication of the amount of blood present within the CSF. Except for a few lym-phocytes, the presence of WBCs in the CSF is abnormal. The presence of polymorphonuclear leukocytes (neutrophils) is in-dicative of bacterial meningitis or cerebral abscess. When mononuclear leukocytes are present, viral or tubercular meningitis or encephalitis is suspected.

Culture and sensitivity

The organisms that cause meningitis or brain abscess can be cultured from the CSF. Organisms found also may include atypical bacteria, fungi, or *Mycobacterium tuberculosis.* A Gram stain of the CSF may give the clinician preliminary information about the causative infectious agent. This may allow appropriate antibiotic therapy to be initiated before the 24 hours necessary to complete the culture and sensitivity report.

Protein

Normally, very little protein is found in CSF from the subarachnoid space. The amount of protein is usually lower in CSF obtained from the cisterna magna and even lower in the ventricle. Only small amounts of protein are found in CSF, because protein is a large molecule that does not cross the blood-brain barrier. Disease processes can alter the permeability of this protective membrane, however, allowing protein to leak into the CSF.

The protein content within CSF is increased in patients who have infectious or inflammatory processes such as meningitis, encephalitis, or myelitis. Tumors also may cause an increase in protein content. CSF protein electrophoresis is very important in the detection of multiple sclerosis. Normally, less than 12% of the total protein consists of gamma globulin. The proportion of albumin to globulin is higher in CSF than in blood plasma (see p. 670), because albumin is smaller in size than globulin and therefore can pass more easily through the blood-brain barrier. Patients with multiple sclerosis, neurosyphilis, or degenerative cord or brain disease have an elevated globulin fraction of total protein. An increase in the CSF level of immunoglobulin G (IgG), an increase in the ratio of IgG to other proteins (e.g., albumin), and the detection of *oligoclonal gamma globulin bands* are highly suggestive of inflammatory and autoimmune diseases of the central nervous system, especially multiple sclerosis.

Glucose

The glucose level is decreased when the cells within the CSF increase in number and use the glucose. These cells may be inflammatory cells in response to infection, shedded tumors, or bacterial cells. A blood sample for glucose (see p. 424) is usually drawn before the spinal tap is performed. A CSF glucose level less than 60% of the blood glucose may indicate meningitis or neoplasm.

Chloride

The chloride concentration in CSF may be decreased in patients with meningeal infections, tubercular meningitis, and conditions of low blood chloride levels. An increase in the chloride level in CSF is not neurologically significant; it correlates with the blood levels of chloride (see p. 225). CSF is not routinely evaluated for chloride; this test is done only if specifically requested.

Lactic dehydrogenase

Quantitation of LDH (specifically, fractions 4 and 5; see p. 501) is helpful in diagnosing bacterial meningitis. The source of LDH is the neutrophils that fight the invading bacteria. When the LDH level is elevated, infection or inflammation is suspected.

Lactic acid

Elevated levels indicate anaerobic metabolism associated with decreased oxygenation of the brain. CSF lactic acid is increased in both bacterial and fungal meningitis but not in viral meningitis. Lactic acid is also increased when CSF glucose is very low or CSF WBC is elevated.

Cytology

Examination of the cells in the CSF can determine if they are malignant or benign. Tumors in the central nervous system may shed cells from their surface. These cells can float freely in CSF. Their presence suggests neoplasm as the cause of any neurologic symptoms.

Serology for syphilis

Latent syphilis is diagnosed by performing one of many presently available serologic tests on CSF. These include (1) the Wasserman test, (2) the Venereal Disease Research Laboratory test (see p. 776), and (3) the fluorescent treponemal antibody (FTA) test (see p. 776). The FTA test is presently considered to be the most sensitive and specific. When test results are positive, the diagnosis of neurosyphilis is made and appropriate antibiotic therapy is initiated.

Glutamine

The CSF can be evaluated for the presence of glutamine. Elevated glutamine levels are helpful in the detection and evaluation of hepatic encephalopathy and coma. Levels of glutamine are also often increased in patients with Reye's syndrome.

Contraindications

- Patients with increased intracranial pressure
  The LP may induce cerebral or cerebellar herniation through the foramen magnum.
- Patients who have severe degenerative vertebral joint disease
  It is very difficult to pass the needle through the degenerated arthritic interspinal space.
- Patients with infection near the LP site
  Meningitis can result from contamination of CSF with infected material.

Potential complications

- Persistent CSF leak, causing severe headache
- Introduction of bacteria into CSF, causing suppurative meningitis
- Herniation of the brain through the tentorium cerebelli or herniation of the cerebellum through the foramen magnum
  In patients with increased intracranial pressure, the quick reduction of pressure in the spinal column by the LP may induce herniation of the brain, causing compression of the brainstem. This results in deterioration of the patient's neurologic status and death.
- Inadvertent puncture of the spinal cord, caused by inappropriately high puncture of the spinal cord
- Puncture of the aorta or vena cava, causing serious retroperitoneal hemorrhage
- Transient back pain and pain or paresthesia in the legs

Procedure and patient care

Before

- Explain the procedure to the patient. Many patients have misconceptions regarding LP. Allay the patient's fears and allow time to verbalize concerns.
- Obtain informed consent if required by the institution.
- Perform a baseline neurologic assessment of the legs by assessing the patient's strengths, sensation, and movement.
- Tell the patient that no fasting or sedation is required.
- Instruct the patient to empty the bladder and bowels before the procedure.
- Explain to the patient that he or she must lie very still throughout this procedure. Movement may cause traumatic injury. Encourage the patient to relax and take deep, slow breaths with the mouth open.

During
- Note the following procedural steps:
  1. This study is a sterile procedure that can be easily performed at the bedside. The patient is usually placed in the lateral decubitus (fetal) position (Figure 19).
  2. The patient is instructed to clasp the hands on the knees to maintain this position. Someone usually helps the patient maintain this position. (A sitting position also may be used.)
  3. A local anesthetic is injected into the skin and subcutaneous tissues after the site has been aseptically cleaned.
  4. A spinal needle containing an inner obturator is placed through the skin and into the spinal canal.
  5. The subarachnoid space is entered.
  6. The insert (obturator) is removed, and CSF can be seen slowly dripping from the needle.
  7. The needle is attached to a sterile manometer, and the pressure (opening pressure) is recorded.
  8. Before the pressure reading is taken, the patient is asked to relax and straighten the legs to reduce the intraabdominal pressure, which causes an increase in CSF pressure.

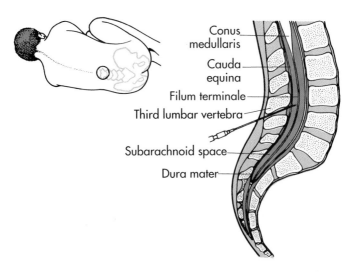

Conus medullaris
Cauda equina
Filum terminale
Third lumbar vertebra
Subarachnoid space
Dura mater

Figure 19 Patient position for a lumbar puncture (LP).

9. Three sterile test tubes are filled with 5 to 10 ml of CSF.
10. The pressure (closing pressure) is measured.

- Note that if blockage in CSF circulation in the spinal sub-arachnoid space is suspected, a *Queckenstedt-Stookey* test may be performed. For this test, the jugular vein is occluded either manually by digital pressure or by a medium-sized blood pressure cuff inflated to approximately 20 mm Hg. Within 10 seconds after jugular occlusion, CSF pressure should increase from 15 to 40 cm H_2O and then promptly return to normal within 10 seconds after release of the pressure. A sluggish rise or fall of CSF pressure suggests partial blockage of CSF circulation. No rise after 10 seconds suggests a complete obstruction within the spinal canal.
- Note that this procedure is performed by a physician in approximately 20 minutes.
- Inform the patient that this procedure is described as uncomfortable or painful by most patients. Some patients complain of feeling pressure from the needle. Some patients complain of a shooting pain in their legs.

After

- Apply digital pressure and an adhesive dressing to the puncture site.
- Place the patient in the prone position with a pillow under the abdomen to increase the intraabdominal pressure, which will indirectly increase the pressure in the tissues surrounding the spinal cord. This retards continued CSF flow from the spinal canal.
- Encourage the patient to drink increased amounts of fluid with a straw to replace the CSF removed during the lumbar puncture. Drinking with a straw will enable the patient to keep the head flat.
- Usually, keep the patient in a reclining position for up to 12 hours to avoid the discomfort of potential postpuncture spinal headache. Allow the patient to turn from side to side as long as the head is not raised.
- Label and number the specimen jars appropriately and deliver them immediately to the laboratory after the test. Refrigeration will alter test results. A delay between collection time and testing can invalidate results, especially cell counts.
- Assess the patient for numbness, tingling, and movement of the extremities; pain at the injection site; drainage of blood

or CSF at the injection site; and the ability to void. Notify the physician of any unusual findings.

Abnormal findings

Brain neoplasm
Spinal cord neoplasm
Cerebral hemorrhage
Encephalitis
Myelitis
Tumor
Neurosyphilis
Degenerative brain disease
Autoimmune disorder
Hepatic encephalopathy
Coma
Meningitis
Encephalitis
Viral or tubercular meningitis
Cerebral abscess
Degenerative cord or brain disease
Multiple sclerosis
Acute demyelinating polyneuropathy
Subarachnoid bleeding
Reye's syndrome

notes

lung biopsy

Type of test   Microscopic examination of tissue

Normal findings   No evidence of pathology

Test explanation and related physiology

This invasive procedure is used to obtain a specimen of pulmonary tissue for a histologic examination by using either an open or a closed technique. The *open method* involves a limited thoracotomy. The *closed technique* includes methods such as transbronchial lung biopsy, transbronchial needle aspiration biopsy, transcatheter bronchial brushing, and percutaneous needle aspiration biopsy.

Lung biopsy is indicated to determine the pathology of pulmonary parenchymal disease. Carcinomas, granulomas, infections, and sarcoidosis can be diagnosed with this procedure. This procedure is also useful in detecting environmental exposures, infections, or familial disease, which may lead to better prevention and treatment.

Contraindications

- Patients with bullae or cysts of the lung
- Patients with suspected vascular anomalies of the lung
- Patients with bleeding abnormalities
- Patients with pulmonary hypertension
- Patients with respiratory insufficiency

Potential complications

- Pneumothorax
- Pulmonary hemorrhage
- Empyema

Procedure and patient care

Before

- Explain the procedure to the patient.
- Ensure that informed and signed consent is obtained.
- Instruct the patient that fasting is usually ordered. The patient may be kept NPO after midnight on the day of the test.
- Administer the preprocedural medications 30 to 60 minutes before the test as ordered. Atropine is usually given to de-

crease bronchial secretions. Meperidine (Demerol) may be used to sedate anxious patients.

- Instruct the patient to remain still during the lung biopsy. Any movement or coughing could cause laceration of the lung by the biopsy needle.

During

- Note that the patient's position depends on the method used and that the histologic lung specimen may be obtained by several different methods:

Transbronchial lung biopsy

1. This technique is performed via flexible fiberoptic bronchoscopy using cutting forceps.
2. Fluoroscopy is used to ensure proper opening and positioning of the forceps on the lesions.
3. Fluoroscopy also permits visualization of the "tug" of the lung as the specimen is removed.

Transbronchial needle aspiration

1. The specimen is obtained via a fiberoptic bronchoscope using a needle.
2. The bronchoscope is inserted, and the target site is identified by fluoroscopy.
3. The needle is inserted through the bronchoscope and into the tumor or desired area, where aspiration is performed with the attached syringe.
4. The needle is retracted within its sheath, and the entire catheter is withdrawn from the fiberoptic scope.

Transcatheter bronchial brushing

1. This is also performed via a fiberoptic bronchoscope.
2. During bronchoscopy, a small brush is moved back and forth over the suspicious area in the bronchus or its branches.
3. The cells adhere to the brush, which is then removed and used to make microscopic slides.

Percutaneous needle biopsy

1. In this method for obtaining a closed specimen, the biopsy is obtained after using fluoroscopic x-ray determination of the desired site.
2. The procedure is carried out by using a cutting needle or by aspiration with a spinal-type needle to obtain a specimen.
3. The main problem with this procedure is potential damage to major blood vessels.

Open lung biopsy

1. The patient is taken to the operating room, and general anesthesia is provided.
2. The patient is placed in the supine or lateral position, and an incision is made into the chest wall.
3. After a piece of lung tissue is removed, the lung is sutured.
4. Chest tube drainage is used for approximately 24 hours after an open lung biopsy.

- Note that this procedure is performed by a surgeon in less than 30 minutes.
- During the lung biopsy procedure, assess the patient carefully for signs of respiratory distress (e.g., shortness of breath, rapid pulse, cyanosis).
- Tell the patient that most patients describe this procedure as painful.

After

- Place biopsy specimens in appropriate containers for histologic and microbiologic examination.
- Observe the patient's vital signs frequently for signs of bleeding (increased pulse, decreased blood pressure) and for shortness of breath.
- Assess the patient's breath sounds and report any decrease on the biopsy side.
- If ordered, obtain a chest x-ray film to check for complications (e.g., pneumothorax).
- Observe the patient for signs of pneumothorax (e.g., dyspnea, tachypnea, decrease in breath sounds, anxiety, restlessness).

Abnormal findings

Carcinoma

Granuloma

Exposure lung diseases (e.g., black lung, asbestosis)

Sarcoidosis

Infection

notes

lung scan (Ventilation/perfusion scanning [VPS], Pulmonary scintiphotography, V/Q scan)

Type of test Nuclear scan

Normal findings Diffuse and homogeneous uptake of nuclear material by the lungs

Test explanation and related physiology

This nuclear medicine procedure is used to identify defects in blood *perfusion* of the lung in patients with suspected pulmonary embolism. Blood flow to the lungs is evaluated using a macroaggregated albumin (MAA) tagged with technetium (Tc), which is injected into the patient's peripheral vein. Because the diameter of the radionuclide aggregates is larger than that of the pulmonary capillaries, the aggregates become temporarily lodged in the pulmonary vasculature. A gamma-ray detector passed over the patient records the distribution of particles within the lung microvasculature.

A homogeneous uptake of particles that fills the entire pulmonary vasculature conclusively rules out pulmonary embolism. If a defect in an otherwise smooth and diffusely homogeneous pattern is seen, a perfusion abnormality exists. This can indicate pulmonary embolism. Unfortunately, many other serious pulmonary parenchymal lesions (e.g., pneumonia, pleural fluid, emphysematous bullae) also cause a defect in pulmonary blood perfusion. Therefore, although the scan may be sensitive, it is not specific, because many different pathologic conditions can cause the same abnormal results.

The chest x-ray film aids in assessing the perfusion scan, because a defect on the perfusion scan seen in the same area as an abnormality on the chest x-ray film does not indicate pulmonary embolism. Rather, the defect may represent pneumonia, atelectasis, effusion, and so on. When a perfusion defect occurs in an area of the lung that is normal on a chest x-ray study, however, pulmonary embolus is likely.

Specificity of a perfusion scan also can be enhanced by performance of a *ventilation scan* (V/Q), which detects abnormalities in ventilation (e.g., pneumonia, pleural fluid, emphysematous bullae). The ventilation scan reflects the patency of the pulmonary airways using krypton gas or Tc-diethylenetriamine pentaacetic acid (DTPA) as an aerosol. When vascular obstruction (embolism) is present by perfusion scan, ventilation scans will demonstrate a normal wash-in and a normal wash-out of radioactivity from the embolized lung area. If parenchymal disease (e.g., pneumonia) is responsible for the perfusion abnormality, however, wash-in or wash-out will be abnormal. Therefore the "mismatch" of perfusion and ventilation is characteristic of embolic disorders, whereas the "match" is indicative of parenchymal disease.

Contraindications

- Patients who are pregnant

Interfering factors

- Patients with known pulmonary parenchymal problems (e.g., pneumonia, emphysema, pleural effusion, tumors)
  These problems will give the picture of a perfusion defect and simulate pulmonary embolism.

Procedure and patient care

Before

- Explain the procedure to the patient.
- Obtain informed consent if required by the institution.
- Assure the patient that he or she will not be exposed to large amounts of radioactivity, because only tracer doses of isotopes are used.
- Although rarely done, if iodine-131 will be administered, give the patient 10 drops of Lugol's solution several hours before the test as a blocking agent for the thyroid gland. This will prevent iodine uptake by the thyroid gland.
- Tell the patient that no fasting is required.
- Note that a recent chest x-ray film should be available.
- Instruct the patient to remove jewelry around the chest area.

During

- Note the following procedural steps:
  1. The unsedated, nonfasting patient suspected of having a pulmonary embolism is taken to the nuclear medicine department.

Perfusion scan
  2. The patient is given a peripheral IV injection of radionuclide-tagged MAA.
  3. While the patient lies in the appropriate position, a gamma ray detector is passed over the patient and records radionuclide uptake on Polaroid or x-ray film.

4. The patient is placed in the supine, prone, and various lateral positions, which allows for anterior, posterior, lateral, and oblique views, respectively.

5. The results are interpreted by a physician trained in diagnostic nuclear medicine.

Ventilation scan

6. The patient breathes the tracer through a face mask with a mouthpiece.

7. Less patient cooperation is needed with a krypton tracer. Ventilation scans can even be performed on comatose patients using krypton. Krypton images can be obtained before, during, or after perfusion images.

8. In contrast, Tc-DTPA images are usually done before perfusion images and require patient cooperation with deep breathing and appropriate use of breathing equipment to prevent contamination.

- Note that this test is usually performed by a physician in approximately 30 minutes.
- Tell the patient that no discomfort is associated with this test other than the peripheral venipuncture.

After

- Inform the patient that no radiation precautions are necessary.

Abnormal findings

Pulmonary embolism
Pneumonia
Tuberculosis
Emphysema
Tumor

Asthma
Atelectasis
Bronchitis
Chronic obstructive pulmonary disease

notes

luteinizing hormone assay (LH assay, Lutropin, Follicle-stimulating hormone [FSH])

Type of test Blood

Normal findings

Male: 7-24 ImU/ml
Female: >6-30 ImU/ml
   Midcycle peak: >3 times the baseline
   Postmenopause: >30 ImU/ml
Child: up to 12 ImU/ml

Test explanation and related physiology

A gonadotropin secreted by the anterior pituitary gland, LH, along with follicle-stimulating hormone (FSH), is necessary for ovulation. FSH is usually measured along with the LH in most bioassay methods. With immunoassay methods, these two hormones can be measured separately.

Performing an LH assay is an easy way to determine if ovulation has occurred. An LH surge in blood levels indicates that ovulation has taken place. Under the influence of LH, the corpus luteum develops from the ruptured graafian follicle. Daily samples of serum LH around the woman's midcycle can detect the LH surge, which is believed to occur on the day of maximal fertility.

These assays also determine whether a gonadal insufficiency is primary (problem with the ovary/testicle) or secondary (because of insufficient stimulation by the pituitary hormones, e.g., LH). Elevated levels in patients with suspected gonadal insufficiency are compatible with primary gonadal failure, as may be seen in women with polycystic ovaries or menopause. In secondary gonadal failure, LH and FSH levels are low as a result of pituitary hypothalamic impairment, stress, malnutrition, or physiologic delay in growth and sexual development. LH hormones are also used to study testicular dysfunction in men and to evaluate endocrine problems related to precocious puberty in children.

Interfering factors

- Recent use of radioisotopes may affect test results.
- HCG and TSH may interfere with some immunoassay methods. Therefore patients with HCG-producing tumors and hypothyroid patients should be expected to have falsely high LH levels.

☛ Drugs that may *increase* LH levels include anticonvulsants, clomiphene, naloxone, and spironolactone.

☛ Drugs that may *decrease* LH levels include estrogens, progesterones, testosterone, digoxin, oral contraceptives, and phenothiazines.

Procedure and patient care

Before

- Explain the procedure to the patient.
- Tell the patient that no food or fluid restrictions are needed.

During

- Collect approximately 7 to 10 ml of venous blood in a red-top tube.
- Note that the patient may also perform LH assays at home using a home urine test or a 24-hour urine test.
- Indicate the date of the last menstrual period on the laboratory slip. Note if the woman is postmenopausal.

After

- Apply pressure or a pressure dressing to the venipuncture site.
- Assess the venipuncture site for bleeding.

Abnormal findings

▲ **Increased levels**
  Gonadal failure
  Polycystic ovaries
  Precocious puberty
  Complete testicular femi-
    nization syndrome
  Hypogonadism
  Anorchia
  Menopause
  Pituitary adenoma

▼ **Decreased levels**
  Pituitary failure
  Hypothalamic failure
  Stress
  Anorexia nervosa
  Malnutrition

notes

Lyme disease test

Type of test Blood

Normal findings Negative (low titers of IgM and IgG antibodies)

Test explanation and related physiology

Lyme disease was first recognized in Lyme, Connecticut, in 1975. The disease usually begins in the summer with a skin lesion called erythema chronicum migrans (ECM), which occurs at the site of a bite by a tick, usually *Ixodes dammini*. Ticks are the best documented vectors of this spirochete, which is the causative agent for Lyme disease.

Weeks to months after the insect bite, some patients develop fatigue, meningoencephalitis, cranial or peripheral neuropathies, myocarditis, atrioventricular nodal block, or arthritis. The last manifestation is joint involvement, which often occurs intermittently in a few large joints for several years.

Currently, the *enzyme-linked immunosorbent assay* (ELISA) is the best diagnostic test for Lyme disease. This test determines titers of specific immunoglobulin M (IgM) and specific IgG antibodies to the *I. dammini* spirochete. Levels of specific IgM antibody peak during the third to sixth week after disease onset and then gradually decline.

Titers of specific IgG antibodies are generally low during the first several weeks of illness, reach maximal levels months later during arthritis, and often remain elevated for years. Early in the illness, the diagnosis usually can be determined from the gross appearance of ECM and known exposure to an endemic area. These patients do not require antibody determination. In the absence of ECM lesions, however, Lyme disease can be confused with various viral infections. In these patients, a single titer of specific IgM antibody may suggest the correct diagnosis. Acute and convalescent sera can be tested to be certain. Later in the illness, determination of specific IgG antibodies can separate Lyme disease from aseptic meningitis or unexplained cranial or peripheral nerve palsies.

Because of the high incidence of false-positive ELISA tests for Lyme disease, it is now recommended that the diagnoses of all patients who have positive serologies for Lyme disease using the ELISA test be confirmed by a Western Blot specific Lyme disease test. (This is very similar to the situation with human immunodeficiency virus [HIV] infection, wherein all positive ELISA tests are confirmed by the more specific and sensitive Western Blot test.)

Procedure and patient care

Before
- Explain the procedure to the patient.
- Tell the patient that no fasting or special preparation is required.

During
- Collect approximately 7 to 10 ml of venous blood in a red-top tube.

After
- Apply pressure or a pressure dressing to the venipuncture site.
- Assess the venipuncture site for bleeding.

Abnormal finding

Lyme disease

notes

lymphangiography (Lymphangiogram, Lymphography)

Type of test X-ray with contrast dye

Normal findings Normal-sized lymph nodes containing no filling defects

Test explanation and related physiology

Lymphangiography provides an x-ray examination of the lymphatic system after the injection of contrast medium into a lymphatic vessel in the foot or hand. The lymphatic system consists of lymph vessels and lymph nodes. Assessment of this system is important, because cancer often spreads via the lymphatic system.

Lymphangiography is especially useful in patients suspected of having lymphatic pathology (lymphoma or metastatic tumor). The test allows one to demonstrate the extent and level of lymphatic metastasis. The lymphangiogram is also useful in staging lymphoma patients and in evaluating the results of chemotherapy or radiation therapy. Because the contrast medium remains in the lymph nodes for 6 months to 1 year, repeat plain x-ray films may be done for continued follow-up of disease progression or response to treatment.

Contraindications

- Patients with an allergy to iodine dye or shellfish
- Patients with severe chronic lung diseases, cardiac disease, or advanced kidney or liver disease

Potential complications

- Lipoid (lipid) pneumonia
  This occurs if the contrast medium flows into the thoracic duct and causes micropulmonary emboli. These small emboli usually disappear after several weeks or months.
- Allergic reaction or allergy to iodine dye
  Allergic reactions vary from flushing, itching, and urticaria to severe, life-threatening anaphylaxis (evidenced by respiratory distress, drop in blood pressure, shock). In the event of anaphylaxis, the patient may be treated with diphenhydramine (Benadryl), steroids, and epinephrine. Oxygen and endotracheal equipment should be on hand for immediate use.

Procedure and patient care

Before

- Explain the procedure to the patient.
- Obtain informed consent if required by the institution.
- Tell the patient that no fasting or sedation is required.
- Inform the radiologist if an allergy to iodinated contrast is suspected. The radiologist may prescribe a Benadryl-and-steroid preparation to be administered before testing. Usually, a hypoallergenic, non-ionic contrast will be used during the test.
- Inform the patient that if a blue-colored dye is used, he or she may note a bluish tinge in the urine. Excessive infiltration or IV administration of the lymphatic stain may create a transient bluish tint to a portion of or the entire skin surface.

During

- Note the following procedural steps:
  1. In the radiology department, the patient is placed on an x-ray table in the supine position.
  2. A lymphatic stain is injected into the subcutaneous tissue between each of the first three toes in each foot to outline the lymphatic vessels. (The stain can also be injected into the web of the skin between the fingers.)
  3. After the stain is taken up by the lymphatic vessels, they can be easily seen.
  4. A local anesthetic is injected.
  5. A small incision is made on the top of the foot (or hand).
  6. The lymphatic vessel is identified and cannulated to infuse the iodine contrast agent.
  7. The dye is slowly infused into the vessel. Usually, a low-rate infusion pump is used. The patient must lie very still during the injection.
  8. The flow of iodine dye is followed by fluoroscopy.
  9. When the dye reaches the upper lumbar level, the flow of dye is discontinued.
  10. X-ray films are taken of the chest, abdomen, and pelvis to demonstrate the filling of the lymph nodes. Often, the patient is asked to return in 24 hours to have additional x-ray studies done.

11. On completion of the injection, the cannula is removed and the incision is sutured closed.

- Note that this procedure is performed by a radiologist in approximately 3 hours. Additional x-ray films are usually taken 24 to 48 hours later.
- Inform the patient that discomfort may be felt when the blue stain is injected subcutaneously and the feet are locally anesthetized.

After

- Observe the injection and incision sites for evidence of cellulitis. If the patient will be returning home, instruct him or her to evaluate the site for redness, pain, and swelling.
- Inform the patient that the sutures should be removed 7 to 10 days after the test.

Abnormal findings

Metastatic tumor involving the lymph glands
Lymphoma

notes

magnesium

Type of test Blood

Normal findings

Adults: 1.2-2.0 mEq/L
Newborn: 1.4-2.0 mEq/L

Possible critical values <0.5 mEq/L or >3.0 mEq/L

Test explanation and related physiology

Most of the magnesium found within the body exists intracellularly. Most of the magnesium is bound to an ATP; therefore this electrolyte is critical in nearly all metabolic processes. Furthermore, magnesium acts as a cofactor that modifies the activity of many enzymes. Carbohydrate, protein, and nucleic acid metabolism depends on magnesium. Most organ functions, including neuromuscular tissue, also depend on magnesium. Symptoms of magnesium depletion are weakness, irritability, tetany, electrocardiographic changes, delerium, and convulsions. Hypermagnesemia can retard the cardiac conduction system, deep-tendon reflexes, and respiration.

As intracellular elements, magnesium, calcium, and potassium are intimately tied together in their body levels. Therefore a reduction in one of those elements creates a comparable reduction in the others. Magnesium deficiency occurs in patients who are malnourished because of malabsorption or maldigestion. Alcohol abuse increases magnesium loss in the urine. Because most of the serum magnesium is reabsorbed in the renal tubule, chronic renal diseases impair magnesium reabsorption and cause reduced magnesium levels. Moderate hypomagnesemia occurs with diabetes, hypoparathyroidism, hyperthyroidism, and hyperaldosteronism. Toxemia of pregnancy is also felt to be associated with reduced magnesium levels.

Increased magnesium levels most commonly are associated with ingestion of magnesium-containing antacids. Several drug interactions also can result in decreased or increased magnesium levels. Because magnesium is an intracellular cation, hemolysis of the collected blood sample should be avoided. Hemolysis will create falsely elevated levels of magnesium.

M

Interfering factors

- Hemolysis should be avoided when collecting this specimen.
- Drugs that *increase* magnesium levels include thyroid medication, antacids, laxatives, calcium-containing medication, lithium, loop diuretics, and aminoglycosides antibiotics.
- Drugs that *decrease* magnesium levels include diuretics, some antibiotics, and insulin.

Procedure and patient care

Before

- Explain the procedure to patient.
- Tell the patient that no special diet or fasting is required.

During

- Collect approximately 5 to 7 ml of venous blood in a red- or green-top tube.
- Avoid hemolysis.
- Indicate on the laboratory slip any drugs that may affect test results.

After

- Apply pressure or a pressure dressing to the venipuncture site.
- Assess the venipuncture site for bleeding.

Abnormal findings

▲ **Increased levels**
Renal insufficiency
Uncontrolled diabetes
Addison's disease
Hypothyroidism
Ingestion of magnesium-
  containing antacids or
  salts

▼ **Decreased levels**
Malnutrition
Malabsorption
Hypoparathyroidism
Alcoholism
Chronic renal disease
Hyperparathyroidism
Diabetic acidosis

notes

magnetic resonance imaging (MRI, Nuclear magnetic resonance [NMRI])

Type of test Magnetic field study

Normal findings No evidence of pathology

Test explanation and related physiology

Magnetic resonance imaging is a noninvasive diagnostic scanning technique that provides valuable information about the body's biochemistry by placing the patient in a magnetic field. MRI is based on how hydrogen atoms behave when placed in a magnetic field and then disturbed by radiofrequency signals. The unique feature about MRI is that is does not require exposure to ionizing radiation. MRI has several advantages over CT scanning, including the following:

1. MRI provides better contrast between normal tissue and pathologic tissue.
2. Obscuring bone artifacts that occur in CT scanning do not occur in MRI scanning.
3. Because rapidly flowing blood appears dark, which results from its quick motion, many blood vessels appear as dark lumens. This provides a natural contrast to the blood vessels when using MRI.
4. Because spatial information depends only on how the magnetic fields are varied in space, it is possible to image the transverse, sagittal, and coronal planes directly with MRI.

Although the full usefulness of MRI is yet to be determined, it shows promise in the evaluation of the following areas:

1. Head and surrounding structures
2. Spinal cord and surrounding structures
3. Face and surrounding structures
4. Neck
5. Mediastinum
6. Heart and great vessels
7. Liver
8. Kidney
9. Prostate
10. Bone and joints
11. Breast
12. Extremities and soft tissues

M

An important advantage of MRI imaging is that serial studies can be performed on the patient without any risk. This is useful in assessing the response of cancer to radiotherapy and chemotherapy. A major disadvantage of MRI is that patient eligibility is reduced as compared with CT scanning. For example, examination of patients requiring cardiac monitoring or having metal implants, pacemakers, or cerebral aneurysm clips will result in MRI image degradation and may endanger the patient.

Contraindications

- Patients who are extremely obese (over 300 pounds)
- Patients who are pregnant, because the long-term effects of MRI are not known at this time
- Patients who are confused or agitated
- Patients who are claustrophobic
- Patients who are unstable and require continuous life-support equipment, because monitoring equipment cannot be used inside the scanner room
- Patients with implantable metal objects such as pacemakers, infusion pumps, aneurysm clips, inner ear implants, and metal fragments in one or both eyes, because the magnet may move the object within the body and may injure the patient

Interfering factor

- Movement during the scan may cause artifacts on MRI.

Procedure and patient care

Before

- Explain the procedure to the patient. Inform the patient that there is no exposure to radiation.
- Obtain informed consent if required by the institution.
- Tell the patient that he or she can drive without assistance after the procedure.
- Tell patients that they may read or talk to a child in the scanning room during the procedure, because no risk of radiation from the procedure exists.
- Assess the patient for any contraindications for testing (e.g., aneurysm clips).
- If possible, show the patient a picture of the scanning machine and encourage verbalization of anxieties. Some patients may experience claustrophobia. Antianxiety medications may be helpful for those with mild claustrophobia.

- Instruct the patient to remove all metal objects (e.g., dental bridges, jewelry, hair clips, belts, credit cards), because they will create artifacts on the scan. The magnetic field can damage watches and credit cards. Also, movement of metal objects within the magnetic field can be detrimental to anyone within the field.
- Inform the patient that he or she will be required to remain motionless during this study. Any movement can cause artifacts on the scan.
- Tell the patient that during the procedure, he or she may hear a thumping sound. Earplugs are available if the patient wishes to use them.
- Inform the patient that no fluid or food restrictions are necessary before MRI.
- For comfort, instruct the patient to empty his or her bladder before the test.

During
- Note the following:
  1. The patient lies on a platform that slides into a tube containing the doughnut-shaped magnet.
  2. The patient is instructed to lie very still during the procedure.
  3. During the scan, the patient can talk to and hear the staff via microphone or earphones placed in the scanner.
  4. A contrast medium called gadolinium (Magnevist) has been approved by the U.S. Food and Drug Administration. This is a paramagnetic enhancement agent that crosses the blood-brain barrier. It is especially useful for distinguishing edema from tumors. If this is to be administered, approximately 10 to 15 ml is injected in the vein. Imaging can begin shortly after the injection. No dietary restrictions are necessary before using this new agent.
- Note that this procedure is performed by a qualified radiologic technologist in approximately 30 to 90 minutes.
- Tell the patient that the only discomfort associated with this procedure may be lying still on a hard surface and a possible tingling sensation in teeth containing metal fillings. Also, an injection is needed for administration of Magnevist.

After
- Inform the patient that no special postprocedural care is needed.

M

Abnormal findings

Brain

Cerebral tumor
Cerebral infarction
Aneurysm
Arteriovenous malformation

Hemorrhage
Subdural hematoma
Multiple sclerosis

Other

Tumor (primary or meta-
   static)
Myocardial infarction
Atherosclerotic plaques
Aortic dissection
Aortic occlusion and stenosis
Abscess

Edema
Congenital heart disease
Dementia
Bone destructive lesion
Joint disorder
Degenerative vertebral disks

notes

mammography (Mammogram)

Type of test X-ray

Normal findings Negative (no tumor noted)

Test explanation and related physiology

Mammography is an x-ray examination of the breast. Careful interpretation of these x-ray films can identify cancers. In many cases, these cancers can be detected before they become palpable lesions. It is believed that early detection of breast cancer may improve patient survival. Radiographic signs of breast cancer include fine, stippled, clustered calcifications (white specks on the breast x-ray films); a poorly defined spiculated mass; asymmetric density; and skin thickening.

Although mammography is not a substitute for breast biopsy, it is reliable and accurate when interpreted by a skilled radiologist. The accuracy of detection of breast cancer with mammography has been approximately 85%. Usually, cancers that are not detected by mammography are in areas of the breast not well imaged by x-ray films (the high axillary tail of the breast). Almost 35% of breast cancers are not palpable and are detected only by mammography. Therefore the combination of mammography and close physical examination provides the best approach to detect breast cancer at its earliest stage.

Some controversy surrounds the role of a mammogram in screening asymptomatic patients. Several large U.S. studies have encouraged mammography yearly after age 40 years. Women over age 50 should have a mammogram yearly. Women who are at great risk for breast cancer (e.g., those who have had a cancer on the opposite side) should have mammograms yearly regardless of age.

Mammography also can detect other diseases of the breast. These include acute suppurative mastitis, abscess, fibrocystic changes, gross cysts, benign tumors (e.g., fibroadenoma), and intraglandular lymph nodes.

In the past, radiation exposure was quite significant with mammography. Today, however, because of fast-speed film, little radiation is required to expose mammogram film. Therefore the patient receives minimal radiation exposure during this test.

A *xeromammogram* provides the same information as routine mammography and has the same risks. Unlike regular x-ray films, which are negative films, xeromammograms are positive prints. The form of mammography used depends on the preference of the radiologist who must interpret the mammogram; however, the use of xeroradiography is decreasing. Newer, "dedicated" mammogram units provide more accurate and easily interpretable x-ray films.

Contraindications
- Patients who are pregnant, because of the risk of fetal damage

Interfering factors
- Talc powder can give the impression of calcification within the breast.
- Jewelry worn around the neck can preclude total visualization of the breast.
- Breast augmentation implants prevent total visualization of the breast.

Procedure and patient care

Before
- Explain the procedure to the patient. Inform the patient that some discomfort may be experienced during breast compression. This compression allows better visualization of the breast tissue. Assure the patient that the breast will not be harmed by the compression.
- Tell the patient that no fasting is required.
- Explain to the patient that a minimal radiation dose will be used during the test.
- Instruct the patient to disrobe above the waist and put on an x-ray gown.

During
- Note the following procedural steps:
  1. The patient is taken to the radiology department and seated in front of a mammogram machine.
  2. One breast is placed on the x-ray plate.
  3. The x-ray cone is brought down on the top of the breast to compress it gently between the broadened cone and the x-ray plate.
  4. The x-ray film is exposed. This is the craniocaudal view.
  5. The x-ray plate is turned about 45 degrees medially and placed on the inner aspect of the breast.
  6. The broadened cone is brought in medially and again

eral view.

gently compresses the breast. This creates the mediolateral view.

7. Occasionally, other views, such as direct lateral (90-degree) or magnified spot views, are obtained to more clearly visualize an area of suspicion.

- Note that mammography is performed by a radiologic technologist in approximately 10 minutes. The x-ray films are interpreted by a radiologist.
- Tell the patient that very little discomfort is associated with mammography. Remind the patient that some pain may be caused by the pressure required to compress the breast tissue while the x-ray films are being taken. If the patient has very tender breasts, this may be painful.

After

- Take this opportunity to instruct the patient in breast self-examination.

Abnormal findings

Breast cancer
Benign tumor (e.g., fibroadenoma)
Breast cyst

Fibrocystic changes
Breast abscess
Suppurative mastitis

M

notes

Meckel's diverticulum nuclear scan

Type of test Nuclear medicine

Normal findings No increased uptake of radionuclide in the right lower quadrant of the abdomen

Test explanation and related physiology

Meckel's diverticulum is the most common congenital abnormality of the intestinal tract. It is a persistent remnant of the omphalomesenteric tract. The diverticulum usually occurs in the ileum, approximately 2 feet proximal to the ileocecal valve. Approximately 20% to 25% of Meckel's diverticulum is lined internally by ectopic gastric mucosa. This gastric mucosa can secrete acid and cause ulceration of the intestinal mucosa nearby. Bleeding, inflammation, and intussusception are other potential complications of this congenital abnormality. The majority of these complications occur by 2 years of age.

Both normal gastric mucosa within the stomach and ectopic gastric mucosa in Meckel's diverticulum concentrate ^{99m}Tc pertechnetate. When this radionuclide is injected intravenously, it is concentrated in the ectopic gastric mucosa of Meckel's diverticulum. One can then expect to see a hot spot in the right lower quadrant of the abdomen at about the same time as the normal stomach mucosa is visualized. This is a very sensitive and specific test for this congenital abnormality.

It is possible that Meckel's diverticulum is present but contains no ectopic gastric mucosa within. Usually, these are not symptomatic. No concentration of radionuclide will occur within the diverticulum. This test is not helpful in these cases.

Other conditions can simulate a hot spot compatible with Merkel's diverticulum containing ectopic gastric mucosa. Usually, these are associated with inflammatory processes within the abdomen (e.g., appendicitis or ectopic pregnancy).

Procedure and patient care

Before

- Explain the procedure to the patient.
- Advise the patient to refrain from eating or drinking anything for 6 to 12 hours before the examination.
- A histamine H_2-receptor antagonist is usually given for 1 to 2 days before the scan. This blocks secretion of the radionu-

clide from the ectopic gastric mucosa and improves visualization of Meckel's diverticulum.

During

- The patient lies in a supine position, and a large-view nuclear detector camera is placed over the patient's abdomen to identify concentration of nuclear material after intravenous injection.
- Images are taken at 5-minute intervals for 1 hour.
- Patients may be asked to lie on their left side to minimize the excretion of the radionuclide from the normal stomach and flood the intestine with radionuclide, precluding visualization of Meckel's diverticulum.
- Occasionally, glucagon is provided to prolong intestinal transit time and avoid downstream contamination with the radionuclide.
- Occasionally, gastrin is given to increase the uptake of the radionuclide by the ectopic gastric mucosa.
- There is no pain associated with this test.

After

- The patient is asked to void, and a repeat image is obtained. This is to ensure that Meckel's diverticulum has not been hidden by a distended bladder.
- Because only tracer doses of radioisotopes are used, inform the patient that no precautions need to be taken by others against radiation.

Abnormal findings

Increased uptake in the right lower quadrant is compatible with Meckel's diverticula containing ectopic gastric mucosa.

notes

mediastinoscopy

Type of test Endoscopy

Normal findings No abnormal mediastinal lymph node tissue

Test explanation and related physiology

Mediastinoscopy is a surgical procedure in which a mediastinoscope (a lighted instrument scope) is inserted through a small incision made at the suprasternal notch. The scope is passed into the superior mediastinum to inspect the mediastinal lymph nodes and to remove biopsy specimens. Because these lymph nodes receive lymphatic drainage from the lungs, their assessment can provide information on intrathoracic diseases such as carcinoma, granulomatous infections, and sarcoidosis; therefore mediastinoscopy is used in establishing the diagnosis of various intrathoracic diseases. This procedure is also employed to "stage" patients with lung cancer and to assess whether they are surgical candidates. Evidence of metastasis is usually a contraindication to thoracotomy because the tumor is considered inoperable. Tumors occurring in the mediastinum (e.g., thymoma or lymphoma) can also be biopsied through the mediastinoscope.

Potential complication

- Puncture of the esophagus, trachea, or blood vessels

Procedure and patient care

Before

- Explain the procedure to the patient.
- Ensure that the physician has obtained the informed consent for this procedure.
- Check whether the patient's blood needs to be typed and crossmatched.
- Provide preoperative care as with any other surgical procedure.
- Keep the patient NPO after midnight on the day of the test.
- Administer preprocedural medication approximately 1 hour before the test as ordered.

During

- Note the following procedural steps:
  1. The patient is taken to the operating room for this surgical procedure.

2. The patient is placed under general anesthesia.
3. An incision is made in the suprasternal notch.
4. The mediastinoscope is passed through this neck incision and into the superior mediastinum.
5. The lymph nodes are biopsied.
6. The scope is withdrawn, and the incision is sutured closed.

- Note that this procedure is performed by a surgeon in approximately 1 hour.
- Inform the patient that he or she is asleep during the procedure.

After

- Provide postoperative care as with any other surgical procedure.

Abnormal findings

Lung cancer
Metastasis
Sarcoidosis
Thymoma

Tuberculosis
Hodgkin's disease
Lymphoma

M

notes

metyrapone

Type of test Blood; urine (24-hour)

Normal findings

24-hour urine: baseline excretion of urinary 17-
   hydroxycorticosteroid (OCHS) more than doubled
Blood: 11-deoxycortisol increased to >7 µg/dl and cortisol
   <10 µg/dl

Test explanation and related physiology

This test is useful in differentiating adrenal hyperplasia from a
primary adrenal tumor by determining whether the pituitary-
adrenal feedback mechanism is intact. Metyrapone (Metopirone)
is a potent blocker of an enzyme involved in cortisol production. Cortisol production is therefore reduced. When this drug
is given, the resulting fall in cortisol production should stimulate pituitary secretion of adrenocorticotropic hormone (ACTH)
by way of a negative feedback system. Cortisol itself cannot be
synthesized because of the metyrapone inhibition of the 11-beta-
hydroxylation step, but an abundance of cortisol precursors (11-
deoxycortisol and OCHS) will be formed. These cortisol precursors can be detected in the urine or in the blood. This test is
similar to the ACTH stimulation test (see p. 16).

In patients with adrenal hyperplasia, the cortisol precursors are
greatly increased, more than expected in normal patients. No response to metyrapone occurs in patients with Cushing's syndrome resulting from adrenal adenoma or carcinoma, because
the tumors are autonomous and therefore insensitive to changes
in ACTH secretion. This test has no significant advantage over
the ACTH stimulation test in the differential diagnosis of Cushing's disease.

This test is also used to document that adrenal insufficiency
exists as a result of pituitary disease (secondary adrenal insufficiency). This test should not be performed if primary adrenal insufficiency is likely. Severe, life-threatening adrenal crisis could
be precipitated. A normal response to ACTH should be demonstrated before metyrapone is given.

Contraindications

- Patients with possible adrenal insufficiency

Potential complications

- Addison's disease and Addisonian crisis, because metyrapone inhibits cortisol production

Interfering factors

- Recent administration of radioisotopes will interfere with test results.
- Chlorpromazine (Thorazine) interferes with the response to metyrapone and should not be administered during the testing.

Procedure and patient care

Before

- Explain the procedure to the patient.
- Obtain a baseline 24-hour urine specimen for 17-OCHS level (see p. 469) for the urine test.
- Obtain a baseline cortisol level (see p. 285) for the blood test.

During

Blood

- Administer 2 to 3 g of metyrapone at 11 PM the night before the blood specimen is to be collected. Collect a blood specimen in the morning.

Urine

- Obtain a 24-hour urine specimen for 17-OCHS level as a baseline. Then collect a 24-hour urine specimen for 17-OCHS level during and again 1 day after the oral administration of 500 to 750 mg of metyrapone, which is given every 4 hours for 24 hours.

After

- Assess the patient for impending signs of Addisonian crisis (muscle weakness, mental and emotional changes, anorexia, nausea, vomiting, hypotension, hyperkalemia, vascular collapse).
- Note that Addisonian crisis is a medical emergency that must be treated vigorously. Basically, the immediate treatment includes replenishing steroids, reversing shock, and restoring blood circulation.

Abnormal findings

Adrenal hyperplasia
Adrenal tumor
Ectopic ACTH syndrome
Secondary adrenal insufficiency

mononucleosis spot test (Mononuclear heterophil test, Heterophil antibody test, Monospot test)

Type of test Blood

Normal findings Negative (<1:28 titer)

Test explanation and related physiology

The mononucleosis test is performed to aid in the diagnosis of infectious mononucleosis, a disease caused by the Epstein-Barr virus (EBV). An EBV titer may also be done (see p. 360). Usually, young adults are affected by mononucleosis. The clinical presentation is fever, pharyngitis, lymphadenopathy, and splenomegaly. Approximately 2 weeks after the onset of the disease, many patients are found to have immunoglobulin M (IgM) antibodies in their serum that react against warm red blood cells (RBCs). When these antibodies are present in serial dilutions of greater than 1:56, infectious mononucleosis can be strongly considered. However, false-positive results occur, and patients with lymphoma or systemic lupus erythematosus occasionally also may have this antibody. Patients with Burkitt's lymphoma, leukemia, and some gastrointestinal cancers also have false-positive test results. Burkitt's lymphoma is strongly associated with EBV.

Several heterophil agglutination tests are available, but the most frequently performed is the spot test for infectious mononucleosis (monospot test). Heterophil antibodies produced by humans react with RBCs of another species. The test is performed by placing the serially diluted patient's serum on one side of the slide and mixing it with guinea pig kidney antigen (containing only Forssman antigen). On the other side of the slide, the patient's serum is mixed with beef RBCs (containing only infectious mononuclear antigen). Horse RBCs (containing Forssman and infectious mononucleosis antigens) are then applied to each slide. Agglutination of the beef RBCs indicates the presence of the infectious mononuclear heterophil antibody-antigen complexes and thus confirms the diagnosis of infectious mononucleosis.

Procedure and patient care

Before

- Explain the procedure to the patient.

- Tell the patient that no fasting or special preparation is required.

During

- Collect approximately 7 to 10 ml of venous blood in a red-top tube.

After

- Apply pressure or a pressure dressing to the venipuncture site.
- Observe the venipuncture site for bleeding.

Abnormal findings

Infectious mononucleosis
Chronic EBV infection
Chronic fatigue syndrome
Burkitt's lymphoma
Some forms of chronic hepatitis

notes

M

myelography (Myelogram)

Type of test X-ray with contrast dye

Normal findings Normal spinal canal

Test explanation and related physiology

By placing radiopaque dye (or air) into the subarachnoid space of the spinal canal, the contents of the canal can be fluoroscopically outlined. Cord tumors, meningeal tumors, metastatic spinal tumors, herniated intravertebral disks, and arthritic bone spurs can be readily detected by this study. These lesions appear as canal narrowing or as varying degrees of obstruction to the flow of the dye column within the canal. The entire canal (from lumbar to cervical areas) can be examined. This test is indicated in patients with severe back pain or localized neurologic signs that suggest the canal as the location of these injuries. Because this test is usually performed by lumbar puncture (LP, see p. 526), all the potential complications of that procedure exist.

Different types of contrast material can be used for myelography. Pantopaque is most often used as the *oil-based* medium. An oil-based dye must be aspirated as much as possible after the procedure before removing the spinal needle, because the dye persists indefinitely. The patient's head is then kept elevated above the level of the spine to prevent upward dispersion of the dye, which could cause meningeal irritation. Because the oil base is heavier than cerebrospinal fluid (CSF), it stays in the lower canal. After the dye is completely removed, the patient may be kept flat for up to 12 hours.

A *water-soluble* contrast material, metrizamide (Amipaque), is now frequently used for myelography. This dye is absorbed by the blood and excreted by the kidneys. Metrizamide has two advantages over the oil-based medium. First, metrizamide does not need to be removed at the end of the procedure, because it is water soluble and will be completely reabsorbed. This feature reduces the length of the procedure and minimizes the discomfort associated with dye removal. Second, metrizamide is less viscous than the iodine, oil-based dye and therefore permits better visualization of small areas (e.g., nerves, nerve roots, nerve sheaths). Also, metrizamide can flow freely through narrow canals and afford better differentiation of complete and incomplete spinal blockages. The disadvantage associated with metrizamide is that it may precipitate seizure activity after the procedure. To prevent this, the patient should be well hydrated and should avoid medications (e.g., phenothiazines, tricyclic antidepressants, central nervous system [CNS] stimulants, amphetamines) that could decrease the seizure threshold. A water-soluble contrast agent, Omnipaque, has a significantly lower risk of CNS toxicity than does metrizamide and is now more routinely used.

After the procedure, the patient's head and thorax should be elevated 30 to 50 degrees for approximately 6 to 8 hours to reduce upward dispersion of the dye and to prevent contact of the water-soluble agent with the cerebral meninges, which could precipitate a seizure. Bed rest may be ordered for up to 24 hours.

To avoid some of the side effects associated with radiopaque substances, some neurosurgeons prefer to use *air-contrast myelography*. After air myelography, the patient is positioned with the head lower than the trunk to prevent air from gravitating to the cerebral space and causing headaches. This position is usually maintained for approximately 48 hours. Most of the air will be absorbed by this time, and the head can then be elevated.

Contraindications

- Patients with multiple sclerosis, because exacerbation may be precipitated by myelography
- Patients with increased intracranial pressure, because LP may cause herniation of the brain
- Patients with infection near the LP site, because this may precipitate a bacterial meningitis
- Patients who are allergic to shellfish or iodinated dye

Potential complications

- Headache
- Meningitis
- Herniation of the brain
- Seizures
- Allergic reaction to iodinated dye
  Allergic reactions vary from mild flushing, itching, and urticaria to severe, life-threatening anaphylaxis (evidenced by respiratory distress, drop in blood pressure, shock). In the unusual event of anaphylaxis, the patient may be treated with diphenhydramine (Benadryl), steroids, and epinephrine.

Oxygen and endotracheal equipment should be on hand for immediate use.

Procedure and patient care

Before

- Explain the procedure to the patient.
- Ensure that the physician has obtained written and informed consent for this procedure.
- Assess the patient for allergies to iodinated contrast dye or shellfish.
- Inform the radiologist if an allergy to iodinated contrast is suspected. The radiologist may prescribe a Benadryl-and-steroid preparation to be administered before testing. Usually, a hypoallergenic, non-ionic contrast will be used during the test.
- Ascertain whether the patient has recently taken phenothiazines, tricyclic antidepressants, CNS stimulants, or amphetamines if a water-soluble contrast (metrizamide) will be used. These medications should be avoided, because they could decrease the seizure threshold.
- Have the patient empty the bladder and bowel before myelography if possible.
- Explain to the patient that he or she must lie very still during the procedure.
- Note that food and fluid restrictions vary according to the type of dye used. Check with the radiology department for specific restrictions.
- Inform the patient that he or she will be tilted into an up-and-down position on the table so that the dye can properly fill the spinal canal and provide adequate visualization in the desired area.

During

- Note the following procedural steps:
  1. A lumbar puncture (see p. 526) or cisternal puncture (see p. 242) is performed.
  2. Fifteen ml of CSF is withdrawn, and 15 ml or more of radiopaque dye or air is injected into the spinal canal. Because the specific gravity of the dye is greater than that of the CSF, the direction of dye flow will depend on the tilt of the table and the patient's position.
  3. With the needle in place, the patient is placed in the prone position on the tilt table with the head tilted

down. A foot support and shoulder brace or harness will keep the patient from sliding.

4. The lights are turned off, and the column of dye is followed in a cephalad direction with fluoroscopy.
5. Representative x-ray films are taken.
6. Obstructions to the flow of the dye are evident, and the level of the lesion is easily detected.
7. After myelography is performed, the needle is removed and a dressing is applied.
8. The patient is returned to the unit on a stretcher and is kept on bed rest.

- Note that this procedure is done by a radiologist in approximately 45 minutes.
- Keep in mind that patient response varies from mild discomfort to severe pain.

After

- Note that nursing interventions after the procedure depend on the type of contrast used.
- Usually, place the patient on bed rest for several hours afterward as indicated. Position the patient as specifically ordered by the physician in consultation with the radiologist. The head position varies with the dye used. For example, the head is usually elevated after using oil-based and water-soluble contrast agents. After an air-contrast study, the head is positioned lower than the trunk.
- Observe the patient for signs and symptoms of meningeal irritation (e.g., fever, stiff neck, occipital headache, photophobia).
- Observe the patient for seizure activity if metrizamide dye was used.
- If metrizamide was used, do *not* administer medications (e.g., phenothiazines) that may precipitate seizure activity.
- Monitor the patient's vital signs and ability to void.
- Encourage the patient to drink fluids to enhance excretion of the dye and to hasten replacement of CSF.
- Evaluate the patient for delayed reaction to dye (dyspnea, rashes, tachycardia, hives). This usually occurs within the first 2 to 6 hours after the test. Treat with antihistamines or steroids.

M

Abnormal findings

Cord tumor
Meningeal tumor
Metastatic spinal tumor
Meningioma
Cervical ankylosing spondylo-
    sis
Arthritic lumbar stenosis

Herniated intravertebral disks
Arthritic bone spurs
Neurofibroma
Avulsion of nerve roots
Cysts
Astrocytoma

notes

myoglobin

Type of test Blood

Normal findings 0-85 ng/ml or 0-85 nmol/L (SI units)

Test explanation and related physiology

Myoglobin is an oxygen-binding protein found in cardiac and skeletal muscle. Measurement of myoglobin is an index of damage to the myocardium, such as occurs in myocardial infarction (MI) or reinfarction. Increased levels, which indicate cardiac muscle injury or death, occur in about 3 hours. Although this test is more sensitive than creatine phosphokinase isoenzymes (see p. 293), it is not as specific, because trauma, inflammation, or ischemic changes to the noncardiac skeletal muscles also can cause elevated levels of myoglobin. The benefit of myoglobin over CPK-MB (see p. 293) is that it may become elevated earlier in some patients. This may prove beneficial, since thrombolytic therapy is to be started within the first 6 hours after an MI. As already indicated, disease or trauma of the skeletal muscle also causes elevations in myoglobin. With sudden and severe muscle injury, myoglobin levels can get very high. Because myoglobin is excreted in the urine and is nephrotoxic, the levels must be monitored in these types of patients. Myoglobin can also be measured in the urine. To screen for myoglobin, the routine urine dipstick for hemoglobin will also react for myoglobin.

Interfering factors

- Recent administration of radioactive substances may affect test results.
- Increased myoglobin levels can occur after IM injections.

Procedure and patient care

Before

- Explain the procedure to the patient.
- Tell the patient that no fasting is required.

During

- Collect approximately 5 ml of venous blood in a red-top tube.

After
- Apply pressure or a pressure dressing to the venipuncture site.
- Observe the venipuncture site for bleeding.

Abnormal findings

▲ **Increased levels**

Myocardial infarction
Skeletal muscle inflammation (myositis)
Malignant hyperthermia

Muscular dystrophy
Skeletal muscle ischemia
Skeletal muscle trauma
Rhabdomyolysis

notes

nonstress fetal test (NST, Fetal activity determination)

Type of test Fetal activity study

Normal findings "Reactive" fetus (heart rate acceleration associated with fetal movement)

Test explanation and related physiology

The NST is a noninvasive study that monitors acceleration of the fetal heart rate (FHR) in response to fetal movement. This FHR acceleration reflects the integrity of the central nervous system and fetal well-being. Fetal activity may be spontaneous, induced by uterine contraction, or induced by external manipulation. Oxytocin stimulation is not used. Fetal response is characterized as "reactive" or "nonreactive." The NST indicates a reactive fetus when, with fetal movement, two or more FHR accelerations are detected, each of which must be at least 15 beats/min for 15 seconds or more within any 10-minute period. The test is 99% reliable in indicating fetal viability and negates the need for the contraction stress test (CST, see p. 277). If the test detects a nonreactive fetus (i.e., no FHR acceleration with fetal movement) within 40 minutes, the patient is a candidate for the CST. A 40-minute test period is used, because this is the average duration of the sleep-wake cycle of the fetus. The cycle may vary considerably, however.

The NST is useful in screening high-risk pregnancies and in selecting those patients who may require the CST. An NST is now routinely performed before the CST to avoid the complications associated with oxytocin administration. No complications are associated with the NST.

Procedure and patient care

Before

- Explain the procedure to the patient.
- Encourage verbalization of the patient's fears. The necessity for the study usually raises realistic fears in the expectant mother.
- If the patient is hungry, instruct her to eat before the NST is begun. Fetal activity is enhanced with a high maternal serum glucose level.

N

During

- After the patient empties her bladder, place her in Sims' position.
- Place an external fetal monitor on the patient's abdomen to record the FHR. The mother can indicate fetal movement by pressing a button on the fetal monitor whenever she feels the fetus move. FHR and fetal movement are concomitantly recorded on a two-channel strip graph.
- Observe the fetal monitor for FHR accelerations associated with fetal movement.
- If the fetus is quiet for 20 minutes, stimulate fetal activity by external methods, such as rubbing or compressing the mother's abdomen, ringing a bell near the abdomen, or placing a pan on the abdomen and hitting the pan.
- Note that a nurse performs the NST in approximately 20 to 40 minutes in the physician's office or a hospital unit.
- Tell the patient that no discomfort is associated with NST.

After

- If the results detect a nonreactive fetus, inform the patient that she is a candidate for the CST.

Abnormal finding

Nonreactive fetus

notes

5'-nucleotidase

Type of test Blood

Normal findings 0.0-1.6 U or 27-233 nmol/sec/L (SI units)

Test explanation and related physiology

5'-Nucleotidase is an enzyme specific to the liver. The 5'-nucleotidase level is elevated in patients with liver diseases, especially those associated with cholestasis. Although levels of other enzymes such as alkaline phosphatase (ALP), alanine aminotransferase (ALT), and aspartate aminotransferase (AST) are elevated with liver diseases, diseases in other organs also may cause elevations of these enzymes. However, when levels of these enzymes *and* 5'-nucleotidase are elevated, the disease is located specifically within the liver. When the ALT, AST, and ALP levels are elevated and the 5'-nucleotidase level is normal, disease exists in organs that make these enzymes other than the liver (e.g., bone, spleen, kidney).

Interfering factors

✠ Drugs that may cause *increased* 5'-nucleotidase levels include hepatotoxic agents.

N

Procedure and patient care

Before
- Explain the procedure to the patient.
- Tell the patient that no fasting is required.

During
- Collect approximately 7 to 10 ml of venous blood in a red-top tube.
- Indicate on the laboratory slip any medication the patient may be taking to aid in the interpretation of test results.

After
- Apply pressure or a pressure dressing to the venipuncture site.
- Assess the venipuncture site for bleeding. Patients with liver dysfunction often have prolonged clotting times.

Abnormal findings

▲ **Increased levels**

Bile duct obstruction
Cholestasis
Hepatitis
Cirrhosis

Hepatic necrosis
Hepatic ischemia
Hepatic tumor
Hepatotoxic drugs

notes

obstruction series (KUB, Flat plate of the abdomen, Plain film of the abdomen, Scout film)

Type of test X-ray

Normal findings

No evidence of bowel obstruction
No abnormal calcifications
No free air

Test explanation and related physiology

The obstruction series is a group of x-ray films performed on the abdomen of patients with suspected bowel obstruction, paralytic ileus, perforated viscus, abdominal abscess, kidney stones, appendicitis, or foreign body ingestion. This series of films usually consists of at least two x-ray studies. The first is an erect abdominal film that should include visualization of both diaphragms. The film is examined for evidence of free air under either diaphragm, which is pathognomonic for a perforated viscus. This view is also used to detect air-fluid levels within the intestine; the presence of an air-fluid level is compatible with bowel obstruction or paralytic ileus. Occasionally, patients are too ill to stand erect. In this case, an x-ray film can be taken with the patient in the left lateral decubitus position. If free air is present, it will be seen between the liver and the right side of the abdominal wall. As with the erect-position film, air-fluid levels also can be detected.

The second view in the obstruction series is usually a supine abdominal x-ray study. This is very similar to the kidney, ureter, and bladder x-ray study (see p. 499). An abdominal abscess may be seen as a cluster of tiny bubbles within one localized area. A calcification within the course of the ureter could indicate a kidney ureteral stone. A small calcification in the right lower quadrant on the film of a patient complaining of pain in this quadrant may be an appendicolith. A gas-filled, distended bowel is compatible with bowel obstruction or paralytic ileus.

The obstruction series can also be used to monitor the clinical course of patients with gastrointestinal (GI) disease. For example, repeated obstruction series on patients who have a par-

O

tial small bowel obstruction or paralytic ileus can indicate worsening or improvement of the clinical situation.

Frequently, a cross-table lateral view of the abdomen is included in an obstruction series to detect abdominal aorta calcification, which often occurs in older patients. The calcification represents the anterior wall of the aorta. If an aortic aneurysm exists, this calcification will be seen to protrude from the spine.

Finally, the supine abdominal x-ray study can be used as a "scout film" before performing GI or abdominal x-ray studies that use contrast, such as a barium enema (see p. 120) or intravenous pyelogram (see p. 487).

Contraindications

- Patients who are pregnant

Interfering factor

- Previous GI barium contrast study

  Although at times barium within the GI tract can preclude the identification of other important calcifications (e.g., kidney stones), barium can be helpful in outlining the GI anatomy.

Procedure and patient care

Before

- Explain the procedure to the patient.
- Ensure that all radiopaque clothing has been removed.
- Remind the patient that no GI contrast will be used.

During

- Although the procedure varies from facility to facility, note that usually a supine abdominal x-ray film, erect abdominal film, and perhaps a lower erect chest film are taken. Often, a cross-table, lateral x-ray film is also included.
- Note that the obstruction series is performed in minutes in the radiology department by a radiologic technologist; however, it can be performed at the bedside with a portable x-ray machine. A radiologist interprets the films.
- Tell the patient that no discomfort is associated with this study.

After

- Note that no special aftercare is needed.

Abnormal findings

Kidney stone
Bowel obstruction
Organomegaly
Presence of a foreign body
Bladder distention
Abdominal abscess
Perforated viscus

Abdominal aortic calcification
Appendicolithiasis
Paralytic ileus
Abdominal aortic aneurysm
Peritoneal effusion
Abnormal position of the kidneys

notes

o

oculoplethysmography (OPG)

Type of test Manometric

Normal findings Normal and equal blood flow in both carotid arteries

Test explanation and related physiology

OPG is a noninvasive study used to indirectly measure blood flow in the ophthalmic artery. Because the ophthalmic artery is the first major branch of the internal carotid artery, its blood flow reflects the carotid blood flow and the alternative blood flow to the brain.

For this study, eye pressures are measured through suction cups placed on the eyes for the recording. OPG is indicated in patients who have symptoms of carotid occlusive disease (e.g., transient ischemic attacks, carotid bruits, neurologic symptoms [e.g., dizziness, fainting]). If indicated, this procedure may be followed by cerebral angiography. This test is often performed as a follow-up after carotid endarterectomy to prove patency of the carotid artery. Carotid Doppler flow studies (see p. 211) are more easily performed and are therefore being used more frequently.

Contraindications

- Patients who have had eye surgery within the last 2 to 6 months
- Patients who have a lens implant
- Patients who have had retinal detachment
- Patients with cataracts
- Patients who are allergic to local anesthetics

Potential complications

- Conjunctival hemorrhage
- Corneal abrasions
  If corneal abrasions occur, the patient's eye is patched and a lubricant (e.g., Dacriose solution) is applied.
- Transient photophobia

Procedure and patient care

Before
- Explain the procedure to the patient.
- Instruct the patient to remove contact lenses if applicable.

- Inform patients with glaucoma to take their usual medications and eye drops.
- Tell the patient that no fasting or sedation is necessary.

During

- Note the following procedural steps:
  1. The patient is asked to lie on his or her back on a table or bed.
  2. Blood pressure in both arms is taken before the test.
  3. Electrocardiographic (EKG) electrodes are applied to the patient's extremities to detect abnormal cardiac rhythms.
  4. Anesthetic eye drops are instilled in both eyes to minimize discomfort.
  5. Small detectors are attached to the earlobes to detect blood flow to the ear through the external carotid artery.
  6. Tracings for both ears are taken and compared.
  7. Suction cups resembling contact lenses are applied directly to the eyeball.
  8. Tracings of the pulsations within each eye are recorded.
  9. A vacuum source is applied to the suction cup. This increased pressure causes the pulse in both eyes to disappear temporarily, because all blood flow to the eye is stopped.
  10. When the suction source is stopped, the blood flow returns to the eyes. Both pulses should return simultaneously.
  11. The time difference in the pulse rate from one eye to the other, one ear to the other, and one ear to the eye on the other side is measured in milliseconds. If internal carotid stenosis is present, blood flow to the eye will be delayed.
- Note that a trained technologist performs this test in approximately 20 to 30 minutes.
- Tell the patient that eyes usually burn slightly when the ophthalmic drops are applied.
- Inform the patient that when suction is applied, he or she may feel a pulling sensation and vision may temporarily be lost.

After

- Inform the patient that the eye anesthesia usually wears off in approximately 30 minutes.

O

- Instruct the patient not to rub his or her eyes for at least 2 hours. If tears appear, the eye should be blotted dry.
- Inform the patient that contact lenses should not be inserted for at least 2 hours after OPG.
- Tell the patient that the eyes may appear bloodshot for several hours after the test. Artificial tears may be instilled to soothe any irritation in the eyes.
- Inform the patient to wear sunglasses if photophobia is present.

Abnormal finding

Carotid atherosclerotic stenosis

notes

oncoscint scan (Immunoscintigraphy)

Type of test Nuclear medicine

Normal findings No increased uptake of radionuclide in the body

Test explanation and related physiology

Immunoscintigraphy is a new procedure. At present, it is used to detect recurrent metastatic colorectal or ovarian cancer. The radionuclide indium chloride-111 is attached to a monoclonal antibody that is commonly on the cell surface of colorectal and ovarian cancer cells. When injected, this radionuclide-antibody conjugate attaches to the cancer cells. With the use of a nuclear counter camera, whole-body images are obtained. Areas of increased uptake may represent tumor.

This scan is not 100% accurate and can be incorrectly negative up to 30% of the time. When positive, however, its accuracy meets or exceeds the accuracy of a computed tomography (CT) scan. This new diagnostic procedure can assist in the decision making of patients with metastatic or recurrent colorectal or ovarian adenocarcinoma. It is very helpful in determining the source of a rising tumor marker (see CEA, p. 194, or CA-125, p. 179) in patients with an otherwise normal diagnostic evaluation. It is particularly helpful in determining extrahepatic abdominal and pelvic recurrent tumors. Also, it is very helpful in differentiating postsurgical or postradiation anatomic changes from recurrent cancer. The former do not take up tracer; the latter does.

Contraindications

- Nursing mothers

Procedure and patient care

Before

- Explain the procedure to the patient.
- Explain that no fasting is required before the test.
- Because the radionuclide can be concentrated in areas of degenerated joint disease, abdominal aortic aneurysms, abdominal inflammatory processes, or inflammatory bowel disease, a careful history should be obtained before scanning.

During

- The patient is injected with the radiolabeled monoclonal antibody.
- Initial images are obtained 48 to 72 hours after IV infusion.
- The patient is asked to lie on a padded table.
- A nuclear counter camera is placed over the anterior or posterior surface of the chest, abdomen, and pelvis. Approximately 10 minutes is required for each view.
- The patient may be asked to return the following day or the day after that for repeated images.
- Little or no discomfort is associated with this procedure.
- The procedure takes approximately 1 hour each day for at least 1 to 4 days.
- This procedure is performed in the nuclear medicine department.

After

- Because only tracer doses of radioisotopes are used, inform the patient that no precautions need to be taken by others against radiation exposure.

Abnormal findings

▲ **Increased uptake**
Recurrent colorectal cancer
Ovarian cancer

notes

osmolality, blood (Serum osmolality)

Type of test Blood

Normal findings
Adult/elderly: 285-295 mOsm/kg H_2O
Child: 275-290 mOsm/kg H_2O

Possible critical values
<265 mOsm/kg H_2O
>320 mOsm/kg H_2O

Test explanation and related physiology

Osmolality measures the concentration of particles in blood. As the amount of free water in the blood increases or the amount of particles decreases, osmolality decreases. As the amount of water in the blood decreases or the amount of particles increases, osmolality increases. Osmolality increases with dehydration and decreases with overhydration. Increased osmolality will stimulate secretion of antidiuretic hormone (ADH); this will result in increased water reabsorption, more concentrated urine, and less concentrated serum. A low serum osmolality will suppress the release of ADH, resulting in decreased water reabsorption and large amounts of dilute urine.

The serum osmolality test is useful in evaluating fluid and electrolyte imbalance and in evaluating the presence of organic acids, sugars, or ethanol. The test is very helpful in the evaluation of seizures, liver disease, hydration status, acid-base balance, and ADH function. Osmolality also has an important role in toxicology and workups for coma patients. Values of 385 mOsm/kg of water are associated with stupor in patients with hyperglycemia. When values of 400 to 420 are detected, grand mal seizures can occur. Values greater than 420 can be lethal.

Interfering factors

- Diseases such as cerebrovascular accident (stroke) or brain tumors may interfere with test results through inappropriate secretion of ADH.

Procedure and patient care

Before
- Explain the procedure to the patient.
- Tell the patient that no fasting is required.

During
- Collect approximately 5 to 10 ml of venous blood in a red-top tube.
- For pediatric patients, draw blood from a heel stick.

After
- Apply pressure or a pressure dressing to the venipuncture site.
- Observe the venipuncture site for bleeding.

Abnormal findings

▲ **Increased levels**
Hypernatremia
Dehydration
Hyperglycemia
Mannitol therapy
Azotemia
Uremia
Ingestion of ethanol, methanol, or ethylene glycol
Hyperosmolar nonketotic hyperglycemia
Diabetes inspidus
Hypercalcemia
Renal tubular necrosis
Severe pyelonephritis
Ketosis
Shock

▼ **Decreased levels**
Hyponatremia
Overhydration
Syndrome of inappropriate ADH secretion
Paraneoplastic syndromes associated with lung carcinoma
Excess fluid intake

notes

osmolality, urine (Urine osmolality)

Type of test Urine

Normal findings

12- to 14-hour fluid restriction: >850 mOsm/kg H_2O
(SI units)
Random specimen: 50-1400 mOsm/kg H_2O, depending on
fluid intake (SI units)

Possible critical values

<100 mOsm/kg H_2O in overhydration
>800 mOsm/kg H_2O in dehydration

Test explanation and related physiology

Osmolality is the measurement of the number of dissolved particles in a solution. It is a more exact measurement of urine concentration than specific gravity, because specific gravity depends
on the number and precise nature of the particles in the urine.
Specific gravity also requires correction for the presence of glucose or protein, as well as for temperature; in contrast, osmolality depends only on the number of particles of solute in a unit
of solution. Osmolality also can be measured over a wider range
than specific gravity and with greater accuracy.

Osmolality is used in the precise evaluation of the concentrating ability of the kidney (e.g., in acute and chronic renal failure). To measure the concentrating capability of the kidney, the
patient is usually asked to fast for 14 hours. This test is also used
to monitor electrolyte and water balance and to evaluate dehydration. In evaluating fluid status, a random urine specimen may
be adequate. Osmolality is valuable in the workup of patients
with renal disease, the syndrome of inappropriate antidiuretic
hormone (ADH) secretion, and diabetes insipidus. Osmolality
may be used as part of the urinalysis when the patient has glycosuria or proteinuria or has had tests that use radiopaque substances.

Procedure and patient care

Before
- Explain the procedure to the patient.
- Tell the patient that no special preparation is necessary for a
  random urine specimen.

- Inform the patient that preparation for a fasting urine specimen may require a high-protein diet for 3 days before the test. Instruct the patient to eat a dry supper the evening before the test and to drink no fluids until the test is completed the next morning.

During

- Collect a first-voided urine specimen for a random sample.
- For a fasting specimen, instruct the patient to empty the bladder at approximately 6 AM and to discard the urine. Collect the test urine at 8 AM.
- Indicate on the laboratory slip the patient's fasting status.

After

- Send the specimen to the laboratory.
- Provide food and fluids for the patient.

Abnormal findings

▲ **Increased levels**

Syndrome of inappropriate ADH secretion
Acidosis
Shock
Hypernatremia
Hepatic cirrhosis
Congestive heart failure
Addison's disease

▼ **Decreased levels**

Diabetes insipidus
Hypercalcemia
Excess fluid intake
Renal tubular necrosis
Aldosteronism
Hypokalemia
Severe pyelonephritis

notes

oximetry (Pulse oximetry, Ear oximetry, Oxygen saturation)

Type of test Photodiagnostic

Normal findings ≥95% or higher

Possible critical values ≤75%

Test explanation and related physiology

Oximetry is a noninvasive method of monitoring arterial blood oxygen saturation (Sao_2). The Sao_2 is the ratio of oxygenated hemoglobin to the total amount of hemoglobin. The Sao_2 is expressed as a percentage; for example, a saturation of 95% indicates that 95% of the total hemoglobin attachments for oxygen have oxygen attached to them. The Sao_2 is an accurate approximation of oxygen saturation obtained from arterial blood gas study (see p. 146). By correlating the Sao_2 and the patient's physiologic status, a close estimate of the partial oxygen pressure (Po_2) can be obtained.

Oximetry is typically used for monitoring the patient's oxygenation status during the perioperative period and for patients receiving mechanical ventilation. This test is also frequently used in many clinical situations, such as pulmonary rehabilitation programs, stress testing, and sleep laboratories. Oximetry can be used to assess the body's response to various drugs, such as theophylline, which causes bronchodilation, and methacholine, which evokes bronchospasm in people with asthma. Pulse oximetry is constantly monitored during the perioperative period. This test is one of the factors used to determine when the patient is discharged from the recovery room.

Procedure and patient care

Before

- Explain the procedure to the patient.
- Tell the patient that no fasting is required.

During

- Rub the patient's earlobe, pinna (upper portion of the ear), or fingertip to increase blood flow.
- Clip the monitoring probe or sensor to the ear or finger. The sensor warms and increases blood flow to the tissue. A beam of light passes through the tissue, and the sensor measures the amount of light the tissue absorbs (Figure 20).

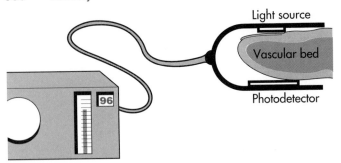

Figure 20 Oximetry. The pulse oximeter passes a beam of light through the tissue. The amount of light absorbed by the oxygen-saturated hemoglobin is measured by the sensor.

- Note that this study is usually performed by a respiratory therapist or nurse at the patient's bedside in a few minutes.
- Tell the patient that no discomfort is associated with this study.

After

- Note that no special aftercare is needed.

Abnormal findings

Impaired cardiopulmonary function
Abnormal gas exchange

notes

Papanicolaou smear (Pap smear, Pap test, Cytologic test for cancer)

Type of test Microscopic examination

Normal findings No abnormal or atypical cells

Test explanation and related physiology

A Pap smear is taken to detect neoplastic cells in cervical and vaginal secretions. This test is based on the fact that normal cells and abnormal cervical and endometrial neoplastic cells are shed into the cervical and vaginal secretions. By examining these secretions microscopically, one can detect early cellular changes compatible with premalignant conditions or an existing malignant condition. The Pap smear is 95% accurate in detecting cervical carcinoma; however, its accuracy in detection of endometrial carcinoma is only approximately 40%. The cells are classified as follows:

Class 1: absence of atypical or abnormal cells (normal)

Class 2: atypical cells but no evidence of malignancy (worrisome but most frequently caused by inflammation of the cervix)

Class 3: cytologic findings suggestive of but not conclusive concerning malignancy (should be evaluated more extensively)

Class 4: cytologic findings strongly suggestive of malignancy (requires more extensive evaluation)

Class 5: cytologic findings conclusive of malignancy (requires treatment)

Abnormal smears in classes 2 to 4 do not necessarily indicate that the patient has a malignancy. Additional procedures are indicated for these women.

A general movement has occurred over the last 10 years to reclassify Pap smear reporting in terms of cervical intraepithelial neoplasia (CIN). This is a simple designation of the spectrum of intraepithelial dysplasia, which usually occurs before invasive cervical cancer. In contrast to the rigid original classification, CIN reporting recognizes the continuum of cervical dysplasia and allows for some overlap. The subclasses of CIN are defined as follows:

CIN 1: mild and mild-to-moderate dysplasia

CIN 2: moderate and moderate-to-severe dysplasia

CIN 3: severe dysplasia and carcinoma in situ

Basically, CIN 1 includes classes 2 and 3, CIN 2 includes class 3, and CIN 3 includes classes 4 and 5.

Most recently, the Bethesda System for reporting cervical/vaginal cytologic diagnoses was developed and revised by the National Cancer Institute. This system includes the following:

Adequacy of specimen
    Satisfactory for evaluation
    Satisfactory for evaluation but limited by (specify disease)
    Unsatisfactory for evaluation (specify reason)
General categorization (optional)
    Within normal limits
    Benign cellular changes: see descriptive diagnosis
    Epithelial cell abnormality: see descriptive diagnosis
Descriptive diagnosis
    Benign cellular changes
    Infection
        Trichomonas
        Fungal organisms
        Coccobacilli
        Herpes simplex
        Other
    Reactive changes
        Inflammation
        Atrophy
        Radiation
        IUD
        Other
Epithelial cell abnormalities
    Squamous cell
        Atypical squamous cells
        Low-grade squamous intraepithelial lesion
        High-grade squamous intraepithelial lesion
        Squamous cell carcinoma
    Glandular cell
        Endometrial cells, cytologically benign
        Atypical glandular cell
        Endocervical adenocarcinoma
        Endometrial adenocarcinoma
        Extrauterine adenocarcinoma
        Adenocarcinoma

A Pap smear also may be performed to follow some abnormalities (e.g., infertility). An abnormal maturation index is characteristic of an estrogen-progesterone imbalance.

Pap smears should be part of the routine pelvic examination, which is usually performed once a year on women over 18 years of age (or even earlier when the patient is sexually active). Opinions differ regarding the necessity for annual Pap smears. The American Cancer Society recommends that a Pap smear be taken annually for two negative examinations, then repeated once every 3 years until age 65 in asymptomatic women. More frequent testing may be indicated for patients with venereal infections, those with a family history of cervical cancer, and those whose mothers had ingested diethylstilbestrol during their pregnancies. A routine cervical culture for gonorrhea is obtained during the Pap smear examination.

Contraindications

- Patients presently having routine, normal menses, because this can alter test interpretation.

Interfering factors

- A delay in fixing a specimen allows the cells to dry, destroys effectiveness of the stain, and makes cytologic interpretation difficult.
- Using lubricating jelly on the speculum can alter the specimen.
- Douching and tub bathing may wash away cellular deposits and interfere with the test results.
- Menstrual flow may alter test results.
- Infections may interfere with hormonal cytology.
- Drugs such as digitalis and tetracycline may alter the test results by affecting the squamous epithelium.

Procedure and patient care

Before

- Explain the procedure to the patient.
- Instruct the patient not to douche or tub bathe during the 24 hours before the Pap smear. (Some physicians prefer that patients refrain from sexual intercourse for 24 to 48 hours before the test.)
- Instruct the patient to empty her bladder before the examination.
- Tell the patient that no fasting or sedation is required.

During

- Note the following procedural steps:
  1. The patient is placed in the lithotomy position.
  2. A vaginal speculum is inserted to expose the cervix.

3. Material is collected from the cervical canal by rotating a moist, saline cotton swab or spatula within the cervical canal and in the squamocolumnar junction.

4. The cells are immediately wiped across a clean glass slide and fixed either by immersing the slide in equal parts of 95% alcohol and ether or by using a commercial spray (e.g., Aqua Net hair spray). The secretions must be fixed before drying, because drying will distort the cells and make interpretation difficult.

5. The slide is labeled with the patient's name, age, and parity, and with the date of her last menstrual period.

6. The patient's medication history (e.g., oral contraceptives) and the reason for the examination should be written on the laboratory request form.

- Note that a Pap smear is obtained by a nurse or a physician in approximately 10 minutes.
- Tell the patient that no discomfort, except for insertion of the speculum, is associated with this procedure.

After

- Inform the patient that usually she will not be notified unless further evaluation is necessary.

Abnormal findings

Cancer	Fungal infection
Infertility	Parasitic infection
Venereal disease	Herpes infection
Reactive inflammatory changes	

notes

---

paracentesis (Peritoneal fluid analysis, Abdominal
paracentesis, Ascitic fluid cytology, Peritoneal tap)

Type of test Fluid analysis

Normal findings
Gross appearance: Clear, serous, light yellow, <50 ml
Red blood cells (RBCs): None
White blood cells (WBCs): <300/μl
Protein: <4.1 g/dl
Glucose: 70-100 mg/dl
Amylase: 138-404 U/L
Ammonia: <50 μg/dl
Alkaline phosphatase
   Adult male: 90-240 U/L
   Female <45 years: 76-196 U/L
   Female >45 years: 87-250 U/L
Lactate dehydrogenase (LDH): Similar to serum lactate dehy-
   drogenase
Cytology: No malignant cells
Bacteria: None
Fungi: None
Carcinoembryonic antigen (CEA): Negative

Test explanation and related physiology

Paracentesis is an invasive procedure entailing the insertion of
a needle into the peritoneal cavity (Figure 21) for removal of
ascitic fluid. Peritoneal fluid is removed for diagnostic and therapeutic purposes. Diagnostically, paracentesis is performed to remove and analyze fluid to determine the etiology of the peritoneal effusion. Therapeutically, this procedure is done to remove
large amounts of ascitic fluid from the abdominal cavity. Usually, these patients experience transient relief of their symptoms
(shortness of breath, distention, and early satiety).

The peritoneal fluid is usually evaluated for gross appearance,
RBCs, WBCs, protein, glucose, amylase, ammonia, alkaline
phosphatase, LDH, cytology, bacteria, fungi, and other tests such
as CEA levels. Each is discussed separately. Urea and creatinine
may be measured if there is a question of bladder perforation or
rupture.

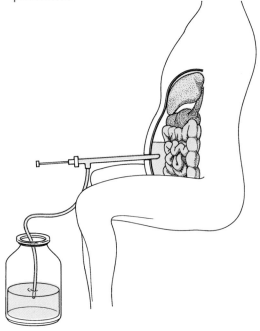

Figure 21 Paracentesis. (From Beare PG, Myers JL: *Principles and practice of adult health nursing,* ed 2, St Louis, 1994, Mosby.)

Gross appearance

While the presence of peritoneal fluid is pathologic, it may be clear, serous, and light yellow, especially in patients with hepatic cirrhosis. Milk-colored peritoneal fluid may result from the escape of chyle from blocked thoracic lymphatic ducts. Conditions that may cause this problem include lymphoma, carcinoma, and tuberculosis.

Cloudy or turbid fluid may result from inflammatory conditions such as peritonitis, pancreatitis, and appendicitis. Bloody fluid may be the result of a traumatic tap, tumor, or hemorrhagic pancreatitis. Bile-stained, green fluid may result from a ruptured gallbladder, acute pancreatitis, or perforated intestines.

Cell counts

Normally, no RBCs should be present. The presence of RBCs may indicate neoplasms, tuberculosis, or intraabdominal bleeding. Increased WBC counts may be seen with peritonitis, cirrhosis, and tuberculosis.

Protein count

Levels greater than 3 g/dl are characteristic of *exudates*, whereas *transudates* usually have a protein content of less than 3 g/dl. Transudates are most frequently caused by congestive heart failure, cirrhosis, nephrotic syndrome, myxedema, peritoneal dialysis, hypoproteinemia, and acute glomerulonephritis. Exudates are most often found in infectious or neoplastic conditions. However, collagen vascular disease, pulmonary infarction, gastrointestinal diseases, trauma, and drug hypersensitivity also may cause an exudative effusion.

It is now thought that the *albumin gradient* between serum and ascitic fluid can differentiate better between the transudate and exudate nature of ascites than can the protein content. This gradient is obtained by subtracting the ascitic albumin value from the serum albumin value. Values of 1.1 g/dl or more suggest a transudate, which is usually caused by portal hypertension due to cirrhosis. Values less than 1.1 g/dl suggest an exudate but will not differentiate malignancy from infection or inflammation.

Glucose

Usually, peritoneal glucose levels approximate serum glucose levels. Decreased levels may indicate tuberculous peritonitis or peritoneal carcinomatosis.

Amylase

Increased amylase levels may be seen in patients with pancreatic trauma, pancreatic pseudocyst, acute pancreatitis, and intestinal necrosis, perforation, or strangulation.

Ammonia

High ammonia levels occur in ruptured or strangulated intestines and also with a ruptured appendix or ulcer.

Alkaline phosphatase

Levels of alkaline phosphatase are greatly increased in infarcted or strangulated intestines.

Lactate dehydrogenase

A peritoneal fluid/serum LDH ratio of greater than 0.6 is typical of an exudate. An exudate is identified with a higher degree of accuracy if the peritoneal fluid/serum protein ratio is greater than 0.5 and the peritoneal fluid/serum LDH ratio is greater than 0.6.

Cytology

A cytologic study is performed to detect tumors. The tumors most often seen are ovarian, pancreatic, colon, and gastric.

Bacteria

The presence of bacteria may indicate a ruptured intestine, primary peritonitis, or infections such as appendicitis, pancreatitis, or tuberculosis.

Fungi

Fungi may indicate infections with histoplasmosis, candidiasis, or coccidioidomycosis.

Carcinoembryonic antigen

Peritoneal fluid levels for CEA are associated with abdominal malignancy, usually arising from the gastrointestinal tract.

Contraindications

- Patients with coagulation abnormalities or bleeding tendencies
- Patients with only a small amount of fluid and extensive previous abdominal surgery

Potential complications

- Hypovolemia if a large volume of peritoneal fluid was removed
- Hepatic coma in a patient with chronic liver disease
- Peritonitis

Procedure and patient care

Before

- Explain the procedure to the patient.
- Obtain informed consent for this procedure.
- Tell the patient that no fasting or sedation is necessary.
- Have the patient urinate or empty the bladder before the test. This will help to prevent accidental bladder trauma.
- Measure abdominal girth.
- Obtain the patient's weight.
- Obtain baseline vital signs.

During

- Note the following procedural steps:
  1. Position the person in a high Fowler's position in bed or

in a chair with the back supported and the feet on a stool.

2. Paracentesis is performed under strict sterile technique. A paracentesis tray usually contains all necessary supplies.

3. The needle insertion site is aseptically cleansed and anesthetized locally.

4. A scalpel may be used to make a stab wound into the peritoneal cavity approximately 1 to 2 inches below the umbilicus.

5. A trocar, cannula, or needle is threaded through the incision.

6. A plastic tubing is attached to the cannula. The other end of the tubing is placed in the collection receptacle (usually a container with a pressurized vacuum).

- Note that this procedure is performed by a physician at the patient's bedside, in a procedure room, or in the physician's office in less than 30 minutes. Usually, the volume removed is limited to about 4 L at any one time to avoid hypovolemia if the ascites is rapidly reaccumulated.

- Although local anesthetics eliminate pain at the insertion site, tell the patient that he or she will feel a pressure-like pain as the needle is inserted.

After

- Place a small bandage over the needle site.
- Label the specimen with the patient's name, date, source of fluid, and diagnosis.
- Send the specimen promptly to the laboratory.
- Observe the puncture site for bleeding, continued drainage, or signs of inflammation.
- Measure the abdominal girth and weight of the patient; compare with baseline values.
- Monitor vital signs for evidence of hemodynamic changes. Watch for signs of hypotension if a large volume of fluid was removed.
- Write any recent antibiotic therapy on the laboratory requisition slip.
- Because of the high protein content of ascitic fluid, albumin infusions may be ordered after paracentesis to compensate for protein loss. Monitor serum protein and electrolyte (especially sodium) levels.

P

Abnormal findings

Lymphoma
Carcinoma
Tuberculosis
Hepatic cirrhosis
Peritonitis
Pancreatitis

Appendicitis
Abdominal trauma
Ruptured viscus
Neoplasm
Peritoneal bleeding

notes

parathyroid hormone (PTH, Parathormone)

Type of test Blood

Normal findings <2000 pg/ml (vary according to individual laboratory)

Test explanation and related physiology

The serum PTH test measures the quantity of PTH within the blood. PTH is the only hormone secreted by the parathyroid gland and is one of the major factors in calcium metabolism. This test is useful in establishing a diagnosis of hyperparathyroidism and distinguishing nonparathyroid from parathyroid causes of hypercalcemia. Increased PTH levels are seen in patients with hyperparathyroidism; in patients with nonparathyroid, ectopic PTH-producing tumors; or as a normal compensatory response to hypocalcemia in patients with renal failure or vitamin D deficiency. Decreased levels are seen in patients with hypoparathyroidism or as a compensatory response to hypercalcemia in patients with metastatic bone tumors, sarcoidosis, vitamin D intoxication, or milk-alkali syndrome.

Interfering factors

- Recent injection of radioisotopes may interfere with this test.
- ⚕ Drugs that *increase* PTH include anticonvulsants, steroids, isoniazid, lithium, and rifampin.
- ⚕ Drugs that *decrease* PTH include cimetidine and propranolol.

Procedure and patient care

Before

- Explain the procedure to the patient.
- Keep the patient NPO except for water after midnight on the day of the test.

During

- Obtain a morning blood specimen, because diurnal rhythm affects PTH levels. (Check with the laboratory if the patient works at night.)
- Collect 5 to 10 ml of venous blood in a red-top tube. Note that some laboratories require 15 ml of blood in an iced plastic syringe.

- Obtain a serum calcium level determination at the same time if ordered. The serum PTH and serum calcium levels are important in the differential diagnosis.

After

- Indicate the time the blood was drawn on the laboratory slip, because a diurnal rhythm affects test results.
- Apply pressure or a pressure dressing to the venipuncture site.
- Check the venipuncture site for bleeding.

Abnormal findings

▲ **Increased levels**

Hyperparathyroidism sec-
ondary to adenoma or
carcinoma of the para-
thyroid gland
Non–PTH-producing
tumors (paraneoplastic
syndrome)
  Lung carcinoma
  Kidney carcinoma
Hypocalcemia
Chronic renal failure
Malabsorption syndrome
Vitamin D deficiency
Rickets
Osteomalacia

▼ **Decreased levels**

Hypoparathyroidism
Hypercalcemia
Metastatic bone tumor
Sarcoidosis
Autoimmune destruction
of the parathyroid
glands
Vitamin D intoxication
Milk-alkali syndrome
Graves' disease
Hypomagnesemia

notes

partial thromboplastin time, activated (APTT, Partial thromboplastin time [PTT])

Type of test Blood

Normal findings

APTT: 30-40 seconds
PTT: 60-70 seconds
Patients receiving anticoagulant therapy: 1.5-2.5 times control
  value in seconds

Possible critical values

APTT: >70 seconds
PTT: >100 seconds

Test explanation and related physiology

The PTT test is used to assess the intrinsic system and the common pathway of clot formation. PTT evaluates factors I (fibrinogen), II (prothrombin), V, VIII, IX, X, XI, and XII. When any of these factors exists in inadequate quantities, as in hemophilia A and B or consumptive coagulopathy, the PTT is prolonged. Because factors II, IX, and X are vitamin K-dependent factors, biliary obstruction, which precludes gastrointestinal absorption of fat and fat-soluble vitamins (e.g., vitamin K), can reduce their concentration and thus prolong the PTT. Because coagulation factors are made in the liver, hepatocellular diseases will also prolong the PTT.

Heparin has been found to inactivate prothrombin (factor II) and to prevent the formation of thromboplastin. These actions prolong the intrinsic clotting pathway for approximately 4 to 6 hours after each dose of heparin. Therefore heparin is capable of providing therapeutic anticoagulation. The appropriate dose of heparin can be monitored by the PTT. PTT test results are given in seconds along with a control value. The control value may vary slightly from day to day because of the reagents used.

Recently, activators have been added to the PTT test reagents to shorten normal clotting time and provide a narrow normal range. This shortened time is called the activated PTT (APTT). The normal APTT is 30 to 40 seconds. Desired ranges for therapeutic anticoagulation are 1.5 to 2.5 times normal (e.g., 70 seconds). The APTT specimen should be drawn 30 to 60 minutes before the patient's next heparin dose is given. If the APTT is less than 50 seconds, the patient may not be receiving therapeutic anticoagulation and needs more heparin. An APTT greater than 100 seconds indicates that too much heparin is being given; the risk of serious spontaneous bleeding exists when the APTT is this high. The effects of heparin can be reversed immediately by the administration of 1 mg of protamine sulfate for every 100 units of the heparin dose.

Heparin's effect, unlike that of warfarin, is immediate and short-lived. When a thromboembolic episode (e.g., pulmonary embolism, arterial embolism, thrombophlebitis) occurs, immediate and complete anticoagulation is most rapidly and safely achieved by heparin administration. This drug is often given during cardiac and vascular surgery to prevent intravascular clotting during clamping of the vessels. Often, small doses of heparin (5000 U subcutaneously every 12 hours) are given to prevent thromboembolism in high-risk patients. This dose alters the PTT very little, and the risk of spontaneous bleeding is minimal.

Interfering factors

✗ Drugs that may prolong PTT test values include antihistamines, ascorbic acid, chlorpromazine, heparin, and salicylates.

Procedure and patient care

Before

- Explain the procedure to the patient.
- If the patient is receiving heparin by intermittent injection, plan to draw the blood specimen for the APTT 30 minutes to 1 hour before the next dose of heparin.
- If the patient is receiving continuous heparin, draw the blood at any time.

During

- Collect 5 to 14 ml of venous blood in one or two blue-top tubes.

After

- Apply pressure or a pressure dressing to the venipuncture site.
- Assess the venipuncture site for bleeding. Remember, if the patient is receiving anticoagulants or has coagulopathies, the bleeding time will be increased.
- Assess the patient to detect possible bleeding. Check for

blood in the urine and all other excretions and assess the patient for bruises, petechiae, and low back pain.

- If severe bleeding occurs, note that the anticoagulant effect of heparin can be reversed by parenteral administration of protamine sulfate.

Abnormal findings

▲ **Increased levels**

Acquired or congenital clotting factor deficiencies

Cirrhosis of the liver

Vitamin K deficiency

Leukemia

Disseminated intravascular coagulation

Heparin administration

Hypofibrinogenemia

von Willebrand's disease

Hemophilia

▼ **Decreased levels**

Early stages of disseminated intravascular coagulation

Extensive cancer

notes

P

parvovirus B19 antibody

Type of test Blood

Normal findings Negative for IgM and IgG specific antibodies to parvovirus B19

Test explanation and related physiology

The parvovirus group includes several species-specific viruses of animals. The parvovirus B19 is known to be a human pathogen. Many of the severe manifestations of B19 viremia relate to the ability of the virus to infect and lyse red blood cell precursors in the bone marrow. The name B19 was derived from the code number of the human serum in which the virus was discovered.

Erythema infectiosum is the most common manifestation of B19 infection and occurs predominantly in children. This pathogen is also referred to as "fifth disease" because it was classified in the late nineteenth century as the fifth in a series of six exanthems of childhood. This infection is also sometimes referred to as "academy rash." The typical presentation is a self-limiting, mild illness with a low-grade fever, a malor rash, and occasionally arthralgia. Normally, the rash begins on the face and may also develop on the arms and legs. Outbreaks of erythema infectiosum appear most often during the winter and spring months.

Recently, parvovirus B19 has been associated with a number of other clinical problems, including:

Flu-like illness associated with joint inflammation, rash, and occasionally purpura in young adults

Hydrops fetalis and fetal loss in ≤10% of infected pregnant women

Transient aplastic crisis in patients with chronic hemolytic anemia

Chronic severe anemia in patients with immunodeficiency related to infection with human immunodeficiency virus (HIV), congenital immunodeficiency, acute lymphocytic leukemia during maintenance chemotherapy, and recipients of bone marrow transplants

Because of the recently discovered spectrum of disease caused by parvovirus B19, laboratory diagnosis has come into great demand. Serologic testing for parvovirus B19 specific IgM and IgG antibodies can be detected by enzyme-linked immunosorbent assay (ELISA) and indirect fluorescent antibody immunofluorescence (IFA) methods. Acute infections can be determined by B19 compatible symptoms and the presence of IgM antibodies that remain detectable up to a few months. Past infection or immunity is documented by IgG antibodies that persist indefinitely. Fetal infection may be recognized by hydrops fetalis and the presence of B19 DNA in amniotic fluid or fetal blood.

Procedure and patient care

Before

- Explain the procedure to the patient.
- Tell the patient that no fasting or special preparation is necessary.

During

- Collect a venous blood sample according to the laboratory protocol.

After

- Apply a pressure or pressure dressing to the venipuncture site.
- Assess the venipuncture site for bleeding.
- Inform the patient that it normally requires approximately 2 to 3 days to get test results.

Abnormal findings

▲ **Increased levels**

Erythema infectiosum (fifth disease)
Joint arthralgia and arthritis
Hydrops fetalis

Fetal loss
Transient aplastic anemia
Chronic anemia in immunodeficient patients
Bone marrow failure

notes

pelvic floor sphincter electromyography (Pelvic floor sphincter EMG, Rectal EMG procedure)

Type of test Electrodiagnostic

Normal findings
Increased EMG signal during bladder filling
Silent EMG signal on voluntary micturition
Increased EMG signal at the end of voiding
Increased EMG signal with voluntary contraction of the anal
  sphincter

Test explanation and related physiology
This urodynamic test uses the placement of electrodes on or in the pelvic floor musculature to evaluate the neuromuscular function of the urinary or anal sphincter. The main benefit of this study is to evaluate the external sphincter (skeletal muscle) activity during voiding. This test is also used to evaluate the bulbocavernous reflex and voluntary control of external sphincter or pelvic floor muscles. The pelvic floor sphincter EMG also aids in the investigation of "functional" or "psychologic" disturbances of voiding. Fecal incontinence caused by muscular dysfunction can also be identified by rectal sphincter EMG.

Three electrodes are used for this procedure. Recordings may be made from surface electrodes or needle electrodes within the muscle; surface electrodes are most often used. These electrodes allow for observation of and change in the muscle activity before and during voiding.

Patient cooperation is essential. If the patient does not cooperate, the interpretation of the test results will be difficult.

Contraindications
- Patients who cannot cooperate during the procedure

Procedure and patient care
Before
- Explain the procedure to the patient.
- Inform the patient that cooperation is essential.

During
- Note the following procedural steps:
  1. Two electrodes are placed at the 2 o'clock and 10 o'clock

positions on the perianal skin to monitor the pelvic floor musculature during voiding.

2. The third electrode is usually placed on the thigh and serves as a ground.

3. Electrical activity is recorded with the bladder empty and the patient relaxed.

4. Reflex activity is evaluated by asking the patient to cough and by stimulating the urethra and trigone by gently tugging on an inserted Foley catheter (bulbocavernous reflex).

5. Voluntary activity is evaluated by asking the patient to contract and relax the sphincter muscle.

6. The bladder is filled with sterile water at room temperature at a rate of 100 ml/min.

7. The EMG responses to filling and detrusor hyperreflexia (if present) are recorded.

8. Finally, when the bladder is full and with the patient in a voiding position, the filling catheter is removed and the patient is asked to urinate. In the normal patient, the EMG signals build during bladder filling and cease promptly on voluntary micturition, remaining silent until the pelvic floor contracts at the end of voiding.

9. The electrical waves produced are examined for their number and form.

- Note that a urologist performs this study in less than 30 minutes.
- Explain to the patient that this study is slightly more uncomfortable than urethral catheterization.

P

After

- If needle electrodes were used, observe the needle site for hematoma or inflammation.

Abnormal findings

Neuromuscular dysfunction of lower urinary sphincter
Pelvic floor muscle dysfunction of the anal sphincter

notes

pelvic ultrasonography (Obstetric echography, Pregnant
uterus ultrasonography, Pelvic ultrasonography in pregnancy,
Obstetric ultrasonography, Vaginal ultrasound)

Type of test Ultrasound

Normal findings Normal fetal and placental size and position

Test explanation and related physiology

Ultrasound examination of the female patient has proved to
be a harmless, noninvasive method of evaluating the female genital tract and fetus. In diagnostic ultrasound, harmless, high-
frequency sound waves are emitted from the transducer and penetrate the structure (uterus, ovaries, parametria, placenta, fetus)
to be studied. These sound waves are bounced back to a sensor
within the transducer and by electronic conversion are arranged
into a pictorial image of the desired organ. A realistic Polaroid
picture is taken of the pattern.

It should be noted that pelvic ultrasonography can be
performed with the transducer placed on the anterior abdomen
or in the vagina with a specially designed vaginal probe. The view
obtained from both transducers complements the information
gained from either one alone. Vaginal ultrasound adds significant accuracy in identifying paracervical, endometrial, and ovarian pathology that otherwise may not be detected with the anterior abdominal probe. Occasionally, abdominal organs fall into
the pelvis and preclude good pelvic visualization with the anterior abdominal probe. Vaginal ultrasound provides better visualization under these circumstances. The anterior abdominal
probe, however, does provide better visualization of the upper
pelvis than does the vaginal probe.

Pelvic ultrasonography may be useful in the *obstetric patient*
to diagnose the following circumstances:
1. Making an early diagnosis of normal pregnancy and abnormal pregnancy (e.g., tubal pregnancy)
2. Identifying multiple pregnancies
3. Differentiating a tumor (e.g., hydatidiform mole) from
   a normal pregnancy
4. Determining the age of the fetus by the diameter of the
   head
5. Measuring the rate of fetal growth

6. Identifying placental abnormalities such as abruptio placentae and placenta previa
7. Determining the position of the placenta (Ultrasound localization of the placenta is done before amniocentesis.)
8. Making differential diagnoses of various uterine and ovarian enlargements (e.g., polyhydramnios, neoplasms, cysts, abscesses)
9. Determining fetal position
10. Ectopic pregnancy

Pelvic ultrasound is used in the *nonpregnant woman* to monitor the endometrium in patients who take tamoxifen and to aid in the diagnosis of:

1. Ovarian cyst
2. Ovarian tumor
3. Tubo-ovarian abscess
4. Uterine fibroids
5. Uterine cancer
6. Pelvic inflammatory disease (PID)

See rectal ultrasonography, p. 666.

Interfering factors

- Patients who have had recent GI contrast studies, because barium creates severe distortion of reflective sound waves
- Patients with air-filled bowels, because gas does not transmit the sound waves well
- Failure to fill the bladder or obesity, which may make the image uninterpretable

P

Procedure and patient care

Before

- Explain the procedure to the patient.
- Assure the patient that this study has no known deleterious effect on maternal or fetal tissues, even when it is repeated several times.
- Give the patient three to four glasses (200 to 350 ml) of water or other liquid 1 hour before the examination, and instruct her *not* to void until after the procedure is completed. This will permit visualization of the bladder, which is used as a reference point in pelvic anatomy.
- Tell the patient that no fasting or sedation is required.

During

- Note the following procedural steps:
  1. The patient is taken to the ultrasound room and placed in the supine position on the examining table.
  2. The ultrasonographer, usually a radiologist, applies a greasy, conductive paste to the abdomen to enhance sound transmission and reception.
  3. A transducer is passed vertically and horizontally over the skin.
  4. If a vaginal probe is used, it is inserted via the vagina and angled to identify the various parts of the pelvis.
  5. Pictures are taken of the reflections.
  6. During the examination, fetal structures are pointed out to the mother.
- Note that this procedure is performed in approximately 20 minutes.
- Inform the patient that no discomfort is associated with this study other than having a full bladder and the urge to void. Some patients may be uncomfortable lying on a hard x-ray table.

After

- Remove the lubricant from the patient's skin.
- Provide an opportunity for the patient to void.

Abnormal findings

Tubal pregnancy
Abdominal pregnancy
Hydatidiform mole
Intrauterine growth retardation
Multiple fetuses
Fetal death
Abruptio placentae
Abnormal fetal position (e.g., breech, transverse)

Placenta previa
Polyhydramnios
Neoplasm of the ovaries, uterus, or fallopian tubes
Cysts
Abscesses
Hydrocephalus of the fetus

notes

pelvimetry (Radiographic pelvimetry)

Type of test X-ray

Normal findings Transverse diameter of the midpelvis >10.5 cm

Testing explanation and related physiology

Although most abnormalities of the pelvis can be suspected by using clinical measurements, x-ray pelvimetry is the most accurate means of determining adequacy of the pelvic bony structures for a normal vaginal delivery. With pelvimetry, one can compare the capacity of the pelvis with the size of the infant and discover any cephalopelvic disproportion.

Radiographic pelvimetry is not used often in modern obstetrics because of the risks associated with radiation; however, this study may be indicated in:

1. Patients suspected of having fetuses in abnormal positions when a vaginal delivery is anticipated
2. Patients who have had injury or disease of the bony pelvis or hips that may have caused pelvic distortion
3. Patients with clinically abnormal pelvic measurements
4. Patients with a debilitating disease and a clinically small or unfavorable pelvis
5. Patients with a history of difficult delivery
6. Patients in early labor with the fetus's head unengaged
7. Patients admitted for trial labor to rule out a contracted pelvis
8. Patients having dysfunctional labor, especially when the physician is considering oxytocin administration

Although measuring the pelvis clinically is less accurate than x-ray determination, it is adequate for most patients. Radiographic pelvimetry is only important late in pregnancy or during labor. If pelvimetry indicates a difficult or dangerous vaginal delivery, cesarean birth is recommended. Cesarean section is now more frequently performed when vaginal delivery is clinically suspected to be difficult. As a result, x-ray pelvimetry rarely affects the physician's decision concerning the type of delivery. In those rare situations in which vaginal delivery is attempted despite an anticipated difficult delivery, radiographic pelvimetry is performed more for legal purposes than for medical benefits. Ultra-

P

sound measurements of fetal size in comparison to pelvic measurements are another method of pelvimetry.

Contraindications

- Patients in early pregnancy, because x-ray films at this time may injure the fetus.

Procedure and patient care

Before

- Explain the procedure to the patient.
- Tell the patient that no fasting or sedation is required.
- Instruct the patient to remove all clothing and don a long x-ray gown.

During

- Note the following procedural steps:
  1. In the radiology department, a lateral x-ray film is taken with the patient standing to detect the effect of gravity on engagement and to indicate the position of the fetal head when it reaches the lower level of the birth canal.
  2. The patient may then be placed in the supine, lateral, and semirecumbent positions.
  3. During the x-ray exposure, the patient is asked to stop breathing.
  4. Generally, the patient is instructed to hyperventilate and then stop breathing while the film is taken.
- Note that a radiologic technologist performs this study in approximately 15 minutes.
- Tell the patient that no discomfort is associated with this study.

After

- Provide emotional support for the patient at this difficult time. Most patients are concerned that some problem exists.

Abnormal findings

Cephalopelvic disproportion
Abnormal fetal position

notes

percutaneous transhepatic cholangiography (PTC, PTHC)

Type of test X-ray with contrast dye

Normal findings Normal gallbladder and biliary ducts

Test explanation and related physiology

By passing a needle through the liver and into an intrahepatic bile duct, the biliary system can be directly injected with iodinated x-ray contrast dye. The intrahepatic and extrahepatic biliary ducts, and occasionally the gallbladder, can be visualized and studied for partial or total obstruction caused by gallstones, benign strictures, malignant tumors, congenital cysts, and anatomic variations. This is especially helpful in jaundiced patients. If the jaundice is found to result from extrahepatic obstruction, a catheter can be left in the bile duct and used for external drainage of bile. Furthermore, a stent can be placed across a stricture and decompress the biliary system internally.

Both PTC and endoscopic retrograde cholangiopancreatography (ERCP, see p. 356) are the only methods available to visualize the biliary tree in jaundiced patients. ERCP is used more frequently because of its lower complication rate.

Contraindications

- Patients with allergies to iodine or shellfish
- Patients with evidence of mild cholangitis
  Dye injections increase biliary pressure and cause bacteremia, which may lead to septicemia and shock.
- Patients who cannot cooperate and remain still
- Patients with prolonged clotting times

Potential complications

- Allergic reaction to iodinated dye
  Allergic reactions may vary from mild flushing, itching, and urticaria to severe, life-threatening anaphylaxis (evidenced by respiratory distress, drop in blood pressure, shock). In the unusual event of anaphylaxis, the patient may be treated with diphenhydramine (Benadryl), steroids, and epinephrine. Oxygen and endotracheal equipment should be on hand for immediate use.

- Peritonitis caused by bile extravasation from the liver after the needle has been removed
- Bleeding caused by inadvertent puncture of a large hepatic blood vessel
- Sepsis and cholangitis resulting from injection of the dye into an already infected and obstructed bowel duct
  The pressure of injection pushes the bacteria into the bloodstream, causing a bacteremia.

Interfering factor

- The presence of barium from a previous upper GI series or barium enema x-ray study may preclude visualization of the biliary tree.

Procedure and patient care

Before

- Explain the procedure to the patient.
- Obtain informed consent for this procedure.
- Assess the patient for allergies to iodinated dye or shellfish.
- Inform the radiologist if an allergy to iodinated contrast is suspected. The radiologist may prescribe a Benadryl-and-steroid preparation to be administered before testing. Usually, a hypoallergenic, non-ionic contrast will be used during the test.
- Type and crossmatch the patient's blood. The patient may bleed and require a transfusion or surgery.
- Check to make sure that the patient's coagulation studies are within the normal ranges.
- Keep the patient NPO after midnight on the day of the test. A laxative may be ordered.
- Premedicate the patient as indicated, usually with atropine and meperidine.

During

- Note the following procedural steps:
  1. The patient is placed in the supine position on an x-ray table in the radiology department.
  2. The abdominal wall or lower chest wall (over the liver) is anesthetized with lidocaine (Xylocaine).
  3. With the use of televised fluoroscopic monitoring, the needle is advanced through the skin and into the liver (Figure 22).
  4. When bile flows freely through the needle, radiographic dye is injected.
  5. X-ray films are taken immediately.

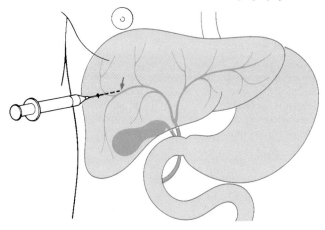

Figure 22 Percutaneous transhepatic cholangiography (PTHC).

6. If an obstruction is found, a catheter or stent is placed over a guide wire and left temporarily in the biliary tract to establish drainage and decompression of the biliary tract.

- Note that PTC is performed by a radiologist in approximately 1 hour, during which time the patient must lie still.
- Inform the patient that abdominal pain may be felt for several hours after the test. Occasionally, the patient also may have right shoulder-top pain because of diaphragmatic irritation of leaking bile or blood.

P

After
- Keep the patient on bed rest for several hours.
- If indicated, place a sandbag over the insertion site.
- Observe the patient for hemorrhage or bile leakage. A small amount of bleeding is usually present.
- Keep the patient NPO for a few hours after the test in the event he or she has any intraabdominal bleeding or bile extravasation that requires surgery.
- Repeatedly assess the patient's vital signs for evidence of hemorrhage.
- Assess the patient for signs of bacteremia or sepsis.
- If a catheter is left in the biliary tract, establish a sterile, closed drainage system.

- Withhold pain medications to avoid blunting the abdominal signs associated with hemorrhage or bile extravasation.

Abnormal findings

Tumors, strictures, or gallstones of the hepatic or common bile duct

Sclerosing cholangitis

Biliary sclerosis

Cysts of the common bile duct

Tumors, strictures, inflammation, or pseudocysts of the pancreatic duct

Anatomic biliary or pancreatic duct variations

notes

pericardiocentesis

Type of test Fluid analysis

Normal findings Minimal amount of clear, straw-colored fluid without evidence of any bacteria, blood, or malignant cells

Test explanation and related physiology

Pericardiocentesis, which involves the aspiration of fluid from the pericardial sac with a needle, may be performed for therapeutic and diagnostic purposes. Therapeutically, the test is performed to relieve cardiac tamponade by removing fluid and improving diastolic filling. Diagnostically, pericardiocentesis is performed to remove a sample of pericardial fluid for laboratory examination in order to determine the cause of the fluid. This is similar to the evaluation described for pleural fluid on p. 784.

Contraindications

- Patients who are uncooperative because of the risk of lacerations to the epicardium or coronary artery
- Patients with a bleeding disorder
  Inadvertent puncture of the myocardium may create uncontrollable bleeding into the pericardial sac, leading to tamponade.

Potential complications

- Laceration of the coronary artery or myocardium
- Needle-induced ventricular arrhythmias (dysrhythmias)
- Myocardial infarction
- Pneumothorax caused by inadvertent puncture of the lung
- Liver laceration caused by inadvertent puncture
- Pleural infection
- Vasovagal arrest

Procedure and patient care

Before

- Explain the procedure to the patient.
- Obtain informed consent for this procedure.
- Restrict fluid and food intake for at least 4 to 6 hours (if this is an elective procedure).
- Obtain IV access for infusion of fluids and cardiac medications if required.

- Administer pretest medication. Atropine is frequently given to prevent the vasovagal reflex of bradycardia and hypotension.

During

- Note the following procedural steps:
  1. The patient is placed in the supine position.
  2. An area in the fifth to sixth intercostal space at the left sternal margin (or subxyphoid) is prepared and draped.
  3. After skin anesthesia is performed, a large-bore, pericardiocentesis needle is placed on a 50-ml syringe and introduced into the pericardial sac (Figure 23).
  4. An electrocardiographic lead is often attached by a clip to the needle to identify any ST-segment elevations, which may indicate penetration into the epicardium.

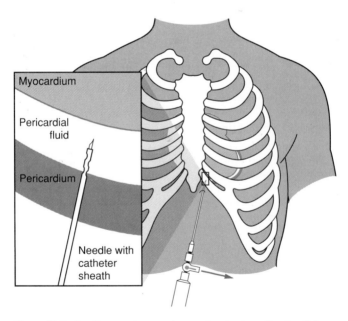

Myocardium

Pericardial fluid

Pericardium

Needle with catheter sheath

Figure 23 Pericardiocentesis procedure and aspiration of pericardial fluid. For recurrent cardiac tamponade and large pericardial effusion, the indwelling catheter may remain.

5. Pericardial fluid is aspirated and placed in multiple specimen containers.
6. Some patients who have recurring cardiac tamponade may require placement of an indwelling pericardial catheter for continuous draining for 1 to 3 days.
7. With certain types of pericarditis, medications (e.g., antibiotics, antineoplastic drugs, corticosteroids) may be instilled during pericardiocentesis.

- Note that a physician usually performs this procedure in the cardiac catheterization laboratory, operating room, or emergency room in approximately 10 to 20 minutes.
- Tell the patient that this procedure is associated with very little discomfort. Most patients feel pressure as the needle is inserted into the pericardial sac.

After

- Closely monitor the patient's vital signs. An increased temperature may indicate infection. Pericardial bleeding would be marked by hypotension or pulsus paradoxus (abnormal decrease in systolic blood pressure during inspiration).
- Label and number the specimen tubes that contain the pericardial fluid and deliver them to the appropriate laboratories for examination. Note the following possibilities:
  1. Usually, the fluid is taken to the chemistry laboratory where the color, turbidity, glucose, albumin, protein, and lactic dehydrogenase levels are obtained (see discussion of thoracentesis, p. 784).
  2. A tube of blood often goes to the hematology laboratory, where the quantities of red and white blood cells are recorded.
  3. The bacteriology laboratory performs routine cultures, Gram stains, fungal studies, acid-fast bacilli smears, and cultures.
  4. When malignancy is suspected, the fluid should be sent for cytology.
- Apply a sterile dressing to the catheter if one has been left for continuing pericardial drainage.
- Establish a closed system if continued pericardial drainage is required. This is usually performed via the straight drainage method.
- Note that to minimize infection, pericardial catheters, if used, are usually removed after 2 days, although there are exceptions. After the sutures are cut and the catheter is removed, apply a sterile dressing to the puncture site.

P

Abnormal findings

Pericarditis
Uremia
Hypoproteinemia
Congestive heart failure

Metastatic cancer
Blunt or penetrating cardiac trauma
Rupture of ventricular aneurysm

notes

phenylketonuria test (PKU test, Guthrie test, Phenylalanine screening)

Type of test Blood; urine

Normal findings

Blood: negative (<2 mg/dl) (Guthrie technique)
Urine: no green coloration

Possible critical values ≥4 mg/dl (Guthrie technique)

Test explanation and related physiology

An inherited disease, PKU is characterized by deficiency of the enzyme phenylalanine hydroxylase, which converts phenylalanine to tyrosine. Phenylalanine is an essential amino acid necessary for growth; however, any excess must be degraded by conversion to tyrosine. An infant with PKU lacks the ability to make this necessary conversion. Thus phenylalanine accumulates in the body and spills over into the urine. If the amount of phenylalanine is not restricted in infants with PKU, progressive mental retardation results. Dietary control must begin early to avoid brain damage; therefore diagnosis must be made early.

Routine screening of newborn infants for PKU is now mandatory in most of the United States. It is important to note that this test is not valid until the newborn has ingested an ample amount (for 2 or 3 days) of the amino acid phenylalanine, which is a constituent of both human and cow's milk. The urine PKU test is normally done after 4 to 6 weeks of age. If the tests are positive, a blood phenylalanine test should be performed.

Interfering factors

- Premature infants may have false-positive results because of delayed development of the liver enzymes.
- Ketonuria can produce an altered urine color reaction.
- Infants tested before 24 hours of age may have false-negative results.
- Feeding problems (e.g., vomiting) may cause false-negative results.
- Drugs that may influence screening results include antibiotics, aspirin, and salicylates.

Procedure and patient care

Before

- Inform the mother about the purpose of the test and the method of performance.
- Assess the infant's feeding patterns before performing the PKU test. An inadequate amount of protein ingested before performing the test can cause false-negative results.

During

- Place a few drops of a heel stick of blood on filter paper for the *Guthrie test.* This test is performed after the newborn has ingested an ample amount (for 2 to 3 days) of the amino acid phenylalanine.
- Indicate on the laboratory slip the present date and time, date and time of birth, and time of first milk-feeding.
- Note that urine tests also may be used to detect PKU in infants who are at least 6 weeks of age. These tests are usually done at the infant's first checkup:
  1. For the *diaper test,* drop 10% ferric chloride on a diaper that contains fresh urine. A green spot indicates probable PKU.
  2. For the *Phenistix test,* press a test stick against a diaper containing urine or dip the stick in the urine. A green color reaction indicates probable PKU.

After

- If test results are positive, inform the mother that dietary control must begin immediately to prevent brain damage to the infant. This is done by substituting Lofenalac for milk. Later, strained foods low in protein are added to the infant's diet. The dietary treatment is monitored by blood and urine testing.
- Instruct women with PKU who wish to have children to begin a low-phenylalanine diet before conception and continue throughout the pregnancy. The risk of producing a mentally retarded infant is very high if the mother remains on a general diet.

Abnormal findings

PKU
Low-birth-weight infants

Galactosemia
Hepatic encephalopathy

phosphorus (P, Phosphate, PO₄)

Type of test Blood

Normal findings
Adult: 3.0-4.5 mg/dl or 0.97-1.45 mmol/L (SI units)
Elderly: values slightly lower than adult
Child: 4.5-6.5 mg/dl or 1.45-2.10 mmol/L (SI units)
Newborn: 4.3-9.3 mg/dl or 1.4-3.0 mmol/L (SI units)

Possible critical values <1 mg/dl

Test explanation and related physiology
Most of the body's phosphorus is combined with calcium within the skeleton; however, approximately 15% of the phosphorus exists in the blood as a phosphate salt. Dietary phosphorus is absorbed in the small bowel. The absorption is very efficient, and only rarely is hypophosphatemia caused by gastrointestinal malabsorption. Antacids, however, can bind phosphorus and decrease intestinal absorption. Renal excretion of phosphorus should equal dietary intake to maintain a normal serum phosphate level.

Phosphorus levels are determined by calcium metabolism, parathormone (parathyroid hormone [PTH]), and to a lesser degree by intestinal absorption. Because an inverse relationship exists between calcium and phosphorus, a decrease of one mineral results in an increase in the other. Serum phosphorus levels therefore depend on calcium metabolism, and vice versa.

Regulation of phosphate by PTH is such that PTH tends to decrease phosphate reabsorption in the kidney. PTH and vitamin D, however, tend to stimulate phosphate absorption weakly within the gut.

Interfering factors
- Laxatives or enemas containing sodium phosphate can increase phosphorus levels.
- Recent carbohydrate ingestion, including IV glucose administration, causes decreased phosphorus levels, because phosphorus enters the cell with glucose.
- Drugs that may cause *increased* levels include methicillin and vitamin D (excessive).
- Drug that may cause *decreased* levels include antacids and mannitol.

P

Procedure and patient care

Before

- Explain the procedure to the patient.
- Keep the patient NPO after midnight on the day of the test.
- If indicated, discontinue IV fluids with glucose for several hours before the test.

During

- Collect approximately 5 to 10 ml of venous blood in a red-top tube.
- Avoid hemolysis. Handle the tube carefully.
- Use a heel stick to draw blood from infants.

After

- Take the specimen to the laboratory immediately.
- Indicate on the laboratory slip the time the blood was obtained.
- Apply pressure or a pressure dressing to the venipuncture site.
- Check the venipuncture site for bleeding.

Abnormal findings

▲ **Increased levels (hyperphosphatemia)**

Renal failure
Increased dietary or IV intake of phosphorus
Acromegaly
Hypoparathyroidism
Bone metastasis
Sarcoidosis
Hypocalcemia
Liver disease
Renal failure

▼ **Decreased levels (hypophosphatemia)**

Inadequate dietary ingestion of phosphorus
Chronic antacid ingestion
Hyperparathyroidism
Hypercalcemia
Chronic alcoholism
Vitamin D deficiency
Diabetic acidosis
Hyperinsulinism
Rickets (childhood)
Osteomalacia (adult)
Malnutrition

notes

plasminogen (Fibrinolysin)

Type of test Blood

Normal findings 2.5-4.5 mmol/ml or 6.1 ± 2.3 Committee on Thrombolytic Agents (CTA) units

Test explanation and related physiology

Plasminogen is a protein involved in the fibrinolytic process of intravascular blood clot dissolution (see Figure 9, p. 251). Plasminogen is converted to plasmin by proteolytic cleavage. This reaction can be catalyzed by urokinase, streptokinase, or tissue plasminogen activator (t-PA). Plasmin can destroy fibrin and dissolve clots. This fibrinolytic system is a normal part of normal homeostatic balance between coagulation and anticoagulation.

Plasminogen levels are occasionally measured during fibrinolytic therapy (for coronary and peripheral arterial occlusion) and are diminished. Decreased levels of plasminogen are also found in hyperfibrinolytic states (e.g., disseminated intravascular coagulation [DIC], primary fibrinolysis). Because plasminogen is made in the liver, patients with cirrhosis or other severe liver diseases can be expected to have decreased levels. There are rare cases of hereditary deficiencies of this protein. Pregnancy and especially eclampsia are associated with increased levels of plasminogen. Inflammatory conditions that may be associated with increased levels of C-reactive protein also may concomitantly have mild elevations of plasminogens.

Procedure and patient care

Before
- Explain the procedure to the patient.
- Tell the patient that no fasting is required.

During
- Collect a venous blood sample in a blue-top tube containing sodium citrate.
- Avoid excessive agitation of the blood sample.

After
- Apply pressure or a pressure dressing to the venipuncture site.
- Assess the venipuncture site for bleeding, especially if the patient is suspected to have a hyperfibrinolytic process (e.g., DIC).

P

Abnormal findings

▲ **Increased levels**
Pregnancy

▼ **Decreased levels**
Hyperfibrinolytic state (e.g., disseminated intravascular coagulation, fibrinolysis)
Primary liver disease
Syndrome associated with hypercoagulation (e.g., venous and arterial clotting)
Rare congenital deficiencies
Malnutrition

notes

platelet aggregation test

Type of test Blood

Normal findings Depend on the platelet agonist used

Test explanation and related physiology

Platelet aggregation is an important part of hemostasis. Surrounding an area of acute blood vessel endothelial injury is a clump of platelets. Normal platelets adhere to this area of injury, and through a series of chemical reactions, they attract other platelets to the area. This is platelet aggregation, the first step of hemostasis. After this step, the normal coagulation factor waterfall occurs. Certain diseases that affect either platelet number or function can inhibit platelet aggregation and thereby prolong bleeding times. Congenital syndromes, uremia, myeloproliferative disorders, and drugs are associated with abnormal platelet aggregation. If blood is passed through a heart-lung or dialysis pump, the platelet injury can occur and aggregation can be reduced.

There are many agonists used to stimulate platelet aggregation in the laboratory. Platelet aggregation is measured by determining the turbidity of platelet-rich plasma. As platelet aggregation is stimulated in vitro, turbidity decreases and light transmission through the specimen increases. This test is performed with an optical device called an *aggregometer*. Usually, the patient's blood specimen is spun to a platelet-rich component. Next, an agonist such as adenosine diphosphate, collagen, epinephrine, or ristocetin is added. Turbidity is then measured within the aggregometer, and a curve indicating light transmission per unit of time is plotted. Normal curves have been identified for any one agonist that is used.

This is a very sensitive test, and it can be significantly affected by a number of variables, including:

1. Concentration of sodium citrate
2. Platelet count
3. Storage temperature
4. Concentration of the agonists
5. Reaction temperature
6. Degrees of lipemia, hemoglobinemia, or bilirubinemia

Interfering factors

- Factors that may cause *increased* levels include blood storage temperature, hyperbilirubinemia, hemoglobinemia, hyperlipidemia, and platelet count.
- Drugs that may cause *decreased* levels include aspirin, antibiotics, sodium warfarin (Coumadin), and heparin.

Procedure and patient care

Before

- Explain the procedure to the patient.
- Tell the patient that no fasting is required.

During

- Collect 5 to 7 ml of venous blood in a blue-top tube.
- If the patient is receiving any drugs that may interfere with platelet aggregation or has any diseases such as jaundice, hyperlipidemia, or hemolysis, this should be listed on the laboratory request slip.

After

- Apply pressure or a pressure dressing to the venipuncture site.
- Assess the venipuncture site for bleeding.
- Remember that abnormalities in platelet aggregation can prolong bleeding time, and a significant hematoma at the venipuncture site may occur.

Abnormal findings

Prolonged platelet aggregation

Various congenital disorders (e.g., Wiskott-Aldrich syndrome, Bernard-Soulier syndrome, glycogen storage)

Connective tissue disorder (e.g., lupus erythematosus)

Recent cardiopulmonary or dialysis bypass

Various myeloproliferative diseases

Primary protein disease

von Willebrand's disease

Uremia

notes

platelet antibody detection (Antiplatelet antibody detection)

Type of test Blood

Normal findings No antiplatelet antibodies identified

Test explanation and related physiology

Immune-mediated destruction of platelets may be caused by autoantibodies directed against antigens located on the platelet membrane. Many different laboratory techniques can be used to demonstrate the antiplatelet antibodies. These tests can directly identify the immunoglobulin with use of radioimmunoassay or immunofluorescence. Quantitative measurements are possible with cytofluorometry. Other tests identify complement binding on the affected platelet membrane. Most antiplatelet antibody testing is now performed using immunologic assays.

Antibodies directed to platelets will cause early destruction of the platelets and subsequent thrombocytopenia. Idiopathic thrombocytopenia purpura is a term that describes a group of disorders characterized by immune-mediated destruction of the platelets within the spleen or other reticuloendothelial organs. The development of these antibodies cannot be identified. Even so, other immunologic causes of thrombocytopenia can be clearly related to induction of antiplatelet antibodies by drugs, previous blood transfusions, or maternal-fetal platelet antigen incapability. Posttransfusion purpura is a rare syndrome characterized by the sudden onset of severe thrombocytopenia a few weeks after transfusion of red blood cells or platelets. This is usually associated with an autoantibody to one of the platelet-specific antigens. Neonatal thrombocytopenia is associated with fetal platelet counts of below 50,000 that persist for the first 2 to 3 weeks of the newborn's life. This is caused by transplacental passage of maternal antiplatelet antibody against the newborn's platelet-specific antigen.

A host of drugs are known to induce autoimmune-mediated thrombocytopenia. They are analgesics (salicylates, acetaminophen), antibiotics (cephalosporins, penicillin, sulfa drugs), quinidine-like drugs, hypnotics (phenobarbital), oral hypoglycemic agents (e.g., chlorpropamide), heavy metals (e.g., gold, organic arsenicals), diuretics (e.g., chlorothiazide), and others (e.g., digoxin, propylthiouracil, Antabuse, heparin).

P

Interfering factor

- Blood transfusion may cause the development of isoantibodies to HLA antigens on the platelets or red blood cells.

Procedure and patient care

Before

- Explain the procedure to the patient.
- Tell the patient that no fasting is required.

During

- Collect 10 to 30 ml of blood in a red-top tube. The amount of blood required depends on the initial platelet count.

After

- Apply pressure or a pressure dressing to the venipuncture site.
- Assure adequate hemostasis in all patients who are suspected to have thrombocytopenia.

Abnormal findings

Immune thrombocytopenia
Idiopathic thrombocytopenia purpura
Neonatal thrombocytopenia

Posttransfusion purpura
Drug-induced thrombocytopenia
Paroxysmal hemoglobinuria

notes

platelet count (Thrombocyte count)

Type of test Blood

Normal findings

Adult/elderly: 150,000-400,000/mm³ or 150 to 400 × 10⁹/L (SI units)
Premature infant: 100,000-300,000/mm³
Newborn: 150,000-300,000/mm³
Infant: 200,000-475,000 mm³
Child: 150,000-400,000/mm³

Possible critical values <50,000 or >1 million/mm³

Test explanation and related physiology

The platelet count is an actual count of the number of platelets (thrombocytes) per cubic milliliter of blood. Platelet activity is essential to blood clotting. Because platelets can clump together, automated counting is subject to at least a 10% to 15% error. Low levels are often hand counted. Counts of 150,000 to 400,000/mm³ are considered normal. Counts less than 100,000/mm³ are considered to indicate thrombocytopenia; thrombocytosis is said to exist when counts are greater than 400,000/mm³. Vascular thrombosis with organ infarction is the major complication of thrombocytosis; spontaneous hemorrhage may occur with thrombocytopenia.

Spontaneous bleeding is a serious danger when platelet counts fall below 20,000/mm³. With counts above 40,000/mm³, spontaneous bleeding rarely occurs, but prolonged bleeding from trauma or surgery may occur at this level.

Causes of *thrombocytopenia* (decreased number of platelets) include:

1. Reduced production of platelets (secondary to bone marrow failure or infiltration of fibrosis, tumor, and so on)
2. Sequestration of platelets (secondary to hypersplenism)
3. Accelerated destruction of platelets (secondary to antibodies, infections, drugs, prosthetic heart valves)
4. Consumption of platelets (secondary to disseminated intravascular coagulation)
5. Platelet loss from hemorrhage

Thrombocytosis (increased number of platelets) may occur as a compensatory response to severe hemorrhage. Other conditions

P

associated with thrombocytosis include polycythemia vera, leukemia, postsplenectomy syndromes, and various malignant disorders.

Interfering factors

- Living in high altitudes may cause increased platelet levels.
- Strenuous exercise may cause increased levels.
- Decreased levels may be seen before menstruation.
- ✗ Drugs that may cause *increased* levels include oral contraceptives.
- ✗ Drugs that may cause *decreased* levels include acetaminophen, aspirin, chemotherapeutic agents, chloramphenicol, colchicine, H_2-blocking agents (cimetidine, Zantac), hydralazine, indomethacin, isoniazid (INH), quinidine, streptomycin, sulfonamides, thiazide diuretics, and tolbutamide (Orinase).

Procedure and patient care

Before

- Explain the procedure to the patient.
- Tell the patient that no fasting is required.

During

- Collect approximately 5 to 7 ml of peripheral venous blood in a lavender-top tube.
- List on the laboratory slip any drugs or other factors that may affect test results.

After

- Apply pressure or a pressure dressing to the venipuncture site.
- Assess the venipuncture site for bleeding.
- If the results indicate that the patient has a serious platelet deficiency:
  1. Observe the patient for signs and symptoms of bleeding.
  2. Check for blood in the urine and all excretions.
  3. Assess the patient for bruises, petechiae, bleeding from the gums, epistaxis, and low back pain.

Abstract findings

▲ Increased levels (thrombocytosis)

Malignant disorder
Polycythemia vera
Leukemia
Postsplenectomy syn-
 drome
Rheumatoid arthritis
Cirrhosis
Trauma

▼ Decreased levels (thrombocytopenia)

Hypersplenism
Hemorrhage
Idiopathic thrombocyto-
 penic purpura
Leukemia
Liver disease
Kidney disease
Disseminated intravascu-
 lar coagulation
Systemic lupus erythema-
 tosus
Sequela of massive blood
 transfusion
Pernicious anemia
Hemolytic anemia
Cancer chemotherapy
Consumption of platelets
Platelet destruction

notes

platelet volume, mean (Mean platelet volume [MPV])

Type of test Blood

Normal findings 25 μm in diameter

Test explanation and related physiology

The MPV is a measure of the volume of a large number of platelets determined by an automated analyzer. MPV is to platelets as mean corpuscular volume (see p. 697) is to the red blood cell.

The MPV varies with total platelet production. In cases with a nonmarrow cause of reduced platelet count, the MPV increases as the normal bone marrow produces (younger and larger) platelets to compensate for the ongoing loss. When lack of bone marrow function is the cause of a low platelet count, the megakaryocytes are small, and therefore the platelets are small. This will be reflected as a low MPV; thus MPV is very useful in the differential diagnosis of thrombocytopenic disorders.

Interfering factor

- Blood collection tubes with ethylenediaminetetraacetic acid can create a variation of as much as 25% in the size of the platelets.

Procedure and patient care

Before
- Explain the procedure to the patient.
- Tell the patient that no fasting is required.

During
- Collect 5 to 7 ml of venous blood in a lavender-top tube.

After
- Apply pressure or a pressure dressing to the venipuncture site.
- Assess the venipuncture site for bleeding.
- If the patient is known to have a low platelet count:
  1. Observe the patient for signs and symptoms of bleeding.
  2. Check for blood in the urine and all excretions.
  3. Assess the patient for bruises, petechiae, bleeding of the gums, epistaxis, and low back pain.

Abnormal findings

▲ **Increased levels**
  Bernard-Soulier syn-
    drome
  May-Hegglin anomaly
  Valvular heart disease
  Myeloproliferative disor-
    der

▼ **Decreased levels**
  Aplastic anemia
  Chemotherapy-induced
    myelosuppression
  Megaoblastic anemia
  Hypersplenism
  Wiskott-Aldrich syn-
    drome

Normal MPV in thrombocytopenic patients
Eclampsia
Idiopathic thrombocytopenia purpura

notes

P

plethysmography, arterial

Type of test Manometric

Normal findings
<20 mm Hg difference in systolic blood pressure of the lower extremity compared with the upper extremity

Normal pulse wave amplitude showing a steep upswing, an acute narrow peak, and a more gentle downslope containing a dicrotic notch (normal arterial pulse wave)

Test explanation and related physiology
Plethysmography is usually performed to rule out occlusive disease of the lower extremities; however, it also can identify arteriosclerotic disease in the upper extremity. This test does require one normal extremity against which the other extremities may be compared.

Arterial plethysmography is performed by applying three blood pressure cuffs to the proximal, middle, and distal portions of the extremity. These are then attached to a pulse volume recorder (plethysmograph), and each pulse wave can be displayed. A reduction in amplitude of a pulse wave in any of the three cuffs indicates arterial occlusion immediately proximal to the area where the decreased amplitude is noted. Also, measurements of arterial pressures are performed at each cuff site. A difference in pressure greater than 20 mm Hg indicates a degree of arterial occlusion in the extremity. A positive result is reliable evidence of arteriosclerotic peripheral vascular occlusion. A negative result, however, does not definitely exclude this diagnosis, because extensive vascular collateralization can compensate for even a complete arterial occlusion.

Although it is not as accurate as arteriography (see p. 100), plethysmography is performed without serious complications and can be done for seriously ill patients who cannot be transported to the arteriography laboratory.

Interfering factors
- Arterial occlusion proximal to the extremity
- Cigarette smoking, because nicotine can cause transient arterial constriction

Procedure and patient care

Before

- Explain the procedure to the patient.
- Inform the patient that this test is painless.
- Tell the patient that he or she must lie still during the testing procedure.
- Remove all clothing from the patient's extremities.
- Instruct the patient to avoid smoking for at least 30 minutes before the test. Nicotine creates constriction of the peripheral arteries and alters the test results.
- Tell the patient that no fasting is required.

During

- Note the following procedural steps:
  1. The patient is placed in the semirecumbent position.
  2. The cuffs are applied to the extremities and then inflated to 65 mm Hg to increase their sensitivity to pulse waves.
  3. The pulse waves are recorded on the plethysmographic paper.
  4. The amplitudes and form of the pulse wave of each cuff are measured and compared. A marked reduction in wave amplitude indicates arterial occlusive disease.
- Note that this test usually is performed in the noninvasive vascular laboratory or at the patient's bedside by a noninvasive vascular technologist in approximately 30 minutes.
- Inform the patient that results are usually interpreted by a physician and are available in a few hours.
- Remind the patient that no discomfort is associated with this test.

After

- Encourage the patient to verbalize any concerns regarding the test results.

Abnormal findings

Arterial occlusive disease
Arterial trauma
Small vessel diabetic changes
Vascular diseases (e.g., Raynaud's phenomenon)
Arterial embolization

notes

plethysmography, venous (Cuff pressure test)

Type of test Manometric

Normal findings Patent venous system without evidence of thrombosis or occlusion

Test explanation and related physiology

Plethysmography measures changes in the volume of an extremity. Usually, this test is performed on a leg to exclude deep-vein thrombosis. During this test, blood pressure cuffs are placed on the proximal, middle, and distal portions of the extremity and attached to a pulse volume recorder. The leg volume can then be recorded as a baseline value. The venous system is occluded by inflating the most proximal cuff *(occlusion cuff)*; the most distal cuff *(recording cuff)* should record a sudden increase in venous volume. When the occlusion cuff is released, the venous volume of the leg should return to preocclusion baseline levels. In patients with venous obstruction, no initial increase in leg volume is recorded. Because venous outflow is obstructed, the venous volume of the leg will not dissipate quickly.

The results of venous plethysmography are less accurate than those of venography (see p. 870); however, no complications are associated with this noninvasive study. Plethysmography can be performed easily and quickly on any patient with suspected venous disease. Furthermore, with the use of portable plethysmography, this test can be performed at the bedside for extremely ill patients.

Doppler flow studies are now being performed to identify deep-vein thrombosis, but Doppler flow studies are less accurate in evaluating the venous system below the knee.

Interfering factor

- Venous occlusion more proximal to the site of the occlusion cuff

Procedure and patient care

Before

- Explain the procedure to the patient.
- Tell the patient that no fasting is required.
- Assure the patient that no discomfort is associated with the study.

- Instruct the patient to lie still during the testing.
- Remove all clothing from the patient's extremity to be tested.

During

- Note the following procedural steps:
  1. A large, inflatable occlusion cuff is placed on the proximal portion of the extremity, usually a leg.
  2. A second, smaller plethysmographic monitor or recording cuff is placed more distal on the leg. A third cuff may be placed in between the proximal and distal cuffs.
  3. The second cuff is inflated to 10 mm Hg to facilitate recognition of small changes in the leg's venous volume.
  4. The effects of respiration on the leg's venous volume are evaluated. If no significant changes occur with respiration, venous occlusion can be suspected.
  5. The occlusion cuff is inflated to 50 mm Hg. The monitor cuff should demonstrate a rise in venous volume, displayed on the pulse-monitor recorder.
  6. After the highest volume is recorded in the monitor cuff, the occlusion cuff is rapidly deflated. The leg should return to its preocclusion volume within 1 second. If return to preocclusion baseline values is delayed for a long period, venous thrombosis is suspected.
  7. Often, this test is performed concomitantly with Doppler ultrasound of the venous system (see p. 329).
- Note that this test is usually performed in the noninvasive vascular laboratory or at the patient's bedside by a noninvasive vascular technologist in approximately 30 minutes.
- Remind the patient that no discomfort is associated with this test.

After

- Note that no special aftercare is needed.

Abnormal findings

Partial venous obstruction
Total venous obstruction

notes

pleural biopsy

Type of test Microscopic examination of tissue

Normal findings No evidence of pathology

Test explanation and related physiology

Pleural biopsy is the removal of pleural tissue for histologic examination. This test is indicated when the pleural fluid obtained by thoracentesis (see p. 784) is exudative fluid, which suggests infection, neoplasm, or tuberculosis. The pleural biopsy is indicated to distinguish among these disease processes.

Pleural biopsy is usually performed by a percutaneous needle biopsy of the pleura. It also can be performed via thoracoscopy, which is done by inserting a laparoscope into the pleural space for inspection and biopsy of the pleura. Pleural tissue also may be obtained by an *open pleural biopsy*, which involves a limited thoracotomy and requires general anesthesia. For this procedure, a small intercostal incision is made and the biopsy of the pleura is done under direct observation. The advantage of this open procedure is that a larger specimen may be obtained.

Contraindications

- Patients with prolonged bleeding or clotting times

Potential complications

- Bleeding or injury to the lung
- Pneumothorax

Procedure and patient care

Before
- Explain the procedure to the patient.
- Obtain informed consent for this procedure.
- Tell the patient that no fasting or sedation is required.
- Instruct the patient to remain very still during the procedure. Any movement may cause inadvertent needle damage.

During
- Note the following procedural steps for percutaneous needle biopsy:
  1. This procedure is usually performed with the patient in a sitting position with his or her shoulders and arms elevated and supported by a padded overbed table.

2. After the presence of the fluid has been determined by the thoracentesis technique, the skin overlying the biopsy site is anesthetized and pierced with a scalpel blade.

3. A needle is inserted with a cannula until fluid is removed (some fluid is left in the pleural space after the thoracentesis to make the biopsy easier).

4. The inner needle is removed, and a blunt-tipped, hooked biopsy trocar, attached to a three-way stopcock, is inserted into the cannula.

5. The patient is instructed to expire all air and then perform the Valsalva maneuver to prevent air from entering the pleural space.

6. The cannula and biopsy trocar are withdrawn while the hook catches the parietal wall and takes a specimen with its cutting edge.

7. Usually, three biopsy specimens are taken from different sites at the same session.

8. The specimens are placed in a fixative solution and sent to the laboratory immediately.

9. After the specimens are taken, additional parietal fluid can be removed.

- Note that this procedure is performed by a physician at the patient's bedside, in a special procedure room, or in the physician's office in approximately 30 minutes.
- Because of the local anesthetic, tell the patient that little discomfort is associated with this procedure.

P

After

- Apply an adhesive bandage to the biopsy site.
- Note that a chest x-ray film is usually taken to detect the potential complication of pneumothorax.
- Observe the patient for signs of respiratory distress (e.g., shortness of breath, diminished breath sounds) on the side of the biopsy.
- Observe the patient's vital signs frequently for evidence of bleeding (increased pulse, decreased blood pressure).
- Ensure that the biopsy specimen is sent immediately to the laboratory.

Abnormal findings

Neoplasm
Tuberculosis

porphyrins and porphobilinogens

Type of test Urine (fresh and 24-hour)

Normal findings

Porphyrins: <50 μg/24 hr or <60 nmol/day (SI units)
Porphobilinogens: 0-2.0 mg/24 hr or 0-8.8 μmol/day (SI units)

Test explanation and related physiology

Porphyrins are proteins used in the synthesis of heme in hemoglobin. Porphyrias are hereditary metabolic disorders of heme synthesis.

Abnormalities of porphyrin metabolism may be genetic or drug (usually lead) induced. These abnormalities are marked by increased levels of the heme precursors porphyrin and porphobilinogen. Normally, insignificant amounts of porphyrins are excreted in the urine. In most forms of porphyria, increased levels of porphyrins and porphobilinogen are found in the urine. This test is a quantitative analysis of urinary porphyrins. If porphyrins are present, the urine may be colored amber-red or burgundy; the urine may turn even darker after standing in the light. (See also test for uroporphyrinogen-I-synthetase, p. 865.)

Interfering factors

☛ Drugs that may alter test results include aminosalicylic acid (PAS), barbiturates, chloral hydrate, chlorpropamide (Diabinese), ethyl alcohol, griseofulvin, morphine, oral contraceptives, phenazopyridine (Pyridium), procaine, and sulfonamides.

Procedure and patient care

Before
- Explain the procedure to the patient.
- Tell the patient that no fasting is required.

During

Porphobilinogens
- Collect a freshly voided urine specimen.
- Protect the specimen from light.
- For both porphobilinogens and porphyrins, indicate on the laboratory slip any drugs that may affect test results.

Porphyrins

- Instruct the patient to begin a 24-hour urine collection after voiding. Discard the initial specimen and start the 24-hour timing at that point.
- Collect all the urine passed during the next 24 hours.
- Instruct the patient to avoid alcohol during the collection period.
- Show the patient where to store the urine container.
- Keep the specimen on ice or refrigerated during the 24 hours.
- Keep the urine in a light-resistant specimen bottle with a preservative to prevent degradation of the light-sensitive porphyrin.
- Indicate the starting time on the urine container and the laboratory slip.
- Post the times for urine collection in a prominent place to prevent accidental discarding of the specimen.
- Instruct the patient to void before defecating so that urine is not contaminated by feces.
- Remind the patient not to put toilet paper in the collection container.
- Encourage the patient to drink fluids during the 24 hours unless contraindicated for medical purposes.
- Collect the last specimen as close as possible to the end of the 24-hour period. Add this urine to the collection.

After

- Transport the urine specimens promptly to the laboratory.

Abnormal findings

▲ **Increased levels**

Porphyrias	Lead poisoning
Liver disease	Pellagra

notes

positron emission tomography (PET)

Type of test Nuclear scan, x-ray

Normal findings Normal patterns of tissue metabolism

Test explanation and related physiology

PET is a unique technique that combines the early biochemical assessment of pathology achieved by nuclear medicine with the precise localization achieved by CT. PET is able to penetrate the body's metabolism by recording tracers of nuclear annihilations in body tissue. The selected tracers are chemically designed to measure body processes (e.g., blood flow and volume, protein metabolism).

A chemical compound with the desired biologic activity is labeled with a radioactive isotope that decays by emitting a positron (or positive electron). The positron combines with an electron, and the two are mutually annihilated with emission of two gamma rays. The gamma rays penetrate the surrounding tissue and are recorded outside the body by a circular array of detectors. Because the gamma rays travel in almost exactly opposite directions, their source can be established with a high degree of accuracy. A computer reconstructs the spatial distribution of the radioactivity for a selected plane within the patient and displays the resulting image on a cathode ray screen. PET provides noninvasive regional assessment of many biochemical processes essential to the functioning of the organ being studied.

The technology of PET is now well developed, and both its capabilities and limitations are being increasingly understood. Many PET studies are being carried out with results that cannot be obtained by other techniques. These include:

1. Determination of regional metabolism in the heart and brain (e.g., radioactive glucose used to map biochemical activity in the brain)
2. Studies of tissue permeability
3. Measurement of the size of infarcts in the heart from a coronary occlusion
4. Investigation into the physiology of psychosis
5. Assessment of the effects of drugs on diseased or malfunctioning tissues
6. Possibility of measuring the effects of cancer treatment by

changes in malignant tissues and by biochemical reactions in surrounding normal tissues

The dose of radioactive material given to the patient, either a gas or injection, produces a radiation exposure comparable to that of other nuclear medicine studies. The cost of PET technology is high; it requires a cyclotron, appropriate chemical facilities, computer equipment, and effective group work by physicians, chemists, mathematicians, physiologists, and physicists. This procedure, once regarded as exotic, may now be on the threshold of becoming a fundamental tool in diagnostic medicine.

Interfering factors

- Recent use (within 24 hours) of caffeine, alcohol, or tobacco may affect test results.
- Excessive anxiety may affect brain function evaluation.
- Drugs that may influence results include tranquilizers and sedatives.

Procedure and patient care

Before

- Explain the procedure to the patient. Because most patients have not heard of this study, they are often anxious and require emotional support.
- Obtain informed consent if required by the institution.
- Inform the patient that he or she may have two IV lines inserted, one for infusion of the radioisotope and the other for serial blood samples.
- Inform the patient that he or she does not need to restrict food or fluids on the day of the test; however, the patient should refrain from alcohol, caffeine, and tobacco for 24 hours.
- Instruct diabetic patients to take their pretest dose of insulin at a meal 3 to 4 hours before the test.
- Tell the patient that no sedatives or tranquilizers should be taken, because he or she may need to perform certain mental activities during the test.
- Tell the patient to empty the bladder before the test for comfort.

During

- Note the following procedural steps:
  1. The patient is positioned in a comfortable, reclining chair.
  2. Two IV lines are inserted.

3. The radioactive material can be infused through an IV line or be inhaled as a radioactive gas.
4. The gamma rays that penetrate the tissues are recorded outside the body by a circular array of detectors and are displayed by a computer.
5. If the brain is being scanned, the patient may be asked to perform different cognitive activities (e.g., reciting the Pledge of Allegiance) to measure changes in brain activity during reasoning or remembering.
6. Extraneous auditory and visual stimuli are minimized by a blindfold and ear plugs.

- Note that this procedure is performed by a physician or trained technologist in approximately 60 to 90 minutes.
- Tell the patient that the only discomfort associated with this study is insertion of the two IV lines.

After

- Instruct the patient to change position slowly from lying to standing to avoid postural hypotension.
- Encourage the patient to drink fluids and urinate frequently to aid removal of the radioisotope from the bladder.

Abnormal findings

Myocardial infarction
Cerebrovascular accident
  (stroke)
Epilepsy
Parkinson's disease
Dementia
Alzheimer's disease
Schizophrenia

Coronary artery disease
Pulmonary edema
Pneumonia
Brain tumor
Breast tumor
Huntington's disease

notes

potassium, blood (K^+)

Type of test Blood

Normal findings

Adults/elderly: 3.5-5.0 mEq/L or 3.5-5.0 mmol/L (SI units)
Child: 3.4-4.7 mEq/L
Infant: 4.1-5.3 mEq/L
Newborn: 3.9-5.9 mEq/L

Possible critical values

Adult: <2.5 or >6.5 mEq/L
Newborn: <2.5 or >8.0 mEq/L

Test explanation and related physiology

Potassium is the major cation within the cell. The intracellular potassium concentration is approximately 150 mEq/L, whereas the normal serum potassium concentration is approximately 4 mEq/L. This ratio is the most important determinant in maintaining membrane electrical potential in excitable neuromuscular tissue. Because the serum concentration of potassium is so small, minor changes in concentration have significant consequences. The potassium level should be carefully followed in patients taking potassium-depleting diuretics and in those with renal failure or acidosis.

Serum potassium concentration depends on many factors, including:

1. *Aldosterone.* This hormone tends to increase renal losses of potassium.
2. *Sodium reabsorption.* As sodium is reabsorbed, potassium is lost.
3. *Acid-base balance.* Alkalotic states tend to lower serum potassium levels by causing a shift of potassium into the cell. Acidotic states tend to raise serum potassium levels by reversing that shift.

Symptoms of hyperkalemia include irritability, nausea, vomiting, intestinal colic, and diarrhea. The electrocardiogram may demonstrate peaked T waves, a widened QRS complex, and depressed ST segment. Signs of hypokalemia are related to a decrease in contractility of smooth, skeletal, and cardiac muscles, which results in weakness, paralysis, hyporeflexia, ileus, increased

P

cardiac sensitivity to digoxin, cardiac arrhythmias (dysrhythmias), flattened T waves, and prominent U waves.

Interfering factors

- Exercise of the forearm with a tourniquet in place may increase potassium levels.
- Hemolysis of blood during venipuncture causes increased levels.
- Drugs that may cause *increased* potassium levels include aminocaproic acid, antibiotics, antineoplastic drugs, captopril, epinephrine, heparin, histamine, isoniazid (INH), lithium, mannitol, potassium-sparing diuretics, potassium supplements, and succinylcholine.
- Drugs that may cause *decreased* levels include acetazolamide, aminosalicylic acid (PAS), amphotericin B, carbenicillin, cisplatin, diuretics (potassium wasting), glucose infusions, insulin, laxatives, lithium carbonate, penicillin G sodium (high doses), phenothiazines, salicylates (aspirin), and sodium polystyrene sulfonate (Kayexalate).

Procedure and patient care

Before

- Explain the procedure to the patient.
- Tell the patient that no special diet or fasting is required.

During

- Instruct the patient to avoid opening and closing the hand after a tourniquet is applied.
- Collect approximately 5 to 7 ml of venous blood in a red- or green-top tube.
- Avoid hemolysis.
- Indicate on the laboratory slip any drugs that may affect test results.

After

- Apply pressure or a pressure dressing to the venipuncture site.
- Assess the venipuncture site for bleeding.
- Evaluate the patient with increased or decreased potassium levels for cardiac arrhythmias (dysrhythmias).
- Monitor for hypokalemia in patients taking digoxin and diuretics.
- If indicated, administer resin exchanges (e.g., Kayexalate enema) to correct hyperkalemia.

Abnormal findings

▲ **Increased levels (hyperkalemia)**

Increased potassium intake
  Excessive dietary intake
  Excessive IV intake
Decreased potassium loss
  Acute or chronic renal failure
  Addison's disease
  Hypoaldosteronism
  Aldosterone-inhibiting diuretics (e.g., spironolactone, triamterene)
Shift from intracellular space
  Acidosis
  Infection
  Crush injury to tissues
Pseudohyperkalemia
  Poor venipuncture technique, causing hemolysis
  Transfusion of hemolyzed blood

▼ **Decreased levels (hypokalemia)**

Decreased potassium intake
  Deficient dietary intake
  Deficient IV intake
Excessive potassium loss
  Gastrointestinal disorders (e.g., diarrhea, vomiting, villous adenomas)
  Diuretics
  Hyperaldosteronism
  Cushing's syndrome
  Renal tubular acidosis
  Licorice ingestion
Shift to intracellular space
  Alkalosis
  Insulin or glucose administration
  Calcium administration

P

notes

potassium, urine (K⁺)

Type of test Urine (24-hour)

Normal findings

25-120 mEq/L/day or 25-120 mmol/day (SI units)
Values vary greatly with diet

Test explanation and related physiology

Potassium is the major cation within the cell. The electrolyte balance of potassium can be measured in both a spot and a 24-hour urine collection. A 24-hour collection is especially important to evaluate electrolyte (especially hypokalemia) balance, acid-base balance, and renal and adrenal diseases.

The serum potassium concentration depends on many factors. Aldosterone tends to increase the renal losses of potassium. Also, as sodium is reabsorbed, potassium is lost. Acid-base balance affects potassium concentration as well. Alkalotic states tend to lower serum potassium levels, causing a shift of potassium into the cell. Acidotic states tend to raise serum potassium levels by reversing the shift. Because the kidneys cannot reabsorb potassium, the balance of potassium in the body is regulated by kidney excretion of potassium through the urine.

Interfering factors

- Dietary intake affects potassium levels.
- Excessive intake or licorice may cause *increased* levels of potassium in the urine.
- ☛ Drugs that may cause *increased* levels include diuretics, glucocorticoids, and salicylates.

Procedure and patient care

Before

- Explain the procedure to the patient.
- Tell the patient that no special diet is required.

During

- Instruct the patient to begin the 24-hour urine collection after voiding.
- Discard the initial specimen and start the 24-hour timing at that point.
- Collect all urine passed during the next 24 hours.

- Show the patient where to store the urine container.
- Keep the specimen on ice or refrigerated during the entire 24 hours.
- Indicate the starting time on the urine container and the laboratory slip.
- Post the hours for urine collection in a noticeable place to prevent accidental discarding of the specimen.
- Instruct the patient to void before defecating so that the urine is not contaminated by feces.
- Remind the patient not to put toilet paper in the collection container.
- Encourage the patient to drink fluids during the 24 hours.
- Instruct the patient to collect the last specimen as close as possible to the end of the 24-hour collection. Add this urine to the container.

After

- Transport the urine specimen promptly to the laboratory.

Abnormal findings

▲ **Increased levels**

Chronic renal failure
Renal tubular acidosis
Starvation
Cushing's syndrome
Hyperaldosteronism
Alkalosis
Excessive intake of licorice
Diabetic acidosis
Salicylate toxicity
Diuretic therapy

▼ **Decreased levels**

Dehydration
Starvation
Vomiting
Diarrhea
Malabsorption
Excessive intake of licorice
Acute renal failure

P

notes

prealbumin (PAB, Thyroxine-binding prealbumin [TBPA], Thyretin, Transthyretin)

Type of test Blood; urine (24-hour); cerebrospinal fluid (CSF) analysis

Normal findings

Serum

Adult/elderly: 15-36 mg/dl or 150-360 mg/L (SI units)
Child
   Cord: 13 mg/dl or 130 mg/L (SI units)
   1 year: 10 mg/dl or 100 mg/L
   2-36 months: 16-28 mg/dl or 160-280 mg/L

Urine (24-hour)

0.017-0.047 mg/day

Cerebrospinal fluid

Approximately 2% of total CSF protein

Possible critical values Serum prealbumin levels <10.7 mg/dl indicate severe nutritional deficiency.

Test explanation and related physiology

Prealbumin is one of the major plasma proteins. Because prealbumin can bind thyroxine, it is also called "thyroxine-binding prealbumin (TBA)." However, prealbumin is secondary to thyroxine-binding globulin in the transportation of triiodothyronine (T_3) and thyroxine (T_4). Prealbumin also plays a role in the transport and metabolism of vitamin A.

Since prealbumin levels in serum fluctuate more rapidly in response to alterations in synthetic rate than do those of other serum proteins, clinical interest in the quantification of serum prealbumin has centered on its usefulness as a marker of nutritional status. Its half-life of 1.9 days is much less than the 21-day half-life of albumin (see p. 670). Because of prealbumin's short half-life, it is a sensitive indicator of any change affecting protein synthesis and catabolism. Because of this, prealbumin is frequently ordered to monitor the effectiveness of total parenteral nutrition (TPN).

Prealbumin is significantly reduced in hepatobiliary disease because of impaired synthesis. Serum levels of prealbumin serve as a better indicator of liver injury than do albumin levels. Prealbumin is also a negative acute-phase reactant protein; serum levels decrease in inflammation, malignancy, and protein-wasting diseases of the intestines or kidneys. Since zinc is required for synthesis of prealbumin, low levels occur with a zinc deficiency. Increased levels of prealbumin occur in Hodgkin's disease and during chronic kidney disease.

Because of the low level of prealbumin in the serum, this protein is not often visualized on serum protein electrophoresis. However, because prealbumin crosses the blood-brain barrier, it is found in the CSF and can be seen on CSF electrophoresis (see discussion of lumbar puncture, p. 526).

Interfering factors

- Coexistent inflammation may make test result interpretation impossible.
- Drugs that may cause *increased* levels include anabolic steroids, androgens, and prednisolone.
- Drugs that may cause *decreased* levels include amiodarone, estrogens, and oral contraceptives.

Procedure and patient care

Before

- Explain the procedure to the patient.
- Tell the patient that no food or fluid restrictions are needed.
- If the patient is going to collect a 24-hour urine specimen, provide a collection bottle.

During

- Collect a venous blood sample in a red-top tube.

After

- Apply pressure or a pressure dressing to the venipuncture site.
- Observe the venipuncture site for bleeding.
- Transport the 24-hour urine specimen promptly to the laboratory.
- Inform the patient how and when to obtain the results of this study.

Abnormal findings

▲ **Increased levels**
Some cases of nephrotic
  syndrome
Hodgkin's disease
Chronic kidney disease
Pregnancy

▼ **Decreased levels**
Malnutrition
Liver damage
Burns
Salicylate poisoning
Inflammation

notes

pregnancy tests (Human chorionic gonadotropin [HCG])

Type of test Blood; urine

Normal findings Negative, unless pregnant

Test explanation and related physiology

All pregnancy tests are based on the detection of HCG, which is secreted by the trophoblast after the ovum is fertilized. HCG will appear in the blood and urine of pregnant women as early as 10 days after conception.

Methods of pregnancy testing fall into four categories. It is important to know that all these pregnancy studies demonstrate the presence of HCG and do not necessarily indicate a normal pregnancy. Hydatidiform mole of the uterus and choriocarcinoma of the uterus, testes, or ovaries can produce HCG. Because HCG is produced by these tumors, determination of HCG can be a valuable test for tumor activity. When HCG levels are elevated in these patients, tumor progression must be suspected. Decreasing HCG levels indicate effective antitumor treatment.

Biologic tests

Biologic (animal) tests have been used since the 1920s and are primarily of historical interest today. Urine from the patient is injected into an animal (mice, rabbit, toad, frog). If HCG is present, a specific response (usually corpus luteum development in the ovaries) will occur in that animal. The exact response varies according to the animal used. The result is usually positive by the fortieth day after the last menses. These biologic tests have largely been replaced by less expensive, more accurate, and more rapidly performed immunologic tests.

P

Immunologic tests (agglutination inhibition test [AIT])

Immunologic tests are performed using a commercially prepared reagent and can be completed within 2 minutes or 2 hours depending on the method used. Immunologic tests are based on the reaction of HCG with antiserum to chorionic gonadotropin. Previous immunologic tests had a high false-positive rate and were usually not positive until about 28 days after the last menses. Immunologic testing for the beta subunit of HCG greatly improved accuracy and shortened the time for positive testing (18 days). Now, with the development of monoclonal antibodies, immunoassays can identify pregnancy 1 to 2 weeks after conception. Several immunologic tests are now commercially available for testing by the public. Usually, these tests are compared with a standard containing a small amount of HCG. These tests take from 5 to 120 minutes to perform.

Radioimmunoassay (RIA)

The RIA is a highly sensitive and reliable blood test for the detection of the beta unit of HCG. In this test, maternal serum HCG (unlabeled) and HCG that has been radioactively bound to an antibody (labeled) compete for binding sites. The higher the concentration of HCG in the maternal serum, the greater the number of binding sites that will be occupied by the unlabeled HCG.

This study requires a blood sample in a red-top tube; however, RIA also may be performed with a urine test. The test can be done in 1 to 5 hours. This test is so sensitive that pregnancy can be diagnosed *before* the first missed menstrual period.

Radioreceptor assay (RRA)

The RRA for serum HCG is highly sensitive and accurate. This test can be performed in 1 hour. The major advantage of this study is its reliable diagnosis of early gestation in patients requesting an early termination of pregnancy and in cases where infertile couples are anxious to confirm pregnancy. This study is 90% to 95% accurate 6 to 8 days after conception. Even the minute amounts of HCG secreted in an ectopic pregnancy can be measured with this study. This test is also used in determining early spontaneous abortion in patients who desire to maintain the pregnancy. This test measures the ability of the blood sample to inhibit the binding of radiolabeled HCG to receptors.

Interfering factors

- Tests performed too early in the pregnancy, before a significant HCG level exists, may cause false-negative results.
- Hematuria and proteinuria in the urine may cause false-positive results.
- Hemolysis of blood may interfere with test results.
- Drugs that may cause false-negative urine results include diuretics (by causing diluted urine) and promethazine.
- Drugs that may cause false-positive results include anticonvulsants, antiparkinsonian drugs, hypnotics, and tranquilizers (especially promazine and its derivatives).

Procedure and patient care

Before

- Explain the procedure to the patient.
- If a urine specimen will be collected, give the patient a urine container the evening before so that she can provide a first-voided morning specimen. This specimen generally contains the greatest concentration of HCG.

During

- Collect the first-voided urine specimen for urine testing.
- Collect approximately 7 to 10 ml of venous blood in a red-top tube for serum testing. Avoid hemolysis.

After

- Apply pressure or a pressure dressing to the venipuncture site.
- Assess the venipuncture site for bleeding.
- Emphasize to the patient the importance of antepartal health care.

Abnormal findings

▲ **Increased levels**

Pregnancy
Ectopic pregnancy
Hydatidiform mole of the uterus
Choriocarcinoma of the uterus, testes, or ovaries
Tumor

▼ **Decreased levels**

Threatened abortion
Incomplete abortion
Dead fetus

P

notes

pregnanediol

Type of test Urine (24-hour)

Normal findings
Increased excretion after ovulation to >1 mg/24 hr
Values vary according to week of pregnancy

Test explanation and related physiology
Urinary pregnanediol is measured to evaluate progesterone production by the ovaries and placenta. The main effect of progesterone is on the endometrium. It initiates the secretory phase in anticipation of implantation of a fertilized ovum. Normally, progesterone is secreted by the ovarian corpus luteum following ovulation. Both serum progesterone levels and the urine concentration of progesterone metabolites (pregnanediol and others) are significantly increased during the later half of an ovulatory cycle. Pregnanediol is the most easily measured metabolite of progesterone.

Because pregnanediol levels rise rapidly after ovulation, this study is useful in documenting whether ovulation has occurred and, if so, its exact time. During pregnancy, pregnanediol levels normally rise because of the placental production of progesterone. Repeated assays can be used to monitor the status of the placenta.

Hormone assays for urinary pregnanediol are primarily used today to monitor progesterone supplementation in patients with an inadequate luteal phase. Urinary assays may be supplemented by plasma assays (progesterone assay, see p. 660), which are quicker and more accurate.

Interfering factors
- Drugs that may cause *increased* levels include adrenocorticotropic hormone (ACTH).
- Drugs that may cause *decreased* levels include oral contraceptives and progesterones.

Procedure and patient care
Before
- Explain the procedure to the patient.
- Tell the patient that no special diet is usually required.
- Inform the patient that no sedation or fasting is necessary.

During

- Instruct the patient to begin the 24-hour urine collection. Discard the initial specimen and start the 24-hour timing at that point.
- Collect all urine passed for the next 24 hours.
- Show the patient where to store the urine collection.
- Keep the specimen on ice or refrigerated during the 24 hours. Check with the laboratory to see if a preservative is needed.
- Indicate the starting time on the urine container and the laboratory slip.
- Post the hours for urine collection in a noticeable place to prevent accidental discarding of the specimen.
- Instruct the patient to void before defecating so that the urine is not contaminated by feces.
- Remind the patient not to put toilet paper in the collection container.
- Encourage the patient to drink fluids during the 24 hours.
- Instruct the patient to collect the last specimen as close as possible to the end of the 24-hour collection. Add this urine to the container.

After

- Record on the laboratory slip the date of the last menstrual period or the week of gestation during pregnancy.

Abnormal findings

▲ **Increased levels**

Ovulation
Pregnancy
Luteal cysts of ovary
Arrhenoblastoma of ovary
Hyperadrenocorticalism
Choriocarcinoma of ovary
Adrenocortical hyperplasia

▼ **Decreased levels**

Threatened abortion
Fetal death
Toxemia of pregnancy
Amenorrhea
Ovarian hypofunction
Placental failure
Preeclampsia
Ovarian neoplasm
Breast neoplasm

notes

progesterone assay

Type of test Blood

Normal findings

Preovulation: 20-150 ng/dl
Midcycle: 300-2400 ng/dl
Pregnancy: >2400 ng/dl

Test explanation and related physiology

Determination of the progesterone level provides evidence to confirm ovulation and to evaluate the function of the corpus luteum. A series of measurements can help define the day of ovulation. Plasma progesterone levels start to rise after ovulation with the luteinizing hormone (LH) surge, and they continue to rise for approximately 6 to 10 days and then fall. Normally, blood samples drawn at days 8 and 21 of the menstrual cycle will show a large increase in progesterone levels in the latter specimen, indicating that ovulation has occurred. Progesterone levels are also very high in early pregnancy. Certain adrenal and ovarian tumors may produce elevated levels as well.

Urinary pregnanediol levels (see p. 658) are an indirect measurement of progesterone production. Serum progesterone levels can provide comparable information and are sometimes done in place of endometrial biopsy (see p. 354) to determine the phase of the menstrual cycle.

Interfering factors

- Recent use of radioisotopes may affect test results.
- Hemolysis caused by rough handling of the sample may affect test results.
- ▼ Drugs that may interfere with test results include estrogen and progesterone.

Procedure and patient care

Before

- Explain the procedure to the patient.
- Tell the patient that no fasting is required.

During

- Collect approximately 5 to 7 ml of venous blood in a red-top tube.

- Indicate the date of the last menstrual period on the laboratory slip.

After

- Apply pressure or a pressure dressing to the venipuncture site.
- Assess the venipuncture site for bleeding.

Abnormal findings

▲ **Increased levels**
   Pregnancy
   Adrenal neoplasm
   Ovarian neoplasm

▼ **Decreased levels**
   Amenorrhea
   Fetal death
   Threatened abortion
   Toxemia of pregnancy

notes

P

progesterone receptor assay (PR assay, PRA, PgR)

Type of test Tumor-specimen analysis

Normal values

Negative: <10 fmol/g of tissue
Positive: >10 fmol/g of tissue

Test explanation and related physiology

The PR assay is used in determining the prognosis and treatment of breast cancer and, to a lesser degree, other cancers. These assays help to determine whether a tumor is likely to respond to endocrine medical or surgical therapy. The test is done on breast cancer specimens when a primary or recurrent cancer is identified; it is usually done in conjunction with estrogen receptor (ER) assay (see p. 376) to increase the predictability of a tumor response to hormone therapy. PR levels tend to be higher in the breast cancer of postmenopausal women. PR-positive tumors are suspected to be associated with a better prognosis than PR-negative tumors. Tumor response rates to medical or surgical hormonal manipulation are potentiated if the ER assay is positive. Response rates are as follows:

ER positive, PR positive = 75%
ER negative, PR positive = 60%
ER positive, PR negative = 35%
ER negative, PR negative = 25%

The test is performed in one of two ways. The standard method is to send 1 g of the breast cancer specimen to a centralized laboratory, where the PR protein is quantified in the cytoplasm or nucleus of breast cancer cells. Another method, however, is sending the actual, paraffin-embedded microscope slides to that laboratory for immunohistochemical staining for PR proteins. This latter method is now considered to be more accurate.

Other tumors (such as ovarian, melanoma, uterine, or pancreatic) are occasionally studied for ER and PR assay. This is mostly done within clinical trials. To date, hormonal therapy has not been very successful with these tumors.

Interfering factors

- Exogenous hormone use
- ✠ Use of hormones such as progesterone or estrogen may cause false-negative results.

Procedure and patient care

Before

- Prepare the patient for breast biopsy per routine protocol.
- Record the menstrual status of the patient.
- Record any exogenous hormone the patient may have used during the last 2 months.
- Instruct the patient to discontinue exogenous hormones before breast biopsy.

During

- The surgeon obtains at least 1 g of tissue.
- Place the specimen on ice, and send it to the laboratory immediately.
- In the pathology department, part of the specimen is used for routine histology. The other part (at least 1 g) is frozen and sent in dry ice to a central laboratory for PR analysis.
- Results are usually available in 2 weeks.

After

- Provide routine postoperative care.

Abnormal findings

▲ **Increased levels**
Hormonally dependent
cancer

▼ **Decreased levels**
Hormonally independent
cancer

notes

prolactin levels (PRLs)

Type of test Blood

Normal findings

Adult male: 0-20 ng/ml
Adult female: 0-20 ng/ml
Pregnant female: 20-400 ng/ml

Test explanation and related physiology

Prolactin is a hormone secreted by the anterior pituitary gland (adenohypophysis). In humans, prolactin promotes lactation. Prolactin secretion is controlled by prolactin-inhibiting and prolactin-releasing factors secreted by the hypothalamus. During sleep, prolactin levels increase twofold to threefold, to circulating levels equaling those of pregnant women. With breast stimulation, pregnancy, nursing, stress, or exercise, a surge of this hormone occurs. This hormone is elevated in patients with prolactin-secreting pituitary acidophilic or chromophobic adenomas, amenorrhea, galactorrhea, primary hypothyroidism, polycystic ovary syndrome, and anorexia. Paraneoplastic tumors may cause ectopic secretion of prolactin as well. In general, very high prolactin levels are more likely to be due to pituitary adenoma than to other causes.

The prolactin level is helpful in the diagnosis and follow-up of the diseases mentioned earlier. Successful treatment of these diseases can be recognized by a reduction in serum prolactin levels. The success of treatment can be monitored by obtaining repeated prolactin levels. Several stimulation (with TRH or chlorpromazine) and suppression (with levodopa) prolactin tests have been designed to help differentiate the various causes of prolactin deficiency.

Interfering factors

- Drugs that may cause *increased* values include phenothiazines, oral contraceptives, reserpine, opiates, verapamil, histamine antagonists, monoamine oxidase inhibitors, estrogens, and antihistamines.
- Drugs that may cause *decreased* values are ergot alkaloid derivatives, clonidine, levodopa, and dopamine.

Procedure and patient care

Before

- Explain the procedure to the patient.
- Tell the patient no fasting or special preparation is required.
- Inform the patient that this blood sample should be drawn in the morning.
- Record the use of any medication that may affect results.

During

- Obtain 5 to 7 ml of venous blood in a red-top tube.
- Transfer the specimen to the laboratory as soon as possible. If a delay occurs, the specimen should be placed on ice.

After

- Apply pressure or a pressure dressing to the venipuncture site.
- Assess the venipuncture site for bleeding.

Abnormal findings

▲ **Increased levels**
Galactorrhea
Amenorrhea
Prolactin-secreting
  pituitary tumor
Infiltrative diseases
  of the hypothalamus
  and pituitary stalk
  (e.g., granuloma,
  sarcoidosis)
Hypothyroidism
Renal failure
Anorexia nervosa
Perineoplastic ectopic
  production of prolactin
Metastatic cancer to the
  pituitary gland
Polycystic ovary
  syndrome

▼ **Decreased levels**
Pituitary apoplexy
Pituitary destruction
  from tumor (craniopha-
  ryngioma)

notes

prostate/rectal sonogram (Ultrasound prostate)

Type of test Ultrasound

Normal findings Normal size, contour, and consistency of the prostate gland

Test explanation and related physiology

Rectal ultrasound of the prostate is a very valuable tool in the early diagnosis of prostate cancer. When combined with rectal digital examination and prostate-specific antigen (see p. 668), very small prostate cancers can be identified. Rectal prostate sonography is also helpful in evaluating the seminal vessels and other perirectal tissue. Ultrasound is very helpful in guiding the direction of a prostate biopsy and can be very helpful in quantitating the volume of prostate cancer. When radiation therapy implantation is required for treatment, ultrasound is used to map the exact location of the prostate cancer. This test can be performed in the ultrasound section of the radiology department, and it is now being routinely performed in most urologists' offices. Results are available almost immediately.

Rectal ultrasound is very helpful in staging rectal cancers as well. The depth of transmural involvement and presence of extrarectal extension can be accurately assessed.

Ultrasonography requires the emission of high-frequency sound waves from a special transducer placed in the rectum. The sound waves are bounced back to the transducer and electronically converted into a pictoral image. A realistic Polaroid picture or x-ray film is obtained.

Interfering factor

- Stool within the rectum

Procedure and patient care

Before

- Explain the procedure to the patient.
- Instruct the patient that a small-volume rectal enema is required approximately 1 hour before the ultrasound examination.

During

- The patient is placed in the left lateral decubitus position.
- A digital rectal examination may be performed to assess the prostate gland or rectal tumor.

- A draped and lubricated ultrasound probe is placed within the rectum.
- Scans are performed in various spatial planes.

After

- Provide the patient with tissue material to cleanse the peri-anal area.

Abnormal findings

Prostate cancer
Benign prostatic hypertrophy
Prostatitis
Seminal vesicle tumor

Prostate abscess
Perirectal abscess
Intrarectal or perirectal tumor

notes

P

prostate-specific antigen (PSA)

Type of test Blood

Normal findings <4 ng/ml

Test explanation and related physiology

PSA is a glycoprotein (part carbohydrate, part protein) normally found in the cytoplasm of prostatic epithelial cells. This antigen can be detected in all males; however, its level is greatly increased in patients with prostatic cancer. Although PSA was originally measured by histochemical techniques, radioimmunoassay (RIA) techniques have recently increased its accuracy.

Elevated PSA levels are associated with prostate cancer. The higher the levels, the greater the tumor burden. Furthermore, the PSA assay is a sensitive test for monitoring response to therapy. Successful surgery, radiation, or hormone therapy is associated with a marked reduction in the PSA blood level. Subsequent significant elevation in PSA indicates the recurrence of prostatic cancer.

Prostate-specific antigen is more sensitive and specific than other prostatic tumor markers, such as prostatic acid phosphatase (PAP, see p. 8). Also, PSA is more accurate than PAP in monitoring response and recurrence of tumor after therapy.

PSA (and PAP) levels also may be minimally elevated in patients with benign prostatic hypertrophy (BPH) and prostatitis. PSA levels greater than 10 ng/ml indicate a high probability for prostate cancer. Lower values may be compatible with BPH or early prostate cancer. Several formulas have been created to partially correct for BPH, which normally occurs in elderly men (e.g., predicted PSA = 0.12 × gland volume [in cubic centimeters] as determined by ultrasound). A PSA level greater than that predicted would indicate cancer. PSA levels have been age adjusted by some investigators. Levels above those predicted by age would be compatible with cancer. Another way to tell whether moderate elevations in PSA levels are due to cancer or BPH is to repeat the PSA level at 3- to 6-month intervals. A rising trend would indicate cancer.

PSA has been recommended for routine use in screening men over 50 years of age. When combined with direct digital rectal examination, it can detect 80% of prostate cancers.

Procedure and patient care

Before

- Explain the procedure to the patient.
- Tell the patient that no fasting is required.

During

- Collect approximately 5 ml of blood in a red-top tube.

After

- Apply pressure or a pressure dressing to the venipuncture site.
- Observe the venipuncture site for bleeding.

Abnormal findings

▲ **Increased levels**

Prostate cancer
Benign prostatic hypertrophy
Prostatitis

notes

protein, blood (Albumin, blood; Serum albumin; Serum globulin; Total protein)

Type of test Blood

Normal findings

Adult/elderly
   Total protein: 6.4-8.3 g/dl or 64.0-83.0 g/L (SI units)
   Albumin: 3.5-5.0 g/dl or 35-50 g/L (SI units)
   Globulin: 2.3-3.4 g/dl
Total protein
   Premature infant: 4.2-7.6 g/dl
   Newborn: 4.6-7.4 g/dl
   Infant: 6.0-6.7 g/dl
   Child: 6.2-8.0 g/dl
Albumin
   Premature infant: 3.0-4.2 g/dl
   Newborn: 3.5-5.4 g/dl
   Infant: 4.4-5.4 g/dl
   Child: 4.0-5.9 g/dl

Test explanation and related physiology

Proteins are constituents of muscle, enzymes, hormones, transport vehicles, hemoglobin, and several other key functional and structural entities within the body. Proteins are the most significant component contributing to the osmotic pressure within the vascular space. This osmotic pressure keeps fluid within the vascular space, minimizing extravasation of fluid.

Albumin and globulin constitute most of the protein within the body and are measured in the total protein. *Albumin* is a protein that is formed within the liver. This makes up approximately 60% of the total protein. The major effect of albumin within the blood is to maintain colloidal osmotic pressure. Furthermore, albumin transports important blood constituents such as drugs, hormones, and enzymes. *Globulins* are the key building block of antibodies. Their role in maintaining osmotic pressure is far less than that of albumin. Globulins, to a lesser degree, also act as transport vehicles. Both albumin and globulins can be measured separately.

Albumin is synthesized within the liver and is therefore a measure of hepatocyte function. When disease affects the liver cell, the hepatocyte loses its ability to synthesize albumin. The serum albumin level is greatly decreased. Because the half-life of albumin is 12 to 18 days, however, severe impairment of hepatic albumin synthesis may not be recognized until after that period.

Serum albumin and globulin are also measures of nutrition. Malnourished patients, especially after surgery, have a greatly decreased level of serum proteins. Burn patients and patients who have protein-losing enteropathies and uropathies have low levels of protein despite normal synthesis. Pregnancy, especially the third trimester, is usually associated with reduced total proteins.

In some diseases, albumin is selectively diminished and globulins are normal or increased to maintain a normal total protein level. For example, in collagen vascular diseases (e.g., lupus erythematosus), capillary permeability is increased. Albumin, a molecule much smaller than globulin, is selectively lost into the extravascular space. Another group of diseases similarly associated with low albumin, high globulin, and normal total protein levels is chronic liver diseases. In these diseases, the liver cannot produce albumin but globulin is adequately made in the reticuloendothelial system. In both these types of diseases, the albumin level is low but the total protein level is normal because of increased globulin levels. These changes, however, can be detected if one measures the albumin/globulin ratio. Normally, this ratio exceeds 1.0. The diseases just described that selectively affect albumin levels are associated with lesser ratios.

Increased total protein levels, particularly the globulin fraction, occur with multiple myeloma and other gammopathies. The albumin fraction of the total protein can be factitiously elevated in dehydrated patients.

Interfering factors

- Prolonged application of a tourniquet can increase both fractions of total proteins.
- Sampling of peripheral venous blood proximal to an IV administration site can result in an inaccurately low protein level. Likewise, massive IV infusion of crystalloid fluid can result in acute hypoproteinemia.
- Drugs that may cause *increased* protein levels include anabolic steroids, androgens, corticosteroids, dextran, growth hormone, insulin, phenazopyridine, and progesterone.
- Drugs that may cause *decreased* protein levels include ammonium ions, estrogens, hepatotoxic drugs, and oral contraceptives.

Procedure and patient care

Before
- Explain the procedure to the patient.
- Tell the patient that no fasting is usually required.

During
- Collect approximately 5 to 7 ml of blood in a red-top tube.

After
- Apply pressure or a pressure dressing to the venipuncture site.
- Observe the venipuncture site for bleeding. Patients with liver dysfunction often have prolonged clotting times.

Abnormal findings

▲ Increased albumin levels

Hemoconcentration

▼ Decreased albumin levels

Liver disease (e.g., hepatitis, extensive metastatic tumor, cirrhosis, hepatocellular necrosis)

Protein-losing enteropathies (e.g., malabsorption syndromes such as Crohn's disease, sprue, Whipple's disease)

Protein-losing nephropathies (e.g., nephrotic syndrome, glomerulonephritis)

Third-space losses (e.g., ascites, third-degree burns)

Malnutrition

Protein dilution secondary to excessive IV fluids

Increased capillary permeability (e.g., collagen vascular diseases such as lupus erythematosus)

Hemodilution

▲ **Increased globulin levels**
Immunologic tumors (e.g., multiple myeloma)

▲ **Increased total protein levels**
Hemoconcentration

▼ **Decreased globulin levels**
Malnutrition
Immunologic deficiency

▼ **Decreased total protein levels**
See Decreased Albumin Levels

notes

P

protein electrophoresis

Type of test   Blood

Normal findings
Total protein: 6.4-8.3 g/dl or 64.0-83.0 g/L (SI units)
Albumin: 3.5-5.0 g/dl or 35-50 g/L (SI units)
Alpha$_1$ globulin: 0.1-0.3 g/dl or 1-3 g/L (SI units)
Alpha$_2$ globulin: 0.6-1.0 g/dl or 6-10 g/L (SI units)
Beta globulin: 0.7-1.1 g/dl or 7-11 g/L (SI units)

Test explanation and related physiology

Total serum protein is a combination of albumin and globulins. *Albumin* is a small protein molecule that is most important in maintaining the oncotic pressure (the pressure that keeps water within the vascular space) of plasma. Albumin also acts as a carrier protein for drugs and hormones. The second type of protein in the blood, *globulins,* are larger molecules and are subclassified into three main groups: alpha, beta, and gamma. *Alpha$_1$ globulins* include alpha antitrypsin and thyroid-binding globulin. *Alpha$_2$ globulins* include serum haptoglobins (bind hemoglobin during hemolysis), ceruloplasmin (carrier for copper), prothrombin, and cholinesterase (an enzyme used in the catabolism of acetylcholine). *Beta$_1$ globulins* include lipoproteins, transferrin, plasminogen, and complement proteins; *beta$_2$ globulins* include fibrinogen. *Gamma globulins* are the immune globulins (antibodies) (see p. 480).

Serum protein electrophoresis can separate the various components of blood protein and quantify them according to their electrical charge. Several well-established electrophoretic patterns have been identified and can be associated with specific diseases (Table 12).

Interfering factors

✔ Drugs that may alter normal serum electrophoretic patterns include aspirin, bicarbonates, chlorpromazine, corticosteroids, isoniazid, neomycin, phenacemide, salicylates, sulfonamides, and tolbutamide.

Procedure and patient care

Before
- Explain the procedure to the patient.
- Tell the patient that no fasting or preparation is required.

TABLE 12 Protein electrophoresis patterns in specific diseases

Pattern	Electrophoresis	Disease
Acute reaction	$\downarrow$ Albumin $\uparrow$ Alpha$_2$ globulin	Acute infections, tissue necrosis, burns, surgery, stress, myocardial infarction
Chronic inflammatory	sl.$\downarrow$ Albumin sl.$\uparrow$ Gamma globulin N Alpha$_2$ globulin	Chronic infection, granulomatous diseases, cirrhosis, rheumatoid-collagen diseases
Nephrotic syndrome	$\downarrow\downarrow$ Albumin $\uparrow\uparrow$ Alpha$_2$ globulin N$\uparrow$ Beta globulin	Nephrotic syndrome
Far-advanced cirrhosis	$\downarrow$ Albumin $\uparrow$ Gamma globulin Incorporation of beta and gamma peaks	Far-advanced cirrhosis
Polyclonal gamma globulin elevation	$\uparrow\uparrow$ Gamma globulin with a broad peak	Cirrhosis, chronic infection, sarcoidosis, tuberculosis, endocarditis, rheumatoid-collagen disease
Hypogamma-globulinemia	$\downarrow$ Gamma globulin with normal other globulin levels	Light-chain multiple myeloma
Monoclonal gammopathy	Thin spikes in gamma globulin	Myeloma, macroglobulinemia, gammopathies

$\downarrow$, Decreased; $\uparrow$, increased; sl.$\downarrow$, slightly decreased; sl.$\uparrow$, slightly increased; N, normal; $\downarrow\downarrow$, greatly decreased; $\uparrow\uparrow$, greatly increased.

During
- Collect approximately 7 to 10 ml of venous blood in a red-top tube.
- Indicate on the laboratory slip any drugs that may affect test results.

After
- Apply pressure or a pressure dressing to the venipuncture site.
- Observe the venipuncture site for bleeding.

Abnormal findings

▼ **Decreased albumin levels**
Malnutrition
Nephrotic syndrome
Gastrointestinal protein-losing enteropathies

▲ **Increased alpha$_1$ globulin levels**
Chronic inflammatory disease
Malignancy

▼ **Decreased alpha$_1$ globulin levels**
Juvenile pulmonary emphysema

▲ **Increased alpha$_2$ globulin levels**
Nephrotic syndrome
Acute inflammation

▼ **Decreased alpha$_2$ globulin levels**
Hemolysis

▲ **Increased beta$_1$ globulin levels**
Lipoprotein disorder

▼ **Decreased beta$_1$ globulin levels**
Malnutrition
Hypoprotein disorders

▲ **Increased gamma globulin levels**
Multiple myeloma
Chronic inflammatory disease
Malignancy
Hyperimmunization
Dysproteinemia
Acute infection

▼ **Decreased beta$_2$ globulin levels**
Consumptive coagulopathy
Disseminated intravascular coagulation
Congenital coagulation disorder

notes

P

prothrombin time (PT, Pro-time, International normalized ratio [INR])

Type of test Blood

Normal findings

11.0-12.5 seconds; 85% to 100%

Full anticoagulant therapy: 1.5-2.0 times control value; 20% to 30%

Possible critical values

>20 seconds

Full anticoagulant therapy: >3 times control value

Test explanation and related physiology

The PT is used to evaluate the adequacy of the extrinsic system and common pathway in the clotting mechanism. The PT measures the clotting ability of factors I (fibrinogen), II (prothrombin), V, VII, and X. When these clotting factors exist in deficient quantities, the PT is prolonged. Many diseases and drugs are associated with decreased levels of these factors. These include:

1. *Hepatocellular liver disease* (e.g., cirrhosis, hepatitis, neoplastic invasive processes). Factors I, II, V, VII, IX, and X are produced in the liver. With severe hepatocellular dysfunction, synthesis of these factors will not occur and serum concentration of these factors will be decreased. Even a small decrease in factor VII will result in marked prolongation of the PT.

2. *Obstructive biliary disease* (e.g., bile duct obstruction secondary to tumor or gallstones or intrahepatic cholestasis secondary to sepsis or drugs). As a result of the biliary obstruction, the bile necessary for fat absorption fails to enter the gut and fat malabsorption results. Vitamins A, D, E, and K are fat soluble and also are not absorbed. Because the synthesis of factors II, VII, IX, and X depends on vitamin K, these factors will not be adequately produced and serum concentrations will fall. Factor VII is the first to decrease and will result in prolongation of PT.

Parenchymal (hepatocellular) liver disease can be differentiated from obstructive biliary disease by determination of the patient's response to parenteral vitamin K administration. If the PT returns to normal after 1 to 3 days of vitamin K administration (10 mg, IM, twice a day), one can safely assume that the patient has obstructive biliary disease that is causing vitamin K malabsorption. If, on the other hand, the PT does not return to normal with the vitamin K injections, one can assume that severe hepatocellular disease exists and that the liver cells are incapable of synthesizing the clotting factors no matter how much vitamin K is available.

3. *Coumarin ingestion.* The coumarin derivates, dicumarol and warfarin (Coumadin, Panwarfin) are used to prevent coagulation in patients with thromboembolic disease (e.g., pulmonary embolism, thrombophlebitis, arterial embolism). These drugs interfere with the production of vitamin K–dependent clotting factors, which results in a prolongation of PT, as already described. The adequacy of coumarin therapy can be monitored by following the patient's PT. Appropriate coumarin therapy for full anticoagulation should prolong the PT by 1.5 to 2 times the control value (or 20% to 30% of the normal value if percentages are used).

To have uniform PT results for physicians in different parts of the country and the world, the World Health Organization has recommended that PT results now include the use of the *international normalized ratio* (INR) value. The reported INR results are independent of the reagents or methods used, because the standard method of obtaining therapeutic anticoagulation by keeping PT ratios of 1.5 to 2 times the control value in certain clinical indications would be converted to a figure that takes the sensitivity of the thromboplastin used as reagent and the type of instrument into account. These international sensitivity indices are different for various thromboplastins and according to whether mechanical or photo-optical methods and instruments are used. Many hospitals are now reporting PT times in both absolute numbers and INR numbers. Therapeutic INR is usually considered to be 2.0 to 3.5 in most institutions, depending on the clinical situation.

Coumarin derivatives are slow acting, but their action may persist for 7 to 14 days after discontinuation of the drug. The action of a coumarin drug can be reversed in 12 to 24 hours by the parenteral administration of vitamin K (phytonadione) given very slowly. The action of coumarin drugs can be enhanced by drugs such as aspirin, quinidine, sulfa, and indomethacin. Barbiturates, chloral hydrate, and oral contraceptives cause increased coumarin drug binding and therefore may decrease the effects of binding coumarin drugs.

■　■　■

PT test results are usually given in seconds along with a control value. The control value usually varies somewhat from day to day, because the reagents used may vary. The patient's PT should be approximately equal to the control value. Some laboratories report PT values as percentages of normal activity, because the patient's results are compared with a curve representing normal clotting time. Normally, the patient's PT is 85% to 100%.

Interfering factors

- Alcohol intake can increase PT levels.
- A high-fat diet may decrease PT levels.
- Drugs that may cause *increased* levels include allopurinol, aminosalicylic acid, barbiturates, beta-lactam antibiotics, chloral hydrate, cephalothins, chloramphenicol, chlorpromazine (Thorazine), cholestyramine, cimetidine, clofibrate, colestipol, ethyl alcohol, glucagon, heparin, methyldopa (Aldomet), neomycin, oral anticoagulants, propylthiouracil, quinidine, quinine, salicylates, and sulfonamides.
- Drugs that may cause *decreased* levels include anabolic steroids, barbiturates, chloral hydrate, digitalis, diphenhydramine (Benadryl), estrogens, griseofulvin, oral contraceptives, and vitamin K.

Procedure and patient care

Before
- Explain the procedure to the patient.
- Tell the patient that no fasting is required.
- If the patient is receiving warfarin, obtain the blood specimen before the patient is given the daily dose of warfarin. The daily dose may be increased, decreased, or kept the same depending on the PT test results for that day.

During
- Collect approximately 5 to 7 ml of venous blood in a blue-top tube.
- List on the laboratory slip any drugs that may affect test results.

After
- Apply pressure or a pressure dressing to the venipuncture site.
- Assess the venipuncture site for bleeding. Remember, hemostasis will be delayed if the patient is taking warfarin or if the patient has any coagulopathies.
- If the PT is greatly prolonged, evaluate the patient for bleeding tendencies (i.e., check for blood in the urine and

all excretions and assess the patient for bruises, petechiae, and low back pain.

- If severe bleeding occurs, the anticoagulant effect of warfarin can be reversed by the slow parenteral administration of vitamin K (phytonadione).
- Because of drug interactions, instruct the patient not to take any medication unless specifically ordered by the physician.

Abnormal findings

▲ **Increased levels**

Cirrhosis
Hepatitis
Vitamin K deficiency
Salicylate intoxication

Bile duct obstruction
Coumarin ingestion
Disseminated intravascular coagulation
Massive blood transfusion

notes

P

pulmonary angiography (Pulmonary arteriography, Bronchial angiography)

Type of test X-ray with contrast dye

Normal findings Normal pulmonary vasculature

Test explanation and related physiology

Through an injection of a radiographic contrast material into the pulmonary arteries, pulmonary angiography permits visualization of the pulmonary vasculature. Angiography is used to detect pulmonary embolism and a variety of congenital and acquired lesions of the pulmonary vessels.

When pulmonary embolism is suspected, lung scanning should be performed first. If the lung scan is normal, pulmonary embolism is ruled out. If the scan is equivocal, however, the diagnosis of pulmonary embolism is questionable, because pathologic parenchymal processes (e.g., emphysema, pneumonia) also may cause abnormalities on the lung scan. Definitive diagnosis for pulmonary embolism may require pulmonary angiography. This may be especially important in patients with peptic ulcers for whom anticoagulant treatment for pulmonary embolism may be associated with significant risks. Also, in rare instances, pulmonary embolectomy rather than anticoagulation is considered critical for patient survival. In these cases, the angiographic location of the clot is important.

Bronchial angiography is now being done in some facilities to identify bleeding sites in the lungs. For this procedure, catheters are placed transarterially into the orifice of bronchial arteries. Radiopaque material is then injected, and the arteries are visualized. If a bleeding site is identified, the site can be injected with a sclerosing agent to prevent further bleeding.

Contraindications

- Patients with allergies to shellfish or iodinated dye
- Patients who are pregnant
- Patients with bleeding disorders

Potential complications

- Allergic reaction to iodinated dye
  Allergic reactions may vary from mild flushing, itching, and urticaria to severe, life-threatening anaphylaxis (evidenced by

respiratory distress, drop in blood pressure, or shock). In the unusual event of anaphylaxis, the patient may be treated with diphenhydramine (Benadryl), steroids, and epinephrine. Oxygen and endotracheal equipment should be immediately available.

- Cardiac arrhythmia (dysrhythmia)
  Premature ventricular contractions during right-sided heart catheterization may lead to ventricular tachycardia and ventricular fibrillation.

Procedure and patient care

Before

- Explain the procedure to the patient.
- Ensure that written and informed consent for this procedure is obtained.
- Inform the patient that a warm flush will be felt when the dye is injected.
- Check the patient for allergies to iodinated dyes and shell-fish.
- Inform the radiologist if an allergy to iodine is suspected. The radiologist may prescribe a Benadryl-and-steroid preparation to be administered before the test. Usually, a hypoallergic, nonionic contrast will be used during the test.
- Determine if the patient has ventricular arrhythmias (dysrhythmias).
- Keep the patient NPO after midnight on the day of the test.
- Administer preprocedural medications as ordered. Atropine is given to decrease secretions. Meperidine is used for sedation and relaxation.

During

- Note the following procedural steps:
  1. The patient is placed on an x-ray table in the supine position.
  2. Electrocardiographic electrodes are attached for cardiac monitoring.
  3. The catheter is placed into the femoral vein and passed into the inferior vena cava.
  4. With fluoroscopic visualization, the catheter is advanced to the right atrium and the right ventricle.
  5. The catheter is manipulated into the main pulmonary artery, where the dye is injected.

P

6. X-ray films of the chest are immediately taken in timed sequence. This allows all vessels visualized by the injection to be photographed. If filling defects are seen in the contrast-filled vessels, pulmonary emboli are present.

- Note that this test is performed by a physician in approximately 1 hour.
- During injection of dye, remind the patient that he or she will feel a burning sensation and flush throughout the body.

After

- Observe the catheter insertion site for inflammation, hemorrhage, and hematoma.
- Assess the patient's vital signs for evidence of bleeding (decreased blood pressure, increased pulse).
- Apply cold compresses to the puncture site if needed to reduce swelling or discomfort.
- Inform the patient that coughing may occur after this study.
- Educate the patient regarding the need for bed rest for 12 to 24 hours after the test.
- Evaluate the patient for delayed reaction to the dye (dyspnea, rashes, tachycardia, hives). This usually occurs within 2 to 6 hours after the test. Treat with antihistamines or steroids.

Abnormal findings

Pulmonary embolism
Congenital and acquired lesions of the pulmonary vessels (e.g., pulmonary hypertension)
Tumor

notes

pulmonary function tests (PFTs)

Type of test Airflow assessment

Normal findings Vary with the patient's age, sex, height, and weight

Test explanation and related physiology

Pulmonary function tests are performed to detect abnormalities in respiratory function and to determine the extent of any pulmonary abnormality. The main reasons for pulmonary function include the following:

1. Preoperative evaluation of the lungs and pulmonary reserve. When planned thoracic surgery will result in loss of functional pulmonary tissue, as in lobectomy (removal of part of a lung) or pneumonectomy (removal of an entire lung), a significant risk of pulmonary failure exists if preoperative pulmonary function is already severely compromised by other diseases such as chronic obstructive pulmonary disease (COPD).

2. Evaluation of response to bronchodilator therapy. Some patients with COPD have a spastic component to their obstructive disease that may respond to long-term use of bronchodilators. Pulmonary function studies performed before and after the use of bronchodilators will identify that group of patients.

3. Differentiation between restrictive and obstructive forms of chronic pulmonary disease. *Restrictive* defects (e.g., pulmonary fibrosis, tumors, chest-wall trauma) occur when ventilation is disturbed by a limitation in chest expansion. Inspiration is primarily affected. *Obstructive* defects (e.g., emphysema, bronchitis, asthma) occur when ventilation is disturbed by an increase in airway resistance. Expiration is primarily affected.

4. Determination of the diffusing capacity of the lungs (D_L). Rates are based on the difference in concentration of gases in inspired and expired air.

5. Performance of inhalation tests in patients with inhalation allergies.

Pulmonary function tests routinely include determination of the following:

1. Forced vital capacity (FVC)
2. Forced expiratory volume in 1 second (FEV_1)

P

   3. Maximal midexpiratory flow (MMEF)
   4. Maximal voluntary ventilation (MVV)
   5. Arterial blood gases (see p. 146)

Forced vital capacity. FVC is the amount of air that can be forcefully expelled from a maximally inflated lung position. This volume is decreased below the expected value in obstructive and restrictive pulmonary diseases.

Forced expiratory volume in 1 second. FEV_1 is the volume of air expelled during the first second of the FVC. In patients with obstructive disease, airways are narrowed and resistance to flow is high. Therefore not as much air can be expelled in 1 second, and FEV_1 will be reduced below the predicted value. In restrictive lung disease, FEV_1 is decreased not because of airway resistance but because the amount of air originally inhaled is less. One should therefore measure the FEV_1/FVC ratio. A normal value of 80% is found in patients with restrictive lung disease. In obstructive lung disease, this ratio is considerably less than 80%. The FEV_1 measurement will reliably improve with bronchodilator therapy if a spastic component to an obstructive disease exists.

Maximal midexpiratory flow. MMEF is the maximal rate of airflow through the pulmonary tree during forced expiration. This is also called *forced midexpiratory flow.* This test is independent of the patient's effort or cooperation. MMFF is reduced below expected values in obstructive diseases and normal in restrictive diseases.

Maximal volume ventilation. MVV, formerly called *maximal breathing capacity,* is the maximal volume of air that the patient can breathe in and out during 1 minute. MVV is decreased below the expected value in both restrictive and obstructive pulmonary disease.

A comprehensive pulmonary function study also may include evaluation of the following lung volumes and lung capacities, many of which are illustrated in Figure 24.

Tidal volume. TV or VT is the volume of air inspired and expired with each normal respiration.

Inspiratory reserve volume. IRV is the maximal volume of air that can be inspired from the end of a normal inspiration. It represents forced inspiration over and beyond the tidal volume.

Expiratory reserve volume. ERV is the maximal volume of air that can be exhaled after a normal expiration.

Residual volume. RV is the volume of air remaining in the lungs following forced expiration.

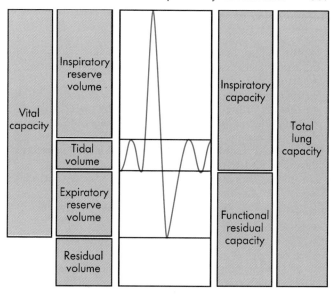

Figure 24 Relationship of lung volumes and capacities.

Inspiratory capacity. IC is the maximal amount of air that can be inspired after a normal expiration (IC = TV + IRV).

Functional residual volume. FRV is the amount of air left in the lungs after a normal expiration (FRV = ERV + RV).

Vital capacity. VC is the maximal amount of air that can be expired after a maximal inspiration (VC = TV + IRV + ERV).

Total lung capacity. TLC is the volume to which the lungs can be expanded with the greatest inspiratory effort (TLC = TV + IRV + ERV + RV).

Minute volume. MV, sometimes called *minute ventilation,* is the volume of air inhaled and exhaled per minute.

Dead space. Dead space is the part of the tidal volume that does not participate in alveolar gas exchange.

Contraindications

- Patients who are in pain because of inability to cooperate by deep inspiration and expiration
- Patients who are unable to cooperate because of age or mental incapability

Procedure and patient care

Before

- Explain the test to the patient.
- Inform the patient that cooperation is necessary to obtain accurate results.
- Instruct the patient not to use any bronchodilators or smoke for 6 hours before this test (if requested by physician).
- Withhold the use of small-dose meter inhalers and aerosol therapy before this study.
- Measure and record the patient's height and weight before this study to determine the predicted values.
- List on the laboratory slip any medications the patient is taking.

During

- Note the following procedural steps:
    1. The unsedated patient is taken to the pulmonary function laboratory.
    2. The patient breathes into a sterile cylinder, which is connected to a computerized machine to measure and record the desired values.
    3. The patient is asked to inhale as deeply as possible and then exhale as much air as possible.
    4. From this the machine computes FVC, FEV_1, FEV_1/FVC, and MMEF.
    5. The patient is asked to breathe in and out as deeply and frequently as possible for 15 seconds. The total volume breathed is recorded and multiplied by 4 to obtain the MVV.

Diffusing capacity of the lung

1. The D_L for any gas can be measured as part of pulmonary function studies. This measures the diffusion of gases per minute across the alveolocapillary membrane. Most laboratories employ carbon monoxide (CO) for measuring D_L, because CO has a great affinity for hemoglobin and only a small concentration is needed in clinical tests. Because of this, the major limiting factor to the transfer of the gas is its rate of diffusion across the alveolocapillary membrane and not pulmonary blood flow.
2. The D_L of CO is usually measured by having the patient inhale a CO mixture.
3. $D_L CO$ is calculated with an analysis of the amount of CO exhaled compared with the amount inhaled. This value is

abnormal in patients with adult respiratory distress syndrome, congestive heart failure, collagen vascular disease, Goodpasture's syndrome, and so on.

Inhalation tests

1. These tests also may be performed during pulmonary function studies to establish a cause-and-effect relationship in some patients with inhalant allergies.
2. The *methacholine* or *histamine challenge test* is typically used to detect the presence of hyperactive airway diseases. This test would not be indicated for a patient known to have asthma. A positive methacholine challenge is a greater than 20% reduction in the patient's FEV_1.
3. Care is taken during this challenge test to reverse any severe bronchospasm with prompt administration of an inhalant bronchodilator (e.g., isoproterenol).

After

- Note that patients with severe respiratory problems are occasionally exhausted after the testing and will need rest.

Abnormal findings

Pulmonary fibrosis
Tumor
Chest wall trauma
Emphysema
Chronic bronchitis
Asthma
Inhalant allergy
Interstitial fibrosis following pneumonectomy

Bronchiectasis
Airway infection
Pneumonia
Neuromuscular disease
Scleroderma
Collagen vascular lung disease

P

notes

rabies-neutralizing antibody test

Type of test Blood

Normal findings <1:16

Test explanation and related physiology

Identification and documentation of the presence of rabies-neutralizing antibody is important for veterinary health care workers and others who may be or may have been exposed to the rabies virus. This test is performed on patients who are at great risk for animal bites and have received the human diploid cell rabies vaccine. A rabies titer of greater than 1:16 is considered to be protective.

In patients who may have been exposed to rabies, immunoglobulin is given. At the same time, these patients are also vaccinated. One can expect to see increases in rabies antibody levels.

The rabies antibody is identified by direct fluorescent antibody method. More recently, immunofluorescence has been used.

Procedure and patient care

Before

- Explain the procedure to the patient.
- Tell the patient that no fasting or special preparation is required.

During

- Collect 7 to 10 ml of venous blood in a red-top tube.

After

- Apply pressure or a pressure dressing to the venipuncture site.
- Assess the venipuncture site for bleeding.

Abnormal findings

Exposure to rabies vaccine
Recent bite exposure to rabies virus
Active rabies in patient or animal

radioactive iodine uptake (RAIU, Iodine uptake test, ^{131}I uptake)

Type of test Nuclear scan

Normal findings

2 hours: 4% to 12% absorbed
6 hours: 6% to 15% absorbed
24 hours: 8% to 30% absorbed

Test explanation and related physiology

The RAIU is a useful guide to thyroid function. This test is based on the ability of the thyroid gland to trap and retain iodine. In this procedure, a known quantity of radioactive iodine is given orally to the patient. A gamma ray detector placed over the thyroid gland determines the quantity or percentage of radioactive iodine taken up by the gland over a specific time.

Performing the measurement at different times after the iodine is given allows several aspects of thyroid function to be evaluated. Uptake determination at 30 minutes reflects the ability of the thyroid gland to trap iodine. When uptake is measured at 6 hours, the ability of the thyroid gland to bind iodine organically is evaluated. Maximal iodine uptake is observed within 24 hours. Determinations of iodine uptake after this time measure the ability of the gland to release iodine in the form of thyroid hormone.

Increased thyroid uptake of radioactive iodine is seen in patients with hyperthyroid states. Decreased uptake occurs in patients with hypothyroid conditions. The RAIU tends to be more accurate for diagnosing hyperthyroidism than hypothyroidism.

Contraindications

- Patients who are allergic to iodine or shellfish
- Patients who are pregnant

Potential complication

- Radioactive exposure to the thyroid gland
  This is minimized when ^{123}I or ^{125}I is used instead of ^{131}I.

Interfering factors

- In patients taking exogenous iodine preparations, the iodine will increase the body's iodine pool and decrease uptake by the thyroid gland.

- Iodine-deficient patients will trap increased amounts of iodine, resulting in increased uptake.
- Rebound thyroid stimulation after discontinuation of suppressive doses of thyroid medications results in falsely elevated RAIU levels.
- Recent x-ray studies using iodinated contrast material will decrease uptake.
- Diarrhea caused by decreased absorption of tracer doses in the GI tract results in decreased RAIU levels.
- Drugs that may cause *increased* levels include barbiturates, estrogen, lithium, phenothiazines, and thyroid-stimulating hormone.
- Drugs that may cause *decreased* levels include adrenocorticotropic hormone, antihistamines, corticosteroids, Lugol's solution, nitrates, saturated solution of potassium iodine, thyroid and antithyroid drugs, and tolbutamide.

Procedure and patient care

Before
- Explain the procedure to the patient.
- Assess the patient for allergies to iodine.
- Note that some laboratories prefer to keep the patient NPO after midnight on the day of the test.
- Restrict iodine and thyroid preparations 1 week before testing if indicated by the institution.
- Evaluate the patient's drug history for interfering factors.

During
- Note the following procedural steps:
  1. A tasteless dose of radioactive iodine, usually ^{123}I, is given by mouth to the patient. If RAIU is to be determined at 2 hours, the iodine is administered IV.
  2. The patient is given written instructions regarding the times to return to the radiology department for scanning.
  3. The patient is informed that he or she may usually eat 45 minutes to 1 hour after the dose of iodine has been given.
  4. For the scanning, the patient is asked to lie in a supine position.
  5. A gamma ray detector is placed over the patient's thyroid gland to determine RAIU.
- List on the laboratory slip the x-ray studies and drugs the patient has received that could affect test results.

- Note that this test is performed in approximately 30 minutes by a radiologic technologist.
- Inform the patient that this test is not uncomfortable.

After

- Inform the patient that the dose of radioactive iodine used in this test is minute and harmless. Tell him or her that no isolation or special urine precautions are necessary.

Abnormal findings

▲ **Increased levels**
Hyperthyroidism

▼ **Decreased levels**
Hypothyroidism

notes

R

red blood cell count (RBC count, Erythrocyte count)

Type of test Blood

Normal findings

Adult/elderly
    Male: 4.7-6.1 million/mm^3
    Female: 4.2-5.4 million/mm^3
Infant/child: 3.8-5.5 million/mm^3
Newborn: 4.8-7.1 million/mm^3

Test explanation and related physiology

This test is a count of the number of circulating RBCs in 1 mm^3 of peripheral venous blood. The RBC is routinely performed as part of a complete blood count. Packed within each RBC are molecules of hemoglobin that permit the transport and exchange of oxygen and carbon dioxide. Normally, RBCs exist in the peripheral blood for approximately 120 days. Toward the end of the RBC's life, the cell membrane becomes less pliable; the aged RBC is then hemolyzed and extracted from the circulation by the spleen. Abnormal RBCs have a shorter life span and are extracted earlier. Intravascular RBC trauma, such as that caused by artificial heart valves or peripheral vascular atherosclerotic plaques, also shortens the RBC's life. An enlarged spleen, such as that caused by portal hypertension or leukemia, may inappropriately destroy and remove normal RBCs from the circulation.

Normal RBC values vary according to gender and age. When the value is decreased by more than 10% of the expected normal value, the patient is said to be anemic. Low RBC values are caused by many factors, including:

1. Hemorrhage (as in gastrointestinal bleeding or trauma)
2. Hemolysis (as in glucose-6-phosphate dehydrogenase deficiency, spherocytosis, or secondary splenomegaly)
3. Dietary deficiency (as of iron or vitamin B$_{12}$)
4. Genetic aberrations (as in sickle cell anemia or thalassemia)
5. Drug ingestion (as of chloramphenicol, hydantoins, or quinidine)
6. Marrow failure (as in fibrosis, leukemia, or antineoplastic chemotherapy)

7. Chronic illness (as in tumor or sepsis)

8. Other organ failure (as in renal disease)

RBC counts greater than normal can be physiologically induced as a result of the body's requirements for greater oxygen-carrying capacity (e.g., at high altitudes). Diseases that produce chronic anoxia (e.g., congenital heart disease) also provoke this physiologic increase in RBCs. Polycythemia vera is a neoplastic condition involving uncontrolled production of RBCs.

Interfering factors

- Normal decreases are seen in the RBC during pregnancy because of normal body fluid increases and dilution of the RBCs.
- Persons living at high altitudes have increased RBCs.
- Hydration status: Dehydration factitiously increases the RBC count, and overhydration decreases the RBC count.
- Drugs that may cause *increased* RBC levels include gentamicin and methyldopa.
- Drugs that may cause *decreased* RBC levels include chloramphenicol, hydantoins, and quinidine.

Procedure and patient care

Before

- Explain the procedure to the patient.
- Tell the patient that no fasting is required.

During

- Collect approximately 5 to 7 ml of blood in a lavender-top tube.
- Thoroughly mix the blood with the anticoagulant by tilting the tube.
- Avoid hemolysis.
- List on the laboratory slip any drugs or other patient factors that may affect RBC levels.

After

- Apply pressure or a pressure dressing to the venipuncture site.
- Observe the venipuncture site for bleeding.

R

Abnormal findings

▲   **Increased levels**
High altitude
Congenital heart disease
Polycythemia vera
Dehydration/
hemoconcentration
Cor pulmonale
Pulmonary fibrosis
Severe diarrhea

▼   **Decreased levels**
Hemorrhage
Hemolysis
Anemia
Hemoglobinopathy
Advanced cancer
Bone marrow fibrosis
Leukemia
Antineoplastic chemo-
therapy
Chronic illness
Organ failure (e.g., renal)
Overhydration
Multiple myeloma
Pernicious anemia
Rheumatic disease
Subacute endocarditis
Pregnancy
Dietary deficiency

notes

red blood cell indices (RBC indices, MCV, MCH, MCHC, Blood indices, Erythrocyte indices, Red cell distribution width [RDW])

Type of test Blood

Normal findings

Mean corpuscular volume (MCV)
Adult/elderly/child: 80-95 μm^3
Newborn: 96-108 μm^3

Mean corpuscular hemoglobin (MCH)
Adult/elderly/child: 27-31 pg
Newborn: 32-34 pg

Mean corpuscular hemoglobin concentration (MCHC)
Adult/elderly/child: 32-36 g/dl (or 32% to 36%)
Newborn: 32-33 g/dl (or 32% to 33%)

Red blood cell distribution (RDW)
Adult: 11% to 14.5%

Test explanation and related physiology

The RBC indices provide information about the size (MCV and RDW), weight (MCH), and hemoglobin concentration (MCHC) of RBCs. This test is routinely performed as part of a complete blood count (CBC). The results of the RBC, hematocrit, and hemoglobin tests are necessary to calculate the RBC indices. When investigating anemia, it is helpful to categorize the anemia according to the RBC indices, as shown in Table 13. Cell size is indicated by the terms *normocytic*, *microcytic*, and *macrocytic*. Hemoglobin content is indicated by the terms *normochromic*, *hypochromic*, and *hyperchromic*. Additional information about the RBC size, shape, color, and intracellular structure is described in the blood smear study (see p. 151).

Mean corpuscular volume

The MCV is a measure of the average volume, or size, of a single RBC and is therefore used in classifying anemias. MCV is derived by dividing the hematocrit by the total RBC count. Normal values vary according to age and gender. When the MCV value is increased, the RBC is said to be abnormally large, or *macrocytic*. This is most frequently seen in megaloblastic anemias (e.g., vitamin B_{12} or folic acid deficiency). When the MCV value

TABLE 13 Categorization of anemia according to RBC indices

Normocytic,[1] normochromic[2] anemia

Iron deficiency (detected early)
Chronic illness (e.g., sepsis, tumor)
Acute blood loss
Aplastic anemia (e.g., chloramphenicol toxicosis)
Acquired hemolytic anemias (e.g., from a prosthetic cardiac
  valve)

Microcytic,[3] hypochromic[4] anemia

Iron deficiency (detected late)
Thalassemia
Lead poisoning

Microcytic, normochromic anemia

Renal disease (because of the loss of erythropoietin)

Macrocytic,[5] normochromic anemia

Vitamin B_{12} or folic acid deficiency
Hydantoin ingestion
Chemotherapy

---

[1]Normocytic—normal RBC size.
[2]Normochromic—normal color (normal hemoglobin content).
[3]Microcytic—smaller than normal RBC size.
[4]Hypochromic—less than normal color (decreased hemoglobin content).
[5]Macrocytic—larger than normal RBC size.

is decreased, the RBC is said to be abnormally small, or *micro-cytic*. This is associated with iron deficiency anemia or thalasse-mia.

Mean corpuscular hemoglobin

The MCH is a measure of the average amount (weight) of he-moglobin within an RBC. MCH is derived by dividing the total hemoglobin concentration by the number of RBCs. Because macrocytic cells generally have more and microcytic cells have less hemoglobin, the causes for these values closely resemble those for the MCV value.

Mean corpuscular hemoglobin concentration

The MCHC is a measure of the average concentration or percentage of hemoglobin within a single RBC. MCHC is derived by dividing the total hemoglobin concentration by the hematocrit. When values are decreased, the cell has a deficiency of hemoglobin and is said to be *hypochromic* (frequently seen in iron deficiency anemia and thalassemia). When values are normal, the anemia is said be *normocytic* (e.g., hemolytic anemia).

Red blood cell distribution width

The RDW is an indication of the variation in RBC size. It is calculated by a machine using the MCV and RBC values. Variations in the width of the RBCs may be helpful when classifying certain types of anemia. The RDW is essentially an indicator of the degree of anisocytosis, a blood condition characterized by RBCs of variable and abnormal size.

Interfering factors

- Abnormal RBC size may affect indices.
- Extremely elevated white blood cell counts may affect RBC indices.

Procedure and patient care

Before

- Explain the procedure to the patient.
- Tell the patient that no fasting is required.

During

- Collect approximately 5 to 7 ml of venous blood in a lavender-top tube.
- Avoid hemolysis.
- Transport the specimen to the hematology laboratory, where the blood is passed through automated machines that calculate the RBC indices.

R

After

- Apply pressure or a pressure dressing to the venipuncture site.
- Assess the venipuncture site for bleeding.

Abnormal findings

▲ **Increased MCV**
Liver disease
Antimetabolite therapy
Alcoholism
Pernicious anemia (vitamin B_{12} deficiency)
Folic acid deficiency

▼ **Decreased MCV**
Iron deficiency anemia
Thalassemia

▲ **Increased MCH**
Macrocytic anemia

▼ **Decreased MCH**
Microcytic anemia
Hypochromic anemia

▲ **Increased MCHC**
Spherocytosis

▼ **Decreased MCHC**
Iron deficiency anemia
Thalassemia

notes

red blood cell survival study (RBC survival study, Splenic sequestration study)

Type of test Nuclear scan

Normal findings

Half-life of RBC: 26-30 days
Spleen/liver ratio: 1:1
Spleen/pericardium ratio: <2:1

Test explanation and related physiology

In patients with hemolytic anemia, the RBCs are destroyed and normally sequestered in the spleen. As a result of this ongoing RBC destruction, the RBC life span will be significantly reduced. This reduction in RBC survival indicates that active hemolysis is occurring and is the cause of the patient's anemia.

Although hemolysis can be identified by determination of the catabolic products of hemoglobin (which are increased) or by measuring the level of circulating haptoglobin—the transport protein that binds hemoglobin (which is decreased)—the nuclear determination of the RBC life span can provide a semiquantitative measurement of the degree of hemolysis. This quantitation can be best performed by determining the half-life of the RBC within the circulation. This portion of the test is performed by extracting some of the patient's RBCs, labeling them with chromium-51 (^{51}Cr), and reinjecting them into the patient. Subsequent blood levels of ^{51}Cr indicate the half-life of the labeled RBCs.

The second portion of the test is the imaging of the spleen, liver, and pericardium. In patients with hemolytic anemia associated with abnormal splenic sequestration, the spleen/liver ratio is in excess of 1:1. However, this abnormally high ratio can occur in patients who have splenomegaly caused by a disease other than hemolytic anemia. Therefore spleen/pericardium ratios are performed; those greater than 2:1 indicate abnormal splenic sequestration of hemolyzed RBCs. A normal spleen/pericardium ratio with an increased spleen/liver ratio indicates splenomegaly.

This second portion of the splenic sequestration study is also helpful in determining which patients with hemolytic anemia will benefit from splenectomy. Patients with increased splenic sequestration can be expected to improve greatly as a result of splenectomy.

R

Contraindications

- Patients who are pregnant because of the risk of fetal damage

Interfering factors

- Factors that can decrease RBC survival include recent RBC transfusion, increased RBC production, active bleeding, high white blood cell (WBC) counts in excess of 25,000, and high platelet counts greater than 500,000.
- Splenomegaly can increase spleen/pericardium ratios.
- Splenic infarctions can decrease spleen/pericardium ratios.

Procedure and patient care

Before

- Explain the procedure to the patient.
- Assure the patient that he or she will not be exposed to large amounts of radioactivity, because only tracer doses of the isotope are used.
- Tell the patient that no preparation or sedation is required.
- Notify the nuclear medicine technologist or physician if blood transfusion or hemorrhage has occurred shortly before or during the study.
- Note that usually, a hematocrit, WBC count, platelet count, and reticulocyte count are performed before testing.

During

- Note the following procedural steps:
  1. Approximately 20 ml of blood is withdrawn from the patient, and the RBCs are labeled with ^{51}Cr.
  2. The RBCs are immediately reinjected into the patient.
  3. On the first day of testing, 10 ml of blood is withdrawn by a peripheral venipuncture into a red-top tube.
  4. The RBCs are quantitated for ^{51}Cr counts per minute.
  5. Nuclear imaging of the spleen, liver, and pericardium is carried out.
  6. This process is repeated three times a week for 3 weeks.
  7. The peripheral venous blood ^{51}Cr counts are plotted on a graph, and the half-life is determined.
  8. The spleen/liver and spleen/pericardium ratios and nuclear counts are determined.
- Note that this test takes place over 2 to 3 weeks. The results are available on the day after the study is completed. The study is performed by a nuclear medicine technologist or physician.

- Tell the patient that no pain or discomfort is associated with this procedure. The patient must lie still during the nuclear imaging portion of the test.

After

- Inform the patient that because only tracer doses of radioisotopes are used, no precautions need to be taken against radioactive exposure.

Abnormal findings

▲ **Increased splenic sequestration**
Hemolysis
Splenomegaly

▼ **Decreased RBC survival**
Hemolysis
Hemorrhage
Abnormally increased erythropoiesis

notes

R

renal biopsy (Kidney biopsy)

Type of test Microscopic examination of tissue

Normal findings No pathologic conditions

Test explanation and related physiology

Biopsy of the kidney affords microscopic examination of renal tissue. Renal biopsy is performed for the following purposes:

1. To diagnose the cause of renal disease (e.g., poststreptococcal glomerulonephritis, Goodpasture's syndrome, lupus nephritis)
2. To detect primary and metastatic malignancy of the kidney in patients who may not be candidates for surgery
3. To evaluate the degree of rejection that occurs after kidney transplantation, which enables the physician to determine the appropriate dose of immunosuppressive agents

Renal biopsy is most often obtained percutaneously (Figure 25). During this procedure, a needle is inserted through the skin and into the kidney to obtain a sample of kidney tissue. The biopsy needle is more accurately placed when guided by ultrasonography or fluoroscopy. These techniques allow more precise localization of the desired kidney tissue.

Occasionally, open renal biopsy is performed. This involves an incision through the flank and dissection to expose the kidney surgically.

Contraindications

- Patients with coagulation disorders because of the risk of excessive bleeding
- Patients with operable kidney tumors, because tumor cells may be disseminated during the procedure
- Patients with hydronephrosis, because the enlarged renal pelvis can be easily entered and cause a persistent urine leak requiring surgical repair
- Patients with urinary tract infections, because the needle insertion may disseminate the active infection throughout the retroperitoneum

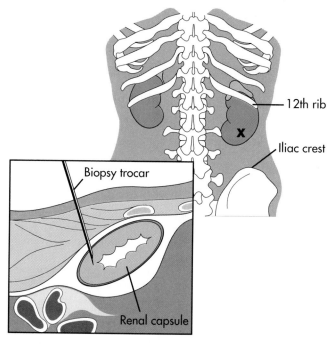

Figure 25 Renal biopsy.

Potential complications
- Hemorrhage from the highly vascular renal tissue
- Inadvertent puncture of the liver, lung, bowel, aorta, and inferior vena cava
- Infection when an open biopsy is performed

Procedure and patient care

Before
- Explain the procedure to the patient.
- Ensure that written and informed consent for this procedure is obtained by the physician.
- Keep the patient NPO after midnight on the day of the test in the event that bleeding or inadvertent puncture of an abdominal organ may necessitate surgical intervention.
- Assess the patient's coagulation studies (prothrombin time, partial thromboplastin time).

- Check the patient's hemoglobin and hematocrit values.
- Note that the patient may need to be typed and cross-matched for blood in the event of severe hemorrhage requiring transfusions.
- Tell the patient that no sedative is required.
- Note that the needle stick may be done at the bedside.
- If fluoroscopic or ultrasound guidance is to be used, note that the needle stick is performed in the radiology or ultrasonography department.

During
- Note the following procedural steps:
  1. The patient is placed in a prone position with a sandbag or pillow under the abdomen to straighten the spine.
  2. Under sterile conditions the skin overlying the kidneys is infiltrated with a local anesthetic (lidocaine).
  3. While the patient holds his or her breath to stop kidney motion, the physician inserts the biopsy needle into the kidney and takes a specimen.
  4. After this procedure is completed, the needle is removed and pressure is applied to the site for approximately 20 minutes.
- Note that this procedure is performed by a physician in approximately 10 minutes.
- Tell the patient that this procedure is uncomfortable, but only minimally if enough lidocaine is used.

After
- After the test, apply a pressure dressing.
- Turn the patient on his or her back and keep on bed rest for approximately 24 hours.
- Check the patient's vital signs, puncture site, and hematocrit values frequently during the 24-hour period.
- Instruct the patient to avoid any activity that increases abdominal venous pressure (e.g., coughing).
- Assess the patient for signs and symptoms of hemorrhage (e.g., decrease in blood pressure, increase in pulse, pallor, backache, flank pain, shoulder pain, lightheadedness).
- Evaluate the patient's abdomen for signs of bowel or liver penetration (e.g., abdominal pain and tenderness, abdominal muscle guarding and rigidity, decreased bowel sounds).
- Inspect all urine specimens for gross hematuria. Usually, the patient's urine will contain blood initially, but this generally will not continue after the first 24 hours. Urine samples may

be placed in consecutive chronologic order to facilitate comparison for evaluation of hematuria. This is referred to as *rack* or *serial* urine samples.

- Encourage the patient to drink large amounts of fluid to prevent clot formation and urine retention.
- Frequently obtain blood for hemoglobin and hematocrit determination after the biopsy specimen to assess for active bleeding. One purple-top tube of blood is needed.
- Instruct the patient to avoid, for at least 2 weeks, strenuous exercise (e.g., heavy lifting, contact sports, horseback riding) or any activity that could cause jolting of the kidney.
- Teach the patient the signs and symptoms of renal hemorrhage, and instruct him or her to call the physician if any of these symptoms occur.
- Instruct the patient to report burning on urination or any temperature elevations. These could indicate a urinary tract infection.

Abnormal findings

Renal disease (e.g., poststreptococcal conditions, Goodpasture's syndrome, lupus nephritis)

Primary and metastatic malignancy of the kidney
Rejection of kidney transplant

notes

R

---

renal scanning (Kidney scan, Radiorenography, Renography, Radionuclide renal imaging, Nuclear imaging of the kidney, DMSA renal scan, DTPA renal scan, Captopril renal scan)

Type of test Nuclear scan

Normal findings Normal size, shape, and function of the kidney

Test explanation and related physiology

This nuclear medicine procedure provides visualization of the urinary tract after IV administration of a radioisotope. The distribution of the radioactive material is scanned or mapped. Scans do not interfere with the normal physiologic process of the kidney. The resultant image (scan) indicates distribution of the radionuclide within the kidney and ureters.

Each radioactive tracer is handled by the kidney in a different manner. For example, technetium-99m diethylenetriamine pentaacetic acid (^{99m}Tc DTPA) is excreted by glomerular filtration. ^{99m}Tc disodium monomethanearsonate (DMSA) is taken up by the tubular cells and not appreciably excreted. Iodine-131 (^{131}I) is both filtered by the glomerulus and secreted by the tubules.

Various agents can be used for the scanning. ^{99m}Tc can be tagged to compounds such as DTPA or DMSA to permit static views of the kidney *structures* or to assess dynamic *perfusion* of the kidneys. Orthoiodohippurate can be tagged with ^{131}I to evaluate *excretory function* by measuring the time necessary for the radioisotope to travel through the cortex and pelvis of each kidney. A second injection may be given to evaluate perfusion, structure, and excretory function of the kidney. This is sometimes called a *triple renal study*.

The time of uptake, transit, and excretion of the radioisotope by each kidney is plotted on a graph called a *renogram curve* (isotope renography). This can be compared with a normal reference curve to aid in the detection of abnormalities in either kidney (e.g., tubular disease, urinary obstruction, pyelonephritis, renal vascular hypertension, absence of kidney function).

The *captopril scan* (captopril renography/scintigraphy) is a new test for the diagnosis of renovascular disease. This scan uses angiotensin-converting enzyme (ACE) inhibitors, such as captopril, to determine the functional significance of a stenosis. After the administration of captopril, the glomerular filtration rate

(GFR) in kidneys with a partial vascular obstruction is reduced despite the preservation of renal plasma flow. The GFR in the contralateral kidney is maintained. Scans after captopril administration may enable the prediction of blood pressure response after angioplasty or surgery.

Renal scanning is used to:

1. Detect renal infarctions. The infarcted area is shown as a nonperfused defect in an otherwise homogenous renal pattern.
2. Detect renal arterial atherosclerosis or trauma. The renal uptake of the radionucleated material will be delayed or absent on the affected side or sides.
3. Monitor rejection of a transplanted kidney. In chronic rejection, the uptake and excretion of the nuclear material are delayed.
4. Detect primary renal disease (e.g., glomerulonephritis, acute tubular necrosis). The uptake and excretion of the nuclear material are delayed.
5. Detect pathologic renal or ureteral conditions in patients who cannot have intravenous pyelography (IVP, see p. 487) because of dye allergies or poor renal function.
6. Detect renal tumors, abscesses, or cysts. These appear as "cold spots" because of the nonfunctioning tissue.
7. Detect and monitor renovascular hypertension.

Contraindications

- Patients who are pregnant because of the risk of fetal damage

Procedure and patient care

R

Before

- Explain the procedure to the patient.
- Do not schedule a renal scan within 24 hours after an IVP.
- Assure the patient that he or she will not be exposed to large amounts of radioactivity, because only tracer doses of isotopes are used.
- Note that Lugol's solution (10 drops) may be ordered if ^{131}I orthoiodohippurate will be used. This minimizes thyroid uptake of the radioisotope.
- Remind the patient to void before the scan.
- Tell the patient that no sedation or fasting is required but that good hydration is essential.

- Instruct the patient to drink two to three glasses of water before the scan.

During

- Note the following procedural steps:
  1. The unsedated, nonfasting patient is taken to the nuclear medicine department.
  2. A peripheral IV injection of radionuclide is given. It takes only minutes for the radioisotopes to be concentrated in the kidneys.
  3. While the patient assumes a supine, prone, or sitting position, a gamma ray detector is passed over the kidney area and records the radioactive uptake on Polaroid or x-ray film.
  4. For a *Lasix renal scan* or a *diuretic renal scan,* the patient is imaged with DTPA. Images are obtained for 20 minutes; then 40 mg of Lasix is administered IV, and another 20 minutes of images are obtained.
  5. For the *captopril renal scan,* the patient is scanned after the administration of angiotensin-converting enzyme (ACE) inhibitors, such as captopril.
  6. Scans may be repeated at different intervals after the initial isotope injection.
- Note that the duration of this test varies from 1 to 4 hours depending on the specific information required. Perfusion scans are done in approximately 20 minutes, and functional scans in less than 1 hour. Static structure scans require 20 minutes to 4 hours for completion.
- Note that this study is performed by a nuclear medicine technologist or physician.
- Tell the patient that no pain or discomfort is associated with this procedure.
- Inform the patient that he or she must lie still during this study.

After

- Because only tracer doses of radioisotopes are used, inform the patient that no precautions need to be taken against radioactive exposure.
- Tell the patient that the radioactive substance is usually excreted from the body within 6 to 24 hours. Encourage the patient to drink fluids.

Abnormal findings

Urinary obstruction
Pyelonephritis
Renovascular hypertension
Absence of kidney function
Renal infarction
Renal arterial atherosclerosis
Glomerulonephritis

Renal tumor
Congenital abnormalities
Renal trauma
Transplant rejection
Acute tubular necrosis
Renal abscess
Renal cyst

notes

R

renin assay, plasma (Plasma renin activity [PRA])

Type of test Blood

Normal findings

Adult/elderly
  Upright position, *sodium depleted* (sodium-restricted diet)
    Ages 20-39 years: 2.9-24.0 ng/ml/hr
    >40 years: 2.9-10.8 ng/ml/hr
  Upright position, *sodium repleted* (normal sodium diet)
    Ages 20-39 years: 0.1-4.3 ng/ml/hr
    >40 years: 0.1-3.0 ng/ml/hr
Child
  0-3 years: <16.6 ng/ml/hr
  3-6 years: <6.7 ng/ml/hr
  6-9 years: <4.4 ng/ml/hr
  9-12 years: <5.9 ng/ml/hr
  12-15 years: <4.2 ng/ml/hr
  15-18 years: <4.3 ng/ml/hr

Test explanation and related physiology

Renin is an enzyme released by the juxtaglomerular apparatus of the kidney into the renal veins in response to sodium depletion and hypovolemia. Renin activates the renin-angiotensin system, which results in angiotensin II, a powerful vasoconstrictor that also stimulates aldosterone production from the adrenal cortex. Angiotensin and aldosterone increase the blood pressure (Figure 26).

The PRA test is a screening procedure for the detection of essential, renal, or renovascular hypertension. The PRA may be supplemented by other tests such as the renal vein renin assay (see p. 715). A determination of the PRA and a measurement of the plasma aldosterone level (see p. 32) are used in the differential diagnosis of primary versus secondary hyperaldosteronism. Patients with primary hyperaldosteronism will have increased aldosterone production associated with decreased renin activity. Patients with secondary hyperaldosteronism caused by renovascular occlusion or primary renal disease will have increased levels of plasma renin.

The PRA is assessed as part of the *captopril test*, a new screening test for renovascular hypertension (RVH). Patients with RVH have greater falls in blood pressure and increases in PRA

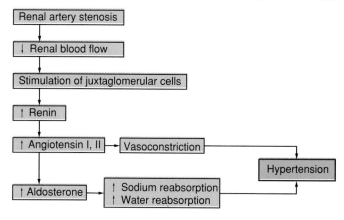

Figure 26 Physiology of renovascular hypertension.

after administration of angiotensin-converting enzyme (ACE) inhibitors than do those with essential hypertension. For the captopril test, the patient receives an oral dose of captopril (ACE inhibitor) after baseline PRA and blood pressure measurements are taken. Subsequent blood pressure measurements and a repeat PRA at 60 minutes are used for test interpretation. This is an excellent screening procedure to determine the need for a more invasive radiographic evaluation (such as digital subtraction renal arteriography or bilateral renal arteriography; see p. 100).

Interfering factors

- Renin levels are affected by pregnancy, salt intake, and licorice ingestion.
- Values are higher early in the day, in patients on low-salt diets, and when the patient is in an upright position.
- Posture affects renin levels. Renin is increased in the erect position and decreased in the recumbent position.
- Drugs that may affect test results include antihypertensives, diuretics, estrogens, oral contraceptives, and vasodilators.

Procedure and patient care

Before

- Explain the procedure to the patient.
- Instruct the patient to maintain a normal diet with a restricted amount of sodium (approximately 3 g/day) for 3

days before the test. A high-sodium diet causes a decrease in renin.
- Instruct the patient to discontinue medications (e.g., diuretics, steroids, antihypertensives, vasodilators, oral contraceptives) and licorice for 2 to 4 weeks before the test.
- Usually, draw a fasting blood sample, because renin values are higher in the morning.

During
- Usually, perform the test with the patient in an upright position.
- Ensure that the patient stands or sits upright for 2 hours before the blood is drawn.
- If a recumbent sample is ordered, have the patient remain in bed in the morning until the blood sample has been obtained.
- Collect approximately 7 to 12 ml of venous blood and place it in a chilled lavender-top tube with ethylenediaminetetraacetic acid (EDTA) as an anticoagulant.
- Gently invert the blood tube to allow adequate mixing of the blood sample and the anticoagulant.
- Record the patient's position, dietary status, and time of day on the laboratory slip. Also, note any medication that the patient is currently taking.
- Place the tube of blood on ice, and immediately send it to the laboratory.

After
- Apply pressure or a pressure dressing to the venipuncture site.
- Observe the venipuncture site for bleeding.
- Tell the patient that usually a normal diet may be resumed.
- Note that medications that were withheld may be reordered.

Abnormal findings

▲ **Increased levels**
Essential hypertension
Malignant hypertension
Renovascular hypertension
Addison's disease
Renin-producing renal tumor (Bartter's syndrome)
Cirrhosis
Hypokalemia
Hemorrhage

▼ **Decreased levels**
Salt-retaining steroid therapy
Antidiuretic hormone therapy

renin assay, renal vein

Type of test Blood

Normal findings Renin ratio of involved kidney to uninvolved kidney <1.4

Test explanation and related physiology

Renin is an enzyme secreted by the kidneys that activates the renin-angiotensin system and causes vasoconstriction and the release of aldosterone. These mechanisms can cause hypertension (see Figure 26, p. 713). Renal vein assays for renin are used to diagnose renovascular hypertension. By injection of a radiopaque dye into the inferior vena cava, the renal veins can be identified. A catheter is placed into each renal vein, and blood is withdrawn from each vein. Radioimmunoassay is used to determine the renin quantity in each sample. If hypertension is caused by renal artery stenosis, the renal vein renin level of the affected kidney should be 1.4 or more times greater than that of the unaffected kidney. If the levels are the same, the hypertension is not caused by renal artery stenosis (any stenosis identified on an arteriogram would not be considered severe enough to cause renin-related hypertension); another cause for the patient's elevated blood pressure must be investigated.

Contraindications

- Patients who are allergic to shellfish or iodinated dye

Potential complications

- Allergic reaction to iodinated dye
  Allergic reactions may vary from mild flushing, itching, and urticaria to severe, life-threatening anaphylaxis (evidenced by respiratory distress, drop in blood pressure, shock). In the unusual event of anaphylaxis, the patient may be treated with diphenhydramine (Benadryl), steroids, and epinephrine. Oxygen and endotracheal equipment should be on hand for immediate use.

Procedure and patient care

Before

- Explain the procedure to the patient.
- Ensure that written and informed consent for this procedure is obtained by the physician.

R

- Assess the patient for allergies to iodine.
- Inform the radiologist if an allergy to iodinated contrast is suspected. The radiologist may prescribe a Benadryl-and-steroid preparation to be administered before testing. Usually, a hypoallergenic, nonionic contrast will be used during the test.
- Place the patient on a "no added salt" diet and diuretics for 3 days before the examination.
- Keep the patient NPO after midnight on the day of the study.
- Instruct the patient to remain in the upright position for 2 hours before the test.
- Premedicate the fasting patient as ordered. Meperidine and atropine are typically used.

During

- Note the following procedural steps:
  1. The patient is taken to the radiology department and placed on the fluoroscopy table in a supine position.
  2. The patient's groin is prepared and draped in a sterile manner and then anesthetized.
  3. The femoral vein is punctured, and a catheter is placed into the vein and advanced into the inferior vena cava.
  4. Fluoroscopy is used to monitor the catheter placement.
  5. Dye is injected, and the renal veins are identified.
  6. The catheter is placed into one renal vein at a time, and separate blood specimens are withdrawn and labeled.
  7. The catheter is removed, and a pressure dressing is applied to the puncture site.
- Note that this procedure is usually performed by a radiologist in less than 1 hour.
- Inform the patient that the groin puncture needed for this study is uncomfortable.

After

- Usually, place the patient on bed rest for several hours.
- Monitor the patient's vital signs.
- Usually, send the blood to a commercial laboratory for analysis.
- Assess the patient for renal vein thrombosis, which may occur 1 to 7 days after the procedure. This will be manifested by costovertebral tenderness, hematuria, and elevated creatinine levels.

- Observe the venous puncture site frequently for hematoma or hemorrhage.
- Apply cold compresses to the puncture site if needed to reduce discomfort and swelling.
- Evaluate the patient for delayed reaction to the dye (dyspnea, rashes, tachycardia, hives). This usually occurs within the first 2 to 6 hours after the test. Treat with antihistamines or steroids.

Abnormal finding

▲   **Increased levels**
Renal artery stenosis

notes

R

reticulocyte count (Retic count)

Type of test Blood

Normal findings

Reticulocyte count
    Adult/elderly/child: 0.5% to 2%
    Infant: 0.5% to 3.1%
    Newborn: 2.5% to 6.5%
Reticulocyte index: 1.0

Test explanation and related physiology

The reticulocyte count is a test for determining bone marrow function and evaluating erythropoietic activity. This test is also useful in identifying anemias. A reticulocyte is an immature red blood cell (RBC) that can be readily identified under a microscope by the staining of a peripheral blood smear with a supravital stain. The reticulocyte count represents a direct measurement of RBC production by the bone marrow. Increased reticulocyte counts are expected as physiologic compensation in patients who are anemic. A normal or low reticulocyte count in a patient with anemia indicates that the marrow production of RBCs is inadequate and perhaps the cause of the anemia (as in aplastic anemia, iron deficiency, vitamin B_{12} deficiency, or depletion of iron stores). An elevated reticulocyte count found in patients with a normal hemogram indicates increased RBC production (compensated hemolysis or hemorrhage). To determine if the increased reticulocyte count indicates adequate erythropoiesis in patients with anemia and a decreased hematocrit, one can determine the *reticulocyte index:*

Reticulocyte index =

$$\text{Reticulocyte count (in \%)} \times \frac{\text{Patient's hematocrit}}{\text{Normal hematocrit}}$$

The reticulocyte index in a patient with a good marrow response to the anemia should be 1.0. If it is below 1.0, even though the reticulocyte count is elevated in the patient, the test indicates that the bone marrow response is inadequate in its ability to compensate (as in iron deficiency, vitamin B_{12} deficiency, or marrow failure).

Interfering factor

- Pregnancy may cause an increased reticulocyte count.

Procedure and patient care

Before

- Explain the procedure to the patient.
- Tell the patient that no fasting is required.

During

- Collect approximately 5 to 7 ml of venous blood in a lavender-top tube.

After

- Apply pressure or a pressure dressing to the venipuncture site.
- Observe the venipuncture site for bleeding.

Abnormal findings

▲ Increased levels

Hemolytic anemia
Sickle cell anemia
Hemorrhage (3 to 4 days later)
Postsplenectomy
Erythroblastosis fetalis
Pregnancy
Leukemias

▼ Decreased levels

Pernicious anemia
Folic acid deficiency
Adrenocortical hypofunction
Cirrhosis of the liver
Aplastic anemia
Radiation therapy
Marrow failure
Anterior pituitary hypofunction
Chronic infection

R

notes

retrograde pyelography

Type of test X-ray with contrast dye

Normal findings Normal outline and size of the ureters and bladder

Test explanation and related physiology

Retrograde pyelography refers to radiographic visualization of the urinary tract through ureteral catheterization and the injection of contrast material. The ureters are catheterized during cystoscopy. A radiopaque material is injected into the ureters, and x-ray films are taken. This test can be performed even if the patient has an allergy to IV contrast dye, because none of the dye injected into the ureters is absorbed.

Retrograde pyelography is helpful in radiographically examining the ureters in patients when visualization with intravenous pyelography (IVP, see p. 487) is inadequate or contraindicated. Frequently, in patients with unilateral renal disease, the involved kidney and collecting system are not visualized. To rule out ureteral obstruction as a cause of the unilateral kidney disease, retrograde pyelography must be done to examine the ureters. Tumors, benign strictures, tortuous ureters, stones, scarring, and extrinsic compression may cause ureteral obstruction. Retrograde pyelography provides complete visualization of the ureters.

Potential complications

- Urinary tract infection
  Infections may be caused by the invasive nature of this procedure.
- Sepsis by seeding the bloodstream with bacteria from infected urine
- Perforation of the bladder or ureter
- Hematuria
- Temporary obstruction to ureteral urine flow
  Manipulation of the ureters may cause edema, which can result in temporary, partial obstruction to urine flow.
- Allergic reaction to iodinated dye
  This rarely occurs, because the dye is not administered IV.

Interfering factor

- Retained barium from previous x-ray studies could obscure visualization.

Procedure and patient care

Before
- Explain the procedure to the patient.
- Ensure that informed consent for this procedure is obtained.
- If enemas are ordered to clear the bowel, assist the patient as needed and record the results.
- If procedure will be done with the patient under local anesthesia, allow the patient to have a liquid breakfast.
- If the procedure will be performed with the patient under general anesthesia, follow the routine general anesthesia precautions. Keep the patient NPO after midnight on the day of the test. Fluids may be given IV.
- Administer the preprocedural medications as ordered 1 hour before the study. Sedatives decrease the spasm of the bladder sphincter, thus decreasing the patient's discomfort.
- Check the patient for allergies to iodinated dye.

During
- Note the following procedural steps:
  1. The ureteral catheters are passed into the ureters by means of cystoscopy (see p. 310).
  2. Radiopaque contrast material (Hypaque or Renografin) is injected into the ureteral catheters, and x-ray films are taken.
  3. The entire ureter and pelvis are demonstrated.
  4. As the catheters are withdrawn, more dye is injected and more x-ray films are taken to visualize the complete outline of the ureters.
- Note that retrograde pyelography is performed by a urologist in approximately 1 hour in a cystoscopy room or operating room.
- Inform the patient that this study is uncomfortable. If awake, the patient will feel pressure and an urge to void.
- Occasionally when ureteral obstruction is identified, a ureteral catheter is placed through the obstruction in order to stent and drain the entire ureter.

R

After

- Check and record the patient's vital signs as ordered. Watch for a decrease in blood pressure and increase in pulse as an indication of bleeding.
- Observe the patient for signs and symptoms of sepsis (elevated temperature, flush, chills, decreased blood pressure, increased pulse).
- Assess the patient's ability to void for at least 24 hours. Urinary retention may be secondary to edema caused by instrumentation.
- Note the color of the urine; a pink tinge is typically present. Report bright-red blood or clots to the physician.
- Encourage the patient to increase intake of fluids. A dilute urine decreases dysuria. Fluids also maintain a constant flow of urine to prevent stasis and the accumulation of bacteria in the bladder.
- Monitor the patient for bladder spasms. Often, belladona-and-opium (B&O) suppositories are given to relieve bladder spasms.
- Observe for an allergic reaction to iodine contrast dye by instructing the patient to report symptoms of itching, rash, hives, flushing, shortness of breath, and increased heart rate. Treat with antihistamines or steroids.
- Administer analgesics as needed.

Abnormal findings

Tumor
Strictures
Stones
Ureteral obstruction

Intrinsic or extrinsic tumor
    affecting the ureters
Congenital anomaly

notes

rheumatoid factor (RF)

Type of test Blood

Normal findings
Negative (<60 U/ml by nephelometric testing)
Elderly patients may have slightly increased values

Test explanation and related physiology
The RF test is useful in the diagnosis of rheumatoid arthritis. Other diseases, such as systemic lupus erythematosus (SLE), also may cause a positive RF test. RF is occasionally seen in patients with tuberculosis, chronic hepatitis, infectious mononucleosis, and subacute bacterial endocarditis as well. Elderly patients often have false-positive results.

Rheumatoid arthritis is a chronic inflammatory disease that affects most joints, especially the metacarpal and phalangeal joints, the proximal interphalangeal joints, and the wrists; however, any synovial joint can be involved. In this disease, abnormal immunoglobulin G (IgG) antibodies produced by lymphocytes in the synovial membranes act as antigens. These antigens react with IgG and IgM antibodies to produce immune complexes. These immune complexes may activate the complement system and other inflammatory systems to cause joint damage. The reactive IgM molecule is the RF. Tissues other than the joints, including blood vessels, lungs, nerves, and heart, may be involved in the autoimmune inflammation.

Tests for RF are directed toward identification of the IgM antibodies. Approximately 80% of patients with rheumatoid arthritis have positive RF titers. To be considered positive, RF must be found in a dilution of greater than 1:80; when RF is found in titers less than 1:80, diseases such as SLE, scleroderma, and other autoimmune conditions should be considered. Although the normal value is "no rheumatoid factor identifiable at low titers," a small number of normal patients will have RF present at a very low titer. When the nephelometric testing procedure is used, the normal value is considered to be less than 60 U/ml.

Although there are many ways of detecting RF, the sheep cell agglutination test or the latex fixation test is usually performed. In the *sheep cell agglutination test,* rabbit IgG is placed on the sheep red blood cells. When this is mixed with the patient's serum (which has been serially diluted), visual agglutination occurs if any RF is present. In the *latex fixation test,* human IgG is placed on a synthetic latex particle and mixed with the patient's serum. Visual agglutination is then detected if RF is present.

Interfering factor
- Elderly patients often have false-positive results.

Procedure and patient care

Before
- Explain the procedure to the patient.
- Tell the patient that no fasting or preparation is required.

During
- Collect approximately 7 ml of venous blood in a red-top tube.

After
- Apply pressure or a pressure dressing to the venipuncture site.
- Observe the venipuncture site for bleeding.

Abnormal findings

▲ **Increased levels**

Rheumatoid arthritis
Other autoimmune disease (e.g., systemic lupus erythematosus)
Chronic viral infection
Subacute bacterial endocarditis
Tuberculosis
Chronic hepatitis

Dermatomyositis
Scleroderma
Infectious mononucleosis
Leukemia
Cirrhosis
Syphilis
Renal disease

notes

rubella antibody test (German measles test, Hemagglutination inhibition [HAI])

Type of test Blood

Normal findings Lack of susceptibility to rubella if the HAI titer is >1:10 to 1:20 or if the complement fixation test is negative

Possible critical values Evidence of susceptibility in pregnant women with recent exposure to rubella

Test explanation and related physiology

Screening for rubella antibodies is done to detect immunity to rubella. These tests detect the presence of IgG and IgM antibodies of past and active infections and determine a patient's susceptibility or immunity to the rubella virus, which is the causative agent for German measles. It is vitally important to identify exposure to rubella infection and susceptibility status in pregnant women, because infection in the first trimester of pregnancy is associated with congenital abnormalities, abortion, or stillbirth. All pregnant women should be screened for rubella during the first prenatal test.

If the pregnant woman's titer is greater than 1:10 to 1:20, she is not susceptible to rubella. If the pregnant woman's titer is 1:8 or less, she has little or no immunity to rubella. She should be strongly advised to stay away from any small children, especially those with symptoms of an upper respiratory tract infection (prodromal symptoms of rubella) during her pregnancy. In addition, all health care personnel associated with maternal and child care should be screened for rubella. Immunization, if required, is not done during pregnancy but should be done after delivery for nonimmune mothers.

A change in the HAI titer from the acute to the chronic phase in a patient with a rash is the most useful method of demonstrating that the rash was due to rubella. With a rubella rash, diagnosis of rubella is confirmed by obtaining an acute sample (taken approximately 3 days after the onset of the rash) and a convalescent sample (taken approximately 3 weeks later). A fourfold increase in titer from the acute to the convalescent titer indicates that the rash was caused by rubella. Alternatively, in a pregnant woman with a rash suspected to be from rubella, an

R

IgM antibody titer could be done. If the titer is positive, recent infection has occurred. IgM titers appear 1 to 2 days after onset of the rash and disappear 5 to 6 weeks after infection.

Procedure and patient care

Before

- Explain the purpose of the test to the patient.

During

- Collect approximately 7 ml of venous blood in a red-top tube.

After

- Apply pressure or a pressure dressing to the venipuncture site.
- Assess the venipuncture site for bleeding.
- Inform the patient when to return for a follow-up HAI titer if indicated.

Abnormal finding

Rubella infection

notes

Schilling test (Vitamin B$_{12}$ absorption test)

Type of test Urine (24- to 48-hour)

Normal findings Excretion of 8% to 40% of radioactive vitamin B$_{12}$ within 24 hours

Test explanation and related physiology

The Schilling test is performed to detect vitamin B$_{12}$ absorption. Normally, ingested vitamin B$_{12}$ combines with intrinsic factor, which is produced by gastric mucosa, and is absorbed in the distal part of the ileum. Pernicious anemia results when absorption of vitamin B$_{12}$ is inadequate. This may be caused by a primary malabsorption problem of the intestinal tract or from lack of intrinsic factor.

The two-stage Schilling test can detect a defect in vitamin B$_{12}$ absorption. With normal absorption, the ileum absorbs more vitamin B$_{12}$ than the body needs and excretes the excess into the urine. With impaired absorption, however, little or no vitamin B$_{12}$ is excreted into the urine.

In the Schilling test, urinary B$_{12}$ levels are measured after the ingestion of radioactive vitamin B$_{12}$. The test can be performed in one stage (without intrinsic factor) or two stages (with intrinsic factor). Patients with pernicious anemia from lack of intrinsic factor will have an abnormal first-stage and a normal second-stage Schilling test. Patients with malabsorption from an intestinal source will have an abnormal first- and second-stage Schilling test.

Contraindications

- Patients who are pregnant
- Patients who are lactating

Interfering factors

- Radioactive nuclear material received 10 days before testing may affect results.
- Renal insufficiency may cause reduced excretion of radioactive vitamin B$_{12}$.
- Patients who are elderly, diabetic, or hypothyroid may have reduced excretion of vitamin B$_{12}$.
- ☛ Drugs that may affect test results include laxatives, because they could decrease the rate of vitamin B$_{12}$ absorption.

S

Procedure and patient care

Before
- Explain the procedure to the patient.
- Instruct the patient to remain NPO except for water 8 to 12 hours before the test. Food should not be given until after the patient receives the injections.
- Instruct the patient not to take laxatives during the test period.

During
- Note the following procedural steps:
  1. Radioactive vitamin B_{12} is administered orally to the patient.
  2. Shortly thereafter, nonradioactive vitamin B_{12} is administered to the patient IM to saturate tissue-binding sites and to permit some excretion of radioactive vitamin B_{12} in the urine if it is absorbed.
  3. A 24- to 48-hour urine collection for vitamin B_{12} is obtained.
  4. The patient is encouraged to drink fluids.

Two-stage Schilling test
  1. If indicated, the second stage is performed approximately 1 week after the first stage.
  2. The fasting patient is provided radioactive vitamin B_{12} combined with human intrinsic factor.
  3. As before, an IM injection of nonradioactive vitamin B_{12} is administered.
  4. Again, 24- to 48-hour urine collections are begun.

Combined one-stage and two-stage Schilling test
  1. The fasting patient receives a capsule of cobalt-57–labeled vitamin B_{12} plus intrinsic factor.
  2. A second capsule of cobalt-58–labeled vitamin B_{12} is also given.
  3. One hour later, an IM injection of nonradioactive vitamin B_{12} is administered.
  4. Again, the urine for vitamin B_{12} is collected for 24 to 48 hours.
  5. Percentages of cobalt-57 and cobalt-58 are calculated. Cobalt-57–labeled vitamin B_{12} only will be present in patients with pernicious anemia secondary to lack of intrinsic factor. No vitamin B_{12} will be present in the urine of patients whose pernicious anemia is caused by primary bowel malabsorption.

After
- Ensure that the urine specimens are promptly transported to the laboratory.

Abnormal findings

▼ **Decreased levels**

Pernicious anemia	Hypothyroidism
Intestinal malabsorption	Liver disease

notes

scrotal nuclear imaging (Scrotal scan, Testicular imaging)

Type of test Nuclear medicine

Normal findings Symmetric and prompt blood flow to both testicles

Test explanation and related physiology

Scrotal imaging is helpful in the diagnosis of patients with a sudden onset of unilateral testicular swelling and pain. Scrotal imaging can differentiate unilateral testicular torsion from other causes of testicular pain (e.g., acute epididymitis, torsion of the testicular appendage, orchitis, strangulated hernia, testicular hemorrhage). Testicular torsion is a surgical emergency requiring prompt surgical exploration to salvage the involved testicle. The other causes of painful testicular swelling, however, do not require surgery. Use of radionuclide scrotal imaging enables the surgeon to diagnose testicular torsion. This study is usually performed on an emergency basis and in the nuclear medicine department.

The patient is positioned under the gamma ray camera with the scrotum supported between the abducted thighs. Technetium-99m pertechnetate is administered, and a dynamic radionuclide angiogram is obtained. Static images are obtained immediately afterward. An area of decreased perfusion corresponding to the involved testes indicates a high probability of torsion of the testicle. If the clinically involved testes is normally perfused or hypervascular, a disease other than torsion of the testicle (as described earlier) exists. In 95% of all cases of testicular torsion, the scrotal image will make the diagnosis. This information can be obtained in 10 to 15 minutes after injection of the nuclear material.

Procedure and patient care

Before

- Explain the procedure to the patient.
- Tell the patient that no fasting or premedication is required.
- Assure the patient that he will not be exposed to large amounts of radiation, because only tracer doses of isotope are used.
- If the patient is a child, encourage the parent(s) to be present.

During
- The patient is placed on a padded table in the supine position.
- The patient's legs are abducted, and the testicles are supported with tape or a lead shield. The penis is taped to the lower abdomen.
- A small IV injection of technetium-99m pertechnetate is administered.
- Radionuclide imaging is then immediately performed over both testicles. Both dynamic and static images are obtained.

After
- Because only tracer doses of radioisotopes are used, inform the patient that no precautions need to be taken by others against radiation exposure.
- If the patient is identified as having torsion of the testicle, prepare the patient for surgery.

Abnormal findings

▲ **Increased testicular blood flow**

Epididymitis
Torsion of the testicular appendage
Orchitis
Trauma

▼ **Decreased testicular blood flow**

Testicular torsion of the spermatic cord

notes

scrotal ultrasound (Ultrasound of testes)

Type of test Ultrasound

Normal findings Normal size, shape, and configuration of the testicles

Test explanation and related physiology

With the advent of scrotal ultrasound, a noninvasive, nonionizing, rapid method for scrotal examination was developed. Through the use of reflected sound waves, ultrasonography provides accurate visualization of the scrotum and its contents. Ultrasonography requires the emission of high-frequency sound waves from the transducer to penetrate the organ being studied. The sound waves are bounced back to the transducer and electronically converted into a pictorial image. A realistic Polaroid picture or x-ray film of the testicle is obtained.

Present uses for scrotal ultrasound include:

1. Evaluation of scrotal masses
2. Measurement of testicular size
3. Evaluation of scrotal trauma
4. Evaluation of scrotal pain
5. Evaluation of occult testicular neoplasm
6. Surveillance of patients with prior primary or metastatic testicular neoplasms
7. Follow-up for testicular infections
8. Location of undescended testicles

With the real-time ultrasound transducer, the scrotum is examined. The testicle and extratesticular intrascrotal tissues are examined. The accuracy of scrotal ultrasound is 90% to 95%. Both benign and malignant tumors (primary and metastatic) can be identified with ultrasound. Benign abnormalities such as testicular abscess, orchitis, testicular infarction, and testicular torsion also can be identified. Extratesticular lesions such as hydrocele, hematocele (blood in the scrotum), and pyocele (pus in the scrotum) can be identified as well. Scrotal and groin ultrasound has been very helpful in locating cryptorchid (undescended) testicles.

There is very little discomfort associated with testicular ultrasound. It is usually performed by an ultrasound technologist and interpreted by an ultrasound physician.

Procedure and patient care

Before

- Explain the procedure to the patient.
- Tell the patient that no fasting is required.

During

- Note the following procedural steps:
  1. Careful examination of the scrotum is performed by the physician. Usually, a short history is obtained.
  2. The scrotum is supported by a towel or cradled by the examiner's gloved hand.
  3. A greasy, conductive paste is applied to the scrotum before scanning. This paste enhances sound wave transmission and reception.
  4. Thorough scanning in the sagittal, transverse, and oblique projections is performed.
- The test takes approximately 20 to 30 minutes.

After

- Remove the coupling agent (grease) from the patient's scrotum.

Abnormal findings

Benign testicular tumor
Malignant testicular tumor
Occult testicular tumor
Testicular infection (orchitis)
Hydrocele
Hematocele
Pyocele

Varicocele
Epididymitis
Spermatocele
Scrotal hernia
Cryptorchidism
Hematoma
Testicular torsion

notes

S

secretin-pancreozymin (Pancreatic enzymes)

Type of test Fluid analysis

Normal findings
Volume: 2-4 ml/kg body weight
HCO_3^- (bicarbonate): 90-130 mEq/L
Amylase: 6.6-35.2 U/kg

Test explanation and related physiology

Children with cystic fibrosis have mucous plugs that obstruct their pancreatic ducts. The pancreatic enzymes (e.g., amylase, lipase, trypsin, chymotrypsin) cannot be expelled into the duodenum and therefore are either completely absent or present only in diminished quantities within the duodenal aspirate. Secretin and pancreozymin are used to stimulate pancreatic secretion of these enzymes. The duodenal contents are aspirated and examined for pH, bicarbonate, and enzyme levels; amylase is the most frequently measured enzyme. Diminished values are suggestive of cystic fibrosis.

Procedure and patient care

Before
- Explain the procedure to the patient and/or parents.
- Instruct the adult patient to fast for 12 hours before testing.
- Determine pediatric fasting times according to the patient's age.

During
- Note the following procedural steps:
  1. With the use of fluoroscopy, a Dreiling tube is passed through the patient's nose and into the stomach.
  2. The distal lumen of the tube is placed within the duodenum.
  3. The proximal lumen of the tube is placed within the stomach.
  4. Both lumens are aspirated. The gastric lumen is continually aspirated to avoid contamination of the gastric contents in the duodenum aspirate.
  5. A control specimen of the duodenal juices is collected for 20 minutes.

6. The patient is tested for sensitivity to secretin and pancreozymin by low-dose intradermal injection.
7. If no sensitivity is present, these hormones are administered IV. Secretin can be expected to stimulate pancreatic water and bicarbonate secretion. Pancreozymin can be expected to stimulate pancreatic enzyme (lipase, amylase, trypsin, chymotrypsin) secretion.
8. Four duodenal aspirates are collected at 20-minute intervals and placed in the specimen container.
9. Each specimen is analyzed for pH, volume, bicarbonate, and amylase levels.

- Note that a physician performs this test in approximately 2 hours in the laboratory or at the patient's bedside.
- Tell the patient that he or she may have discomfort and gagging during placement of the Dreiling tube.

After

- Place the aspirated specimens on ice. Send them to the chemistry laboratory as soon as the test is completed.
- Remove the Dreiling tube after completion of the test. Give appropriate nose and mouth care.
- Allow the patient to resume a normal diet.

Abnormal findings

Cystic fibrosis
Sprue

notes

sella turcica x-ray

Type of test X-ray

Normal findings No abnormalities

Test explanation and related physiology

This study involves taking x-ray films of the sella turcica, an area of the bony cranium at the base of the skull. The sella turcica contains the pituitary gland. Pituitary tumors that produce adrenocorticotropic hormone may cause Cushing's syndrome. One can diagnose these tumors easily by detecting erosion and destruction of the normal sella turcica. Computed tomography (CT) scanning is usually done if a pituitary tumor is suspected.

Procedure and patient care

Before

- Explain the procedure to the patient.
- Tell the patient that all objects above the neck must be removed.
- If a glass eye is present, note this on the x-ray examination request, because it will present a confusing shadow.

During

- Note that axial (submentovertical), half-axial (Towne), posteroanterior, and lateral views of the skull are usually taken.
- Tell the patient that this test is painless.
- Note that a radiologic technologist performs this test in a few minutes.

After

- Note that no special aftercare is needed.

Abnormal findings

Pituitary tumor
Destruction of the sella turcica

notes

semen analysis (Sperm count, Sperm examination, Seminal cytology, Semen examination)

Type of test Fluid analysis

Normal findings

Volume: 2-5 ml
Liquification time: 20 to 30 minutes after collection
pH: 7.12-8.00
Sperm count (density): 50-200 million/ml
Sperm motility: 60% to 80% actively motile
Sperm morphology: 70% to 90% normally shaped

Test explanation and related physiology

Semen analysis is one of the most important aspects of the fertility workup, because the cause of a woman's inability to conceive often lies with the man. After 2 to 3 days of sexual abstinence, sperm is collected and examined for volume, sperm count, motility, and morphology.

The freshly collected semen is first measured for volume. After liquification of the white, gelatinous ejaculate, a sperm count is done. Men with very low or very high counts likely are infertile. The motility of the sperm is then evaluated; at least 60% should show progressive motility. Morphology is studied by staining a semen preparation and calculating the number of normal versus abnormal sperm forms.

A simple sperm analysis, especially if it indicates infertility, is inconclusive, because the sperm count varies from day to day. A semen analysis should be done at least twice. Men with *aspermia* (no sperm) or *oligospermia* (20 million/ml) should be evaluated endocrinologically for pituitary, thyroid, adrenal, or testicular aberrations.

A normal semen analysis alone does not accurately assess the male factor unless the effect of the partner's cervical secretion on sperm survival is also determined (see Sims-Huhner test, p. 747). In addition to its value in infertility workups, semen analysis is also helpful in documenting adequate sterilization after a vasectomy. It is usually performed 6 weeks after the surgery. If any sperm are seen, the adequacy of the vasectomy must be questioned.

S

Interfering factors

☒ Drugs that may cause *decreased* semen levels include antineo-plastic agents (e.g., nitrogen mustard, procarbazine, vincris-tine, methotrexate), cimetidine, estrogens, and methyltestos-terone.

Procedure and patient care

Before
- Explain the procedure to the patient.
- Instruct the patient to abstain from sexual activity for 2 to 3 days before collecting the specimen. Prolonged abstinence before the collection should be discouraged, because the quality of the sperm cells, and especially their motility, may diminish.
- Give the patient the proper container for the sperm collec-tion.
- Instruct the patient to avoid alcoholic beverages for several days before the collection.
- For evaluation of the adequacy of vasectomy, the patient should ejaculate once or twice before the day of examina-tion.

During
- Note that semen is best collected by ejaculation into a clean container. For best results, the specimen should be collected in the physician's office or laboratory by masturbation.
- Note that less satisfactory specimens can be obtained in the patient's home by coitus interruptus or masturbation. Note the following procedural steps:
  1. Instruct the patient to deliver these home specimens to the laboratory within 1 hour after collection.
  2. Tell the patient to avoid excessive heat and cold during transportation of the specimen.

After
- Record the date of the previous semen emission along with the collection time and date of the fresh specimen.
- Tell the patient when and how to obtain the test results. Re-member that abnormal results may have a devastating effect on the patient's sexuality.

Abnormal findings

Infertility
Vasectomy (obstruction of vas
   deferens)
Orchitis

Testicular atrophy
Testicular failure
Hyperpyrexia

notes

sialography

Type of test X-ray

Normal findings No evidence of pathology in the salivary ducts and related structures

Test explanation and related physiology

Sialography is an x-ray procedure used to examine the salivary ducts (parotid, submaxillary, submandibular, sublingual) and related glandular structures after injection of a contrast medium into the desired duct. This procedure is used to detect calculi, strictures, tumors, or inflammatory disease in patients who complain of pain, tenderness, or swelling in these areas.

Contraindications

- Patients with mouth infections

Potential complication

- Allergic reaction to the iodinated dye
  This rarely occurs, because the dye is not administered IV.

Procedure and patient care

Before

- Explain the procedure to the patient. The thought of a dye injection in the mouth is frightening to many patients. Provide emotional support.
- Obtain informed consent if required by the institution.
- Instruct the patient to remove jewelry, hairpins, and dentures, which could obscure x-ray visualization.
- Instruct the patient to rinse his or her mouth before the procedure with an antiseptic solution to reduce the possibility of introducing bacteria into the ductal structures.

During

- Note the following procedural steps:
  1. X-ray studies are taken before the dye injection to ensure that stones are not present, which could prevent the contrast material from entering the ducts.
  2. The patient is placed in a supine position on an x-ray table.
  3. The contrast medium is injected directly into the desired orifice via a cannula or a special catheter.

4. X-ray films are taken with the patient in various positions.
5. The patient is given a sour substance (e.g., lemon juice) orally to stimulate salivary excretion.
6. Another set of x-ray studies is taken to evaluate ductal drainage.

- Note that a radiologist performs this procedure in the radiology department in less than 30 minutes.
- Tell the patient that he or she may feel a little pressure as the contrast medium is injected into the ducts.

After

- Encourage the patient to drink fluids to eliminate the dye.

Abnormal findings

Calculi
Strictures

Tumor
Inflammatory disease

notes

S

sickle cell test (Sickle cell preparation, Sickledex, Hgb S test)

Type of test Blood

Normal findings No sickle cells present

Test explanation and related physiology

Both sickle cell disease (homozygous for hemoglobin [Hgb] S) and sickle cell trait (heterozygous for Hgb S) can be detected by this study. Sickle cell anemia results from a genetic homozygous defect and is caused by the presence of Hgb S instead of Hgb A. When Hgb S becomes deoxygenated, it tends to bend in a way that causes the red blood cell (RBC) to assume a sickle shape. These sickled RBCs cannot freely pass through the capillaries, and thus they cause plugging of the microvascular tree. This may compromise the blood supply to various organs. Hgb S is found in varying quantities in 8% to 10% of the black population.

The routine peripheral blood smear of patients with sickle cell disease does not contain sickled RBCs unless hypoxemia is present. In the sickle cell test, a deoxygenating agent is added to the patient's blood. If 25% or more of the patient's hemoglobin is of the S variation, the cells will assume the crescent (sickle) shape and the test is positive. If no sickling occurs, the test is negative. A negative test indicates that the patient has no or very little Hgb S. Other less common hemoglobin variants also may cause sickling.

This test is only a screening test, and its sensitivity varies according to the method used by the laboratory. The definitive diagnosis is made by hemoglobin electrophoresis (see p. 456), in which Hgb S can be identified and quantified.

Interfering factors

- Any blood transfusions within 3 to 4 months before the sickle cell test may cause false-negative results, because the donor's normal hemoglobin may dilute the recipient's abnormal Hgb S.
- Polycythemia may cause false-negative results.
- Infants less than 3 months of age may have false-negative results.
- Drugs that may cause false-negative results include phenothiazines.

Procedure and patient care

Before
- Explain the procedure to the patient.
- Tell the patient that no fasting is required.

During
- Collect approximately 7 ml of venous blood in a lavender-top tube.

After
- Apply pressure or a pressure dressing to the venipuncture site.
- Check the venipuncture site for bleeding.
- If the test is positive, offer the family genetic counseling. A patient with one recessive gene (heterozygous) is said to have sickle cell *trait*. A patient with two recessive genes (homozygous) has sickle cell *anemia*.
- Inform patients with sickle cell anemia that they should avoid situations in which hypoxia may occur (e.g., strenuous exercise, air travel in unpressurized aircraft, travel to high-altitude regions).

Abnormal findings

Sickle cell trait
Sickle cell anemia

notes

S

sigmoidoscopy (Proctoscopy, Anoscopy)

Type of test Endoscopy

Normal findings Normal anus, rectum, and sigmoid colon

Test explanation and related physiology

Endoscopy of the lower gastrointestinal (GI) tract allows one to visualize and perform biopsies of tumors, polyps, hemorrhoids, or ulcers of the anus, rectum, and sigmoid colon. *Anoscopy* refers to examination of the anus; *proctoscopy* to examination of the anus and rectum; and *sigmoidoscopy* (the most frequent procedure) to examination of the anus, rectum, and sigmoid colon. This test can be performed with a rigid or flexible sigmoidoscope. Because the lower GI tract is difficult to visualize radiographically, direct visualization by sigmoidoscopy is helpful.

Furthermore, sigmoidoscopy, as with colonoscopy, can be therapeutic. Reduction of sigmoid volvulus, removal of polyps, and obliteration of hemorrhoids can be performed through the sigmoidoscope.

Contraindications

- Patients who are uncooperative
- Patients with diverticulitis
- Patients with painful anorectal conditions (e.g., fissures, fistulas, hemorrhoids)
- Patients with severe bleeding
  Blood clots obstruct the view of the scope.
- Patients suspected of having perforated colon lesions

Potential complications

- Perforation of the colon
- Bleeding from biopsy sites

Interfering factors

- Poor bowel preparation may obscure visualization of the bowel mucosa.
- Rectal bleeding may obstruct the lens system and preclude adequate visualization.

Procedure and patient care

Before

- Explain the procedure to the patient.
- Obtain informed consent for this procedure.
- Assist the patient with the bowel preparation. In most cases, two Fleet enemas are sufficient.
- Instruct the patient to ingest only a light breakfast on the morning of the endoscopy.
- Assure patients that they will be properly draped to avoid unnecessary embarrassment.

During

- Note the following procedural steps:
  1. The patient is placed on the endoscopy table or bed in the left lateral decubitus position. Physicians often prefer the knee-chest position; many operating and examining tables are easily converted to make the knee-chest position more comfortable. This procedure also can be performed with the patient in the lithotomy position.
  2. Usually, no sedation is required.
  3. The anus is mildly dilated with a well-lubricated finger.
  4. The rigid or flexible sigmoidoscope is placed into the rectum and advanced to its point of maximal penetration.
  5. Air is insufflated during the procedure to distend more fully the lower intestinal tract.
  6. The sigmoid, rectum, and anus are visualized.
  7. Biopsies can be obtained and polypectomy performed at the time of sigmoidoscopy.
- Note that a physician trained in GI endoscopy usually performs this procedure in the GI laboratory, operating room, patient's bedside, or outpatient clinic setting in approximately 15 to 20 minutes.
- Tell the patient that he or she probably will feel discomfort and the urge to defecate as the sigmoidoscope is inserted.

After

- Inform the patient that because air has been insufflated into the bowel during the procedure, he or she may have flatulence or gas pains. Ambulation may help.
- Observe the patient for signs of abdominal distention, increased tenderness, or rectal bleeding.
- Tell the patient that slight rectal bleeding may occur if biopsies have been taken.

S

Abnormal findings

Tumor (benign or malignant)
Polyps
Ulcerative colitis
Pseudomembranous colitis

Crohn's disease (regional enteritis)
Intestinal ischemia
Irritable bowel syndrome

notes

Sims-Huhner test (Postcoital test, Postcoital cervical mucus test, Cervical mucus sperm penetration test)

Type of test Fluid analysis

Normal findings

Cervical mucus adequate for sperm transmission, survival, and penetration

6 to 20 active sperm per high-power field

Test explanation and related physiology

The Sims-Huhner test consists of a postcoital examination of the cervical mucus to measure the ability of the sperm to penetrate the mucus and maintain motility. This study evaluates interaction between the sperm and the cervical mucus. It also measures the quality of the cervical mucus. This test can determine the effect of vaginal and cervical secretions on the activity of the sperm. This procedure is only performed after a previously performed semen analysis has been determined to be normal.

This test is performed during the middle of the ovulatory cycle, because at this time, the secretions should be optimal for sperm penetration and survival. During ovulation, the quantity of cervical mucus is maximal whereas the viscosity is minimal, thus facilitating sperm penetration. The endocervical mucus sample is examined for color, viscosity, and tenacity (spinnbarkeit). The fresh specimen is then spread on a clean glass slide and examined for the presence of sperm. Estimates of the total number and of the number of motile sperm per high-power field are reported. Normally, 6 to 20 active sperm cells should be seen in each microscopic high-power field; if the sperm are present but not active, the cervical environment is unsuitable (e.g., abnormal pH) for their survival. After the specimen has dried on the glass slide, the mucus can be examined for ferning (see cervical mucus test, p. 214). The Sims-Huhner study is invaluable in fertility examinations; however, it is not a substitute for the semen analysis. If the results of the Sims-Huhner test are less than optimal, the test is usually repeated during the same or next ovulatory cycle.

This analysis is also helpful in documenting cases of suspected rape by testing the vaginal and cervical secretions for sperm.

Procedure and patient care

Before

- Explain the procedure to the patient.
- Inform the patient that basal body temperature recordings should be used to indicate ovulation.
- Tell the patient that no vaginal lubrication, douching, or bathing is permitted until after the vaginal cervical examination, because these factors will alter the cervical mucus.
- Inform the patient that this study should be performed after 3 days of sexual abstinence.
- Instruct the patient to remain in bed for 10 to 15 minutes after coitus to ensure cervical exposure to the semen. After resting, the patient should report to her physician for examination of her cervical mucus within 2 hours after coitus.

During

- Note that with the patient in the lithotomy position, the cervix is then exposed by an unlubricated speculum. The specimen is aspirated from the endocervix and delivered to the laboratory for analysis.
- Note that this procedure is performed by a physician in approximately 5 minutes.
- Tell the patient that the only discomfort associated with this study is insertion of the speculum.

After

- Tell the patient how and when she may obtain the test results.

Abnormal findings

Infertility
Suspected rape

notes

skull x-ray

Type of test X-ray

Normal findings Normal skull and surrounding structures

Test explanation and related physiology

An x-ray film of the skull allows for visualization of the bones making up the skull, the nasal sinuses, and any cerebral calcification. This study is indicated for patients in whom a pathologic condition is suspected in any of these structures.

Skull fractures are easily seen as abnormal radiolucent lines in an otherwise radiopaque skull bone. Metastatic tumors of the skull can easily be seen as radiolucent spots in an otherwise normal skull. Opacification of the nasal sinuses may indicate sinusitis, hemorrhage, or tumor.

Located in the middle of the brain, the pineal gland is thought to regulate the biorhythms of mammals. This gland may become calcified after puberty. When calcified, the pineal gland is a very useful marker and allows the midline of the brain to be easily identified on the skull x-ray film. Conditions such as unilateral hematoma or tumor will cause a shift of the midline structures (and the calcified pineal gland) to the side opposite the site of the pathologic condition. Simple skull x-ray films therefore allow for the easy detection of these unilateral, space-occupying lesions.

The sella turcica is the bony structure surrounding and protecting the pituitary gland (see p. 736). Tumors of the pituitary gland may cause an increase in size or an erosion of the sella turcica. These changes can be detected by skull x-ray films.

S

Procedure and patient care

Before

- Explain the procedure to the patient.
- Instruct the patient to remove all objects above the neck, because metal objects and dentures will prevent x-ray visualization of the structures they cover.
- Avoid hyperextension and manipulation of the head if surgical injuries are suspected.
- Tell the patient that no sedation or fasting is required.

During
- Note that the patient is taken to the radiology department and placed on an x-ray table. Axial (submentovertical), half-axial (Towne), posteroanterior, and lateral views of the skull are usually taken.
- Note that a radiologic technologist takes skull films in a few minutes.
- Tell the patient that this test is painless.

After
- If a glass eye is present, note this on the x-ray examination request, because it can present a confusing shadow on x-ray film.

Abnormal findings

Skull fracture
Metastatic tumor
Sinusitis
Hemorrhage

Tumor
Hematoma
Congenital anomaly

notes

small bowel follow-through (SBF, Small bowel enema)

Type of test X-ray with contrast dye

Normal findings

Normal positioning, motility, and patency of the small intestine
No evidence of intrinsic obstruction or extrinsic compression

Test explanation and related physiology

The SBF study is performed to identify abnormalities in the small bowel. Usually, the patient is asked to drink barium; in patients who cannot drink, barium can be injected through a nasogastric tube. X-ray films are then taken at timed intervals (usually 30 minutes) to follow the progression of barium through the small intestine. Significant delays in transit time of the barium may occur with both benign and malignant forms of obstruction or diminished intestinal motility (ileus). On the other hand, the flow of barium is faster in patients who have hypermotility states of the small bowel (malabsorption syndromes). Failure of the progression through the small bowel can be seen in patients with partial mechanical small bowel obstruction or diminished intestinal motility, as seen in patients with diabetes. Furthermore, SBF series are helpful in identifying and defining the anatomy of small bowel fistulas (abnormal connections between the small bowel and other abdominal organs or skin).

A more accurate radiographic evaluation of the small intestine is provided by the *small bowel enema*. Unlike the SBF, in which the barium is swallowed by the patient, during the small bowel enema the barium is injected into a tube previously passed to the small bowel. This small bowel enema provides better visualization of the entire small bowel, because the barium is not diluted by gastric and duodenal juices, as occurs when the patient drinks barium. This test is especially useful in the evaluation of patients with partial small bowel obstruction of unknown etiology. Tumors, ulcers, and small bowel fistulas are more easily identified and defined with the enema.

Contraindications

- Patients with a complete small bowel obstruction
  The introduction of barium into an obstructed bowel may create a stonelike impaction; however, this is extremely rare.
- Patients suspected of having a perforated viscus

S

Barium should not be used in these patients, because it may cause prolonged and recurrent abscesses if it leaks out of the bowel. Gastrografin, a water-soluble contrast medium, can be used if perforation is suspected. Unfortunately, Gastrografin becomes diluted very rapidly, minimizing the accuracy of the SBF with this contrast medium.

- Patients with unstable vital signs
These patients should be supervised during the time required for this study.

Potential complication

- Barium-induced small bowel obstruction

Interfering factors

- Barium within the intestinal tract from a previous barium x-ray film
This may obstruct adequate visualization of the small bowel.
- Food or fluid within the gastrointestinal (GI) tract

Procedure and patient care

Before

- Explain the procedure to the patient.
- Instruct the patient not to eat anything for at least 8 hours before the test. Usually, keep the patient NPO after midnight on the day of the test.
- Inform the patient that the SBF series may take several hours. Suggest that the patient bring reading material or some paperwork to occupy his or her time.
- Accompany the patient to the radiology department if his or her vital signs are not stable.
- Arrange for transportation of the hospitalized patient back to the nursing unit between serial films.

During

- Note the following procedural steps:
  1. A specially prepared drink containing barium sulfate is mixed as a milkshake, which the patient drinks through a straw.
  2. Usually, an upper GI series is performed concomitantly (see p. 834).
  3. The barium flow is followed through the upper GI tract fluoroscopically.
  4. At frequent intervals (15 to 60 minutes), repeat x-ray films are taken to follow the flow of barium through the

small intestine. These films are repeated until barium is seen flowing into the right colon. This usually takes 60 to 120 minutes, but in patients with delayed progression of the barium, the test may take as much as 24 hours to complete.

Small bowel enema
1. This is usually performed by placing a long, weighted tube transorally; however, a tube also can be placed into the upper small bowel endoscopically.
2. After the tube is in place, a thickened barium mixture is injected through the tube and x-ray films are serially performed as described for the SBF.

- Note that this procedure is performed by a radiologist in the radiology department in approximately 30 minutes.
- Tell the patient that this test is not uncomfortable.

After

- Inform the patient of the need to evacuate adequately all the barium. Cathartics (e.g., magnesium citrate) are recommended. Initially, stools will be white and should return to normal color with complete evacuation.

Abnormal findings

Small bowel tumor

Small bowel obstruction from intrinsic tumors

Small bowel obstruction from adhesions, extrinsic tumors, or hernia

Inflammatory small bowel disease (e.g., Crohn's disease)

Malabsorption syndromes (e.g., Whipple's disease, sprue)

Congenital anatomic anomaly (e.g., malrotation)

Congenital abnormalities (e.g., small bowel atresia, duplication, Meckel's diverticulum)

Small bowel intussusception

Small bowel perforation

S

notes

sodium (Na$^+$), blood

Type of test Blood

Normal findings

Adult/elderly: 136-145 mEq/L or 136/145 mmol/L
(SI units)
Child: 136-145 mEq/L
Infant: 134-150 mEq/L
Newborn: 134-144 mEq/L

Possible critical values <120 or >160 mEq/L

Test explanation and related physiology

Sodium is the major cation in the extracellular space, where serum levels of approximately 140 mEq/L exist. The concentration of sodium intracellularly is only 5 mEq/L. Therefore sodium salts are the major determinants of extracellular osmolality. The sodium content of the blood is a result of a balance between dietary sodium intake and renal excretion. Normally, individual nonrenal (e.g., sweat) sodium losses are minimal.

Many factors regulate homeostatic sodium balance. For example, aldosterone causes conservation of sodium by decreasing renal losses. Natriuretic hormone, or third factor, increases renal losses of sodium. Antidiuretic hormone (ADH), which controls the reabsorption of water at the distal tubules of the kidney, also affects sodium serum levels.

Physiologically, water and sodium are very closely interrelated. As free body water is increased, serum sodium is diluted and the concentration may decrease. The kidney compensates by conserving sodium and excreting water. If free body water were to decrease, the serum sodium concentration would rise; the kidney would then respond by conserving free water. Aldosterone, ADH, and natriuretic factor all assist in these compensatory actions of the kidney.

An average dietary intake of approximately 90 to 250 mEq/day is needed to maintain sodium balance in adults. Symptoms of hyponatremia may include weakness, confusion, lethargy, stupor, and coma. Symptoms of hypernatremia include dry mucous membranes, thirst, agitation, restlessness, hyperreflexia, mania, and convulsions.

Interfering factors

- Recent trauma, surgery, or shock may cause increased levels.
- Drugs that may cause *increased* levels include anabolic steroids, antibiotics, clonidine, corticosteroids, cough medicines, laxatives, methyldopa, carbenicillin, estrogens, and oral contraceptives.
- Drugs that may cause *decreased* levels include carbamazepine, diuretics, sodium-free IV fluids, sulfonylureas, triamterene, ACE inhibitors, captopril, haloperidol, heparin, nonsteroidal antiinflammatory drugs (NSAIDs), tricyclic antidepressants, and vasopressin.

Procedure and patient care

Before

- Explain the procedure to the patient.
- Tell the patient that no food or fluid is restricted.

During

- Collect 5 to 10 ml of venous blood in a red- or green-top tube.
- If the patient is receiving an IV infusion, obtain the blood from the opposite arm.
- List on the laboratory slip any drugs that may affect test results.

After

- Apply pressure or a pressure dressing to the venipuncture site.
- Assess the venipuncture site for bleeding.

S

Abnormal findings

▲ **Increased levels
(hypernatremia)**

Increased sodium intake
  Excessive dietary intake
  Excessive sodium in IV
    fluids
Decreased sodium loss
  Cushing's syndrome
  Hyperaldosteronism
Excessive free body water
  loss
  Excessive sweating
  Extensive thermal burns
Diabetes insipidus
Osmotic diuresis

▼ **Decreased levels
(hyponatremia)**

Decreased sodium intake
  Deficient dietary intake
  Deficient sodium in IV
    fluids
Increased sodium loss
  Addison's disease
  Diarrhea
  Vomiting or nasogastric
    aspiration
  Diuretic administration
  Chronic renal insuffi-
    ciency
Increased free body water
  Excessive oral water
    intake
  Excessive IV water in-
    take
  Congestive heart failure
  Syndrome of inappro-
    priate secretion of
    ADH (SIADH)
  Osmotic dilution
Third-space losses of so-
  dium
Ascites
Peripheral edema
Pleural effusion
Intraluminal bowel loss
  (ileus or mechanical
  obstruction)

notes

sodium (Na$^+$), urine

Type of test Urine (24-hour)

Normal findings

40-220 mEq/L/day or 40-220 mmol/L (SI units)
Values vary greatly with dietary intake

Test explanation and related physiology

This test evaluates sodium balance in the body by determining the amount of sodium excreted in urine over 24 hours. Sodium is the major cation in the extracellular space. Measuring the amount of sodium in the urine is useful for evaluating patients with volume depletion, acute renal failure, adrenal disturbances, and acid-base imbalances. This test is important, especially when the serum sodium concentration is low. For example, in patients with hyponatremia caused by inadequate sodium intake, the urine sodium will be low. In patients with hyponatremia caused by chronic renal failure, however, the urine sodium concentration will be high.

The sodium content in urine is the result of the balance between the dietary sodium and renal excretion of sodium. In the normal individual, nonrenal sodium losses are minimal. Many factors affect this delicate homeostatic sodium balance. For example, aldosterone tends to decrease urine sodium levels by stimulating conservation of sodium. Antidiuretic hormone (ADH), which increases the reabsorption of water in the distal tubules of the kidney, tends to increase urine sodium levels.

Interfering factors

- Dietary salt intake may increase sodium levels.
- Altered kidney function may affect levels.
- ✔ Drugs that may cause *increased* levels include antibiotics, cough medicines, laxatives, and steroids.
- ✔ Drugs that may cause *decreased* levels include diuretics (e.g., Lasix) and steroids.

Procedure and patient care

Before

- Explain the procedure to the patient.
- Tell the patient that no fasting is required.

During

- Instruct the patient to begin the 24-hour urine collection after urinating. Discard the initial specimen and start the 24-hour timing at that point.
- Collect all urine passed during the next 24 hours.
- Show the patient where to store the urine specimen.
- Keep the specimen on ice or refrigerated during the 24 hours.
- Indicate the starting time on the urine container and on the laboratory slip.
- Post the hours for urine collection in a noticeable place to prevent accidental discarding of the specimen.
- Instruct the patient to void before defecating so that urine is not contaminated by feces.
- Remind the patient not to put toilet paper in the collection container.
- Encourage the patient to drink fluids during the 24 hours.
- Instruct the patient to collect the last specimen as close as possible to the end of the 24-hour period. Add this urine to the container.

After

- Transport the urine specimen promptly to the laboratory.

Abnormal findings

▲ **Increased levels**

Dehydration
Starvation
Adrenocortical insufficiency
Diuretic therapy
Hypothyroidism
Syndrome of inappropriate ADH secretion (SIADH)
Diabetic ketoacidosis
Toxemia of pregnancy

▼ **Decreased levels**

Congestive heart failure
Malabsorption
Diarrhea
Renal failure
Cushing's disease
Aldosteronism
Diaphoresis
Pulmonary emphysema
Inadequate sodium intake

notes

somatomedin C (Insulin-like growth factors I, IGF-1)

Type of test Blood

Normal findings

Adults: 42-110 ng/ml

Children:	Ages (yr)	Girls (ng/ml)	Boys (ng/ml)
	0-8	7-110	4-87
	9-10	39-186	26-98
	11-13	66-215	44-207
	14-16	96-256	48-255

Test explanation and related physiology

Because growth hormone (see p. 442) secretion is episodic, random measurements of plasma growth hormone are not adequate tests of growth hormone deficiency. Measuring somatomedin C is a good screening test for growth hormone deficiency, because most patients with growth hormone deficiency have low somatomedin levels. The amount of somatomedin provides an indirect measure of the amount of growth hormone present. Somatomedins (also known as *insulin-like growth factors*) are the "middlemen" in the growth process. The majority of growth-producing actions are mediated by somatomedin. Growth hormone stimulates the liver and other body tissues to produce somatomedin, which then induces growth.

Because somatomedin peptides are tightly bound to plasma proteins and have half-lives of hours rather than minutes, a random measurement provides an accurate reflection of mean growth hormone plasma concentrations. Therefore measurement of somatomedin C provides a reasonable screening test for growth hormone deficiency. Low levels of somatomedin C should lead to a more extensive evaluation, such as growth hormone stimulation tests (see p. 445).

Interfering factors

- A radioactive scan performed within the week before the test may affect test results.
- Drugs that may cause *decreased* levels include high doses of estrogens.

Procedure and patient care

Before
- Explain the procedure to the patient.
- Tell the patient that an overnight fast is preferred.

During
- Collect one lavender- or red-top tube of venous blood.

After
- Apply pressure or a pressure dressing to the venipuncture site.
- Assess the venipuncture site for bleeding.

Abnormal findings

▲ **Increased levels**
   Acromegaly
   Gigantism
   Hyperpituitarism
   Obesity
   Pregnancy
   Precocious puberty

▼ **Decreased levels**
   Growth hormone deficiency
   Laron dwarfism
   Inactive growth hormone
   Resistance to somatomedins
   Nutritional deficiency
   Delayed puberty
   Pituitary tumor
   Hypopituitarism
   Cirrhosis of the liver

notes

spinal x-rays (Cervical, thoracic, lumbar, sacral, or coccygeal x-ray studies)

Type of test X-ray

Normal findings Normal spinal vertebrae

Test explanation and related physiology

Spinal x-ray studies may be performed to evaluate any area of the spine. They usually include anteroposterior, lateral, and oblique views of these structures. These x-ray films are often done to assess back pain, degenerative arthritic changes, traumatic fractures, tumor invasion, spondylosis (stress fracture of the vertebrae), and spondylolisthesis (slipping of one vertebral disk on the other). Cervical spine x-ray studies are routinely performed in cases of multiple trauma.

Contraindications

- Patients who are pregnant

Procedure and patient care

Before

- Explain the procedure to the patient.
- Instruct the patient to remove any metal objects covering the area to be visualized.
- Immobilize the patient if a spinal fracture is suspected. Apply a neck brace if a cervical spine fracture is suspected.
- Tell the patient that no fasting or sedation is required; however, if a fracture is suspected, the patient may be kept NPO.

During

- Note that the patient is placed on an x-ray table. Anterior, posterior, lateral, and oblique x-ray films are taken of the desired area on the spinal cord.
- Note that a radiologic technologist takes spinal x-ray films in a few minutes.
- Tell the patient that no discomfort is associated with this study.

After

- Note that positioning and patient activity depend on test results.

S

Abnormal findings

Degenerative arthritis changes

Traumatic or pathologic fracture

Spondylosis

Spondylolisthesis

Metastatic tumor invasion

notes

sputum culture and sensitivity (C&S, Culture and Gram stain)

Type of test Sputum

Normal findings Normal upper respiratory tract

Test explanation and related physiology

Sputum cultures are obtained to determine the presence of pathogenic bacteria in patients with respiratory infections, such as pneumonia. *Gram staining* is the first step in the microbiologic analysis of sputum. Through sputum staining, bacteria are classified as gram positive or gram negative. This may be used to guide drug therapy until the C&S report is complete. The sputum sample is then applied to a series of bacterial culture plates. The bacteria that grow on those plates 1 to 3 days later are then identified. Determinations of bacterial sensitivity to various antibiotics are done to identify the most appropriate antimicrobial drug therapy. This is done by observing a ring of growth inhibition around an antibiotic plug in the culture medium. Sputum for C&S should be collected before antimicrobial therapy is initiated, unless the test is being performed to evaluate the effectiveness of medications already being given. Preliminary reports are usually available in 24 hours. Cultures require at least 48 hours for completion. Sputum cultures for fungus and *Mycobacterium tuberculosis* may take 6 to 8 weeks.

Procedure and patient care

Before

- Explain the procedure for sputum collection to the patient.
- Remind the patient that sputum must be coughed up from the lungs and that saliva is not sputum.
- Hold antibiotics until after the sputum has been collected.
- If an elective specimen is to be obtained, give the patient a sterile sputum container on the night before the sputum is to be collected so that the morning specimen may be obtained on arising.
- Instruct the patient to rinse out his or her mouth with water before the sputum collection to decrease contamination of the sputum by particles in the oropharynx.

S

During

- Note that sputum specimens are best when the patient awakes in the morning before eating or drinking.
- Collect at least 1 teaspoon of sputum in a sterile sputum container.
- Usually, obtain sputum by having the patient cough after taking several deep breaths.
- If the patient is unable to produce a sputum specimen, stimulate coughing by lowering the head of the patient's bed or giving the patient an aerosol administration of a warm, hypertonic solution.
- Note that other methods to collect sputum include endotracheal aspiration, fiberoptic bronchoscopy, and transtracheal aspiration.

After

- Inform the patient to notify the nurse as soon as the sputum is collected.
- Label the sputum, and send it to the laboratory as soon as possible.
- Note any current antibiotic therapy on the laboratory slip.

Abnormal findings

Bacterial infection (e.g., pneumonia)
Viral infection

Atypical bacterial infection (e.g., tuberculosis)

notes

sputum cytology

Type of test Sputum

Normal findings Normal epithelial cells

Test explanation and related physiology

Tumors within the pulmonary system frequently slough cells into the sputum. When the sputum is gathered, the cells are examined. If the cytologic test is positive, malignant cells are seen, indicating a lung tumor. If only normal epithelial cells are seen, either no malignancy exists or any existing tumor is not shedding cells. Therefore a positive test indicates malignancy; a negative test means nothing. This test is rarely performed, because actual tissue can be obtained by bronchoscopic biopsy (see p. 171).

Procedure and patient care

Before

- Explain the procedure for sputum collection to the patient.
- Remind the patient that sputum must be coughed up from the lungs and that saliva is not sputum.
- Give the patient a sterile sputum container on the night before the sputum is to be collected so that the morning specimen may be obtained on arising.
- Instruct the patient to rinse out her or his mouth with water to decrease contamination of the sputum by particles in the oropharynx.

During

- Note that sputum specimens are best collected when the patient awakes in the morning.
- Collect at least 1 teaspoon of sputum in the sterile sputum container.
- Usually, obtain sputum by having the patient cough after taking several deep breaths.
- If the patient is unable to produce a sputum specimen, stimulate coughing by lowering the head of the patient's bed or giving the patient an aerosol administration of a warm, hypertonic solution.
- Note that other methods to collect sputum include endotracheal aspiration, fiberoptic bronchoscopy, and transtracheal aspiration.

S

- Usually, collect sputum for cytology on three separate occasions.

After

- Instruct the patient to notify the nurse as soon as the sputum is collected.
- Label the specimen, and send it to the laboratory as soon as possible.

Abnormal findings

Malignancies

notes

stool culture (Stool for culture and sensitivity [C&S], Stool for ova and parasites [O&P])

Type of test Stool

Normal findings Normal intestinal flora

Test explanation and related physiology

Normally, stool contains many bacteria and fungi. The more common bacteria include *Enterococcus, Escherichia coli, Proteus, Pseudomonas, Staphylococcus aureus, Candida albicans, Bacteroides,* and *Clostridium* Bacteria are indigenous to the bowel; however, several bacteria act as pathogens within the bowel. These include *Salmonella, Shigella, Campylobacter, Yersinia,* pathogenic *Escherichia coli, Clostridium,* and *Staphylococcus.* Parasites also may affect the stool. Common parasites are *Ascaris* (hookworm), *Strongyloides* (tapeworm), and *Giardia* (protozoans). Identification of any of these pathogens in the stool incriminates that "bug" as the etiology of the infectious enteritis.

Infections of the bowel from bacteria, virus, or parasites usually present as acute diarrhea, excessive flatus, and abdominal discomfort.

Interfering factors

- Urine may inhibit the growth of bacteria. Therefore urine should not be mixed with the feces during collection of a stool sample.
- Recent barium studies may obscure the detection of parasites.
- ✠ Drugs that may affect test results include antibiotics, bismuth, and mineral oil.

Procedure and patient care

Before

- Explain the method of stool collection to the patient. Be matter-of-fact to avoid any embarrassment to the patient.
- Instruct the patient not to mix urine or toilet paper with the stool specimen.
- Instruct the patient to use an appropriate collection container.

During

- Ask the patient to defecate into a clean bedpan.
- Place a small amount of stool in a sterile collection container.
- Send mucus and blood streaks with the specimen.
- If a rectal swab is to be used, wear gloves and insert the cotton-tipped swab at least 1 inch into the anal canal. Then, rotate the swab for 30 seconds and place it into the clean container.

Tape test
- Use this test when pinworms *(Enterobius)* are suspected.
- Place a clear tape in the patient's perianal region. (This is especially helpful in children.)
- Because the female worm lays her eggs at night around the perianal area, apply the tape before bedtime and remove it in the morning before the patient gets out of the bed.
- Press the sticky surface of the tape directly to a glass slide and examine microscopically for pinworm ova.

After

- Handle the stool specimen carefully, as though it were capable of causing infection. Wear gloves when obtaining and handling the specimen.
- Indicate on the laboratory slip any antibiotics that the patient may be taking.
- Promptly send the stool specimen to the laboratory. Delays in transfer of the specimen may affect viability of the organism. If long delays are necessary, obtain a buffered glycerol-saline solution to be combined with the stool and use as a preservative.
- Note that some enteric pathogens occasionally take as long as 6 weeks to isolate.
- When pathogens are detected, maintain isolation of the patient's stool until therapy is completed.

Abnormal findings

Bacterial enterocolitis
Protozoan enterocolitis
Parasitic enterocolitis

stool for occult blood testing (Stool for OB)

Type of test Stool

Normal findings No occult blood within stool

Test explanation and related physiology

Normally, only minimal quantities of blood are passed into the gastrointestinal (GI) tract. Usually, this bleeding is not significant enough to cause a positive result in stool for occult blood (OB) testing. Tumors of the intestine grow into the lumen and are subjected to repeated trauma by the fecal stream. Eventually, the friable tumor ulcerates and bleeding occurs. Most often, bleeding is so slight that gross blood is not seen in the stool. The blood can only be detected by chemical assay through the OB testing of the stool.

Benign and malignant GI tumors, ulcers, inflammatory bowel disease, arteriovenous malformations, diverticulosis, and hematobilia (hemobilia) can all cause OB within the stool. Other more common abnormalities (e.g., hemorrhoids, swallowed blood from oral or nasal pharyngeal bleeding) may also cause OB within the stool.

It has been well documented that vigorous exercise can create OB within the stool. It is important to note that many drugs and the ingestion of hemoglobin contained in red meats such as beef and pork may cause a false-positive OB stool test. The more sensitive the test, the more false positives will be obtained.

When OB testing is properly performed, a positive result should be an indication for a thorough GI evaluation.

Interfering factors

- Bleeding gums following a dental procedure.
- Ingestion of red meat within the 3 days before testing.
- Ingestion of fish, turnips, and horseradish.
- Drugs that may cause GI bleeding include anticoagulants, aspirin, colchicine, iron preparations (large doses), nonsteroidal antiarthritics, and steroids.
- Drugs that may cause false-positive results include colchicine, iron, oxidizing drugs (e.g., iodine, bromides, boric acid), and rauwolfia derivatives.
- Drugs that may cause false-negative results include vitamin C.

Procedure and patient care

Before

- Explain the procedure to the patient.
- Instruct the patient to refrain from eating any red meat for at least 3 days before the test.
- Instruct the patient to refrain from drugs known to interfere with OB testing.
- Instruct the patient as to the method of obtaining appropriate stool specimens. Many procedures are available (e.g., specimen cards, tissue wipes, test paper). Tests may be done at home with specimen cards (Hemoccult) and mailed when collected.
- Instruct the patient not to mix urine with the stool specimen.
- Inform the patient as to the need for multiple specimens obtained on separate days to increase the test's accuracy.
- Note that in some centers, a high-residue diet is recommended to increase the abrasive effect of the stool.
- Note on the laboratory slip any anticoagulant medications that the patient may be taking.
- Be gentle in obtaining stool by digital rectal examination. Traumatic digital examination can cause a false-positive stool, especially in patients with prior anorectal disease such as hemorrhoids.

During

Hemoccult slide test

- Place a stool sample on one side of guaiac paper.
- Place two drops of developer on the other side.
- Note that a bluish discoloration indicates OB in the stool.

Tablet test

- Place a stool sample on the developer paper.
- Place a tablet on top of the stool specimen.
- Put two or three drops of tap water on the tablet and allow to flow onto the paper.
- Note that a bluish discoloration indicates OB in the stool.

After

- Inform the patient as to the results.
- If the tests are positive, inquire whether the patient violated any of the preparation recommendations.

Abnormal findings

GI tumor
Polyps
Ulcer
Varices
Inflammatory bowel disease
Diverticulosis

Ischemic bowel disease
GI trauma
Recent GI surgery
Hemorrhoids
Esophagitis
Gastritis

notes

S

swallowing examination (Videofluoroscopy swallowing examination)

Type of test X-ray with contrast dye

Normal findings Normal swallowing function and complete clearing of radiographic material through the upper digestive tract

Test explanation and related physiology

This test is performed to identify the exact problems that exist in a patient who is unable to swallow. Problems in swallowing may result from local structural diseases such as tumors, upper esophageal diverticula, inflammation, extrinsic compression of the upper gastrointestinal (GI) tract, or surgery to the oropharyngeal tract. Motility disorders of the upper GI tract such as Zenker's diverticulum and neurologic disorders such as stroke syndrome, Parkinson's disease, and neuropathies also may cause difficulty in swallowing. Videofluoroscopy of the swallowing function allows the speech pathologist to delineate more clearly the exact pathology in the swallowing mechanism. This videofluoroscopy then can be used to determine the most appropriate treatment and teach the patient proper swallowing technique.

This test is performed by asking the patient to swallow barium or a barium-containing meal. With the use of videofluoroscopy, the swallowing function is visualized and documented. Morphologic abnormalities and functional impairment can be identified easily using the slow-framed progression and reversal that is available with videofluoroscopy. While this test is similar to the barium swallow (see p. 124), finer details of swallowing can be evaluated with the use of videofluoroscopy.

Contraindications

- Patients who obviously aspirate their saliva and are not candidates for swallowing, because they will require nonswallowing methods of alimentation

Procedure and patient care

Before

- Explain the procedure to the patient.
- Explain to the patient that no preparation is required.

During

- In the radiology department, the patient is asked to swallow a barium-containing meal. The consistency of the meal will be determined by the speech therapist and radiologist. The meal consistency is to simulate foods to which the patient is to be initially reintroduced. The food may be in the form of a liquid, semisoft (e.g., applesauce), or solids (e.g., a tea biscuit). While the patient is swallowing, videofluoroscopy is recorded in both the lateral and the anterior positions.
- The video is then repeatedly examined and reexamined by the radiologist and speech pathologist.

After

- No catharsis is required.

Abnormal findings

Oral pharyngeal inflammation
Cancer
Extrinsic compression
Neuromuscular disorder
Achalasia

Upper GI motility disorder (e.g., stroke syndrome, Parkinson's disease, peripheral neuropathy)
Diffuse esophageal spasms
Zenker's diverticulum

notes

S

sweat electrolytes test (Iontophoretic sweat test)

Type of test Fluid analysis

Normal findings

Sodium values in children
Normal: <70 mEq/L
Abnormal: >90 mEq/L
Equivocal: 70-90 mEq/L

Chloride values in children
Normal: <50 mEq/L
Abnormal: >60 mEq/L
Equivocal: 50-60 mEq/L

Test explanation and related physiology

Patients with cystic fibrosis have increased sodium and chloride contents in their sweat. That forms the basis of this test, which is both sensitive and specific for cystic fibrosis. Cystic fibrosis is an inherited disease characterized by abnormal secretion by exocrine glands within the bronchi, small intestines, pancreatic ducts, bile ducts, and skin (sweat glands). Sweat, induced by electrical current *(pilocarpine iontophoresis),* is collected, and its sodium and chloride contents are measured. The degree of abnormality is no indication of the severity of cystic fibrosis; it merely indicates that the patient has the disease.

In children with recurrent respiratory tract infections, malabsorption syndromes, or failure to thrive, this test is indicated to diagnose cystic fibrosis. Almost all patients with cystic fibrosis have sweat sodium and chloride contents 2 to 5 times greater than normal values. In patients with suspicious clinical manifestations, these levels are diagnostic of cystic fibrosis.

The sweat test is not reliable during the first few weeks of life. High serum concentrations of immunoreactive trypsin may be a better test for this age group.

Procedure and patient care

Before
- Explain the procedure to the patient and/or parents.
- Tell the patient and/or parents that no fasting is required.

During

- Note the following procedural steps:
  1. For iontophoresis, a low-level electrical current is applied to the test area (the thigh in infants, the forearm in older children).
  2. The positive electrode is covered by gauze and saturated with pilocarpine hydrochloride, a stimulating drug that induces sweating.
  3. The negative electrode is covered by gauze saturated with a bicarbonate solution.
  4. The electrical current is allowed to flow for 5 to 12 minutes.
  5. The electrodes are removed, and the arm is washed with distilled water.
  6. Paper disks are placed over the test site with the use of clean, dry forceps.
  7. These disks are covered with paraffin to obtain an air-tight seal, preventing evaporation of sweat.
  8. After 1 hour, the paraffin is removed. The paper disks are transferred immediately by forceps to a weighing jar and sent for sodium and chloride analysis.
  9. A *screening test* may be done to detect sweat chloride levels. For screening, a test paper containing silver nitrate is pressed against the child's hand for several seconds. The test is positive when the excess chloride combines with the silver nitrate to form white-silver chloride on the paper. That is, the child with cystic fibrosis will leave a "heavy" handprint on the paper.
  10. A positive screening test is usually validated by iontophoresis.
- Note that an experienced technologist performs the sweat test in approximately 90 minutes in the laboratory or at the patient's bedside.
- Inform the patient that the electrical current is small and no discomfort or pain is generally associated with this test.

After

- Initiate extensive education and counseling for the patient and/or parents if the results indicate cystic fibrosis.

Abnormal finding

Cystic fibrosis

syphilis detection test (Serologic test for syphilis [STS], Venereal Disease Research Laboratory [VDRL], Rapid plasma reagin [RPR], Fluorescent treponemal antibody test [FTA])

Type of test Blood

Normal findings Negative, or nonreactive

Test explanation and related physiology

The serologic tests for syphilis (STS) are used to detect antibodies to *Treponema pallidum,* the causative agent of syphilis. There are two groups of antibodies. The first is a nontreponemal antibody (reagin) directed against a lipoidal agent that results from the *T. pallidum* infection. The second is an antibody directed against the *Treponema* organism itself. The nontreponemal antibody test is relatively nonspecific. These antibodies are most often detected by the *Wassermann test* or the *Venereal Disease Research Laboratory* (VDRL) *test.* A new, more sensitive nontreponemal test is the *rapid plasma reagin* (RPR) *test.* The VDRL and RPR tests, by virtue of their testing for nonspecific antibody, have a high false-positive rate. The VDRL test becomes positive approximately 2 weeks after the patient's inoculation with *Treponema* and returns to normal shortly after adequate treatment is given. The test is positive in nearly all primary and secondary stages of syphilis and in two thirds of patients with tertiary syphilis.

If the VDRL or RPR test is positive, the diagnosis may be confirmed by the *Treponema* test, such as the *fluorescent treponemal antibody absorption test* (FTA-ABS). This second test is much more specific. The FTA test, which tests for a more specific antibody, is more accurate than the VDRL and RPR tests.

False-positive and false-negative results are rare in all stages of the disease. The FTA test is required before the diagnosis of syphilis can be made with certainty.

Screening for syphilis is usually done during the first prenatal checkup for pregnant women. Syphilis, if untreated, may cause abortion, stillbirth, and premature labor. The effect on the fetus can be central nervous system damage, hearing loss, and possible death.

Interfering factors

- Excessive hemolysis and gross lipemia may affect test results.
- Excess chyle in the blood may interfere with the test results.

- Many conditions cause false-positive results when VDRL and RPR tests are used. Some of these conditions include *Mycoplasma* pneumonia, malaria, acute bacterial and viral infections, autoimmune diseases, and pregnancy.
- Recent ingestion of alcohol may alter the test results.

Procedure and patient care

Before

- Explain the procedure to the patient.
- Check with the laboratory regarding fasting requirements. Some prefer collecting the specimen before meals. Some laboratories request that the patient refrain from alcohol for 24 hours before the blood test.

During

- Collect approximately 7 ml of blood in a red-top tube.

After

- Apply pressure or a pressure dressing to the venipuncture site.
- Check the venipuncture site for bleeding.
- If the test is positive, instruct the patient to inform recent sexual contacts so they can be evaluated.
- If the test is positive, be sure the patient receives the appropriate antibiotic therapy.

Abnormal finding

Syphilis

notes

S

testosterone (Total testosterone serum level)

Type of test Blood

Normal findings

Adolescent male: 75-400 ng/dl
Adolescent female: 20-64 ng/dl
Adult male: 300-1000 ng/dl or 10.4-34.7 nmol/L (SI units)
Adult female: 20-75 ng/dl or 0.69-2.6 nmol/L (SI units)

Test explanation and related physiology

Testosterone is made in the male by the Leydig cells in the testicle; this accounts for 95% of the circulating testosterone in men. In women, the ovary and adrenal gland secrete small amounts of testosterone; the majority of the testosterone in the female is made as a derivative of metabolism of androstenedione (see p. 57). Approximately 60% of circulating testosterone binds strongly to sex hormone–binding globulin. Most of the remaining testosterone is bound loosely to albumin, and approximately 2% is unbound.

Physiologically, testosterone affects spermatogenesis and influences the development of male secondary sexual characteristics. Overabundance of this hormone in the young male may cause precocious puberty. Overabundance can be caused by testicular, adrenal, or pituitary tumors. Overproduction of this hormone in females causes masculinization, which is demonstrated by amenorrhea and excessive growth of body hair (hirsutisim). Ovarian and adrenal tumors/hyperplasia and medications (e.g., danazol) are all potential causes of masculinization in the female.

Reduced levels of testosterone in the male suggest hypogonadism or Klinefelter's syndrome.

Interfering factors

* Drugs that may cause *increased* testosterone levels include anticonvulsants, barbiturates, estrogens, and oral contraceptives.
* Drugs that may cause *decreased* testosterone levels include androgens, dexamethasone, diethylstilbestrol, digoxin, alcohol, steroids, ketoconazole, phenothiazine, and spironolactone.

Procedure and patient care

Before

- Explain the procedure to the patient.
- Tell the patient that no fasting is required.
- Because testosterone levels are highest in the early morning hours, blood should be drawn in the morning.

During

- Collect 7 ml of peripheral venous blood in a red-top tube.

After

- Apply pressure or a pressure dressing to the venipuncture site.
- Assess the venipuncture site for bleeding.

Abnormal findings

▲ **Increased levels (male)**
Idiopathic sexual precocity
Adrenal hyperplasia
Adrenocortical tumor
Testicular or extragonadal tumor

▲ **Increased levels (female)**
Ovarian tumor
Adrenocortical tumor
Adrenocortical hyperplasia
Trophoblastic tumor during pregnancy
Polycystic ovaries
Idiopathic hirsutism
Arrhenoblastoma

▼ **Decreased levels (male)**
Klinefelter's syndrome
Cryptorchidism
Primary and secondary hypogonadism
Down's syndrome
Corticosteroid use
Uremia

T

notes

therapeutic drug monitoring

Type of test   Blood

Normal findings   See Table 14.

Test explanation and related physiology

Therapeutic drug monitoring entails taking measurements of blood drug levels to determine effective drug dosages and to prevent toxicity. Drug monitoring is especially important in patients taking medications (e.g., antiarrhythmics, bronchodilators, antibiotics, anticonvulsants, cardiotonics) when the margin of safety between therapeutic and toxic levels is narrow.

Table 14 lists the therapeutic and toxic ranges for most patients. These ranges may not apply to all patients, because clinical response is influenced by many factors (e.g., noncompliance, concurrent drug use, other clinical conditions, patient's age and size, extent and rate of drug absorption, metabolism). Also, note that different laboratories use different units for reporting test results and normal ranges. It is important that sufficient time pass between the administration of the medication and the collection of the blood sample to allow for therapeutic levels to occur.

Blood samples can be taken at the drug's *peak level* (the highest therapeutic concentration) or at the *trough level* (the lowest therapeutic concentration). Peak levels are useful when testing for toxicity, and trough levels are useful for demonstrating a satisfactory therapeutic level. Trough levels are often referred to as *residual levels.* The time when the sample should be drawn after the last dose of the medication varies according to whether a peak or trough level is requested and according to the half-life of the drug.

Procedure and patient care

Before

- Explain the procedure to the patient.
- Tell the patient that no food or fluid restrictions are needed.

During

- Collect approximately 7 to 10 ml of venous blood in a tube designated by the laboratory. *Peak* levels are usually obtained 1 to 2 hours after oral intake, approximately 1 hour after IM administration, and approximately 30 minutes after IV ad-

TABLE 14 Therapeutic drug monitoring data

Drug	Use	Therapeutic level*	Toxic level*
Acetaminophen	Analgesic, antipyretic	Depends on use	>250 μg/ml
Amikacin	Antibiotic	15-25 μg/ml	>25 μg/ml
Aminophylline	Bronchodilator	10-20 μg/ml	>20 μg/ml
Amitriptyline	Antidepressant	120-150 ng/ml	>500 ng/ml
Carbamazepine	Anticonvulsant	5-12 μg/ml	>12 μg/ml
Chloramphenicol	Antiinfective	10-20 μg/ml	>25 μg/ml
Desipramine	Antidepressant	150-300 ng/ml	>500 ng/ml
Digitoxin	Cardiac glycoside	15-25 ng/ml	>25 ng/ml
Digoxin	Cardiac glycoside	0.8-2.0 ng/ml	>2.4 ng/ml
Disopyramide	Antiarrhythmic	2-5 μg/ml	>5 μg/ml
Ethosuximide	Anticonvulsant	40-100 μg/ml	>100 μg/ml
Gentamicin	Antibiotic	5-10 μg/ml	>12 μg/ml
Imipramine	Antidepressant	150-300 ng/ml	>500 ng/ml
Kanamycin	Antibiotic	20-25 μg/ml	>35 μg/ml
Lidocaine	Antiarrhythmic	1.5-5.0 μg/ml	>5 μg/ml

*Levels vary according to the institution performing the test.

Continued.

TABLE 14 Therapeutic drug monitoring data—cont'd

Drug	Use	Therapeutic level*	Toxic level*
Lithium	Manic episodes of manic-depression psychosis	0.8-1.2 mEq/L	>2.0 mEq/L
Methrotrexate	Antitumor agent	>0.01 μmol	>10 μmol/24 hr
Nortriptyline	Antidepressant	50-150 ng/ml	>500 ng/ml
Phenobarbital	Anticonvulsant	10-30 μg/ml	>40 μg/ml
Phenytoin	Anticonvulsant	10-20 μg/ml	>30 μg/ml
Primidone	Anticonvulsant	5-12 μg/ml	>15 μg/ml
Procainamide	Antiarrhythmic	4-10 μg/ml	>16 μg/ml
Propranolol	Antiarrhythmic	50-100 ng/ml	>150 ng/ml
Quinidine	Antiarrhythmic	2-5 μg/ml	>10 μg/ml
Salicylate	Antipyretic, antiinflammatory, analgesic	100-250 μg/ml	>300 μg/ml
Theophylline	Bronchodilator	10-20 μg/ml	>20 μg/ml
Tobramycin	Antibiotic	5-10 μg/ml	>12 μg/ml
Valproic acid	Anticonvulsant	50-100 μg/ml	>100 μg/ml

*Levels vary according to the institution performing the test.

ministration. *Residual (trough)* levels are usually obtained shortly before (0 to 15 minutes) the next scheduled dose. Consult with the pharmacy for specific times.

After

- Apply pressure or a pressure dressing to the venipuncture site.
- Assess the venipuncture site for bleeding.
- Clearly mark all blood samples with the following information: patient's name, diagnosis, name of drug, time of last drug ingestion, time of sample, and any other medications the patient is currently taking.
- Promptly send the specimen to the laboratory.

Abnormal findings

Nontherapeutic levels of drugs
Toxic levels of drugs

notes

T

thoracentesis and pleural fluid analysis (Pleural tap)

Type of test Fluid analysis

Normal findings Normal pleural fluid

Test explanation and related physiology

Thoracentesis is an invasive procedure that entails insertion of a needle into the pleural space for removal of fluid (or rarely, air) (Figure 27). Pleural fluid is removed for diagnostic and therapeutic purposes. Therapeutically, it is done to relieve pain, dyspnea, and other symptoms of pleural pressure. Removal of this fluid also permits better radiographic visualization of the lung.

Diagnostically, thoracentesis is performed whenever a pleural effusion (abnormal accumulation of fluid in the pleural space) of unknown etiology is recognized. A decubitus chest x-ray film is obtained before thoracentesis to ensure that the pleural fluid is mobile and therefore accessible to a needle placed within the pleural space.

Pleural fluid is usually evaluated for gross appearance; cell

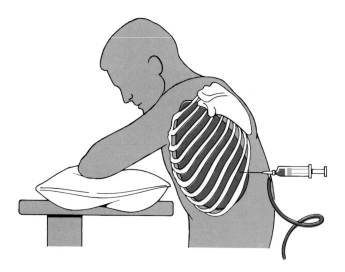

Figure 27 Thoracentesis. (From Beare PG, Myers JL: *Principles and practice of adult health nursing,* ed 2, St Louis, 1994, Mosby.)

counts; protein, lactic dehydrogenase (LDH), glucose, and amylase levels; Gram stain and bacteriologic cultures; *Mycobacterium tuberculosis* and fungus; cytology; carcinoembryonic antigen (CEA) levels; and sometimes for other specific tests. Each is discussed separately.

Gross appearance

The color, optical density, and viscosity are noted as the pleural fluid appears in the aspirating syringe. Empyema is characterized by the presence of a foul odor and thick, puslike fluid. An opalescent, pearly fluid is characteristic of chylothorax (chyle in the pleural cavity).

Cell counts

The white blood cell (WBC) and differential counts are determined. A WBC count exceeding 1000/ml is suggestive of an exudate. The predominance of polymorphonuclear leukocytes usually is an indication of an acute inflammatory condition (e.g., pneumonia, pulmonary infarction, early tuberculosis effusion). When over 50% of the WBCs are small lymphocytes, the effusion is usually caused by tuberculosis or tumor.

Protein content

Levels greater than 3 g/dl are characteristic of exudates, whereas transudates usually have a protein content less than 3 g/dl. Because there is significant overlap in protein values differentiating transudate from exudate, the total protein ratio (fluid/serum) has been considered to be a more accurate criterion. A total protein ratio of fluid to serum of greater than 0.5 is considered to be an exudate. *Transudates* are most frequently caused by congestive heart failure, cirrhosis, nephrotic syndrome, myxedema, peritoneal dialysis, and acute glomerulonephritis. *Exudates* are most often found in infectious disease and in neoplastic conditions; however, collagen vascular disease, pulmonary infarction, gastrointestinal (GI) diseases, trauma, and drug hypersensitivity are also causes of exudative effusions.

Lactic dehydrogenase

A pleural fluid/serum LDH ratio greater than 0.6 is typical of an exudate. An exudate is identified with a high degree of accuracy if the pleural fluid/serum protein ratio is greater than 0.5 and the pleural fluid/serum LDH ratio is greater than 0.6.

Glucose

Usually, pleural glucose levels approximate serum levels. Low values appear to be a combination of glycolysis by the extra cells and impairment of glucose diffusion because of damage to the pleural membrane. Values less than 60 mg/dl are occasionally seen in tuberculosis or malignancy and typically occur in rheumatoid arthritis and empyema.

Amylase

In a malignant effusion, the amylase concentration is slightly elevated. Amylase levels above the normal range for serum or two times the serum level are seen when the effusion is caused by pancreatitis or rupture of the esophagus associated with leakage of salivary amylase.

Triglyceride

Measurement of triglyceride levels is an important part of identifying chylous effusions. These effusions are usually produced by obstruction or transection of the lymphatic system caused by lymphoma, neoplasm, trauma, or recent surgery.

Gram stain and bacteriologic culture

These tests are routinely performed when bacterial pneumonia or empyema is a possible cause of the effusion. If possible, these should be done before initiation of antibiotic therapy.

Cultures for *Mycobacterium tuberculosis* and fungus

Tuberculosis is less often a cause for pleural effusion in the United States today than it was in the past. Fungus may be a cause of pulmonary effusion in patients with compromised immunologic defenses.

Cytology

A cytologic study is performed to detect tumor cells in approximately 50% to 60% of patients with malignant effusions. Breast and lung are the two most frequent tumors; lymphoma is the third.

Carcinoembryonic antigen

Pleural fluid CEA levels are elevated in various malignant (GI, breast) conditions.

Special tests

The pH of pleural fluid is usually 7.4 or greater. The pH is typically less than 7.2 when empyema is present. The pH may be 7.2 to 7.4 in tuberculosis or malignancy.

In some instances, the rheumatoid factor (see p. 723) and the complement levels (see p. 259) are also measured in pleural fluid.

Pleural fluid antinuclear antibody and pleural fluid/ANA ratios are often used to evaluate pleural effusion secondary to systemic lupus erythematosus.

Contraindications

- Patients with significant thrombocytopenia

Potential complications

- Pneumothorax because of puncture of the visceral pleura or entry of air into the pleural space
- Interpleural bleeding because of puncture of tissue or a blood vessel
- Hemoptysis caused by needle puncture of a pulmonary vessel or by inflammation
- Reflex bradycardia and hypotension
- Pulmonary edema
- Seeding of the needle tract with tumor when malignant pleural effusion exists

Procedure and patient care

Before

- Explain the procedure to the patient.
- Obtain informed consent for this procedure.
- Tell the patient that no fasting or sedation is necessary.
- Inform the patient that movement or coughing should be minimized to avoid inadvertent needle damage to the lung or pleura during the procedure.
- Administer a cough suppressant before the procedure if the patient has a troublesome cough.
- Note that an x-ray film or ultrasound scan is often used to assist in location of the fluid. Fluoroscopy also may be used.

During

- Note the following procedural steps:
  1. The patient is usually placed in an upright position with the arms and shoulders raised and supported on a padded overhead table. This position spreads the ribs and enlarges the intercostal space for insertion of the needle.
  2. Patients who cannot sit upright are placed in a side-lying position on the unaffected side with the side to be tapped uppermost.
  3. The thoracentesis is performed under strict sterile technique.

T

4. The needle insertion site, which is determined by percussion, auscultation, and examination of a chest x-ray film, ultrasound scan, or fluoroscopy, is aseptically cleansed and anesthetized locally.

5. The needle is positioned in the pleural space, and the fluid is withdrawn with a syringe and a three-way stopcock.

6. Various mechanisms to stabilize the pleural needle are available to secure the needle depth during the fluid collection.

7. A short polyethylene catheter may be inserted into the pleural space for fluid aspiration; this decreases the risk of puncturing the visceral pleura and inducing a pneumothorax.

8. Also, large volumes of fluid may be collected by connecting the catheter to a gravity-drainage system.

- Note that this procedure is performed by a physician at the patient's bedside, in a procedure room, or in the physician's office in less than 30 minutes.

- Monitor the patient's pulse for reflex bradycardia and evaluate the patient for diaphoresis and the feeling of faintness during the procedure.

- Although local anesthetics eliminate pain at the insertion site, tell the patient that he or she may feel a pressurelike pain when the pleura is entered and the fluid is removed.

After

- Place a small bandage over the needle site. Usually, turn the patient on the unaffected side for 1 hour to allow the pleural puncture site to heal.

- Label the specimen with the patient's name, date, source of fluid, and diagnosis. Send the specimen promptly to the laboratory.

- Obtain a chest x-ray study as indicated to check for pneumothorax.

- Monitor the patient's vital signs.

- Observe the patient for coughing or expectoration of blood (hemoptysis), which may indicate trauma to the lung.

- Evaluate the patient for signs and symptoms of pneumothorax, tension pneumothorax, subcutaneous emphysema, and pyogenic infection (e.g., tachypnea, dyspnea, diminished breath sounds, anxiety, restlessness, fever).

- Assess the patient's lung sounds for diminished breath sounds, which could be a sign of pneumothorax.
- If the patient has no complaints of dyspnea, normal activity usually can be resumed 1 hour after the procedure.

Abnormal findings

Empyema
Chylothorax
Infection
Pneumonia
Pulmonary infarction
Tuberculosis effusion
Cirrhosis
Nephrotic syndrome
Myxedema
Peritoneal dialysis
Acute glomerulonephritis
Collagen vascular disease

Pulmonary infarction
Gastrointestinal disease
Trauma
Drug hypersensitivity
Tuberculosis
Rheumatoid arthritis
Pancreatitis
Ruptured esophagus
Tumors
Lymphoma
Systemic lupus erythematosus

notes

T

throat culture and sensitivity (C&S)

Type of test Microscopic examination

Normal findings Negative

Test explanation and related physiology

Because the throat is normally colonized by many organisms, culture of this area serves only to isolate and identify a few particular pathogens (e.g., streptococci, meningococci, gonococci, *Bordetella pertussis, Corynebacterium diphtheriae*). Recognition of these organisms requires treatment. Streptococci are most often sought, because a beta-hemolytic streptococcal pharyngitis may be followed by rheumatic fever or glomerulonephritis. This type of streptococcal infection most frequently affects children between the ages of 3 and 15 years. Therefore all children with a sore throat and fever should have a throat culture done to attempt to identify streptococcal infections. In adults, however, fewer than 5% of patients with pharyngitis have a streptococcal infection. Therefore throat cultures in adults are only indicated when the patient has severe or recurrent sore throat, often associated with fever and palpable lymphadenopathy. These adults often have a history of streptococcal infections. Rapid immunologic tests *(strep screen)* with antiserum against group A streptococcus antigen are now available and are very accurate. With these newer kits, the streptococcus organism can be identified directly from the swab specimen without culture. These tests can be performed in about 15 minutes. Agglutination on the slide indicates group A streptococci are present. If no agglutination occurs, the specimen is cultured for streptococcus. If that culture is negative, no streptococcus infection exists.

All cultures should be performed before antibiotic therapy is initiated. Otherwise, the antibiotic may interrupt the growth of the organism in the laboratory. More often than not, however, the physician will want to institute antibiotic therapy before the culture results are reported. In these instances, a *Gram stain* of the specimen smeared on a slide is most helpful and can be reported in less than 10 minutes. All forms of bacteria are grossly classified as gram positive (blue staining) or gram negative (red staining). Knowledge of the shape of the organism (e.g., spheric [coccus], rod shaped [bacillus]) also can be very helpful in the tentative identification of the infecting organism. With knowledge of the Gram stain results, the physician can institute a reasonable antibiotic regimen based on past experience as to the organism's possible identity. Most organisms take approximately 24 hours to grow in the laboratory, and a preliminary report can be given at that time. Occasionally, a period of 48 to 72 hours is required for growth and identification of the organism. Cultures may be repeated on completion of appropriate antibiotic therapy to identify resolution of the infection.

Interfering factors

☑ Drugs that may affect test results include antibiotics and antiseptic mouthwashes.

Procedure and patient care

Before

- Explain the procedure to the patient.

During

- Obtain a throat culture by depressing the tongue with a wooden tongue blade and touching the posterior wall of the throat and areas of inflammation, exudation, or ulceration with a sterile cotton swab. Two swabs are preferred. Growth of streptococcus from both swabs is more accurate, and the second swab can also be used in the strept screen.
- Avoid touching any other part of the mouth.
- Wear gloves and handle the specimen as if it were capable of transmitting disease.
- Place the swab in a sterile container and send it to the microbiology laboratory within 30 minutes.
- Indicate on the laboratory slip any medications that the patient may be taking that could affect test results.

After

- Notify the physician of any positive results so that appropriate antibiotic therapy can be initiated.

Abnormal findings

Bacterial pathogens (e.g., streptococci)

notes

thyroid scanning (Thyroid scintiscan)

Type of test Nuclear scan

Normal findings

Normal size, shape, position, and function of the thyroid gland
No areas of decreased or increased uptake

Test explanation and related physiology

Thyroid scanning allows the size, shape, position, and physiologic function of the thyroid gland to be determined with the use of radionuclear scanning. A radioactive substance such as technetium-99m is given to the patient to visualize the thyroid gland. A scanner is passed over the neck area, and an image is recorded.

Thyroid nodules are easily detected by this technique. Nodules are classified as functioning (warm/hot) or nonfunctioning (cold) depending on the amount of radionuclide taken up by the nodule. A functioning nodule could represent a benign adenoma or a localized toxic goiter. A nonfunctioning nodule may represent a cyst, carcinoma, nonfunctioning adenoma or goiter, lymphoma, or localized area of thyroiditis.

Scanning is useful in:

1. Patients with a neck or substernal mass
2. Patients with a thyroid nodule. Thyroid cancers are usually nonfunctioning (cold) nodules.
3. Patients with hyperthyroidism. Scanning will assist in differentiating Graves' disease (diffusely enlarged hyperfunctioning thyroid gland) from Plummer's disease (nodular hyperfunctioning gland).
4. Patients with metastatic tumors without a known primary site. A normal scan excludes the thyroid gland as a possible primary site.
5. Patients with a well-differentiated form of thyroid cancer. Areas of metastasis may show up on subsequent whole-body nuclear scans.

Contraindications

- Patients who are allergic to iodine or shellfish
- Patients who are pregnant

Potential complication

- Radiation-induced oncogenesis
  This complication is eliminated if technetium or low-radioactive iodine isomers are used instead of iodine-131.

Interfering factors

- Iodine-containing foods
- Recent administration of x-ray contrast agents
- ⚑ Drugs that may affect test results include cough medicines, multiple vitamins, oral contraceptives (some), and thyroid drugs.

Procedure and patient care

Before

- Explain the procedure to the patient.
- Check the patient for allergies to iodine.
- Instruct the patient about medications that need to be restricted for weeks before the test (e.g., thyroid drugs, medications containing iodine).
- Obtain a history concerning previous contrast x-ray studies, nuclear scanning, or intake of any thyroid-suppressive or antithyroid drugs.
- Tell the patient that fasting is usually not required. Check with the laboratory.

During

- Note the following procedural steps:
  1. A standard dose of radioactive technetium is usually given to the patient by mouth. The capsule is tasteless.
  2. Scanning is usually performed 24 hours later. If technetium is used, scanning may be performed 2 hours later.
  3. At the designated time, the patient is placed in a supine position and a detector is passed over the thyroid area.
  4. The radioactive counts are recorded and displayed.
- Note that this study is performed by a radiologic technologist in less than 30 minutes.
- Tell the patient that no discomfort is associated with this study.

After

- Assure the patient that the dose of radioactive technetium used in this test is minute and therefore harmless. No isolation and no special urine precautions are needed.

Abnormal findings

Adenoma

Toxic and nontoxic goiter

Cyst

Carcinoma

Lymphoma

Thyroiditis

Graves' disease

Plummer's disease

Metastasis

Hyperthyroidism

Hypothyroidism

Hashimoto's disease

notes

thyroid-stimulating hormone (TSH, Thyrotropin)

Type of test Blood

Normal findings

Adult: 2-10 μU/ml or 2-10 mU/L (SI units)
Newborn: 3-18 μU/L or 3-18 mU/L
Cord: 3-12 μU/L or 3-12 mU/L
Values vary between laboratories

Test explanation and related physiology

The TSH concentration aids in differentiating *primary* from *secondary* hypothyroidism. Pituitary TSH secretion is stimulated by hypothalamic thyroid-releasing hormone (TRH). Low levels of triiodothyronine and thyroxine (T_3, T_4) are the underlying stimuli for TRH and TSH. Therefore a compensatory elevation of TRH and TSH occurs in patients with primary hypothyroid states, such as surgical or radioactive thyroid ablation; patients with burned-out thyroiditis, thyroid agenesis, idiopathic hypothyroidism, or congenital cretinism; or patients taking antithyroid medications.

In secondary hypothyroidism, the function of the hypothalamus or pituitary gland is faulty because of tumor, trauma, or infarction. Therefore TRH and TSH cannot be secreted, and plasma levels of these hormones are near 0 despite low T_3 and T_4 levels.

The TSH test is used as well to monitor exogenous thyroid replacement. The goal of thyroid replacement therapy is to provide an adequate amount of thyroid medication so that TSH secretion is minimal, indicating a euthyroid state. Therefore doses of medication are given to keep the TSH level less than 2.0. Even lower TSH levels are preferred if thyroid suppression is the clinical goal. This test is also done to detect primary hypothyroidism in newborns with low screening T_4 levels. TSH and T_4 levels are frequently measured to differentiate pituitary from thyroid dysfunction. A decreased T_4 and normal or elevated TSH level can indicate a thyroid disorder. A decreased T_4 with a decreased TSH level can indicate a pituitary disorder.

T

Interfering factors

- Recent radioisotope administration may affect test results.
- Severe illness may cause decreased TSH levels.

- Drugs that may cause *increased* levels include antithyroid medications, lithium, potassium iodide, and TSH injection.
- Drugs that may cause *decreased* levels include aspirin, dopamine, heparin, steroids, and T_3.

Procedure and patient care

Before

- Explain the procedure to the patient.
- Tell the patient that no food or drink restrictions are necessary.

During

- Collect approximately 5 ml of venous blood in a red-top tube.
- Use a heel stick to obtain blood from newborns.

After

- Apply pressure or a pressure dressing to the venipuncture site.
- Assess the venipuncture site for bleeding.

Abnormal findings

▲ **Increased levels**

Primary hypothyroidism (thyroid dysfunction)
Thyroiditis
Thyroid agenesis
Congenital cretinism

▼ **Decreased levels**

Secondary hypothyroidism (pituitary dysfunction)
Hyperthyroidism
Pituitary hypofunction

notes

thyroid-stimulating hormone stimulation test
(TSH stimulation test)

Type of test Blood

Normal findings Increased thyroid function with administration of exogenous TSH

Test explanation and related physiology

The TSH stimulation test is used to differentiate *primary* (or thyroidal) hypothyroidism from *secondary* (or hypothalamic-pituitary) hypothyroidism. Normal people and patients with hypothalamic-pituitary hypothyroidism are capable of increasing thyroid function when exogenous TSH is given. Patients with primary thyroidal hypothyroidism, however, are not; their thyroid gland is inadequate and cannot function no matter how much stimulation it receives. Patients with less than a 10% increase in radioactive iodine uptake (RAIU) or less than a 1.5 μg/dl rise in thyroxine (T_4) are considered to have a primary cause for their hypothyroid state. If the initially low uptake is caused by inadequate pituitary stimulation of an intrinsically normal thyroid gland, the RAIU should increase at least 10% and the T_4 level should rise 1.5 μg/dl or more. This is characteristic of secondary hypothyroidism.

Procedure and patient care

Before
- Explain the procedure to the patient.
- Obtain baseline levels of RAIU (see p. 691) or T_4 (see p. 802) as indicated.
- Tell the patient that no fasting is required.

During
- Administer 5 to 10 U of TSH intramuscularly for 3 days.
- Repeat the levels of RAIU or T_4 as indicated.

After
- Apply pressure or a pressure dressing to the venipuncture site.
- Assess the venipuncture site for bleeding.

Abnormal findings

Primary (thyroidal) hypothyroidism
Secondary (hypothalamic-pituitary) hypothyroidism

T

thyroid ultrasound (Thyroid echogram, Thyroid sonogram)

Type of test Ultrasound

Normal findings Normal size, shape, and position of the thyroid gland

Test explanation and related physiology

Ultrasound examination of the thyroid gland is valuable for distinguishing cystic from solid thyroid nodules. If the nodule is found to be purely cystic (fluid filled), the fluid can simply be aspirated (cysts are not cancerous), and surgery is avoided. If the nodule has a mixed or solid appearance, however, a tumor may be present and surgery may be required for diagnosis and treatment.

This study may be repeated at intervals to determine the response of a thyroid mass to medical therapy. This test is also the procedure of choice for studying the thyroid gland of pregnant patients, because no radioactive material is used.

Procedure and patient care

Before

- Explain the procedure to the patient.
- Tell the patient that breathing or swallowing will not be affected by the placement of a transducer on the neck.
- Inform the patient that a liberal amount of lubricant will be applied to the neck to ensure effective transmission and reception of sound waves.
- Tell the patient that no fasting or sedation is required.

During

- Note the following procedural steps:
  1. The patient is taken to the ultrasonography department (usually in the radiology department) and placed in the supine position with the neck hyperextended.
  2. Gel is applied to the patient's neck.
  3. A sound transducer is passed over the nodule.
  4. Photographs are taken of the image displayed.
- Note that an ultrasound technologist usually performs this study in approximately 15 minutes and that a radiologist evaluates the results.

- Tell the patient that no discomfort is associated with this study.

After

- Assist the patient in removing the lubricant from his or her neck.

Abnormal findings

Cyst

Tumor

Thyroid adenoma

Thyroid carcinoma

Goiter

notes

T

thyrotropin-releasing hormone test (TRH test, Thyrotropin-releasing factor test [TRF test])

Type of test Blood

Normal findings Prompt rise in serum TSH level to approximately twice the baseline value in 30 minutes after an IV bolus of TRH (response normally greater in women)

Test explanation and related physiology

The TRH test assesses the responsiveness of the anterior pituitary gland via its secretion of thyroid-stimulating hormone (TSH) to an IV injection of TRH. After the TRH injection, the normally functioning pituitary gland should secrete TSH. In hyperthyroidism, either slight or no increase in the TSH level is seen, because pituitary TSH production is suppressed by the direct effect of excess circulating thyroxine and triiodothyronine (T_4, T_3) on the pituitary gland. A normal result is considered reliable evidence for excluding the diagnosis of thyrotoxicosis. The TRH test is one of the most reliable confirmatory procedures for hyperthyroidism; other tests are often compared with it to determine their accuracy.

In addition to assessing the responsiveness of the anterior pituitary gland, this test aids in the detection of primary, secondary, and tertiary hypothyroidism. In primary hypothyroidism (thyroid gland failure), the increase in the TSH level is two or more times the normal result. With secondary hypothyroidism (anterior pituitary failure), no TSH response occurs. Tertiary hypothyroidism (hypothalamic failure) may be diagnosed by a delayed rise in the TSH level. Multiple injections of TRH may be needed to induce the appropriate TSH response in this case.

The TRH test also may be useful in differentiating primary depression from manic-depressive psychiatric illness and from secondary types of depression. In primary depression, the TSH response is blunted in most patients, whereas patients with other types of depression have a normal TRH-induced TSH response.

Interfering factors

- Pregnancy may increase the TSH response to TRH.
- Drugs that may modify the TSH response include antithyroid drugs, aspirin, corticosteroids, estrogens, levodopa, and T_4.

Procedure and patient care

Before

- Explain the procedure to the patient.
- Instruct the patient to discontinue thyroid preparations for 3 to 4 weeks before the TRH test.
- Assess the patient for medications currently being taken.
- Tell the patient that no fasting or sedation is required.

During

- Administer a 500-μg IV bolus of TRH.
- Obtain venous blood samples at intervals and measure for TSH levels.

After

- Apply pressure or a pressure dressing to the venipuncture site.
- Assess the venipuncture site for bleeding.
- Indicate on the laboratory slip if the patient is pregnant.
- List any medications that the patient is taking.

Abnormal findings

Hyperthyroidism
Hypothyroidism
Psychiatric primary depression

Acute starvation
Old age (especially in men)
Pregnancy

notes

T

thyroxine (T₄, Thyroxine screen)

Type of test Blood

Normal findings

Murphy-Pattee technique
Neonate: 10.1-20.0 μg/dl
1-4 months: 7.5-16.5 μg/dl
4-12 months: 5.5-14.5 μg/dl
1-6 years: 5.6-12.6 μg/dl
6-10 years: 4.9-11.7 μg/dl
Over 10 years: 4-11 μg/dl

Radioimmunoassay
5-12 μg/dl or 65-155 nmol/L (SI units)

Possible critical values
Newborn: <7.0 μg/dl
Adult: <2.0 μg/dl if myxedema coma possible; >20 μg/dl if thyroid storm possible

Test explanation and related physiology
The serum thyroxine (T_4) study is a direct measurement of the total amount of T_4 present in the patient's blood. Greater-than-normal levels indicate hyperthyroid states, and subnormal values are seen in hypothyroid states. Newborns are screened by T_4 tests to detect hypothyroidism. Mental retardation can be prevented by early diagnosis.

This is a very reliable test of thyroid function; however, results are affected by thyroid-binding globulin (TBG). Because T_4 is bound by serum proteins such as TBG, any increase in these proteins (as in pregnant women and patients taking oral contraceptives) will cause factitiously elevated levels of T_4 and, to some extent, triiodothyronine (T_3). Therefore levels of these carrier proteins (e.g., TBG) are concomitantly measured by T_3 resin uptake studies (see p. 823). T_3 resin results must be considered in interpreting the T_4 test results.

Interfering factors
- T_4 levels may be increased after x-ray iodinated contrast studies.
- Pregnancy will cause increased levels.

☛ Drugs that may cause *increased* levels include clofibrate, estrogens, heroin, methadone, and oral contraceptives.
☛ Drugs that may cause *decreased* levels include anabolic steroids, androgens, antithyroid drugs (e.g., propylthiouracil), lithium, phenytoin (Dilantin), and propranolol (Inderal).

Procedure and patient care

Before
- Explain the procedure to the patient.
- Evaluate the patient's medication history.
- If indicated, instruct the patient to stop exogenous T_4 medication 1 month before testing.
- Tell the patient that no fasting is required.

During
Adult
- Collect a venous blood specimen in a red-top tube.
- List on the laboratory slip any drugs that may affect test results.

Newborn
- Perform a heel stick to obtain blood.
- Thoroughly saturate the circles on the filter paper with blood.
- Note that prompt collection and processing are crucial to the early detection of hypothyroidism.
- Note that the optimal collection time is 2 to 4 days after birth. All newborns should be screened before discharge (regardless of age), however, because of the consequences of delayed diagnosis.

After
- Apply pressure or a pressure dressing to the venipuncture site.
- Assess the venipuncture site for bleeding.

Abnormal findings

▲ Increased levels
   Hyperthyroid states (e.g., Graves' disease, Plummer's disease, toxic thyroid adenoma)
   Acute thyroiditis
   Pregnancy

▼ Decreased levels
   Hypothyroid states (e.g., cretinism, myxedema)
   Protein malnutrition
   Renal failure

thyroxine index, free (FTI, FT$_4$ index)

Type of test Blood

Normal findings 0.8-2.4 ng/dl or 10-31 pmol/L (SI units)

Test explanation and related physiology

The FTI study measures the amount of free thyroxine (T$_4$), which is only a fraction of the total T$_4$. Free T$_4$ is the unbound T$_4$ that enters the cell and is metabolically active. The diagnostic value of measuring the FTI is that it is not affected by thyroid-binding globulin (TBG) abnormalities; therefore it correlates more closely with the true hormonal status than do total T$_4$ or triiodothyronine (T$_3$) determinations. To determine the FTI, T$_3$ uptake (see p. 823) is measured and multiplied by the measured T$_4$ (see p. 802). This simple mathematic computation corrects the estimated total T$_4$ assay for the effects of TBG protein alterations.

This index is useful in diagnosing hyperthyroidism and hypothyroidism, especially in patients with abnormalities in TBG levels. High FTI calculations suggest hyperthyroidism; low FTI values suggest hypothyroidism. The FTI study also aids in the evaluation of the thyroid status of pregnant women and patients who have abnormal TBG levels as a result of being treated with certain drugs (e.g., estrogen, phenytoin, salicylates).

Interfering factor

- Recent radionuclear scan

Procedure and patient care

Before

- Explain the procedure to the patient.
- Obtain the T$_4$ value and T$_3$ uptake ratio.

During

- Multiply the T$_3$ uptake value by the T$_4$ value to obtain the FTI.

After

- Apply pressure or a pressure dressing to the venipuncture site.
- Check the venipuncture site for bleeding.

Abnormal findings

▲ **Increased levels**
Hyperthyroidism

▼ **Decreased levels**
Hypothyroidism

notes

tilt-table testing

Type of test Manometric

Normal findings <20 mm Hg decrease in systolic blood pressure and <10 mm increase in diastolic blood pressure. Heart rate increase should be less than 10 beats/min.

Test explanation and related physiology

The tilt-table test is a provocative test used to diagnose vasopressor syncope. Patients with this syndrome usually demonstrate symptomatic hypotension and syncope within a few to 30 minutes of being tilted upright by approximately 60 to 80 degrees. This test is usually performed with an electrophysiologic cardiac study (see p. 351). This test is often used to assess the efficacy of prophylactic pacing in some patients with vasopressor syncope. It is also used to evaluate the impact of posture with some forms of tachyarrhythmias. Normally, a minimal drop in systolic blood pressure, rise in diastolic blood pressure, and increase in heart rate occur in the tilted position. Patients with vasopressor syncope demonstrate these changes in an exaggerated fashion and become lightheaded and dizzy on assuming the tilted position.

Interfering factors

- Patients with dehydration or hypovolemia will demonstrate comparable changes in blood pressure and heart rate. This is especially true in elderly patients.
- Patients on antihypertensive medications or diuretics also may demonstrate similar changes when placed in the tilt position.

Procedure and patient care

Before

- Explain the procedure to the patient.
- Obtain IV access in the event emergency drugs are required.
- Often, an arterial line is placed to accurately monitor blood pressure.
- Inquire as to whether the patient has had excessive fluid loss (diarrhea or vomiting) in the previous 24 hours.
- Record antihypertensive or diuretic medicines that the patient may be taking.

During

- The patient lies supine on a horizontal tilt table.
- Obtain the patient's blood pressure and pulse as baseline values before tilting is carried out.
- Monitor these vital signs during the procedure.
- Question the patient as to the presence of symptoms of dizziness and lightheadedness.
- The table is progressively tilted to 60° to 80° while the patient is being monitored. Alternatively, the patient is asked to sit or stand.

After

- Monitor the arterial IV site for bleeding after removal of the vascular access.
- A pressure dressing should be firmly secured to both sites (arterial and venous).

Abnormal finding

Vasomotor syncope

notes

T

TORCH test

The term *TORCH* (*t*oxoplasmosis, *o*ther, *r*ubella, *c*ytomega-
lovirus, *h*erpes) has been applied to infections with recognized
detrimental effects on the fetus. The effects on the fetus may be
direct or indirect (e.g., precipitating abortion or premature labor). Included in the category of *other* are infections (e.g., syphilis). All of these tests are discussed separately:

Toxoplasmosis, p. 813
Rubella, p. 725
Cytomegalovirus, p. 315
Herpes virus, p. 463

notes

toxicology screening

Type of test Blood; urine

Normal findings See Tables 15 and 16 for blood toxicology and urine toxicology, respectively.

Test explanation and related physiology

Toxicology screening is performed to determine the cause of acute drug toxicity, monitor drug dependency, and detect the presence of narcotics in the body for medicolegal purposes. Toxicology screening is especially important in patients with a drug overdose or poisoning.

Procedure and patient care

Before
- Explain the procedure to the patient or significant others.
- If the specimen is obtained for medicolegal testing, ensure that the patient or family member has signed a consent form.
- Obtain as much information as possible about the drug type, amount, and ingestion time.
- Carefully assess the patient for respiratory distress (a common adverse reaction of drug overdosage).

During
- Collect blood as designated by the laboratory or urine specimens as indicated. Urine specimens are usually collected in the presence of the nurse.
- Collect gastric contents for analysis if indicated.
- Note that hair and nail samples may be used to detect or document exposure to arsenic and mercury.

After
- Apply pressure or a pressure dressing to the venipuncture site.
- Assess the venipuncture site for bleeding.
- Assess the patient for respiratory distress (a common adverse reaction of drug overdosage).
- Refer the patient for appropriate drug and psychiatric counseling.

T

TABLE 15 Blood toxicology screening

Drug	Type	Therapeutic level*	Toxic level*
Acetaminophen	Analgesic, antipyretic	Depends on the use	>250 μg/ml
Alcohol	—	None	80-200 mg/dl (mild to moderate intoxication)
			250-400 mg/dl (marked intoxication)
			>400 mg/dl (severe intoxication)
Amobarbital	Sedative, hypnotic	0.5-3.0 μg/ml	>10 μg/ml
Butabarbital	Sedative, hypnotic	0.5-3.0 μg/ml	>10 μg/ml

Carboxyhemoglobin (COHb, carbon monoxide)	Gas	None	>30% COHb (beginning of coma)
Glutethimide	Sedative	0.5-3.0 µg/ml	>10 µg/ml
Lead	—	None	>40 µg/dl
Lithium	Manic episodes of manic-depression psychosis	0.8-1.2 mEq/l	>2.0 mEq/l
Meprobamate	Antianxiety agent	0.5-3.0 µg/ml	>10 µg/ml
Methyprylon	Hypnotic	0.5-3.0 µg/ml	>10 µg/ml
Phenobarbital	Anticonvulsant	15-30 µg/ml	>40 µg/ml
Phenytoin (Dilantin)	Anticonvulsant	10-20 µg/ml	>20 µg/ml
Salicylate	Antipyretic, anti-inflammatory, analgesic	100-250 µg/ml	>300 µg/ml

*Levels vary according to the institution performing the test.

T

TABLE 16 Urine toxicology screening for amphetamines

Drug	Therapeutic level*	Toxic level*
Amphetamine	2-3 μg/ml	>3 μg/ml
Dextroamphetamine	0.1-1.5 μg/ml	>15 μg/ml
Methamphetamine	3-5 μg/ml	>40 μg/ml
Phenmetrazine	5-30 μg/ml	>50 μg/ml

*Levels vary according to the institution performing the test.

Abnormal finding

Toxicity

notes

toxoplasmosis antibody titer

Type of test Blood

Normal findings

Titers <1:16 indicate no previous infection
Titers 1:16-1:256 are usually prevalent in general population
Titers >1:256 suggest recent infection
Rising titers are of great significance

Test explanation and related physiology

Toxoplasmosis is a protozoan disease caused by *Toxoplasma gondii,* which is found in poorly cooked or raw meat and in the feces of cats. This disease is characterized by central nervous system lesions, which may lead to blindness, brain damage, and death. The condition may occur congenitally or postnatally. Because approximately 25% to 50% of the adult population are asymptomatically affected with toxoplasmosis, the Centers for Disease Control recommends that patients who are pregnant be serologically tested for this disease.

The presence of antibodies before pregnancy probably ensures protection against congenital toxoplasmosis in the child. Chronic toxoplasmosis, which affects a large percentage of adults, will not cause spontaneous abortion or infection of the infant. Fetal infection occurs only if the mother acquires toxoplasmosis after conception. Repeat testing of pregnant patients with low or negative titers may be done before the twentieth week and before delivery to identify antibody converters and determine appropriate therapy (e.g., therapeutic abortion at 20 weeks, treatment during the remainder of the pregnancy, or treatment of the newborn). Hydrocephaly, microcephaly, and chronic retinitis and convulsions are complications of congenital toxoplasmosis. Congenital toxoplasmosis is diagnosed when the test levels are persistently elevated or a rising titer is found in the infant 2 to 3 months after birth.

Procedure and patient care

Before

- Explain the procedure to the patient.

During
- Collect approximately 5 ml of blood in a red-top tube.
- Indicate on the laboratory slip if the patient is pregnant or has been exposed to cats.

After
- Apply pressure or a pressure dressing to the venipuncture site.
- Assess the venipuncture site for bleeding.

Abnormal finding

Toxoplasmosis infection

notes

transesophageal echocardiography (TEE)

Type of test Endoscopy/ultrasound

Normal findings Normal position, size, and movement of the heart muscle, valves, and heart chambers

Test explanation and related physiology

TEE provides ultrasonic imaging of the heart from a retrocardiac vantage point, avoiding interference of the ultrasound by the interposed subcutaneous tissue, bony thorax, and lungs. In this procedure, a high-frequency ultrasound transducer placed in the esophagus by endoscopy provides better resolution than that of images obtained with routine transthoracic echocardiography (see p. 332). For TEE, the distal end of the endoscope is advanced into the esophagus. The transducer is positioned behind the heart (Figure 28). Controls on the handle of the endoscope permit the transducer to be rotated and flexed in both the anteroposterior and right-left lateral planes. TEE images have better resolution than those obtained by routine transthoracic echocardiography because of the higher-frequency sound waves and closer proximity of the transducer to the cardiac structures.

In the evaluation of structures that are inaccessible or poorly visualized by the transthoracic probe approach, TEE is helpful. TEE is especially helpful in patients who are obese or have large lung-air spaces.

This test is performed for the following reasons:
1. To better visualize the mitral valve
2. To differentiate intracardiac from extracardiac masses and tumors
3. To better visualize the atrial septum (for atrial septal defects)
4. To diagnose thoracic aortic dissection
5. To better detect valvular vegetation indicative of endocarditis
6. To determine cardiac sources of arterial embolism
7. To detect coronary artery disease

Also, TEE can be used intraoperatively to monitor high-risk patients for ischemia. Ischemic muscle movement is much different from normal muscle movement; therefore TEE is a very sensitive indicator of myocardial ischemia. TEE can be used to monitor patients undergoing major abdominal, peripheral vas-

T

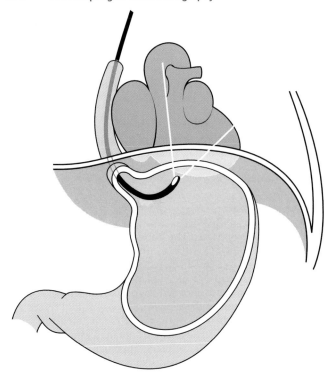

Figure 28 Transesophageal echocardiography (TEE). Diagram illustrates location of the transesophageal endoscope within the esophagus.

cular, and carotid artery procedures who are at high risk for intraoperative ischemia because of coronary artery disease.

Transesophageal echocardiography is more sensitive than electrocardiography (EKG) for detecting ischemia. TEE is also used intraoperatively to evaluate surgical results of valvular or congenital heart diseases. Furthermore, TEE is also the most sensitive technique for detecting air emboli, a serious complication of neurosurgery performed with the patient in the upright position (cervical laminectomy).

Contraindications

- Patients with known upper esophageal pathology
- Patients with known esophageal varices

- Patients with Zenker's diverticulum
- Patients with esophageal abnormalities (e.g., stricture diverticula, scleroderma, esophagitis)
- Patients with bleeding disorders
- Patients who have had prior esophageal surgery
- Patients who cannot cooperate with the procedure

Potential complications

- Esophageal perforation or bleeding
- Cardiac arrhythmias

Procedure and patient care

Before

- Explain the procedure to the patient.
- Instruct the patient to fast for 4 to 6 hours before the test.
- Removal all oral prostheses.
- Obtain intravenous IV access.

During

- Intravenous sedation is commonly provided with a short-acting benzodiazepine. Other sedation may be provided.
- Apply EKG leads, and continually monitor heart rhythm.
- Apply a blood pressure cuff, and monitor blood pressure periodically.
- Occasionally, pulse oximetry is monitored to determine oxygen saturation in heavily sedated patients.
- Note the following procedural steps:
  1. The pharynx is anesthetized with a local topical agent to depress the gag reflex.
  2. The patient is placed in the left lateral decubitus position.
  3. Intubation is carried out through the mouth and into the upper esophagus.
  4. The patient is asked to swallow, and the transducer is advanced into position behind the heart.
  5. The room is darkened, and the ultrasound images are displayed on a monitor. Views can be obtained of the ultrasound image after desired images are visualized.
- The procedure is performed by a cardiologist and/or a GI endoscopist in approximately 20 minutes in the endoscopy suite. It also can be performed at the bedside.
- Very little discomfort is associated with this test.

T

After
- Naloxone or mazicon may be administered to reverse the sedative effects of the narcotics.
- Observe the patient closely for approximately 1 hour after the procedure, until the effects of sedation have worn off.

Abnormal findings

Myocardial ischemia
Myocardial infarction
Valvular heart disease
Intracardiac thrombi
Cardiac valvular vegetation

Ventricular and atrial septal defects
Cardiomyopathy
Marked cardiac chamber dilation
Cardiac tumors

notes

triglycerides (TGs)

Type of test Blood

Normal findings

Adult/elderly
  Male: 40-160 mg/dl or 0.45-1.81 mmol (SI units)
  Female: 35-135 mg/dl or 0.40-1.52 mmol/L (SI units)

Child	*Male*	*Female*
0-5 years:	30-86 mg/dl	32-99 mg/dl
6-11 years:	31-108 mg/dl	35-114 mg/dl
12-15 years:	36-138 mg/dl	41-138 mg/dl
16-19 years:	40-163 mg/dl	40-128 mg/dl

Test explanation and related physiology

TGs are a form of fat that exists within the bloodstream. They are transported by very-low-density lipoproteins (VLDLs) and low-density lipoproteins (LDLs). TGs are produced in the liver by using glycerol and other fatty acids as building blocks. A TG acts as a storage source for energy. When TG levels in the blood are in excess, TGs are deposited into the fatty tissues. TGs are a part of a lipid profile that also evaluates cholesterol (see p. 232) and lipoproteins (see p. 514). A lipid profile is performed to assess the risk of coronary and vascular disease.

Interfering factors

- Ingestion of fatty meals may cause elevated TG levels.
- Ingestion of alcohol may cause elevated levels.
- Pregnancy may cause increased levels.
- ☞ Drugs that may cause *increased* TG levels include cholestyramine, estrogens, and oral contraceptives.
- ☞ Drugs that may cause *decreased* levels include ascorbic acid, asparaginase, clofibrate, and colestipol.

Procedure and patient care

Before
- Explain the procedure to the patient.
- Instruct the patient to fast for 12 to 14 hours before the test. Only water is permitted.
- Tell the patient not to drink alcohol for 24 hours before the test.

T

- Inform the patient that dietary indiscretion for as much as 2 weeks before this test will influence results.

During

- Collect 5 to 10 ml of venous blood in a red-top tube.

After

- Apply pressure or a pressure dressing to the venipuncture site.
- Assess the venipuncture site for bleeding.
- Mark the patient's age and gender on the laboratory slip.
- Instruct the patient with increased TG levels regarding diet, exercise, and appropriate weight.

Abnormal findings

▲ Increased levels

Glycogen storage disease
Hyperlipidemias
Hypothyroidism
High-carbohydrate diet
Poorly controlled diabetes
Risk of arteriosclerotic occlusive coronary disease and peripheral vascular disease
Nephrotic syndrome
Hypertension
Alcoholic cirrhosis
Pregnancy
Myocardial infarction

▼ Decreased levels

Malabsorption syndrome
Malnutrition
Hyperthyroidism

notes

triiodothyronine (T$_3$ radioimmunoassay [T$_3$ by RIA])

Type of test Blood

Normal findings

Adult/elderly: 110-230 ng/dl or 1.2-1.5 nmol/L (SI units)
Newborn: 90-170 ng/dl
Child (6-12 years): 115-190 ng/dl

Test explanation and related physiology

As with the thyroxine (T$_4$) test, the serum T$_3$ test is an accurate measure of thyroid function. T$_3$ is less stable than T$_4$ and occurs in minute quantities in the active form. Generally, when the T$_3$ level is below normal, the patient is in a hypothyroid state. An elevated T$_3$ determination is clinically important in the patient with a normal T$_4$ level but with all the symptoms of hyperthyroidism. In this patient, the test may identify T$_3$ thyrotoxicosis. This test is not the same as the T$_3$ uptake test (see p. 823) and should not be confused with it.

Interfering factors

- Radioisotope administration before the test may alter the results.
- T$_3$ values are increased in pregnancy.
- ⚕ Drugs that may cause *increased* levels include estrogen, methadone, and oral contraceptives.
- ⚕ Drugs that may cause *decreased* levels include anabolic steroids, androgens, phenytoin (Dilantin), propranolol (Inderal), reserpine, and salicylates (high dose).

Procedure and patient care

Before

- Explain the procedure to the patient.
- Determine whether the patient is taking any exogenous T$_3$ medication, because this will affect test results.
- Withhold drugs that may affect results (with physician's approval).
- Tell the patient that no fasting is required.

During

- Collect approximately 5 to 10 ml of venous blood in a red-top tube.

T

- List on the laboratory slip any medications the patient is currently taking.

After

- Apply pressure or a pressure dressing to the venipuncture site.
- Observe the venipuncture site for bleeding.

Abnormal findings

▲ **Increased levels**
  Hyperthyroidism
  T_3 thyrotoxicosis
  Thyroiditis
  Toxic adenoma

▼ **Decreased levels**
  Hypothyroidism
  Starvation
  Chronic illness

notes

triiodothyronine uptake test (T₃ resin uptake test, Resin triiodothyronine uptake test [RT₃U, T₃RU])

Type of test Blood

Normal findings 24% to 34% or 24-34 AU (arbitrary units; SI units)

Test explanation and related physiology

The T_3 resin uptake test indirectly quantifies *thyroid-binding globulin* (TBG) and *thyroid-binding prealbumin* (TBPA) in the blood. Pregnancy, oral contraceptives, and some genetic disorders tend to raise inappropriately the quantity of these carrying proteins. As a result, thyroxine (T_4) and T_3 levels may be artificially elevated, but the patient may be euthyroid. Similarly, androgenic hormones, intercurrent serious illness, and nephrotic syndromes tend to lower the quantity of these proteins, causing falsely low T_3 and T_4 levels in euthyroid patients. Therefore, accurate assessment of the patient's thyroid status requires measurement of the TBG and TBPA levels directly, but the thyroid status can be assessed indirectly by the use of RT_3U testing. Because this is an exchange resin test, high results indicate low TBG and TBPA levels and low results indicate high TBG and TBPA levels.

The T_3 uptake test is useful for the diagnosis of hypothyroidism or hyperthyroidism. This test is also used with the T_4 to provide the free T_4 index (see p. 804). It is important to note that the RT_3U test is *not* a measurement of serum T_3.

Interfering factors

- Recent radioisotope scans before the blood collection may affect test results.
- Drugs that may cause *elevated* TBG and TBPA levels include anabolic steroids, heparin, phenytoin (Dilantin), salicylates (high dose), thyroid agents, and warfarin (Coumadin).
- Drugs that may cause *decreased* levels include antithyroid agents, clofibrate, estrogen, oral contraceptives, and thiazides.

Procedure and patient care

Before
- Explain the procedure to the patient.
- Tell the patient that no fasting is required.

T

During

- Collect approximately 5 to 7 ml of venous blood in a red-top tube.
- List on the laboratory slip any drugs that may affect test results.

After

- Apply pressure or a pressure dressing to the venipuncture site.
- Assess the venipuncture site for bleeding.

Abnormal findings

▲ **Increased levels**
Hyperthyroidism
Protein malnutrition
Nephrotic syndrome
Malnutrition
Renal failure

▼ **Decreased levels**
Hypothyroidism
Pregnancy
Acute hepatitis

notes

T-tube and operative cholangiogram

Type of test X-ray with contrast dye

Normal findings

Normal common bile duct with no dilation or filling defects
Good runoff of dye through the ampulla of Vater and into the
duodenum

Test explanation and related physiology

In *operative cholangiography,* the common bile duct is directly
injected with radiopaque material. This is usually performed during cholecystectomy. Stones appear as radiolucent shadows. Gallstones, tumors, or strictures cause partial or total obstruction of
the flow of dye into the duodenum. By visualization of the biliary duct structures, the surgeon is provided with the surgical
anatomy of the biliary tree. This reduces the possibility of inadvertent common bile duct injury during cholecystectomy. If
common duct stones are demonstrated on operative cholangiography, a common duct exploration is performed. Some surgeons perform operative cholangiography on all patients who
have cholecystectomy. Other surgeons use specific indications for
operative cholangiography, including:

1. Jaundice
2. Abnormal liver enzymes
3. Dilated common bile duct
4. Evidence of pancreatitis
5. Evidence of small stones in the cystic duct during cholecystectomy

T-tube cholangiography is performed postoperatively following
a common duct exploration. Its main purpose is to detect retained common bile duct stones and demonstrate good flow of
contrast dye into the duodenum. This test is performed
through the use of a T-shaped rubber tube that is placed into
the common bile duct at surgery. This test is usually performed
5 to 10 days after surgery. If no stones are evident and there is
good runoff of bile into the duodenum, the T-tube can be removed. If there are residual stones, the T-tube tract can be used
to extract the stones.

Potential complication

- Sepsis caused by increased ductal pressure with dye infusion

Interfering factor

- Barium within the abdomen from a previous upper GI series or barium enema x-ray film precludes visualization of the bile duct.

Procedure and patient care

Before

- Explain the procedure to the patient when obtaining consent for the main biliary procedure.
- Tell the patient that no fasting or sedation is required for T-tube cholangiography. However, routine preoperative NPO status is necessary for the operative cholangiogram.

During

- Note the following procedural steps:

Operative cholangiogram
1. This is performed through catheterization of the cystic duct during cholecystectomy.
2. A needle or catheter is placed in the common bile duct.
3. The dye is injected directly into the common bile duct.
4. X-ray films are taken while the patient is on the operating table and are immediately reviewed by the surgeon.

T-tube cholangiogram
1. The patient is taken to the radiology department.
2. A sterile dye solution is injected into the T-tube previously placed by the surgeon.
3. X-ray films are taken of the right upper quadrant of the abdomen while the patient is placed in various positions.

- Note that a radiologist or surgeon performs these procedures in approximately 10 minutes.
- Tell the patient that no discomfort is associated with these studies.

After

- Observe the patient for signs of sepsis.
- If a T-tube has been surgically placed, establish a sterile, closed drainage system.

Abnormal findings

Common bile duct stones
Anatomic variations
Bile duct cysts
Stricture or tumor obstructing the common bile duct
Bile duct surgical trauma

tuberculin test (PPD skin test)

Type of test Skin

Normal findings Negative; reaction <5 mm

Test explanation and related physiology

Although this test is used to detect tuberculosis (TB) infection, it is unable to indicate whether the infection is active or dormant. For this test, a *purified protein derivative* (PPD) of the tubercle bacillus is injected intradermally. If the patient is infected with TB (whether active or dormant), lymphocytes will recognize the PPD antigen and cause a local reaction; if the patient is not infected, no reaction will occur. If the test is negative and the physician strongly suspects TB, a "second-strength" PPD can be used. If this test is then negative, the patient does not have TB. (See p. 829 for tuberculosis culture.)

The PPD test also can be used as part of a series of skin tests done to assess the immune system. If the immune system is nonfunctioning because of poor nutrition or chronic illness (e.g., neoplasia, infection), the PPD test will be negative despite the patient having had an active or a dormant TB infection. It has been well established that surgery is associated with greater mortality in these patients (with immunocompromise) than in patients whose immune systems are intact.

Laboratory testing for TB is usually performed as part of the routine prenatal evaluation in pregnant women. Often, this may be the mother's first contact with the health care system in several years.

When a patient known to have active TB receives a PPD test, the local reaction may be so severe as to cause a complete skin slough requiring surgical care. When these patients are eliminated from PPD testing, the test has no complications. The PPD test will not cause active TB, because no live organisms exist in the test solution.

Contraindications

- Patients with known active TB
- Patients who have received *bacille Calmette-Guérin* (BCG) immunization against PPD, because these patients will demonstrate a positive reaction to the PPD vaccination even though they have never had TB infection

Procedure and patient care

Before

- Explain the procedure to the patient.
- Assure the patient that she or he will not develop TB from this test.
- Assess the patient for previous history of TB. Report a positive history to the physician.
- Evaluate the patient's history for previous PPD results and BCG immunization.

During

- Prepare the patient's forearm with alcohol, and allow it to dry.
- Intradermally inject the PPD. A skin wheal will occur.
- Circle the area with indelible ink.
- Record the time at which the PPD was injected.

After

- Read the results in 48 to 72 hours.
- Examine the test site for induration (hardening). Measure the area of induration (*not* redness) in millimeters.
- If the test is positive, ensure that the physician is notified and the patient is treated appropriately.
- If the test is positive, check the patient's arm 4 to 5 days after the test to be certain that a severe skin reaction has not occurred.

Abnormal findings

Positive results

TB infection

Negative results

Possible immunoincompetence in chronically ill patients

notes

tuberculosis culture (TB culture, BACTEC method, Polymerase chain reaction)

Type of test Microbiology culture

Normal findings Negative for tuberculosis

Test explanation and related physiology

A diagnosis of TB should be considered in any patient with a persistent productive cough, night sweats, anorexia, weight loss, fever, and hemoptysis. This diagnosis should be especially considered in high-risk patients, such as those who are immunocompromised, are alcoholic, or have had a recent exposure to TB. (See p. 827 for other TB testing.)

Diagnosis can be made only by identification and culture of *Mycobacterium tuberculosis* in the specimen. Conventional culture techniques for growth, identification, and susceptibility of acid-fast mycobacterium take 4 to 6 weeks. Because the patient suspected of having TB cannot be isolated for that duration, the disease may spread to many other people while waiting for the diagnosis. With the resurgence and increasing incidence of TB in the U.S. population (especially among immunocompromised patients with AIDS), newer, more rapid culture techniques have been identified and are now being performed.

The *BACTEC method* is a radiometric culture technique where the growth medium for culturing mycobacteria is supplanted with a substrate labeled with radioactive carbon (^{14}C). This substrate is used by mycobacteria, and during metabolism, radioactive carbon dioxide ($^{14}CO_2$) is produced from the substrate. The $^{14}CO_2$ is detected quantitatively by counting the radioactivity with the Becton Dickinson Diagnostic Instrument System. The rate and amount of CO_2 produced is directly proportional to the rate and amount of growth occurring in the medium. With this technique, very small quantities of $^{14}CO_2$ can be detected. This permits quick identification of mycobacterial growth. This technique is not only used to isolate mycobacteria from clinical specimens but also to differentiate *M. tuberculosis* complex from other mycobacteria and for antimicrobial susceptibility testing.

Polymerase chain reaction culture methods also have recently been developed. With the addition of a DNA polymerase, genetic chromosomal parts can be multiplied. This allows amplification of genomes, which then can be detected by genetic DNA probes. With the newer techniques already described, *M. tuberculosis* can be identified in as little as 36 to 48 hours. With this reduction in diagnostic time, treatment can be started earlier. It is anticipated that the spread of tuberculosis therefore will be greatly reduced. The average detection time, however, is longer for extrapulmonary specimens than for sputum specimens. The time for identification is greatly reduced when numerous mycobacteria are present. Generally, organisms in specimens from patients already receiving antituberculosis treatment take longer to grow.

After identification and growth of mycobacteria, antibiotic susceptibility testing is performed to identify the most effective antimycobacterial drugs. The culture specimen can be performed on sputum, body fluids, cerebrospinal fluid, and even biopsy tissue specimens.

Interfering factors

☛ Antituberculosis drugs

Procedure and patient care

Before

- Explain the procedure to the patient.
- Tell the patient that no fasting is required.

During

- For *sputum,* obtain an early morning specimen. It is best to induce sputum production with an ultrasonic or nebulizing device.
- Collect three to five early morning specimens. All specimens must contain mycobacteria to make the diagnosis of TB.
- For *urine* collection, obtain three to five single, clean-voided specimens early in the morning.
- *Swabs, intestinal washings,* and *biopsy* specimens should be transported to the laboratory immediately for preparation.
- Follow the institution's policy for universal specimen handling.
- Once the specimen is received by the laboratory, a decontamination process is applied to it to kill all nonmycobacteria. The specimen is then cultured in the appropriate medium.
- With the rapid growth techniques, the specimen is evaluated every 24 hours.
- When cultural growth is considered adequate, the organisms are stained for acid-fast bacillus and identified.

- With genetic probes, the *Mycobacterium* species is identified.
- At this point, if *M. tuberculosis* is present, the report will read "culture more positive for mycobacteria." If the species has been identified, this also will be reported.
- Drug-susceptibility testing then will be carried out and subsequently reported.

After

- Instruct the patient as to appropriate isolation of sputum and other body fluids to avoid potential spread of suspected TB.

Abnormal findings

TB
Atypical mycobacterial nontuberculosis disease

notes

T

tubular phosphate reabsorption (TPR, Tubular reabsorption of phosphate [TRP])

Type of test Blood; urine (hourly or 24-hour)

Normal findings 80% to 90%

Test explanation and related physiology

The TPR test indirectly measures parathyroid hormone (PTH) by estimating its effects on renal phosphate reabsorption. TPR is primarily done to detect primary hyperparathyroidism. This test value is calculated using the serum creatinine level (see p. 297), the serum phosphate concentration (see p. 623), and the creatinine clearance rate (see p. 299). Results are based on the ratio of creatinine clearance to phosphate clearance. Values less than 80% indicate diminished renal tubular reabsorption of phosphate and suggest primary hyperparathyroidism. Decreased values also may be associated with sarcoidosis, myeloma, and hypercalcemia caused by malignancy.

Interfering factors

- Low-phosphate diets raise TPR values.
- High-phosphate diets lower TPR values.

Procedure and patient care

Before

- Explain the procedure to the patient.
- Instruct the patient concerning the method that will be used (24-hour urine or hourly samples).
- Instruct the patient that he or she should have a normal phosphate diet (>500 mg/day and <3000 mg/day).

During

24-hour urine test
- Keep the patient NPO, except for water, for 8 hours before drawing the blood sample.
- Collect the 24-hour urine sample using a preservative.
- Draw the blood early in the urine collection.

Hourly urine test
- Instruct the patient to drink several 8-ounce glasses of water and empty the bladder. (This marks the beginning of the test.)

- One hour later, draw a blood specimen for phosphorus and creatinine measurements.
- One hour later (2 hours after beginning the test), instruct the patient to void for determination of the urine volume and urine concentration of creatinine and phosphorus.
- Note that urine may be collected again 1 hour later.

After

- Mark each specimen with the time it was collected.
- Send the specimen to the laboratory as soon as it is collected.

Abnormal findings

▼ **Decreased values**

Primary hyperparathyroidism

Sarcoidosis

Myeloma

Hypercalcemia caused by malignancy

notes

T

upper gastrointestinal x-ray study (Upper GI series, UGI)

Type of test X-ray with contrast dye

Normal findings Normal size, contour, patency, filling, positioning, and transit of barium through the lower esophagus, stomach, and upper duodenum

Test explanation and related physiology

The upper GI study consists of a series of x-ray films of the lower esophagus, stomach, and duodenum, usually using barium sulfate as the contrast medium. When there is concern for leakage of x-ray contrast through a perforation of the GI tract, however, Gastrografin (a water-soluble contrast) is used. This test can be performed in conjunction with a barium swallow (see p. 124), which can precede the upper GI study.

The purpose of this examination is to detect ulcerations, tumors, inflammations, or anatomic malpositions (e.g., hiatal hernia) within these organs. Obstruction of the upper GI tract is also easily detected.

In this test, the patient is asked to drink barium. As the contrast descends, the lower esophagus is examined for position, patency, and filling defects (e.g., tumors, scarring, varices). As the contrast enters the stomach, the gastric wall is examined for benign or malignant ulcerations, filling defects (most often in cancer), and anatomic abnormalities (e.g., hiatal hernia). The patient is placed in a flat or head-down position, and the gastroesophageal area is examined for evidence of gastroesophageal reflux of barium.

As the contrast leaves the stomach, patency of the pyloric channel and the duodenum is evaluated. Benign peptic ulceration is the most common pathologic condition affecting these areas. Extrinsic compression caused by tumors, cysts, or enlarged pathologic organs (e.g., liver) near the stomach also can be identified by anatomic distortion of the outline of the upper GI tract. The small intestine can then be studied if need be (see discussion of small bowel follow-through (p. 751).

Contraindications

- Patients with complete bowel obstructions
- Patients suspected of upper GI perforation

Water-soluble Gastrografin should be used instead of barium.
- Patients with unstable vital signs
  These patients should be supervised during the time required for this test.
- Patients who are uncooperative because of the necessity of frequent position changes

Potential complications
- Aspiration of barium
- Constipation or partial bowel obstruction caused by inspissated barium in the small bowel or colon

Interfering factors
- Previously administered barium
  This may block visualization of the upper GI tract.
- Poor performance status of the patient
  Incapacitated patients cannot assume the multiple positions required for the study.
- Food and fluid in the stomach
  This gives the false impression of filling defects within the stomach, precluding adequate evaluation of the gastric mucosa.

Procedure and patient care

Before
- Explain the procedure to the patient. Allow the patient to verbalize concerns.
- Instruct the patient to abstain from eating for at least 8 hours before the test. Usually, keep the patient NPO after midnight on the day of the test.
- Assure the patient that the test will not cause any discomfort.

During
- Note the following procedural steps:
  1. The patient is asked to drink approximately 16 ounces of barium sulfate. This is a chalky substance usually suspended in milkshake form and drunk through a straw. Usually, the drink is flavored to increase palatability.
  2. After drinking the barium, the patient is moved through several position changes (e.g., prone, supine, lateral) to promote filling of the entire upper GI tract.

U

3. Films are taken at the discretion of the radiologist observing the flow of barium fluoroscopically.
4. The flow of barium is followed through the lower esophagus, stomach, and duodenum.
5. Several films are taken throughout the course of the test.
6. In an *air-contrast upper GI study,* the patient is asked to swallow rapidly some carbonated powder. This creates carbon dioxide in the stomach, providing air contrast to the barium within the stomach and increased visualization of the gastric mucosa.

- Note that a radiologist performs this procedure in approximately 30 minutes.
- Tell the patient that he or she may be uncomfortable lying on the hard x-ray table and occasionally may experience the sensation of bloating or nausea during the test.

After

- Inform the patient that if Gastrografin was used, he or she may have significant diarrhea. Gastrografin is an osmotic cathartic.
- Instruct the patient to use a cathartic (e.g., milk of magnesia) if barium sulfate was used as the contrast medium. Water absorption may cause the barium to harden and create a fecal impaction if catharsis is not carried out.
- Instruct the patient to watch his or her stools to ensure that all of the barium has been removed. The stools should return to normal color after completely expelling the barium, which may take as much as a day and a half.

Abnormal findings

Esophageal cancer
Esophageal varices
Hiatal hernia
Esophageal diverticula
Gastric cancer
Gastric inflammatory disease (e.g., Ménétrier's disease)
Benign gastric tumor (e.g., leiomyoma)
Extrinsic compression by pancreatic pseudocysts, cysts, pancreatic tumors, or hepatomegaly

Perforation of the esophagus, stomach, or duodenum
Congenital abnormalities (e.g., duodenal web, pancreatic rest, malrotation syndrome)
Gastric ulcer (benign and malignant)
Gastritis
Duodenal ulcer
Duodenal cancer
Duodenal diverticulum

urea nitrogen blood test (Blood urea nitrogen [BUN], Serum urea nitrogen)

Type of test Blood

Normal findings

Adult: 10-20 mg/dl or 3.6-7.1 mmol/L (SI units)
Elderly: may be slightly higher than those of adults
Child: 5-18 mg/dl
Infant: 5-18 mg/dl
Newborn: 3-12 mg/dl
Cord: 21-40 mg/dl

Possible critical values >100 mg/dl (indicates serious impairment of renal function)

Test explanation and related physiology

The BUN measures the amount of urea nitrogen in the blood. Urea is formed in the liver as the end product of protein metabolism. During ingestion, protein is broken down into amino acids. In the liver, these amino acids are catabolized and free ammonia is formed. The ammonia is combined to form urea, which is then deposited into the blood and transported to the kidneys for excretion. Therefore, the BUN is directly related to the metabolic function of the liver and the excretory function of the kidney. It serves as an index of the function of these organs.

Nearly all renal diseases cause an inadequate excretion of urea, which causes the blood concentration to rise above normal. If the disease is unilateral, however, the unaffected kidney can compensate for the diseased kidney and the BUN may not become elevated. The BUN also increases in conditions other than primary renal disease. For example, when excess amounts of protein are available for hepatic catabolism (from a high-protein diet or gastrointestinal [GI] bleeding), large quantities of urea are made. BUN levels also may vary according to the state of hydration, with increased levels seen in dehydration and decreased levels seen in overhydration. Finally, one must be aware that the synthesis of urea depends on the liver. Patients with severe primary liver disease will have a decreased BUN. With combined liver and renal disease (as in hepatorenal syndrome), the BUN can be normal not because renal excretory function is good but

U

because poor hepatic functioning resulted in decreased formation of urea.

The BUN is interpreted in conjunction with the creatinine test (see p. 297). These tests are referred to as *renal function studies*.

Interfering factors

- Changes in protein intake may affect BUN levels.
- Advanced pregnancy may cause increased levels.
- Overhydration and underhydration will affect levels.
- Drugs that may cause *increased* BUN levels include allopurinol, aminoglycosides, cephalosporins, chloral hydrate, cisplatin, furosemide, guanethidine, indomethacin, methotrexate, methyldopa, nephrotoxic drugs (e.g., aspirin, amphotericin B, bacitracin, carbamazepine, colistin, gentamicin, methicillin, neomycin, penicillamine, polymyxin B, probenecid, vancomycin), propranolol, rifampin, spironolactone, tetracyclines, thiazide diuretics, and triamterene.
- Drugs that may cause *decreased* levels include chloramphenicol and streptomycin.

Procedure and patient care

Before

- Explain the procedure to the patient.
- Tell the patient that no fasting is required.

During

- Collect approximately 5 ml of blood in a red-top tube.
- Avoid hemolysis.

After

- Apply pressure or a pressure dressing to the venipuncture site.
- Observe the venipuncture site for bleeding.

Abnormal findings

▲ **Increased levels**

Renal disease (e.g., glomerulonephritis, pyelonephritis, acute tubular necrosis)

Urinary obstruction (e.g., from tumors, stones, prostatic hypertrophy)

Hypovolemia

Shock

Congestive heart failure

Burns

Excessive protein catabolism

GI bleeding

Myocardial infarction

Renal failure

Nephrotoxic drugs

Excessive protein ingestion

Dehydration

Starvation

▼ **Decreased levels**

Liver failure

Overhydration

Negative nitrogen balance (e.g., malnutrition)

Pregnancy

notes

U

urethral pressure profile (UPP, Urethral pressure measurements)

Type of test Manometric

Normal findings Maximal urethral pressures in normal patients (cm H_2O):

Age	Male	Female
<25 years	37-126	55-103
25-44 years	35-113	31-115
45-64 years	40-123	40-100
>64 years	35-105	35-75

Test explanation and related physiology

The UPP indicates the intraluminal pressure along the length of the urethra with the bladder at rest. Indications for this urodynamic investigation include the following:

1. Assessment of prostatic obstruction
2. Assessment of stress incontinence in females
3. Assessment of postprostatectomy sequelae of incontinence
4. Assessment of the adequacy of external sphincterotomy
5. Analysis of the effects of drugs on the urethra
6. Analysis of the effects of stimulation on urethral flow
7. Assessment of the adequacy of implanted artificial urethral sphincter devices

Contraindications

- Patients with urinary tract infections

Procedure and patient care

Before
- Explain the procedure to the patient.
- Because many patients are embarrassed by this procedure, assure the patient that he or she will be draped to ensure privacy.
- Tell the patient that no fasting or sedation is required.

During
- Note the following procedural steps:
  1. A catheter is placed into the bladder.
  2. Fluids (or gas) are instilled through the catheter, which is

withdrawn while the pressures along the urethral wall are obtained.

3. A constant infusion of the fluids or gas is maintained by a motorized syringe pump.
4. The catheter is removed, and the test is completed.

- Note that this test is usually performed by a urologist in less than 15 minutes.
- Explain to the patient that this test is slightly more uncomfortable than urethral catheterization.

After

- Give the patient a sitz bath if requested.

Abnormal findings

Prostatic obstruction secondary to benign prostatic hypertrophy or cancer

Urinary incontinence

notes

U

uric acid, blood

Type of test Blood

Normal findings

Adult
  Male: 2.1-8.5 mg/dl or 0.15-0.48 mmol/L
  Female: 2.0-6.6 mg/dl or 0.09-0.36 mmol/L
Elderly: values may be slightly increased
Child: 2.5-5.5 mg/dl or 0.12-0.32 mmol/L
Newborn: 2.0-6.2 mg/dl

Possible critical values >12 mg/dl

Test explanation and related physiology

Uric acid is a nitrogenous compound that is a product of purine (a deoxyribonucleic acid [DNA] building block) catabolism. Uric acid is excreted to a large degree by the kidney and to a smaller degree by the intestinal tract. When uric acid levels are elevated (hyperuricemia), the patient may have gout. Causes of hyperuricemia can be overproduction or decreased excretion of uric acid (e.g., kidney failure). Overproduction of uric acid may occur in patients with a catabolic enzyme deficiency that stimulates purine metabolism or in patients with cancer, in whom purine and DNA turnover is great. Other causes of hyperuricemia may include alcoholism, leukemias, metastatic cancer, multiple myeloma, hyperlipoproteinemia, diabetes mellitus, renal failure, stress, lead poisoning, and dehydration caused by diuretic therapy. Ketoacids (as occur in diabetic or alcoholic ketoacidosis) may compete with uric acid for tubular excretion and may cause decreased uric acid excretion. Many causes of hyperuricemia are undefined and therefore labeled as *idiopathic*.

Interfering factors

- Stress may cause increased uric acid levels.
- Recent use of x-ray contrast agents may cause decreased levels.
- Drugs that may cause *increased* levels include alcohol, ascorbic acid, aspirin (low dose), caffeine, cisplatin, diazoxide, diuretics, epinephrine, ethambutol, levodopa, methyldopa (Aldomet), nicotinic acid, phenothiazines, and theophylline.
- Drugs that may cause *decreased* levels include allopurinol, aspirin (high dose), azathioprine (Imuran), clofibrate, corti-

costeroids, estrogens, glucose infusions, guaifenesin, mannitol, probenecid, and warfarin.

Procedure and patient care

Before
- Explain the procedure to the patient.
- Follow the institution's requirements regarding fasting.
  (Some recommend that the patient fast.)

During
- Collect approximately 5 to 7 ml of venous blood in a red-
  top tube.
- List on the laboratory slip any drugs that may affect test results.

After
- Apply pressure or a pressure dressing to the venipuncture
  site.
- Assess the venipuncture site for bleeding.

Abnormal findings

▲ **Increased levels
  (hyperuricemia)**
  Gout
  Arthritis
  Soft tissue deposits of
    uric acid (tophi)
  Uric acid kidney stones
  Lead poisoning
  Hypothyroidism
  Multiple myeloma
  Metastatic cancer
  Acidosis
  Toxemia of pregnancy
  Alcoholism
  Leukemias
  Hyperlipoproteinemia
  Diabetes mellitus
  Renal failure
  Stress
  Cancer chemotherapy
  Shock
  Strenuous exercise
  Starvation

▼ **Decreased levels**
  Wilson's disease
  Fanconi's syndrome
  Yellow atrophy of the
    liver

U

uric acid, urine

Type of test   Urine (24-hour)

Normal findings   250-750 ml/24 hr or 1.48-4.43 mmol/day (SI units)

Test explanation and related physiology

Uric acid is a nitrogenous compound that is a product of purine (a DNA building block) catabolism. (See p. 842 for blood uric acid level.) Uric acid is excreted to a large degree by the kidney and to a smaller degree by the intestinal tract. When the uric acid levels are elevated, the patient may have gout. Uric acid levels can be measured in both the blood and the urine. Urine levels of uric acid are helpful in evaluating uric acid metabolism in gout and for assessing hyperuricosuria in patients with renal calculus formation. This test also helps to identify people at risk for stone formation.

Interfering factors

- Recent use of x-ray contrast agents may increase uric acid levels in the urine.
- ☤ Drugs that may interfere with test results include alcohol, antiinflammatory preparations, salicylates, thiazide diuretics, vitamin C, and warfarin.

Procedure and patient care

Before

- Explain the procedure to the patient.
- Tell the patient that no special diet is usually required.

During

- Instruct the patient to begin the 24-hour urine collection after voiding. Discard the initial specimen, and start the 24-hour timing at that point.
- Collect all the urine passed during the next 24 hours. A preservative may be used.
- Show the patient where to store the urine container.
- Keep the specimen on ice or refrigerated during the entire 24 hours. (Note that some laboratories do not require refrigeration.)

- Indicate the starting time on the urine container and laboratory slip.
- Post the hours for the urine collection in a noticeable place to prevent accidental discarding of the specimen.
- Instruct the patient to void before defecating so the urine is not contaminated by feces.
- Remind the patient not to put toilet paper in the collection container.
- Encourage the patient to drink fluids during the 24 hours.
- Instruct the patient to collect the last specimen as close as possible to the end of the 24-hour period. Add this urine to the container.

After

- Transport the urine specimen promptly to the laboratory.

Abnormal findings

▲ **Increased levels (uricosuria)**

Gout

Chronic myelogenous leukemia

Polycythemia vera

Ulcerative colitis

Febrile illness

Liver disease

Toxemia of pregnancy

High purine diet

▼ **Decreased levels**

Kidney disease (chronic glomerulonephritis, urinary obstruction)

Eclampsia

Lead toxicity

Chronic alcohol ingestion

notes

U

urinalysis (UA)

Type of test Urine

Normal findings

Appearance: clear
Color: amber yellow
Odor: aromatic
pH: 4.6-8.0 (average 6.0)
Protein
  None or up to 8 mg/dl
  50-80 mg/dl (at rest)
  <250 mg/dl (exercise)
Specific gravity
  Adult: 1.005-1.030 (usually 1.010-1.025)
  Elderly: values decrease with age
  Newborn: 1.001-1.020
Leukocyte esterase: negative
Nitrites: negative
Ketones: negative
Crystals: negative
Casts: none present
Glucose (see urine glucose discussion, p. 429)
  Brand new specimen: negative
  24-hour specimen: <0.5 g/dl or <70 mmol/day (SI units)
White blood cells (WBCs): 0-4 per low-power field
WBC casts: negative
Red blood cells (RBCs): up to 2
RBC casts: none

Test explanation and related physiology

A total urinalysis involves multiple routine tests on a urine specimen. This specimen is not necessarily a clean-catch specimen. However, if urinary tract infection is suspected, often a midstream, clean-catch specimen is obtained. This urine is then split into two portions. One is sent for urinalysis, and the other is held in the laboratory refrigerator and cultured (see p. 860) if the urinalysis indicates infection. Routinely, a urinalysis includes remarks as to the color, appearance, and odor of the urine. The pH is determined. The urine is tested for the presence of proteins, glucose, ketones, blood, and leukocyte esterase. The urine is examined microscopically for RBCs, WBCs, casts, crystals, and bacteria.

Appearance and color

Urine appearance and color are noted as part of routine urinalysis. The appearance of a normal urine specimen should be clear. Cloudy urine may be caused by the presence of pus, RBCs, or bacteria; however, normal urine also may be cloudy because of ingestion of certain foods (e.g., large amounts of fat, ureates, or phosphates). The color of urine ranges from pale yellow to amber because of the pigment urochrome. The color indicates the concentration of the urine and varies with specific gravity. Dilute urine is straw colored, and concentrated urine is deep amber.

Abnormally colored urine may result from a pathologic condition or the ingestion of certain foods or medicines. For example, bleeding from the kidney produces dark-red urine, whereas bleeding from the lower urinary tract produces bright-red urine. Dark-yellow urine may indicate the presence of urobilinogen or bilirubin. *Pseudomonas* organisms may produce green urine. Beets may cause red urine, and rhubarb can color the urine brown. Many frequently used drugs also may affect urine color (Table 17).

Odor

Determination of urine odor is a part of routine urinalysis. The aromatic odor of fresh, normal urine is caused by the presence of volatile acids. Urine of patients with diabetic ketoacidosis has the strong, sweet smell of acetone. In patients with a urinary tract infection, the urine may have a very foul odor. Patients with a fecal odor to their urine may have an enterobladder fistula.

pH

The analysis of the pH of a freshly voided urine specimen indicates the acid-base balance of the patient. An alkaline pH is obtained in a patient with alkalemia. Also, bacteria, urinary tract infection, or a diet high in citrus fruits or vegetables may cause an increased urine pH. Certain medications (e.g., streptomycin, neomycin, kanamycin) are effective in treating urinary tract infections when the urine is alkaline. Acidic urine is generally obtained in patients with acidemia, which can result from metabolic or respiratory acidosis, starvation, dehydration, or a diet high in meat products or cranberries.

The urine pH is useful in identifying crystals in the urine and

TABLE 17 Frequently used drugs that may affect urine color

Generic and brand names	Drug classification	Urine color
Anisindione (Miradon)	Oral anticoagulant	Red-orange in alkaline urine
Cascara sagrada	Stimulant laxative	Red in alkaline urine; yellow-brown in acid urine
Chloroquine (Aralen)	Antimalarial	Rusty yellow or brown
Chlorzoxazone (Paraflex)	Skeletal muscle relaxant	Orange or purple-red
Docusate calcium (Doxidan, Surfak)	Laxative	Pink to red to red-brown
Furazolidone (Furoxone)	Antiinfective, antiprotozoal	Brown
Iron preparations (Ferotran, Imferon)	Hematinic	Dark brown or black on standing
Levodopa	Antiparkinsonian	Dark brown on standing

Methylene blue (Urolene Blue)	Antimethemoglobinemic	Blue-green
Nitrofurantoin (Macrodantin, Nitrodan)	Antibacterial	Brown
Phenazopyridine (Pyridium)	Urinary tract analgesic	Orange to red
Phenindione (Eridione)	Anticoagulant	Red-orange in alkaline urine
Phenolphthalein (Ex-Lax)	Contact laxative	Red or purplish pink in alkaline urine
Phenothiazines (e.g., prochlorperazine [Compazine])	Antipsychotic, neuroleptic, antiemetic	Red-brown
Phenytoin (Dilantin)	Anticonvulsant	Pink, red, red-brown
Riboflavin (vitamin B)	Vitamin	Intense yellow
Rifampin	Antibiotic	Red-orange
Sulfasalazine (Azulfidine)	Antibacterial	Orange-yellow in alkaline urine
Triamterene (Dyrenium)	Diuretic	Pale blue fluorescence

U

determining the predisposition to form a given type of stone. Acidic urine is associated with xanthine, cystine, uric acid, and calcium oxalate stones. To treat or prevent these urinary calculi, urine should be kept alkaline. Alkaline urine is associated with calcium carbonate, calcium phosphate, and magnesium phosphate stones; for these stones, urine should be kept acidic.

Protein

Evaluation of protein is a sensitive indicator of kidney function. Normally, protein is not present in the urine, because the spaces in the normal glomerular filtrate membrane are too small to allow its passage. If the glomerular membrane is injured, as in glomerulonephritis, the spaces become much larger and protein seeps out into the filtrate and then into the urine. If this persists at a significant rate, the patient can become hypoproteinemic because of the severe protein loss through the kidneys. This decreases the normal capillary oncotic pressure that holds fluid within the vasculature and causes severe interstitial edema. The combination of proteinuria and edema is known as the nephrotic syndrome.

Proteinuria is probably the most important indicator of renal disease. The urine of all pregnant women is routinely checked for proteinuria, which can be an indicator of preeclampsia. In addition to screening for nephrotic syndrome, urinary protein also screens for complications of diabetes mellitus, glomerulonephritis, amyloidosis, and multiple melanoma (see test for Bence Jones protein, p. 129).

Specific gravity

The specific gravity is a measure of the concentration of particles (including wastes and electrolytes) in the urine. A high specific gravity indicates a concentrated urine; a low specific gravity indicates dilute urine.

The specific gravity is used to evaluate the concentrating and excretory power of the kidney. Renal disease tends to diminish the concentrating capability of the kidney. As a result, chronic renal diseases are associated with a low specific gravity. The specific gravity must be interpreted in light of the presence or absence of glycosuria and proteinuria. The specific gravity is also a measurement of the hydration status of the patient. An overhydrated patient will have a more dilute urine with a lower specific gravity. The specific gravity of the urine in a dehydrated patient can be expected to be abnormally high. The measurement of urine specific gravity is easier and more convenient than the measurement of osmolality (see p. 585). The specific gravity correlates roughly with osmolality. Knowledge of the specific gravity is needed for interpreting the results of most parts of the urinalysis. Specific gravity is usually evaluated by the use of a refractometer or a dipstick.

Leukocyte esterase (WBC esterase)

Leukocyte (WBC) esterase is a screening test used to detect leukocytes in the urine. When positive, this test indicates a urinary tract infection. This examination employs chemical testing with a leukocyte esterase dipstick; a shade of purple is considered positive. Some laboratories have established screening protocols in which a microscopic examination (see p. 860) is only performed if a leukocyte esterase test is positive.

Nitrites

Like the leukocyte esterase, the nitrite test is a screening test for the identification of urinary tract infections. This test is based on the principle that many bacteria produce an enzyme called *reductase,* which can reduce urinary nitrates to nitrites. Chemical testing is done with a dipstick containing a reagent that reacts with nitrites to produce a pink color, thus indirectly suggesting the presence of bacteria. A positive test result would indicate the need for a urine culture. Nitrite screening enhances the sensitivity of the leukocyte esterase test to detect urinary tract infections.

Ketones

Normally, no ketones are present in the urine; however, a patient with poorly controlled diabetes who is hyperglycemic may have massive fatty acid catabolism. The purpose of this catabolism is to provide an energy source when glucose cannot be transferred into the cell because of an insufficiency of insulin. Ketones (beta-hydroxybutyric acid, acetoacidic acid, and acetone) are the end products of this fatty acid breakdown. As with glucose, ketones spill over into the urine when the blood levels of patients with diabetes are elevated. The excess production of ketones in the urine is usually associated with poorly controlled diabetes. This test for ketonuria is also important in evaluating ketoacidosis associated with alcoholism, fasting, starvation, high-protein diets, and isopropanol ingestion. Ketonuria may occur with acute febrile illnesses, especially in infants and children.

U

Crystals

Crystals found in the urinary sediment on microscopic examination indicate that renal stone formulation is imminent, if not already present. Urea crystals occur in patients with high serum uric acid levels (gout). Phosphate and calcium oxalate crystals occur in the urine of patients with parathyroid abnormalities or malabsorption states. The type of crystal found varies with the disease and the pH of the urine (see above discussion on urinary pH).

Hyaline casts

Casts are clumps of materials or cells. They are found in the renal collecting tubules and have the shape of the tubule, thus the term *cast*. Hyaline casts are conglomerations of protein and indicate proteinuria. A few hyaline casts are normally found—especially after strenuous exercise.

Granular casts

Granular casts result from the disintegration of cellular material in WBCs and epithelial cells into granular particles. Granular casts are found after exercise and in patients with various renal diseases.

Fatty casts

Usually composed of individual fat droplets, fatty casts occur most often in patients with nephrotic syndrome.

Epithelial casts (renal tubular casts)

Epithelial casts are formed from tubular epithelial cells. The presence of occasional epithelial cells is not remarkable. Tubular (epithelial) casts are most suggestive of glomerulonephritis.

Waxy casts

Waxy casts may be cell casts, hyaline casts, or renal failure casts. Waxy casts are found especially in patients with chronic renal diseases and are associated with chronic renal failure. They also occur in patients with diabetic nephropathy, malignant hypertension, and glomerulonephritis.

White blood cells and casts

Normally, few WBCs are found in the urine sediment on microscopic examination. The presence of five or more WBCs in the urine indicates a urinary tract infection. A clean-catch urine culture should be done for further evaluation.

Hence, on microscopic examination of the urine sediment, WBC casts are most frequently found in patients with acute pyelonephritis. WBC casts are also seen in patients with glomerulonephritis and lupus nephritis.

Red blood cells and casts

Any disruption in the blood-urine barrier whether at the glomerular or tubular level will cause RBCs to enter the urine. This is seen in patients with glomerulonephritis, interstitial nephritis, acute necrosis, polynephritis, renal trauma, or renal tumor. Pathologic conditions (e.g., tumors, trauma, stones, infection) that involve the mucous membrane in the collecting system will also cause hematuria. This can be detected easily by routine analysis.

RBC casts suggest glomerulonephritis, which may exist in patients with some acute bacterial endocarditis, renal infarct, Goodpasture's syndrome, vasculitis, sickle cell disease, or malignant hypertension.

Interfering factors

- Certain foods affect urine color. Carrots may cause a dark-yellow color. Beets may cause a red-colored urine. Rhubarb may cause a red or brown discoloration.
- Urine color darkens with prolonged standing.
- Some foods (e.g., asparagus) produce characteristic urine odors.
- When urine stands for a long time and begins to decompose, it has an ammonia-like smell.
- The urine pH becomes alkaline on standing because of the action of urea-splitting bacteria, producing ammonia.
- The urine pH of an uncovered specimen will become alkaline because carbon dioxide will vaporize from the urine and into the air.
- Dietary factors affect urine pH. An alkaline urine is observed in people who eat large quantities of citrus fruits, dairy products, and vegetables. Acidic urine is observed with a diet high in meat and certain foods (e.g., cranberries).
- A transient proteinuria may be associated with severe emotional stress, excess exercise, and cold baths.
- Radiopaque contrast media received within the last 3 days may cause false-positive results for protein in the urine.
- Urine contaminated with vaginal secretions may cause proteinuria.
- Recent use of radiographic dyes in the urine increases specific gravity.
- False-positive leukocyte esterase results may occur in specimens contaminated with vaginal secretions (e.g., heavy menstrual discharge, *Trichomonas* infection, and parasites).

U

- False-negative leukocyte esterase results may occur in specimens containing high levels of protein or ascorbic acid.
- Special diets (carbohydrate-free, high-protein, high-fat) may cause ketonuria.
- Radiographic dyes may cause precipitation of urinary crystals.
- Vaginal discharge may contaminate the urine specimen and factitiously cause WBCs in the urine.
- Strenuous physical exercise may cause RBC casts. Traumatic urethral catheterization may cause RBCs in the urine.
- Many drugs affect urine color and appearance (see Table 17).
- Drugs that may affect urine color include antibiotics and vitamins.
- Drugs that may cause acidic urine include ammonium chloride, chlorothiazide diuretics, and methenamine mandelate.
- Drugs that may cause alkaline urine include acetazolamide, potassium citrate, and sodium bicarbonate.
- Drugs that may cause *increased* protein levels include acetazolamide, aminoglycosides, amphotericin B, cephalosporins, colistin, griseofulvin, lithium, methicillin, nafcillin, nephrotoxic drugs (e.g., arsenicals, gold salts), oxacillin, penicillamine, penicillin G, phenazopyridine, polymyxin B, salicylates, sulfonamides, tolbutamide, and vancomycin.
- Drugs that may cause *increased* specific gravity include dextran and sucrose.
- Drugs that may cause false-positive results for ketones include bromosulfophthalein (BSP), isoniazid, isopropanol, levodopa, paraldehyde, phenazopyridine, and PSP dye.

Procedure and patient care

Before

- Explain the procedure to the patient.

During

- Collect a fresh urine specimen in a urine container.
- If the urine specimen contains vaginal discharge or bleeding, a clean-catch or midstream specimen will be needed. This requires meticulous cleaning of the urinary meatus with an iodine preparation to reduce contamination of the specimen by external organisms. The cleansing agent then must be

completely removed, or it will contaminate the specimen. The midstream collection is obtained by:

1. Having the patient begin to urinate in a bedpan, urinal, or toilet and then stop urinating (this washes the urine out of the distal urethra)
2. Correctly positioning a sterile urine container into which the patient voids 3 to 4 ounces of urine
3. Capping the container
4. Allowing the patient to finish voiding

- For ketones, this test can be performed immediately after collection by placing a drop of urine on an Acetest tablet. If acetone is present, shades of lavender will appear at the designated time.
- With a Ketostix, dip the reagent into the urine specimen and remove it. Read the strip in 15 seconds by comparing it with the color chart.
- For urine specific gravity, a first-voided specimen is best obtained.
- For protein, again the first-voided specimen is best; however, occasionally a 24-hour urine collection (see p. 374) is preferred.

After

- Transport the urine specimen to the laboratory promptly.
- If the specimen cannot be processed immediately, refrigerate it.
- If a 24-hour urine collection is requested, the specimen should be refrigerated or preserved with formalin during the collection time.
- Casts will break up as urine is allowed to sit. Urine examinations for casts should be performed on fresh specimens.

Abnormal findings

Appearance and color

Bacteria
Pus
Red blood cells
Certain foods (e.g., beets, carrots)
Drug therapy (see Table 17)
Pathologic conditions (e.g., bleeding from the kidney)

Dehydration
Overhydration
Diabetes insipidus
Fever
Excessive sweating
Jaundice

U

Odor

Infection
Ketonuria
Urinary tract infection
Rectal fistula

Maple sugar urine disease
Phenylketonuria
Hepatic failure

pH

▲ **Increased levels**

Respiratory alkalosis
Metabolic alkalosis
Urea-splitting bacteria
Vegetarian diet
Renal failure with inability to form ammonia
Gastric suction
Vomiting
Diuretic therapy
Renal tubular acidosis
Urinary tract infection

▼ **Decreased levels**

Metabolic acidosis
Diabetes mellitus
Diarrhea
Starvation
Respiratory acidosis
Emphysema
Sleep
Pyrexia

Protein

▲ **Increased levels**

Nephrotic syndrome
Diabetes mellitus
Multiple myeloma
Preeclampsia
Glomerulonephritis
Congestive heart failure
Malignant hypertension
Polycystic disease
Diabetic glomerulosclerosis

▼ **Decreased levels**

Amyloidosis
Lupus erythematosus
Goodpasture's syndrome
Renal vein thrombosis
Heavy-metal poisoning
Galactosemia
Bacterial pyelonephritis
Nephrotoxic drug therapy
Bladder tumor

Specific gravity

▲ **Increased levels**

Dehydration (because kidneys are reabsorbing all available free water; thus, excreted urine is very concentrated)

Pituitary tumor or trauma that causes syndrome of inappropriate release of excessive antidiuretic hormone (SIADH), resulting in excessive water reabsorption

Decrease in renal blood flow (as in heart failure, renal artery stenosis, or hypotension)

Glycosuria and proteinuria

Water restriction

Fever

Excessive sweating

Vomiting

Diarrhea

X-ray contrast dye

▼ **Decreased levels**

Overhydration

Diabetes insipidus (because of the inadequate antidiuretic hormone secretion, which causes a decrease in water reabsorption)

Renal failure (because the kidney has lost its ability to concentrate urine through water reabsorption)

Diuresis

Hypothermia

Glomerulonephritis

Pyelonephritis

Leukocyte esterase

Possible urinary tract infection

Nitrites

Possible urinary tract infection

Ketones

Uncontrolled diabetes mellitus

Starvation

Excessive aspirin ingestion

Ketoacidosis of alcoholism

Febrile illnesses in infants and children

Weight reduction diets

Following anesthesia

Prolonged vomiting

Anorexia

Fasting

High-protein diets

Isopropanol ingestion

Dehydration

U

Crystals

Renal stone formation
Drug therapy
Urinary tract infection

Granular casts

Acute tubular necrosis
Urinary tract infection
Glomerulonephritis
Pyelonephritis
Nephrosclerosis
Chronic lead poisoning
Reaction after exercise
Stress
Renal transplant rejection

Fatty casts

Nephrotic syndrome
Diabetic nephropathy
Glomerulonephritis
Chronic renal disease

Epithelial casts

Glomerulonephritis
Eclampsia
Heavy-metal poisoning
Ethylene glycol intoxication
Acute renal allograph rejection

Waxy casts

Chronic renal disease
Chronic renal failure
Diabetic nephropathy
Malignant hypertension
Glomerulonephritis
Renal transplant rejection
Nephrotic syndrome

Hyaline casts

Proteinuria
Fever
Strenuous exercise
Stress
Glomerulonephritis
Pyelonephritis
Congestive heart failure
Chronic renal failure

Red blood cells and casts

▲ **Increased RBC levels**

Glomerulonephritis
Interstitial nephritis
Acute tubular necrosis
Pyelonephritis
Renal trauma
Renal tumor
Renal stones
Cystitis
Prostatitis
Traumatic bladder catheterization

▲ **Increased RBC cast levels**

Glomerulonephritis
Subacute bacterial endocarditis
Renal infarct
Goodpasture's syndrome
Vasculitis
Sickling
Malignant hypertension
Systemic lupus erythematosus

White blood cells and casts

▲ **Increased WBC levels**
  Bacterial infection in the urinary tract

▲ **Increased WBC cast levels**
  Acute pyelonephritis
  Glomerulonephritis
  Lupus nephritis

notes

urine culture and sensitivity (C&S)

Type of test Urine

Normal findings Negative

Test explanation and related physiology

Urine cultures and sensitivities are obtained to determine the presence of pathogenic bacteria in patients with suspected urinary tract infections. All cultures should be performed before antibiotic therapy is initiated; otherwise, the antibiotic may interrupt the growth of the organism in the laboratory. More often than not, however, the physician will want to institute antibiotic therapy before the culture results are reported. In these instances, a *Gram stain* of the specimen smeared on a slide is most helpful and can be reported in less than 10 minutes. All forms of bacteria are grossly classified as gram positive (blue staining) or gram negative (red staining). Knowledge of the shape of the organism (e.g., spheric, rod shaped) also can be very helpful in the tentative identification of the infective organism. With knowledge of the Gram stain results, the physician can institute a reasonable antibiotic regimen based on past experience as to the organism's possible identity. Most organisms require approximately 24 hours to grow in the laboratory, and a preliminary report can be given at that time. Occasionally, 48 to 72 hours are required for growth and identification of the organism. Cultures may be repeated after appropriate antibiotic therapy to assess for complete resolution of the infection (especially in urinary tract infections).

To save money in some institutions, urine cultures are only done if the urinalysis suggests a possible infection (e.g., increased number of white blood cells [WBCs], bacteria, high pH, leukocyte esterase). In these institutions, urine is collected and "split." One half is sent for urinalysis, and the other is held in the laboratory refrigerator and evaluated only if the urinalysis indicates a possible infection.

Interfering factors

✶ Drugs that may affect test results include antibiotics.

Procedure and patient care

Before

- Explain to the patient the procedure for collecting a clean-catch (midstream) urine collection.

- Hold antibiotics until after the urine specimen has been collected.
- Provide the patient with the necessary supplies for the collection.

During

- Note that a clean-catch or midstream urine collection is required for culture and sensitivity (C&S) testing. This requires meticulous cleansing of the urinary meatus with an iodine preparation to reduce contamination of the specimen by external organisms. Then, the cleansing agent must be completely removed or it will contaminate the urine specimen. The midstream collection is obtained by:
    1. Having the patient begin to urinate in a bedpan, urinal, or toilet and then stop urinating (This washes the urine out of the distal urethra.)
    2. Correctly positioning a sterile urine container, into which the patient voids 3 to 4 ounces of urine
    3. Capping the container
    4. Allowing the patient to finish voiding
- Note that *urinary catheterization* may be needed for patients unable to void. This procedure is not usually performed, however, because of the risk of inducing organisms and because of patient discomfort.
- For inpatients with an *indwelling urinary catheter,* obtain a specimen by attaching a small-gauge (e.g., 25) needle to a syringe and aseptically inserting the needle into the catheter at a point distal to the sleeve leading to the balloon. Urine is aspirated and then placed in a sterile urine container. (Usually, the catheter tubing distal to the puncture site needs to be clamped for 15 to 30 minutes before the aspiration of urine to allow urine to fill the tubing. After the specimen is withdrawn, the clamp is removed.)
- Note that *suprapubic aspiration* of urine is a safe method of obtaining urine in neonates and infants. The abdomen is prepared with an antiseptic, and a 25-gauge needle is inserted into the suprapubic area 1 inch above the symphysis pubis. Urine is aspirated into the syringe and then transferred to a sterile urine container.
- Collect specimens from infants and young children in a disposable pouch called a *U bag.* This bag has an adhesive backing around the opening to attach to the child.
- Note that for patients with a *urinary diversion* (e.g., an ileal

U

conduit), catheterization should be done through the stoma.
Urine should *not* be collected from the ostomy pouch.

- Indicate on the laboratory slip any medications that may affect test results.

After

- Transport the specimen to the laboratory immediately (at least within 30 minutes). If this is not possible, the specimen may be refrigerated up to 2 hours.
- Notify the physician of any positive results so that appropriate antibiotic therapy can be initiated.

Abnormal finding

Urinary tract infection

notes

urine flow studies (Uroflowmetry, Urodynamic studies)

Type of test Urodynamic

Normal findings Depend on the patient's age, gender, and volume voided

Test explanation and related physiology

Uroflowmetry is the simplest of the urodynamic techniques, being noninvasive and requiring uncomplicated and relatively inexpensive equipment. This study measures the volume of urine expelled from the bladder per second. This test is indicated to investigate dysfunctional voiding or suspicious outflow tract obstruction. It is also done before and after any procedure designed to modify the function of the urologic outflow tract.

The urine flow depends greatly on the volume of urine voided. The flow rates are highest and most predictable in the urine volume range of 200 to 400 ml. When the bladder contains more than 400 ml of urine, the efficiency of the bladder muscle is greatly decreased. Nomograms of maximal flow versus voided volume may be used for accurate test result interpretation, taking into account the patient's gender and age. If the flow rates are abnormally low, the test should be repeated to check for accuracy.

Modern urine flowmeters provide a permanent graphic recording. If flowmeters are not available, the patient can time the urinary stream with a stopwatch and record the voided volume; from this, the average flow is calculated.

In some cases, it is more valuable to analyze several voided volumes and flow rates rather than a single flow rate. If this is to be done, the patient is taught to use a flowmeter. A graph of flow versus volume can be plotted. Together with clinical observation, this provides very valuable information on the severity of outflow obstruction, the likelihood of urinary retention, and the state of compensation or decompensation of the detrusor muscle.

Procedure and patient care

Before

- Explain the procedure to the patient.
- Instruct the patient how to void into the urine flowmeter.
- Determine the number of flow rates that will be needed.

During
- Note that this test should be performed when the patient has a normal desire to void and in conditions suitable for privacy. The bladder should be adequately full. Essentially, all the patient must do is urinate into the flowmeter. Several different types of flowmeters are available.
- Tell the patient that no discomfort is associated with this test.
- Note that the duration of this test is several seconds.

After
- Record the position of the patient, the method of filling the bladder (it should be natural), and whether this study was part of another evaluation.

Abnormal findings

Dysfunctional voiding
Outflow tract obstruction caused by urethral stricture, prostatic cancer, or hypertrophy

notes

uroporphyrinogen-I-synthase

Type of test Blood

Normal findings 1.27-2.00 mU/g of hemoglobin or 81.9-129.6 U/mol Hgb (SI units)

Test explanation and related physiology

Porphyria is a group of disorders characterized by abdominal pain, neuromuscular signs and symptoms, constipation, and, occasionally, psychotic behavior. This group of disorders results from an enzymatic deficiency in anabolism of heme (a portion of hemoglobin). Acute intermittent porphyria is the most common form of these disorders; this is caused by a deficiency in porphobilinogen deaminase. Another name for this enzyme is uroporphyrinogen-I-synthase. This enzyme is necessary for the red blood cell to fabricate heme. While this enzyme is significantly reduced during the acute phase of this disorder, it is still noted to be reduced in the latent (asymptomatic) phase of this disorder. It is important to identify this disease process, because acute bouts of porphyria occasionally may be fatal. See p. 642 for more discussions on the metabolic testing for porphyria.

Procedure and patient care

Before
- Explain the procedure to the patient.
- Tell the patient that no fasting is required.

During
- Collect 7 ml of peripheral venous blood in a purple-top tube.
- Because this test is based on the hemoglobin measurement, concurrently obtain a hemoglobin level on the patient.

After
- Indicate on the laboratory slip if the patient is having symptoms of acute porphyria.
- Apply pressure or a pressure dressing to the venipuncture site.
- Assess the venipuncture site for bleeding.

Abnormal finding

▼ **Decreased levels**
   Acute intermittent porphyria

U

vanillylmandelic acid and catecholamines (VMA and epinephrine, norepinephrine, metanephrine, normetanephrine, dopamine)

Type of test Urine (24-hour)

Normal findings

VMA

Adult/elderly: 2-7 mg/24 hr or 10-35 μmol/24 hr (SI units)
Adolescent: 1-5 mg/24 hr
Child: 1-3 mg/24 hr
Infant: <2.0 mg/24 hr
Newborn: <1.0 mg/24 hr

Catecholamines

Epinephrine
Adult/elderly: 0.5-20.0 μg/24 hr or <275 nmol/24 hr (SI units)
Child
  0-1 years: 0-2.5 μg/24 hr
  1-2 years: 0-3.5 μg/24 hr
  2-4 years: 0.0-6.0 μg/24 hr
  4-7 years: 0.2-10.0 μg/24 hr
  7-10 years: 0.5-14.0 μg/24 hr

Norepinephrine
Adult/elderly: 15-80 μg/24 hr
Child
  0-1 years: 0-10 μg/24 hr
  1-2 years: 0-17 μg/24 hr
  2-4 years: 4-29 μg/24 hr
  4-7 years: 8-45 μg/24 hr
  7-10 years: 13-65 μg/24 hr

Dopamine
Adult/elderly: 65-400 μg/24 hr
Child
  0-1 years: 0-85 μg/24 hr
  1-2 years: 10-140 μg/24 hr
  2-4 years: 40-260 μg/24 hr
  >4 years: 65-400 μg/24 hr

Metanephrine
24-96 μg/24 hr

Normetanephrine
75-375 µg/24 hr

Test explanation and related physiology

This 24-hour urine test for VMA and catecholamines is primarily performed to diagnose hypertension secondary to pheochromocytoma. This test is also used to detect the presence of neuroblastomas and rare adrenal tumors.

A *pheochromocytoma* is an adrenal tumor that frequently secretes abnormally high levels of epinephrine and norepinephrine. These hormones cause episodic or persistent hypertension by causing peripheral arterial vasoconstriction. Dopamine is the precursor of epinephrine and norepinephrine. Metanephrine and normetanephrine are catabolic products of epinephrine and norepinephrine, respectively. VMA is the product of catabolism of both metanephrine and normetanephrine. In patients with pheochromocytoma, one or all of these substances will be present in excessive quantities in a 24-hour collection of urine.

Interfering factors

- Increased levels of VMA may be caused by certain foods (e.g., tea, coffee, cocoa, vanilla, chocolate).
- Vigorous exercise, stress, and starvation may cause increased VMA levels.
- Falsely decreased levels of VMA may be caused by uremia, alkaline urine, and radiographic iodine contrast agents.
- Drugs that may cause *increased* VMA levels include caffeine, epinephrine, levodopa, lithium, and nitroglycerin.
- Drugs that may cause *decreased* VMA levels include clonidine, disulfiram (Antabuse), guanethidine, imipramine, monoamine oxidase (MAO) inhibitors, phenothiazines, and reserpine.
- Drugs that may cause *increased* catecholamine levels include alcohol (ethyl), aminophylline, caffeine, chloral hydrate, clonidine (chronic therapy), contrast media (iodine containing), disulfiram, epinephrine, erythromycin, insulin, methenamine, methyldopa, nicotinic acid (large doses), nitroglycerin, quinidine, riboflavin, and tetracyclines.
- Drugs that may cause *decreased* catecholamine levels include guanethidine, reserpine, and salicylates.

V

Procedure and patient care

Before

- Explain the dietary restrictions and the 24-hour urine collection procedure to the patient.
- For 2 or 3 days before the 24-hour collection for VMA and throughout the collection, place the patient on a VMA-restricted diet. Generally, instruct the patient to avoid coffee, tea, bananas, chocolate, cocoa, licorice, citrus fruit, all foods and fluids containing vanilla, and also aspirin. Obtain specific restrictions from the laboratory.
- Restrict the patient from taking antihypertensive medications, and sometimes all medications, during this period and possibly even longer.

During

- Collect the 24-hour urine specimen using a preservative.
- Instruct the patient to begin the 24-hour urine collection after voiding. Discard the initial specimen and note the time; this is the starting time.
- Collect all urine passed during the next 24 hours. Refrigerate or keep on ice during the collection period.
- Post the hours for the urine collection in a prominent place to avoid accidental discarding of the specimen.
- Remind the patient to void before defecating so that the urine is not contaminated by feces.
- Instruct the patient not to put toilet paper in the collection container.
- Encourage the patient to drink fluids during the 24 hours unless contraindicated for medical purposes.
- Collect the last specimen as close as possible to the end of the 24-hour period. Add this urine to the container.
- Indicate the time of the last specimen collected on the laboratory slip or urine container.
- Identify and minimize factors contributing to patient stress and anxiety. Excessive physical exercise and emotion may alter catecholamine test results by causing an increased secretion of epinephrine and norepinephrine.

After

- Send the specimen to the laboratory as soon as the test is completed.
- Allow the patient to have foods and drugs that have been restricted in preparation for the test.

Abnormal findings

▲ **Increased levels**

Pheochromocytomas	Severe stress
Neuroblastomas	Strenuous exercise
Ganglioneuromas	Acute anxiety
Ganglioblastomas	

notes

V

venography of lower extremities (Phlebography, Venogram)

Type of test X-ray with contrast dye

Normal findings No evidence of venous thrombosis or obstruction

Test explanation and related physiology

Venography is an x-ray study designed to identify and locate thrombi within the venous system of the lower extremities. During this study, dye is injected into the venous system of the affected extremity. X-ray films are then taken at timed intervals to visualize the venous system. Obstruction to the flow of dye or a filling defect within the dye-filled vein indicates that thrombosis exists. A positive study accurately confirms the diagnosis of venous thrombosis; however, a normal study, although not as accurate, does make the diagnosis of venous thrombosis very unlikely. Often, both extremities are studied, even though only one leg is suspected to contain deep-vein thrombosis. The normal extremity is used for comparison with the involved extremity. Unlike venous plethysmography (see p. 638), venography is accurate for thrombi in veins below the knee.

Contraindications

- Patients with severe edema of the legs, making venous access impossible
- Patients who are uncooperative
- Patients who are allergic to iodinated dye or shellfish
- Patients with renal failure, because the iodinated dye is nephrotoxic

Potential complications

- Allergic reaction to iodinated dyes
  Allergic reactions vary from flushing, itching, and urticaria to severe, life-threatening anaphylaxis (evidenced by respiratory distress, drop in blood pressure, shock). In the event of anaphylaxis, the patient may be treated with diphenhydramine (Benadryl), steroids, and epinephrine. Oxygen and endotracheal equipment should be on hand for immediate use.
- Renal failure, especially in elderly people who are chronically dehydrated or may have a mild degree of renal failure

- Subcutaneous infiltration of the dye, causing cellulitis and pain
- Venous thrombophlebitis caused by the dye
- Bacteremia caused by a break in sterile technique
- Venous embolism caused by dislodgment of a deep-vein clot induced by the dye injection

Procedure and patient care

Before

- Explain the procedure to the patient.
- Obtain informed consent for this procedure.
- Assess the patient for allergies to iodinated dyes and shellfish. If a suspected allergy exists and the venogram is absolutely necessary, the patient should receive a steroid-and-antihistamine preparation. Notify the radiologist of the potential for allergic reaction so that hypoallergenic, nonionic contrast may be used.
- If needed, provide appropriate pain medication so the patient is able to lie still during the procedure.
- Ensure that the patient is appropriately hydrated before testing. Injection of the iodinated contrast may cause renal failure, especially in the elderly.

During

- Note the following procedural steps:
  1. The patient is taken to the radiology department and placed in a supine position on the x-ray table.
  2. Catheterization of a superficial vein on the foot is performed. This may require a surgical cutdown.
  3. An iodinated, radiopaque dye is injected into the vein.
  4. X-ray films are taken to follow the course of the dye up the leg.
  5. Frequently, a tourniquet is placed on the leg to prevent filling of the superficial saphenous vein. All of the dye therefore goes to filling the deep venous system, which contains the most clinically significant thrombosis that can embolize.
- Note that a radiologist performs this study in approximately 30 to 90 minutes.
- Tell the patient that the venous catheterization is only as uncomfortable as a cutaneous heel stick or a small incision in the foot.

V

- The dye may cause the patient to feel a warm flush. (This is not as severe as that noted with arteriography.) Inform the patient that occasionally, mild degrees of nausea, vomiting, or skin itching also may occur.

After

- Continue appropriate hydration of the patient to prevent dehydration caused by the diuretic action of the dye.
- Observe the puncture site for infection, cellulitis, or bleeding.
- Assess the patient's vital signs for signs of bacteremia (e.g., high temperature, tachycardia, chills, fever).
- Evaluate the patient for signs of allergic reaction (e.g., rash, chills, fever, irritability). Treat with antihistamines or steroids.

Abnormal findings

Obstructed venous systems caused by thrombosis, tumor, or inflammation
Acute deep-vein thrombosis

notes

white blood cell count and differential count (WBC and differential, Leukocyte count, Neutrophil count, Lymphocyte count, Monocyte count, Eosinophil count, Basophil count)

Type of test Blood

Normal findings

Total WBCs

Adult/child >2 years: 5000-10,000/mm^3 or 5-10.0 × 10^9/L (SI units)
Child ≤2 years: 6200-17,000/mm^3
Newborn: 9000-30,000/mm^3

Differential count

Neutrophils: 55% to 70%
Lymphocytes: 20% to 40%
Monocytes: 2% to 8%
Eosinophils: 1% to 4%
Basophils: 0.5% to 1.0%

Possible critical values WBCs <2500 or >30,000/mm^3

Test explanation and related physiology

The WBC count has two components. One is a count of the total number of WBCs (leukocytes) in 1 mm^3 of peripheral venous blood. The other component, the differential count, measures the percentage of each type of leukocyte present in the same specimen. An increase in the percentage of one type of leukocyte means a decrease in the percentage of another. Neutrophils and lymphocytes make up 75% to 90% of the total leukocytes. These leukocyte types may be identified easily by their morphology on a venous blood smear. The total leukocyte count has a wide range of normal values, but many diseases may induce abnormal values. An increased total WBC count (leukocytosis) usually indicates infection, inflammation, tissue necrosis, or leukemic neoplasia. Trauma or stress, either emotional or physical, may increase the WBC count. Leukopenia (i.e., a decreased WBC count) occurs in many forms of bone marrow failure (e.g., following antineoplastic chemotherapy or radiation therapy, marrow infiltrative diseases, overwhelming infections, dietary deficiencies, and autoimmune diseases).

W

The major function of the WBCs is to fight infection and re-act against foreign bodies or tissues. Five types of WBCs may easily be identified on a routine blood smear. These cells, in or-der of frequency, include neutrophils, lymphocytes, monocytes, eosinophils, and basophils. All these WBCs arise from the same "pluripotent" stem cell within the bone marrow as the red blood cell (RBC) does. Beyond this origin, however, each cell line dif-ferentiates separately. Most mature WBCs are then deposited into the circulating blood.

Polymorphonuclear *neutrophils* are produced in 7 to 14 days and exist in the circulation for only 6 hours. The primary func-tion of the neutrophil is phagocytosis (killing and digestion of bacterial microorganisms). Acute bacterial infections and trauma stimulate neutrophil production, resulting in an increased WBC count. Often, when neutrophil production is stimulated, early immature forms of neutrophils enter the circulation. These im-mature forms are called *band* or *stab cells*. This process, referred to as a "shift to the left" in WBC production, is indicative of an ongoing acute bacterial infection.

Lymphocytes are divided into two types: T cells and B cells. T cells are primarily involved with cellular-type immune reactions, whereas B cells participate in humoral immunity (antibody pro-duction). The primary function of the lymphocytes is fighting chronic bacterial infection and acute viral infections. The differ-ential count does not separate the T and B cells but rather counts the combination of the two.

Monocytes are phagocytic cells capable of fighting bacteria in a way very similar to that of the neutrophil. Monocytes can be pro-duced more rapidly, however, and can spend a longer time in the circulation than the neutrophils.

Basophils, and especially *eosinophils,* are involved in the allergic reaction. Parasitic infestations also are capable of stimulating the production of these cells.

The WBC and differential count are routinely measured as part of the complete blood count (see p. 261). Serial WBC counts and differential counts have both diagnostic and prognostic value. For example, a persistent increase in the WBC count may indicate a worsening of an infectious process (e.g., appendicitis). A dramatic decrease in the WBC count below the normal range may indicate marrow failure and delay further chemotherapy in patients undergoing cancer treatment.

Interfering factors

- Eating, physical activity, and stress may cause an increase in WBC and differential values.
- Pregnancy (final month) and labor may cause increased WBC levels.
- Patients who have had a splenectomy have a persistent, mild elevation of WBC counts.
- ⚔ Drugs that may cause *increased* WBC levels include adrenalin, allopurinol, aspirin, chloroform, epinephrine, heparin, quinine, steroids, and triamterene (Dyrenium).
- ⚔ Drugs that may cause *decreased* WBC levels include antibiotics, anticonvulsants, antihistamines, antimetabolites, antithyroid drugs, arsenicals, barbiturates, chemotherapeutic agents, diuretics, and sulfonamides.

Procedure and patient care

Before
- Explain the procedure to the patient.
- Tell the patient that no fasting is required.

During
- Collect approximately 5 to 7 ml of venous blood in a lavender-top tube.

After
- Apply pressure or a pressure dressing to the venipuncture site.
- Check the venipuncture site for bleeding.

Abnormal findings

▲ **Increased WBC count (leukocytosis)**
Infection
Leukemic neoplasia
Trauma
Stress
Tissue necrosis
Inflammation

▼ **Decreased WBC count (leukopenia)**
Drug toxicity (e.g., chloramphenicol)
Bone marrow failure
Overwhelming infections
Dietary deficiency
Autoimmune disease
Bone marrow infiltration (e.g., myelofibrosis)

▲▼ **Increased/decreased differential count**
See Table 18

W

TABLE 18 Causes for abnormalities in the WBC differential count

Type of WBC	Elevated	Decreased
Neutrophils	*Neutrophilia* Physical or emotional stress Acute suppurative infection Myelocytic leukemia Trauma Cushing's syndrome Inflammatory disorders (e.g., rheumatic fever, thyroiditis, rheumatoid arthritis) Metabolic disorders (e.g., ketoacidosis, gout, eclampsia)	*Neutropenia* Aplastic anemia Dietary deficiency Overwhelming bacterial infection (especially in the elderly) Viral infections (e.g., hepatitis, influenza, measles) Radiation therapy Addison's disease Drug therapy: myelotoxic drugs (as in chemotherapy)
Lymphocytes	*Lymphocytosis* Chronic bacterial infection Viral infection (e.g., mumps, rubella) Lymphocytic leukemia Multiple myeloma Infectious mononucleosis Radiation Infectious hepatitis	*Lymphocytopenia* Leukemia Sepsis Immunodeficiency diseases Lupus erythematosus Later stages of human immunodeficiency virus infection Drug therapy: adrenocorticosteroids, antineoplastics Radiation therapy

TABLE 18 Causes for abnormalities in the WBC differential count—cont'd

Type of WBC	Elevated	Decreased
Monocytes	*Monocytosis* Chronic inflammatory disorders Viral infections (e.g., infectious mononucleosis) Tuberculosis Chronic ulcerative colitis Parasites (e.g., malaria)	*Monocytopenia* Drug therapy: prednisone
Eosinophils	*Eosinophilia* Parasitic infections Allergic reactions Eczema Leukemia Autoimmune diseases	*Eosinopenia* Increased adrenosteroid production
Basophils	*Basophilia* Myeloproliferative disease (e.g., myelofibrosis, polycythemia rubra vera) Leukemia	*Basopenia* Acute allergic reactions Hyperthyroidism Stress reactions

notes

W

wound culture and sensitivity (C&S)

Type of test Microscopic examination

Normal findings Negative

Test explanation and related physiology

Wound cultures are obtained to determine the presence of pathogens in patients with suspected wound infections. Wound infections are most often caused by pus-forming organisms.

All cultures should be performed before antibiotic therapy is initiated. Otherwise, the antibiotic may interrupt the growth of the organism in the laboratory. More often than not, however, the physician will want to institute antibiotic therapy before the culture results are reported. In these instances, a *Gram stain* of the specimen smeared on a slide is most helpful and can be reported in less than 10 minutes. All forms of bacteria are grossly classified as gram positive (blue staining) or gram negative (red staining). Knowledge of the shape of the organism (e.g., spheric, rod shaped) also may be very helpful in the tentative identification of the infecting organism. With knowledge of the Gram-stain results, the physician can institute a reasonable antibiotic regimen based on past experience as to the organism's possible identity. Most organisms require approximately 24 hours to grow in the laboratory, and a preliminary report can be given at that time. Occasionally, 48 to 72 hours are required for growth and identification of the organism. Cultures may be repeated after appropriate antibiotic therapy to assess for complete resolution of the infection.

Interfering factors

☑ Drugs that may alter test results include antibiotics.

Procedure and patient care

Before

- Explain the procedure to the patient.

During

- Aseptically place a sterile cotton swab into the pus of the patient's wound, and then place the swab into a sterile, covered test tube. (Culturing specimens from the skin edge is much less accurate than culturing the suppurative material.)

- If an anaerobic organism is suspected, obtain an anaerobic culture tube from the microbiology laboratory.
- If wound cultures are to be obtained on a patient requiring wound irrigation, obtain the culture *before* the wound is irrigated.
- If any antibiotic ointment or solution has been previously applied, remove it with sterile water or saline before obtaining the culture.
- Handle all specimens as though they were capable of transmitting disease.
- Indicate on the laboratory slip any medications the patient may be taking that could affect test results.

After
- Transport the specimen to the laboratory immediately after testing (at least within 30 minutes).
- Notify the physician of any positive results so that appropriate antibiotic therapy can be initiated.

Abnormal finding
Wound infection

notes

W

D-xylose absorption test (Xylose tolerance test)

Type of test Blood; urine

Normal findings

Adult/elderly
   Blood levels equal to 25-40 mg/dl 2 hours after ingestion
   80% to 95% excreted in urine 5 hours after ingestion
Child
   Blood levels equal to 30 mg/dl 1 hour after ingestion
   16% to 33% excreted in urine 5 hours after ingestion

Test explanation and related physiology

D-Xylose is a monosaccharide that is easily absorbed by the normal intestine. In patients with malabsorption, intestinal D-xylose absorption is diminished, and as a result, blood levels and urine excretion will be reduced. D-Xylose is the monosaccharide chosen for the test, because it is not metabolized by the body. Its serum levels directly reflect intestinal absorption.

Also, this monosaccharide is used because absorption does not require pancreatic or biliary exocrine function. Its absorption is directly determined by the small intestine. This test is used to separate patients with diarrhea caused by maldigestion (pancreatic/biliary dysfunction) from those with diarrhea caused by malabsorption (sprue, Whipple's disease, Crohn's disease).

In this test, the patient is asked to drink a fluid containing a prescribed amount of D-xylose. Blood and urine levels are subsequently evaluated. Excellent gastrointestinal absorption would be documented by high blood levels and a good urine secretion of D-xylose. Poor intestinal absorption would be marked by decreased blood levels and urine excretion.

Contraindications

- Patients with abnormal kidney function
- Patients who are dehydrated

Interfering factors

✘ Drugs that may affect test results include aspirin, atropine, and indomethacin.

Procedure and patient care

Before

- Explain the procedure to the patient.
- Instruct the adult patient to fast for 8 hours before testing.
- Tell the pediatric patient or the parents that the patient should fast for at least 4 hours before testing.

During

- Collect approximately 7 ml of venous blood in a red-top tube before the patient ingests the D-xylose.
- Collect a first-voided morning urine specimen, and send it to the laboratory.
- Ask the patient to drink 25 g of D-xylose dissolved in 8 ounces of water. Record the time of ingestion.
- Calibrate pediatric doses according to the patient's body weight.
- Repeat venipunctures to obtain blood in exactly 2 hours for an adult and 1 hour for a child.
- Collect urine for a designated time, usually 5 hours. Refrigerate the urine during the collection period.
- Observe the patient for nausea, vomiting, and diarrhea, which may occur as side effects of D-xylose.
- Instruct the patient to remain in a restful position. Intense physical activity may alter the digestive process and affect the test results.

After

- Observe the venipuncture site for bleeding.
- Provide the patient with food or drink and inform the patient that normal activity may be resumed after completion of the study.

Abnormal findings

▼ **Decreased levels**

Malabsorption caused by:
Sprue
Lymphatic obstruction
Enteropathy (e.g., radiation)
Crohn's disease
Whipple's disease
Small intestine bacterial overgrowth
Hookworm
Viral gastroenteritis
Giardia lamblia infestation
Short-bowel syndrome

X

Appendix A: List of tests by body system

CANCER STUDIES

Acid phosphatase, 8-10
Bence Jones protein, 129-130
Bone scan, 160-162
CA 15-3 tumor marker, 175-176
CA 19-9 tumor marker, 177-178
CA-125 tumor marker, 179-180
Carcinoembryonic antigen, 194-195

Estrogen-receptor assay, 376-377
Gallium scan, 405-406
Lymphangiography, 544-546
Mammography, 553-555
Papanicolaou smear, 589-592
Progesterone receptor assay, 662-663
Prostate-specific antigen, 668-669
Sputum cytology, 765-766

CARDIOVASCULAR SYSTEM

Adenosine stress test, 203-206
Aldosterone assay, blood, 32-35
Antimyocardial antibodies, 78
Antistreptolysin O titer, 88-89
Apolipoproteins, 95-99
Arteriography, 100-106
Aspartate aminotransferase, 117-119
Cardiac catheterization, 196-202
Cardiac exercise stress testing, 203-206
Cardiac nuclear scanning, 207-210
Carotid duplex scanning, 211

Catecholamines, 866-869
Chest x-ray, 219-221
Cholesterol, 232-234
Computed tomography of chest, 269-271
Creatine phosphokinase, 293-296
Cryoglobulin, 302-303
Digital subtraction angiography, 100-106
Dipyridamole-thallium scan, 203-206
Dobutamine stress test, 203-206
Doppler studies, 329-331
Echocardiography, 332-334
Electrocardiography, 335-339

Tests in this list are grouped by the following body systems: cancer, cardiovascular, endocrine, gastrointestinal, hematologic, hepatobiliary, immunologic, miscellaneous studies, nervous, pulmonary, reproductive, skeletal, and urologic.

ENDOCRINE SYSTEM

GASTROINTESTINAL SYSTEM

HEMATOLOGIC SYSTEM

HEPATOBILIARY SYSTEM

IMMUNOLOGIC SYSTEM

MISCELLANEOUS TESTS

NERVOUS SYSTEM

PULMONARY SYSTEM

REPRODUCTIVE SYSTEM

SKELETAL SYSTEM

UROLOGIC SYSTEM

Appendix B: List of tests by type

BLOOD TESTS

Tests in this list are grouped by the following types: blood, electrodiagnostic, endoscopy, fluid analysis, manometric, microscopic examination, nuclear scan, other studies, sputum, stool, ultrasound, urine, and x-ray.

ELECTRODIAGNOSTIC TESTS

ENDOSCOPY

FLUID ANALYSIS

MANOMETRIC TESTS

MICROSCOPIC EXAMINATIONS

NUCLEAR SCANS

OTHER STUDIES

SPUTUM TESTS

STOOL TESTS

ULTRASOUND TESTS

URINE TESTS

X-RAY EXAMINATIONS

list of tests by type

Appendix C: Typical abbreviations and units of measurement

<	Less than
≤	Less than or equal to
>	Greater than
≥	Greater than or equal to
C	Celsius
cc	Cubic centimeter
cg	Centigram
cm	Centimeter
cm H_2O	Centimeter of water
cu	Cubic
dl	Deciliter (100 ml)
fmol	Femtomole
g	Gram
hr	Hour
IU	International unit
ImU	International milliunit
IµU	International microunit
K	Kilo
kg	Kilogram
L	Liter
m	Meter
m^2	Square meter
m^3	Cubic meter
mEq	Milliequivalent
mEq/L	Milliequivalent per liter
mg	Milligram
min	Minute
ml	Milliliter
mm	Millimeter
mm^3	Cubic millimeter
mM	Millimole
mm Hg	Millimeter of mercury
mm H_2O	Millimeter of water
mol	Mole
mmol	Millimole
mOsm	Milliosmole
mµ	Millimicron

mU	Milliunit
mV	Millivolt
ng	Nanogram
nm	Nanometer
nmol	Nanomole
Pa	Pascal
pg	Picomole (or micromicro-gram)
pl	Picoliter
pm	Picometer
pmol	Picomole
sec	Second
SI units	International System of Units
μ	Micron
μ^3	Cubic micron
μg	Microgram
μIU	Microinternational unit
μl	Microliter
μm	Micrometer
μm^3	Cubic micrometer
μmol	Micromole
μU	Microunit
U	Unit
yr	Year

Bibliography

Aspelin P: Ultrasound examination of soft tissue injury of the lower limb in athletes, *Am J Sports Med* 20(5):601-603, 1992.

Bates SE: Clinical applications of serum tumor markers, *Ann Intern Med* 115(8):623-634, 1991.

Behrman RE et al, editors: *Nelson textbook of pediatrics*, ed 14, Philadelphia, 1992, WB Saunders.

Bordow RA, Moser KM: *Manual of clinical problems in pulmonary medicine*, ed 3, Boston, 1991, Little, Brown.

Braunwald E, editor: *Heart disease: a textbook of cardiovascular medicine*, ed 4, Philadelphia, 1992, WB Saunders.

Brunzel NA: *Fundamentals of urine and body fluid analysis*, Philadelphia, 1994, WB Saunders.

Bubien RS et al: What you need to know about radiofrequency ablation, *Am J Nurs* 93(7):30-36, 1993.

Casperson DS: Focus on oncology: prostatic specific antigen testing, *Urol Nurs* 11(1):31-34, 1992.

Cheney AM, Maquindang ML: Patient teaching for x-ray and other diagnostics, *R N* 56(4):54-56, 1993.

Coulter JS: Red blood cell distribution width and mean corpuscular volume: clinical applications, *Adv Clin Care* 6(6):13, 1991.

Creasy RK, Resnik R: *Maternal-fetal medicine: principles and practice*, ed 3, Philadelphia, 1994, WB Saunders.

Cupp MR, Oesterling JE: Prostate-specific antigen, digital rectal examination, and transrectal ultrasonography: their role in diagnosing early prostate cancer, *Mayo Clin Proc* 68:297-306, 1993.

Dalence CR et al: Amniotic fluid lamellar body count: a rapid and reliable fetal lung maturity test, *Obstet Gynecol* 86(2):235-239, 1995.

De Veciana M et al: Postprandial versus preprandial blood glucose monitoring in women with gestational diabetes mellitus requiring insulin therapy, *N Engl J Med* 333(19):1239-1241, 1995.

Gawlikowski J: White cells at war, *Am J Nurs* 92(3):44-51, 1992.

Gregor CL: Antepartum fetal assessment techniques: an update for today's perinatal nurse, *J Perinatal Neonatal Nurs* 5(4):1-15, 1992.

Greenberg LR, Moore TR, Murphy H: Gestational diabetes mellitus: antenatal variables as predictors of postpartum glucose intolerance, *Gest Diabetes* 86(1):97-101, 1995.

Halfman-Francy M: Recognition and management of bleeding following cardiac surgery, *Crit Care Nurs Clin North Am* 3(4):675-689, 1991.

Hancock RD: Venipuncture vs. arterial catheter activated partial thromboplastin times in heparinized patients, *DCCN* 12(5):238-245, 1993.

Henry JB: *Clinical diagnosis and laboratory management by laboratory methods,* ed 18, Philadelphia, 1991, WB Saunders.

Isselbacher KJ et al, editors: *Harrison's principles of internal medicine,* ed 13, New York, 1994, McGraw-Hill.

Kee JL, Hayes ER: Assessment of patient laboratory data in the acutely ill, *Nurs Clin North Am* 25(4):751-759, 1990.

Kikuchi S et al: Serum anti–*Helicobacter pylori* antibody and gastric carcinoma among young adults, *Cancer* 75(12):2789-2792, 1995.

Koepke JA, editor: *Practical laboratory hematology,* New York, 1991, Churchill Livingstone.

Kuhlman JE: Oral and IV contrast-enhanced abdominal CT, *Appl Radiol* 21(10):20-21, 1992.

Lancaster LE: Immunogenetic basis of tissue and organ transplantation and rejection, *Crit Care Nurs Clin North Am* 4(1):1-24, 1992.

Lavin J: Anergy testing—a vital weapon, *RN* 56(9):31-33, 1993.

Lee GR et al, editors: *Wintrobe's clinical hematology,* ed 9, Philadelphia, 1993, Lea & Febiger.

Littrup PJ, Goodman AC, Mettlin CJ: The benefit and cost of prostate cancer early detection, *CA* 43(3):134-149, 1993.

Lowry WS: Tumor suppressor genes and risk of metastasis in ovarian cancer, *BMJ* 307(6903):542, 1993.

McClatchey KD, editor: *Clinical laboratory medicine,* Baltimore, 1994, Williams & Wilkins.

Melillo KD: Interpretation of laboratory values in older adults, *Nurse Pract* 18(7):59-67, 1993.

Merva J: A closer look at the heart SAECG, *RN* 56(5):50-53, 1993.

Moore S: Screening for prostate cancer: PSA blood test, rectal examination, and ultrasounds, *Urol Nurs* 12(3):106-107, 1992.

Norris MKG: Assessing fibrin-split products, *Nursing* 22(6):29, 1992.

Pagana KD, Pagana TJ: *Diagnostic testing and nursing implications: a case study approach,* ed 4, St Louis, 1994, Mosby.

Rainwater LM et al: Prostate-specific antigen testing in untreated and treated prostatic adenocarcinoma, *Mayo Clin Proc* 65(8):1118-1126, 1990.

Rao JK et al: The role of antineutrophil cytoplasmic antibody (c-ANCA) testing in the diagnosis of Wegener granulomatosis, *Ann Intern Med* 123(12):925-932, 1995.

Resnick ML, Rifkin MD, editors: *Ultrasonography of the urinary tract,* ed 3, Baltimore, 1991, Williams & Wilkins.

Robie BH: Cardiovascular technology: noninvasive diagnosis of cardiovascular disease using ultrasound imaging, *J Cardiovasc Nurs* 6(2):36-42, 1992.

Rudolphi DM: Duplex scanning, *Am J Nurs* 90(4):123-124, 1990.

Ryan KJ, Berkowitz R, Barbieri R, editors: *Kistner's gynecology: principles and practice,* ed 5, St Louis, 1990, Mosby.

Schwartz SL et al, editors: *Principles of surgery,* ed 6, New York, 1994, McGraw-Hill.

Sistrom C: Liver CT for cancer staging, *Appl Radiol* 21(6):19-24, 1992.

Spiro HM: *Clinical gastroenterology,* ed 4, New York, 1993, McGraw-Hill.

Tanagho EA, McAninch JW, editors: *Smith's general urology,* ed 13, Norwalk, Conn, 1992, Appleton & Lange.

Taylor A, Datz FL, editors: *Clinical application of nuclear medicine,* New York, 1991, Churchill Livingstone.

Thompson EJ: Transesophageal echocardiography: a new window on the heart and great vessels, *Crit Care Nurse* 13(10):55-56, 1993.

Thompson S: Ultrasonography: intraoperative diagnosis of choledocholithiasis, *AORN J* 51(4):983-985, 1990.

Tilton RC et al, editors: *Clinical laboratory medicine,* St Louis, 1992, Mosby.

Velos JC: A review of cardiac imaging modalities, *Nurse Pract Forum* 2(4):231-238, 1991.

Wozniak-Petrofsky J: Prostate specific antigen in prostate cancer, *J Urol Nurs* 12(3):104-105, 1992.

Wozniak-Petrofsky J: Basics of urodynamics, *J Urol Nurs* 12(2):434-463, 1993.

Young DS: *Effects of drugs on clinical laboratory tests,* ed 3, Washington, DC, 1990, AACS Press.

Zoloth SR: Anergy compromise screening for tuberculosis in high-risk populations, *Am J Public Health* 83(5):749-751, 1993.

Index